OXFORD MEDICAL PUBLICATIONS

High-Altitude Medicine and Pathology

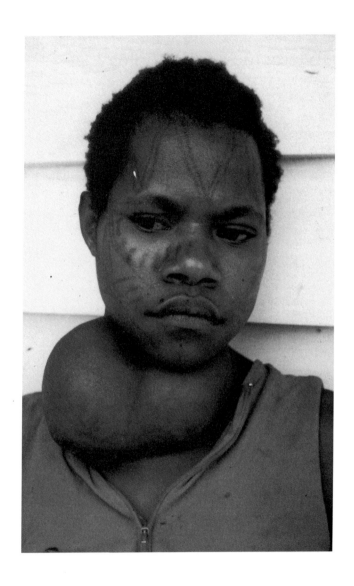

Goitre in a girl from the highlands of New Guinea.

High-Altitude Medicine and Pathology

DONALD HEATH

Emeritus Professor of Pathology, University of Liverpool, UK; Honorary Professor of Pathology, Cayetano Heredia Medical School, Lima, Peru; Honorary Professor of Pathology, San Andres University, La Paz, Bolivia; Member of the National Academy of Medicine of Peru

and

DAVID REID WILLIAMS

Department of Pathology, University of Liverpool, UK

Oxford   New York   Tokyo
OXFORD UNIVERSITY PRESS
1995

Oxford University Press, Walton Street, Oxford OX2 6DP

Oxford   New York
Athens   Auckland   Bangkok   Bombay
Calcutta   Cape Town   Dar es Salaam   Delhi
Florence   Hong Kong   Istanbul   Karachi
Kuala Lumpur   Madras   Madrid   Melbourne
Mexica City   Nairobi   Paris   Singapore
Taipei   Tokyo   Toronto

and associated companies in
Berlin   Ibadan

Oxford is a trade mark of Oxford University Press

Published in the United States
by Oxford University Press Inc., New York

First and second editions published by Churchill Livingstone (1977, 1981) as
'Man at High Altitude'
Third edition published by Butterworths (1989) as 'High-Altitude
Medicine and Pathology'

A catalogue record for this book is available from the British Library

Library of Congress Cataloging in Publication Data
Heath, Donald
High-altitude medicine and pathology/Donald Heath and David Reid Williams.
(Oxford medical publications)
Includes bibliographical references and index.
1. Mountain sickness   2. Altitude, Influence of   3. Adaptation (Physiology)
4. Acclimatization   I. Williams, David Reid.   II. Title.   III. Series.
[DNLM: 1. Altitude.   2. Adaptation, Physiological.   3. Acclimatization.
4. Anoxia–physiopathology.   WD 710 H437m 1994]
RC103.A4H4   1994   616.9'893–dc20   94–24865
ISBN 0 19 262504 7 (Hbk)

Typeset by
EXPO Holdings, Malaysia

Printed in Great Britain by
The Bath Press, Avon

This book is dedicated to
Claudia and Gareth Williams
and to the memory of
Florence Heath

Preface

The publication of the fourth edition of this book only 6 years after the appearance of the third is a measure of the growth of interest in high-altitude medicine and the realization of the importance of the subject. An ever-increasing number of tourists is being attracted to the great mountain ranges and this has stimulated the building of wide new roads in formerly remote areas like Ladakh. This has facilitated the rapid ascent of unacclimatized lowlanders to high altitude with all the attendant risks of developing pulmonary and cerebral oedema. At the time of writing there has been such an influx of high-altitude climbers into areas like the Everest Base Camp that a determined effort at conservation is being made to clear up the litter and latrines of the crowds flocking to scale the great heights. This attraction of the mountains demands that climbers and their medical advisers become more familiar with the avoidance and treatment of the various forms of high-altitude illness some of which may be fatal. The appearance of large holes in the ozone layer is likely to expose native highlanders and sojourners to increased levels of ultraviolet radiation with all its attendant dangers.

In the last 5 years new clinical syndromes of subacute mountain sickness have been described. One form affects infants of Han origin ascending to live on the Tibetan plateau. An understanding of its pathology has shown unexpected and fascinating links with that of brisket disease in calves in the mountains of Utah. A second form occurs in young Indian soldiers in the Himalaya and has stimulated much research into its endocrinological basis.

New treatments have emerged. The introduction of light-weight hyperbaric suits as a temporizing procedure before descent has introduced a new approach to the treatment of acute mountain sickness. Nifedipine has been employed to reduce pulmonary arterial pressure and ameliorate high-altitude pulmonary oedema.

Our understanding of many aspects of high-altitude pathology has deepened. It has become clear that the simplistic view of the pulmonary vascular remodelling attributed to the hypobaric hypoxia of high altitude as comprising muscularization of pulmonary arterioles can no longer be sustained. Instead it seems that one must think in terms of hyperplasia of vascular smooth muscle causing longitudinal muscle to form in the intima and circular muscle to form inner muscular tubes. Our understanding of the carotid bodies, their peptides, and their nerve fibrils has deepened so that we now understand why the enlarged chemoreceptors of the native highlander show a diminished hypoxic ventilatory response. It has become clear that the adrenal glands of healthy, native highlanders are enlarged compared to those of lowlanders. The role of atrial natriuretic hormone in healthy man at high altitude and in acute mountain sickness is becoming clearer. These examples illustrate how our knowledge of high-altitude medicine, physiology, and pathology is expanding in many directions.

The award of a Leverhulme Emeritus Fellowship to Professor Heath to support the writing of this book is gratefully acknowledged. We are glad to take this opportunity to thank Miss Linda Byron for all her expertise and patience in typing the manuscript.

Southport   D.H.
Liverpool   D.R.W.
July 1994

Acknowledgements

We would like to thank Churchill Livingstone, publishers of the two editions of our previous book *Man at high altitude*, for permission to reproduce illustrations and text from those volumes. We also wish to thank Butterworths, publishers of the last edition of *High-altitude medicine and pathology*, for similar permission.

The following colleagues have kindly provided us with clinical and pathological material from which the figures indicated have been prepared, or were co-authors in papers from which the illustrations have been taken:

Dr I.S. Anand
Figs 17.2–17.10, 25.11

Professor J. Arias-Stella
Figs 11.5, 11.6, 15.9, 15.10

Dr K. Ball
Fig. 2.9

Dr R. Behm
Figs 18.10, 18.11

Dr M. Calderon
Figs 10.9, 10.10

Dr Y. Castillo
Figs 11.5, 11.6

Chester Zoo (North of England Zoological Society)
Fig. 29.7

Professor J. Cawley
Fig. 8.2

Dr X.S. Cheng
Figs 17.2–17.5, 17.7

Dr C. Clarke
Fig. 27.5

Dr D.F. Danzl
Fig. 24.2

Dr J. Dickinson
Figs 9.1, 12.4, 13.5, 13.7, 13.8, 14.1–14.3, 36.6

Dr C. Edwards
Figs 7.9, 7.10

Mrs E. Ellison and Mr W. Butt
Fig. 18.5

Dr P.G. Forster
Fig. 19.3

Dr J.R. Gosney
Figs 4.12, 9.1, 10.9, 10.10, 13.5, 13.7, 13.8, 14.1–14.3, 17.6, 17.8, 17.9, 22.6–22.10

Dr E. Gradwell
Figs 22.1, 22.2

Dr E. Harris
Figs 17.2–17.9

Professor P. Harris
Figs 4.9, 7.9, 7.10, 10.7, 11.5, 11.6, 17.2–17.9, 25.11, 35.1

Professor C.A. Hart
Fig. 26.3

Professor H.H. Hecht
Figs 16.1, 16.3, 16.4

Professor A. Hurtado
Figs 11.5, 11.6

Dr F. Jackson
Fig. 19.2

Dr Moira R. Jackson
Fig. 23.5

Dr H. Krüger
Figs 11.5, 11.6, 13.4, 13.6, 15.9, 36.5

Dr Y.H. Liu
Figs 17.2–17.9

Dr K. Marsh
Figs 29.3–29.6

Dr T. Mayhew
Fig. 23.5

Dr C. Monge-C
Figs 15.1, 15.12

Dr H. Moosavi
Fig. 13.9

Dr F. Murphy
Figs 26.8–26.10

Dr C.S. Nath
Fig. 15.9

Dr B.C. Paton
Figs 24.3–24.9

Dr D. Peñaloza
Figs 10.14, 13.2, 15.4, 15.11

Professor P. Pharoah
Figs 22.4, 22.5

Professor J. Rios-Dalenz
Figs 4.12, 10.7, 10.9, 10.10, 22.6–22.8

Professor J. Rüttner
Fig. 29.1

Dr J. Scott
Fig. 21.5

Dr F. Sime
Fig. 13.2

Dr M. Sissons
Fig. 4.11

Dr P. Smith
Figs 4.9, 10.7, 10.12, 10.18, 13.9

Dr G.J. Sui
Figs 17.2–17.9

Miss L. Taggart
Fig. 26.4

Dr D. Weinman
Figs 26.5–26.7

We are indebted to the Editors of the following journals for permission to reproduce the illustrations listed below which were previously published by them:

The Alpine Club
Fig. 19.2

American Journal of Cardiology
Fig. 13.2

Biomedica biochimica acta
Figs 18.10, 18.11

British Heart Journal
Figs 11.5, 11.6, 25.8, 25.9

Cardioscience
Fig. 10.18

Experimental Cell Biology
Fig. 4.9

Histopathology
Figs 10.9, 10.10

International Journal of Biometeorology
Figs 10.11, 10.15, 22.6–22.8

Investigative and Cell Pathology
Fig. 10.21

Journal of Pathology
Figs 7.9, 7.10, 10.12, 17.2–17.5, 17.7

Journal of Virology
Figs 26.8–26.10

Liverpool University Press
Figs 4.11, 35.6–35.8

Popperfoto (Photographic Agency)
Fig. 31.3

Respiratory Medicine
Figs 17.6, 17.8, 17.9

Springer-Verlag
(Diseases of the Human Carotid Body 1992, D. Heath and P. Smith.
Figs 7.1, 7.2, 7.7, 7.8

Thorax
Figs 4.12, 9.1, 10.7, 10.16, 10.17, 13.5, 13.7–13.9, 14.1–14.3, 25.10 (b)

Contents

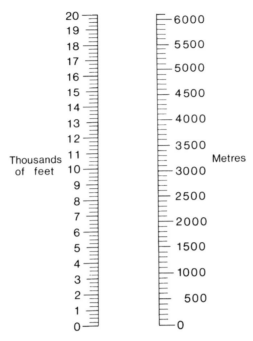

Above: Nomogram relating feet and metres. Throughout the text altitudes are expressed in metric units, but may be readily converted above to the more familiar 'thousands of feet'

Below: To facilitate rapid interpretation of the histograms, the conventions shown in this illustration are employed consistently throughout the book with only one or two exceptions. Conventions other than those shown are used infrequently and do not have a uniform meaning.

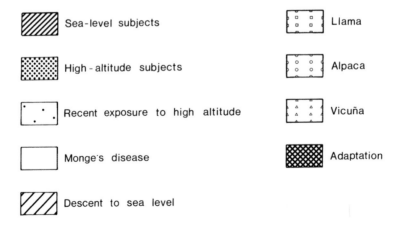

1

The importance of high-altitude studies

Man has always been aware that travels into high mountainous areas commonly lead to illness. It is fascinating in reading reports of travellers in the great mountain ranges in days long since past to discover fleeting references to symptoms that we think we can identify now as distinct clinical entities recognized in modern high-altitude medicine. At the same time it is prudent not to read too much into these ancient writings. Gilbert (1983a) refers to the travels of a certain Too Kin during the years 37 to 32 BC along the silk routes from Kashi in Chinese Turkestan to the area of present-day Kabul in Afghanistan. A report of his journey includes the sentence: 'Next, one comes to Big Headache and Little Headache Mountains.' Gilbert (1983a) believes this to be the first documented report of acute mountain sickness and he is brave enough to suggest that the two mountains referred to are the Kilik pass (4830 m) and the Ulugh Rabat pass (4200 m) in the Karakorams on the borders of Pakistan. Another intriguing report from this area and about this period seems to be the earliest reference to high-altitude pulmonary oedema (Chapter 13), a condition that had to wait another 1500 years before achieving formal medical recognition. About AD 400, Fâ Hsien, a Chinese monk travelling in Kashmir, lost his companion who died after foaming at the mouth as they were ascending a high mountain pass (Fâ Hsien, c. 415).

Western Europe first became aware of the discomforts and dangers of travelling in high mountains with the arrival of Pizzaro and his Conquistadors in Peru in the sixteenth century. To extend their conquest of the country and especially to reach the fabulously rich silver mines of such towns as Potosi (4070 m) the Spaniards had to traverse the High Andes. With the rough soldiery went the priests with the task of conversion of the Indians to the Faith but able to make accurate observations and write clearly. Father José de Acosta was a Jesuit priest who lived in the Viceroyalty of Peru from 1572 to 1587. He wrote a book about the New World. The first part of his work was written in Latin but a further section was composed later in Spanish and contained a reference to symptoms the priest suffered whilst travelling through the Andes.

Robert Boyle (1660), who himself carried out experiments on the effects of high and low barometric pressure on animals, was one of the early authorities to refer to the English translation of the account of the priest's illness, which has traditionally come to be regarded by physiologists as the first description of acute mountain sickness to reach Europe. This reads: 'I therefore perswade myselfe that the element of the aire is there so subtile and delicate, as it is not proportionable with the breathing of man, which requires a more grosse and temperate aire, and I beleeve it is the cause that doth so much alter the stomacke and trouble all the disposition.'

The work of Father de Acosta (1590) was widely circulated in Europe and within 15 years was translated into several languages. Knowledge of mountain sickness thus became available to those who could read and had access to books. However, modern Peruvian authorities (Bonavia et al. 1985) are sceptical about this classical description of acute mountain sickness by de Acosta and are inclined to think it more likely that at least some of the priest's symptoms were due to acute gastroenteritis, probably due to contaminated food.

In his book de Acosta (1590) refers to his illness occurring while he was in the vicinity of a high mountain range called Pariacaca. Gilbert (1983b) suggested that in the sixteenth century this term referred to the Andes as a whole, but this has been refuted by Bonavia et al. (1985) who pin-point Pariacaca as a saddle-shaped mountain looking down on Las Escaleras (staircase) de Pariacaca, which are part of the Inca road used by the Spaniards in their travelling between Lima and Cuzco. The altitudes of the two peaks of the mountain are both in the region of 5750 m, while those of the Inca road are about 4500 m. Thus the priest on his journey would have encountered elevations up to about 4500 m.

It is fascinating that the Conquistadors soon became aware that the illness of the mountains was not restricted to breathlessness with associated headache and nausea. Soon after their arrival in the mountains the Spaniards expanded the ancient silver-mining city of Potosi at an altitude of 4070 m. The historian Antonio de la Calancha (1639) describes how, in the early years, no infant born of Spanish immigrants in that city survived (Monge and Monge 1966). Mothers learned to descend to the neighbouring valleys to give birth and the child would not be brought up to Potosi until it was more than 1 year old. The first Spanish infant to live was born on Christmas Eve in the year 1598, 53 years after the founding of the city. Father Calancha referred to the event as 'the miracle of Saint Nicholas of Tolentino'. The recognition of the existence and nature of this problem had to await until 1988 when a comparable disease of the infants of immigrant Chinese into Tibet was recognized as 'subacute infantile mountain sickness' in Western European medical circles (Sui *et al.* 1988; Chapter 17, this volume).

Europeans hardly needed any intimation that mountains were associated with illness to keep them away from heights. As we note in Chapter 29 a love of mountains and a desire to scale them was not innate in the lowlander. In the Middle Ages the Alps were thought to be infested with dragons and the summits of mountains like the Matterhorn were considered to be populated by djinns and efreets. Only gradually in the eighteenth century did a change in attitude begin. By the middle of the nineteenth century climbing had become a popular pastime culminating in such events as the climbing of the Matterhorn by Edward Whymper and his party in 1865. Whymper opened up the way for the conquest of peaks throughout the world, and was himself to follow de Acosta's ascent into the Andes some three centuries later. He describes (1892) the onset of intense headache, a marked acceleration of the pulse, and 'an indescribable feeling of illness pervading the whole body', while he was 'preoccupied by the paramount necessity of obtaining air'. He was under no illusion that all that was required for successful ascents at high altitude was expertise in climbing and determination. He recognized the physiological problems to be overcome.

HIGH-ALTITUDE CLIMBERS

In the following years even higher peaks were scaled and increasing numbers of climbers became exposed to the altered physiology and medical risks of exposure to high altitude. These activities have exerted a great influence on the study of high-altitude physiology and medicine. Small groups of high-altitude climbers and scientists have now carried out research at the limit of human endurance on peaks exceeding 8000 m. We consider the problems of exposure to such extreme altitudes (Chapter 32), but only in so far as they illustrate the ultimate physiological responses to hypoxia. This book is not primarily concerned with the problems of such climbers striving, as Whymper says, 'to reach the loftiest summits in the earth'. Rather we consider the nature and biological and clinical significance of physiological and structural changes that occur in the human body on acute and chronic exposure to altitudes where people live permanently. This difference of approach has an interesting effect on the definition of 'extreme altitude'. We regard 5800 m as the entrance to this zone for this is the critical elevation above which successful, permanent acclimatization cannot be achieved. Much of the work on high-altitude climbers relates to elevations above 8000 m. Most of the data in this specialized area have been obtained from three large investigations. Two were at natural high altitude. These were the Himalayan Scientific and Mountaineering Expedition of 1960–61 (Pugh 1962) and the American Medical Research Expedition to Everest in 1981 (West *et al.* 1983). A third investigation was carried out at simulated high altitude in Operation Everest II in 1985 (Houston *et al.* 1987). Excellent descriptive accounts of the biological stresses in high-altitude climbers are available (Bonington 1971; Ward 1975; Ward *et al.* 1989).

NATIVE HIGHLANDERS

In this book we are primarily concerned with the many different processes of acclimatization that enable man to survive at high altitude be he a lowlander ascending to mountainous areas or a native highlander. There is no precise, scientific definition of the term 'high altitude' but for our purposes it begins at 3000 m when in the majority of lowlanders symptoms and signs associated with the ascent begin. From a practical standpoint we shall be interested in disordered physiology up to an altitude of about 4500 m. Large native populations in the Andes, the Himalaya, Tibet, and other parts of the world live permanently at such altitudes. Settlements in the Andes are higher than in Asia but even in the South American setting communities above 4500 m are exceptional. These native highlanders exhibit physiological and microanatomical changes, not only in their thoracic organs, where changes might be anticipated under such conditions, but in most systems of the body including the endocrine and reproductive organs. We do not accept these changes in form and function in native highlanders as normal, even though they occur in millions of people throughout the world. We think they are to be regarded as pathophysiological responses to deprivation of oxygen just as occur in lowlanders ascending to high altitude. Indeed, if these responses become exaggerated, as they do in a minority of subjects, they induce disease states that may prove fatal. In native highlanders processes of acclimatization begin in infancy and extend into adult life.

GENETIC ADAPTATION TO HIGH ALTITUDE

While we are primarily concerned with the processes of acclimatization in man to high altitude and the diseases that may be produced by the mountain environment we also consider the features of genetic adaptation to high altitude by indigenous mountain species such as the llama, vicuña, alpaca, mountain-viscacha, yak, and Tibetan snow pig (Chapter 35).

THE TOURIST INDUSTRY

High-altitude studies are of importance to many groups involved in a wide range of activities. Thus, they have a broad application to the increasing numbers of holiday-makers in mountainous areas. Acute mountain sickness is likely to prove an increasing problem for the travel industry, for the introduction in recent years of trekking and 'adventure holidays' in remote mountainous areas raises the likelihood of tourists being suddenly exposed to the hypoxia of high altitude after rapid transit from sea level. There is now a substantial tourist industry based on the Andean empire of the Incas, centred on its capital Cuzco (3400 m) (Figs 1.1 and 1.2) and the 'lost city of the Incas', Majchu Picchu (2440 m) (Fig. 1.3). Every day in July and August about 3600 people visit the summit of Pike's Peak, Colorado, at 4300 m (*Lancet* Annotation 1976). Hackett *et al.* (1976) studied the incidence of acute mountain sickness in tourist-hikers, as opposed to expedition mountaineers, who were ascending through the village of Pheriche (4240 m) in the Himalaya of Nepal to visit the Everest Base Camp at 5500 m. Up this one tiny remote mountain path some 648 tourists hiked in a mere 4 weeks from 10 October to 10 November 1975. There are, moreover, plenty of such peaks from which the tourist may choose. Some 568 Himalayan peaks are higher

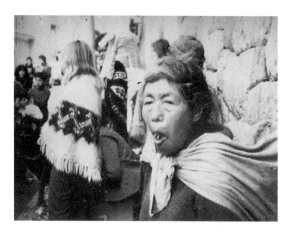

1.1 *A group of American tourists at Cuzco (3400 m), the ancient capital of the Inca empire. In the foreground is an Andean Indian woman chewing coca (see Chapter 34). Cuzco is the Quechua word for 'navel'.*

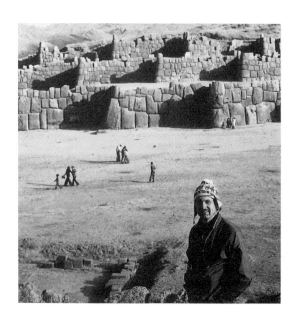

1.2 *Fortification at Sacsayhuaman (3580 m) above Cuzco showing the characteristic features of Inca architecture. Huge blocks of stone have been accurately shaped together to form a wall without the use of any form of cement. It is impossible to insert a knife blade between the blocks of stone. Another remarkable aspect of such building is that the blocks of stone were transported to the building site at great altitudes without the use of the wheel, which was unknown to the Inca people.*

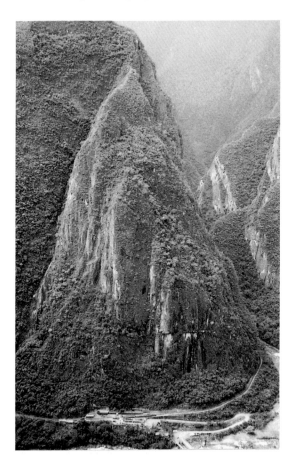

1.3 *Majchu Picchu (2440 m), the 'lost city of the Incas', built on the humid eastern slopes of the Andes which descend into the Amazon. Note the single-track railway and the train for tourists dwarfed by the precipitous hills chosen by the Incas.*

than 6100 m according to Mordecai (1966) and, excluding Antarctica, about 2.5% of the world's land surface lies above 3050 m (*Lancet* Annotation 1976).

The number of tourists visiting high mountain areas is increasing explosively and it seems certain that thousands more people will suffer from acute mountain sickness every year, with increasing mortality. In the opinion of Hackett *et al.* (1976) this should be a matter of concern both to the tourist industry and to the medical profession. We have ourselves, in lecturing at various postgraduate centres throughout the United Kingdom, been disturbed by the reports of illness experienced by many tourists to high altitude, including accounts of life-threatening incidents due to high-altitude pulmonary and cere-

bral oedema. Some tourist operators commonly hardly recognize the hazards, let alone provide simple advice on how to avoid them. General practitioners are often woefully uninformed on the nature of diseases likely to be faced by newcomers to the mountains and rarely give worthwhile advice on prevention. Even physicians who accompany trekking groups into the mountains are often ignorant of the nature and treatment of acute mountain sickness, high-altitude pulmonary oedema, and cerebral mountain sickness. Ignorance of the nature, avoidance, and treatment of diseases facing those who acutely expose themselves to high altitude has been stressed in an annotation in the *Lancet* (1976), grimly entitled 'See Nuptse and die'.

VOLCANOES

Volcanoes are another increasing tourist attraction throughout the world and some of them are high enough to approach the altitude at which symptoms of acute mountain sickness might be anticipated. Mount Fuji (3775 m), the sacred mountain of Japan, is visited each year by more than 100 000 people. However, the great majority of visitors ascend two-thirds of the way up by motor coach and only a few climb to the summit as a novelty or as a pilgrimage. Under these circumstances, the risk of acute mountain sickness is slight.

The situation on Mt Teide (3720 m) on Tenerife is somewhat different. Although the elevation of this volcano is almost identical to that of Mt Fuji, the numerous holidaymakers gain a much closer access to the summit. They are first driven up rapidly in buses from hotels on the coast to the foot of the volcano and are then transported almost to the summit extremely quickly by cable-car, leaving only a final, brisk steep walk to the top. Here they have ascended above the critical altitude of 3000 m where symptoms and signs related to altitude may be expected. The authors have witnessed the summit of this volcano swarming with tourists (Fig. 1.4), some of whom show the clinical features of acute mountain sickness. The one saving grace in this situation is that the time of exposure of the tourists to high altitude is usually insufficient to allow associated disease to develop.

Such is not the case when man has to work on the summit of volcanoes for periods of months or years rather than visit them fleetingly. For example, astronomers operate the United Kingdom infrared telescope on the summit of the volcano Mauna Kea (4210 m) on the island of Hawaii. Here the altitude is of sufficient magnitude to give rise to significant

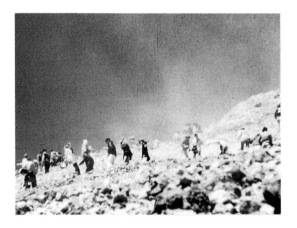

1.4 *Swarms of tourists on the slope of Mt Teide (3720 m) on the island of Tenerife amid the swirling clouds of volcanic ash.*

symptomatology, although the physiological stresses are unique in that the astronomers oscillate every 12 hours from the altitude of the telescope to a lodge for sleeping and acclimatization at Hale Pohaku (2750 m). This problem is considered at length in Chapter 30. A minority of lowlanders has to take up prolonged or even permanent residence in high mountainous areas as, for example, in the employment of mining companies on the Andean altiplano. To such people a knowledge of the presentation and treatment of, and prophylaxis against, acute mountain sickness (Chapter 12), high-altitude pulmonary oedema (Chapter 13), and cerebral mountain sickness (Chapter 14) is of importance.

HIGH-ALTITUDE DISEASES
Acclimatization may be inadequate or it may break down to give rise to diseases peculiar to high altitude. In this respect we shall consider benign acute mountain sickness and its two severe and potentially fatal developments of high-altitude pulmonary oedema and cerebral mountain sickness. We shall also describe the long-term loss of acclimatization called chronic mountain sickness or Monge's disease. Calves may not adjust to ascent to high altitude but instead may develop a condition called brisket disease which we shall analyse. We shall also consider the features of a recently recognized illness in infants of Han origin taken up by their parents to live in Lhasa which is the human counterpart of brisket disease in representing failure of the young to achieve successful acclimatization to the hypobaric hypoxia of high altitude (Chapter 17). Finally,

the extreme cold of high altitude may induce the serious conditions of hypothermia and frostbite.

Diseases at high altitude may be caused not by hypobaric hypoxia but by organisms in the environment. They include the dreaded Oroya fever due to *Bartonella bacilliformis* (Chapter 26). Decreased incidence of bronchial asthma at these elevations is commonly considered to be due to fewer dust-mites, which do not fare well in the cold, dry atmosphere of high altitude (Chapter 26).

ATHLETICS
Diminished barometric pressure and the associated hypobaric hypoxia proved to have deleterious effects on the performance of sea-level athletes who competed in the Olympic Games held in Mexico City (2380 m) in 1968. Here the altitudes were moderate but the penalties were a failure to achieve anticipated world records (Chapter 31).

MILITARY OPERATIONS
The glories and successes of Simon Bolivar, San Martin, and the other great liberators of the South American continent have to be considered in relation to the altitudes at which the battles were fought. From accounts of the battle of Junin (4400 m) in 1824 it would appear that some of the Spanish troops rapidly brought up from the coast to fight the native highlanders frothed at the mouth, almost certainly due to high-altitude pulmonary oedema. These early military lessons in the powerful influence of high altitude in the conduct of battles were lost on the Indian government in 1962 when it was called upon to confront an incursion of Chinese troops into its Himalayan borders. Large numbers of Indian soldiers were flown to the airstrip at Leh (3500 m) in Ladakh and provided the world medical literature with the largest series of cases of acute mountain sickness ever recorded, with much serious illness and many fatalities. We include reference to the experiences gained from this disastrous episode in Chapter 12.

CLINICAL APPLICATIONS
Important as all these applications of high-altitude studies undoubtedly are, they are overshadowed by the wider and deeper implication that an investigation of the processes of acclimatization of man to hypobaric hypoxia is at the same time a study of the responses of living tissues to chronic oxygen deprivation without the complicating factors of superadded disease. Chronic hypoxia and hypoxaemia are not confined to life at high altitude, but are to be found

in common and important heart and lung diseases such as chronic bronchitis and emphysema. Thus the results of investigations into high-altitude physiology and pathology can be applied to much cardiopulmonary disease. It is revealing and rewarding to regard chronically hypoxaemic patients with lung disease as subjects acclimatizing to hypoxia. One example is the enlargement of the carotid bodies that is to be found equally in the Quechua Indians of the Andes and in the hypoxaemic patient with chronic obstructive lung disease (Chapter 7). Another is the muscularization of the terminal portions of the pulmonary arterial tree that is to be found in both groups (Chapter 10).

Since the end of the previous century a large volume of data has been accumulated on high-altitude medicine and pathology. Much of this material is widely scattered in specialist journals and in this book we have attempted to bring some of it together. By integrating clinical, physiological, pathological, and experimental data we have aimed to produce a readable account of the characteristics of man at high altitude.

References

Bonavia, D., León-Velarde, F., Monge-C, C., Sanchez-Griñán, M.I., and Whittembury, J. (1985). Acute mountain sickness: critical appraisal of the Pariacaca story and on-site study. *Respiration Physiology*, **62**, 125.

Bonington, C. (1971). *Annapurna South Face*. London; Cassell.

Boyle, R. (1660). New experiments physico-mechanicall, touching the spring of the air, and its effects (Made, for the most part, in a new pneumatical engine) written by way of a letter to the Right Honourable Charles Lord Viscount of Dungarvan, eldest son to the Earl of Corke: Oxford; Thomas Robinson, pp. 356–8

de Acosta, Father Joseph (1590). The naturall and morall historie of the East and West Indies. Intreating of the remarkable things of heaven, of the elements, mettalls, plants and beasts which are proper to that country: Together with the manners, ceremonies, lawes, governments, and warres of the Indians. (Translated from the Spanish by Edward Grimstone, London; Edward Blount, 1604)

Fâ Hsien (*c.* 415). A record of Buddhistic kingdoms being an account by the Chinese Monk Fâ-Hsien of his travels in India and Ceylon (399–414) in search of the Buddhist books of discipline. (Translated and annotated with a Korean recension of the Chinese text by J. Legge. New York; Dover Publications, 1965, pp. 40–1, and p. 12 of the Korean text)

Gilbert, D.L. (1983*a*). The first documented report of mountain sickness: the China or Headache Mountain story. *Respiration Physiology*, **52**, 315

Gilbert, D.L. (1983*b*). The first documented description of mountain sickness: the Andean or Pariacaca story. *Respiration Physiology*, **52**, 327

Hackett, P.H., Rennie, D., and Levine, H.D. (1976). The incidence, importance and prophylaxis of acute mountain sickness. *Lancet*, **ii**, 1149

Houston, C.S., Sutton, J.R., Cymerman, A., and Reeves, J.T. (1987), Operation Everest II. Man at extreme altitude. *Journal of Applied Physiology*, **63**, 877

Lancet Annotation (1976). See Nuptse and die. *Lancet*, **ii**, 1177

Monge-M, C. and Monge-C, C. (1966). High-altitude animal pathology. In *High Altitude Diseases. Mechanism and Management*, Springfield, Illinois Charles C. Thomas, p. 70

Mordecai, D. (1966). *The Himalayas*. Calcutta; Daw Sen

Pugh, L.G.C.E. (1962). Physiological and medical aspects of the Himalayan Scientific and Mountaineering Expedition 1960–61. *British Medical Journal*, **i**, 621

Sui, G.J., Liu, Y.H., Anand, I.S., Harris, E., Harris, P., and Heath, D. (1988). Subacute infantile mountain sickness. *Journal of Pathology*, **155**, 161

Ward, M. (1975). *Mountain Medicine. A Clinical Study of Cold and High Altitude*. London; Crosby Lockwood Staples

Ward, M.P., Milledge, J.S., and West, J.B. (1989). *High Altitude Medicine and Physiology*. London; Chapman and Hall Medical

West, J.B., Lahiri, S., Maret, K.H., Peters, R.M., and Pizzo, C.J., (1983). Barometric pressures at extreme altitudes on Mt Everest; physiological significance. *Journal of Applied Physiology*, **54**, 1188

Whymper, E. (1892). *Travels Amongst the Great Andes of the Equator*. London; John Murray

2

Physical and climatic factors at high altitude

At high altitude there are significant alterations in several of the physical factors in the environment and these have important medical implications for life in mountainous areas.

THE CONCEPT OF 'HIGH ALTITUDE'

The term 'high altitude' has no precise scientific definition. There is not even a general consensus among the public as to what the term implies. To the tourist in such Alpine resorts as Zermatt (1620 m), the snow-covered summit of the nearby Matterhorn (4480 m) must epitomize great heights reached by the comparatively few after great effort. Yet at the almost identical altitude of 4330 m in the Peruvian Andes lies the thriving mining town of Cerro de Pasco whose Quechua inhabitants daily attend school, shop, play football, or go to the cinema. Throughout this book we shall take 'high altitude' to mean 3000 m or more, for at this elevation most lowlanders ascending mountains show unequivocal signs and symptoms associated with the ascent. Above this height the physiological features of acclimatization or the clinical features of acute mountain sickness become progressively more pronounced. In other words, ours is a medical rather than a physical definition of 'high altitude' and on this account it is inexact because of the considerable individual variation in response to the physical factors at high altitude described in this chapter.

The impact of television and popular books on mountain-climbing leads many members of the public to equate 'high altitude' with assaults on the great Himalayan peaks such as Mt Everest (8850 m). In this book we define elevations exceeding 5800 m as 'extreme altitude' because above this height further successful acclimatization cannot be achieved and survival cannot be maintained permanently (Chapter 32).

BAROMETRIC PRESSURE

The earth is surrounded by a mantle of air composed almost entirely of nitrogen, oxygen, and carbon dioxide. These gases are compressible so that the number of molecules per unit volume is greater at sea level than at high altitude. In other words the barometric pressure, which depends upon the molecular concentration of the air, decreases with increase in altitude. The relation between altitude and barometric pressure is shown in Fig. 2.1.

With the birth and development of the aviation industry it became necessary to define a relation between barometric pressure and altitude for such important matters as the calibration of altimeters on aircraft. There were clear advantages in developing the concept of a model atmosphere that applied approximately to mean conditions over the surface of the earth. This is referred to as the ICAO Standard Atmosphere (International Civil Aviation Organisation 1968) (see also Pugh 1957). It was never meant to be used to produce the actual barometric pressure at a particular location. Nevertheless, it has frequently been used inappropriately by some physiologists to predict barometric pressure at specific points on high mountains. The error in this has been noted nowhere more dramatic-

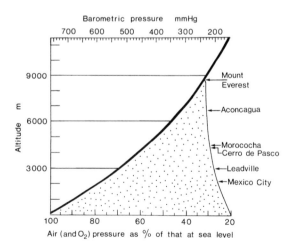

2.1 *Relation between altitude, barometric pressure, and air (and oxygen) pressure as a percentage of that at sea level. (After Frisancho (1975).)*

ally than at the summit of Mt Everest, the precise altitude of which is known as the result of detailed trigonometric surveys to be 8848 m. The standard atmospheric pressure for this elevation is 236 mmHg (Fig. 2.1), but in fact direct measurement of the barometric pressure at the summit was shown to be 253 mmHg by one of the members of the American Medical Research Expedition to the mountain in 1981.

West (1984) points out that, although barometric pressure at the surface of the earth and at an elevation of 24 000 m is essentially independent of latitude, at the lower range of 2000–16 000 m it is in fact influenced by this factor. The reason for this is the presence of a large mass of very cold air in the stratosphere above the equator brought about by complex phenomena of radiation and convection (Brunt 1952). This equatorial bulge converts the mantle of air around the earth into an oblate spheroid elevating barometric pressure near the equator but not at the poles (West *et al.* 1983). The latitude of Mt Everest is 28°N so this mountain is in the zone of influence of this mass of cold air. Barometric pressure at the summit varies considerably with season, being some 11 mmHg higher in midsummer than in midwinter. As we shall see below, this geophysical phenomenon has important implications for high-altitude climbers on mountains near the equator.

HYPOXIA

The amount of oxygen in the atmosphere remains constant at 20.93% up to an altitude of 110 000 m (Frisancho 1975). The percentage of oxygen in the ambient air is the same at high altitude as it is at sea level. Thus, with the diminution of the barometric pressure with increasing altitude, there is a progressive fall of partial pressure of oxygen. At sea level the barometric pressure is 760 mmHg and hence the partial pressure of oxygen in the air is 20.93% of that figure, namely 159 mmHg. When air is breathed into the bronchial tree, it becomes saturated with water vapour that exerts a pressure of 47 mmHg, so that the partial pressure of oxygen in inspired air, as contrasted to ambient air, is 20.93% of (760 – 47) mmHg, that is 149 mmHg. The relation between altitude, barometric pressure, and air (and thus oxygen) pressure as a percentage of that at sea level is shown in Fig. 2.1. As an example, at 3500 m the barometric pressure is 493 mmHg and the partial pressure of oxygen in the ambient air is 103 mmHg which is 65% of the sea-level value. Throughout this book we shall be largely concerned

with the biochemical, physiological, histological, and ultrastructural changes that occur in many organs in response to the chronic hypoxia of high altitude.

The partial pressure of oxygen at the summit of Mt Everest, as calculated from the barometric pressure deduced from the standard atmosphere, is barely enough to sustain human basal metabolism (West and Wagner 1980). This reasoning seemed to be borne out by the experience of high-altitude climbers such as Norton who, during the attempted ascent of the mountain in 1924, was able to reach only 8500 m breathing ambient air (Norton 1925). Mount Everest was not climbed until 1953 and then only with the use of supplementary oxygen, and this seemed to confirm the accepted wisdom at the time. Physiologists were, therefore, surprised when Messner (1979) and Habeler (1979) were able to reach the summit of the mountain without the use of supplementary oxygen, although the margin of physiological reserve was slim. The reason appears to be that the maximal oxygen uptake, only slightly above the requirements to sustain basal metabolism, is exquisitely sensitive to small variations in barometric pressure. The increase in barometric pressure of 17 mmHg brought about by the equatorial bulge described above is enough to improve maximal oxygen uptake and thus make possible the ascent of Mt Everest without supplementary oxygen.

COLD

Another environmental hazard that faces man at high altitude is cold. Temperature falls with increasing altitude to the extent of approximately 1°C for every 150 m and this is independent of latitude. However, latitude does influence the temperature of mountainous areas, for in tropical climes there is very little seasonal change but much diurnal variation in temperature. The reverse is true of areas of higher latitude. At night, a black-bulb thermometer exposed to the sky records a lower temperature than a sheltered instrument. This is a measure of the intense reradiation of heat to the night sky at high altitude. Hence the environment for nocturnal animals is very cold, forcing foxes, snow leopards, and similar animals to shelter in the ground, where the daily temperature variation is much narrower.

In the Andes we have been impressed by the striking difference in temperature that occurs in shadow as contrasted with direct sunlight. This difference has been documented by Swan (1961; see also Fig. 2.2). He recorded a temperature of 33.3°C on the sunlit rock surface at 5490 m; the air temperature in the shade was at the same time 12.8°C. With in-

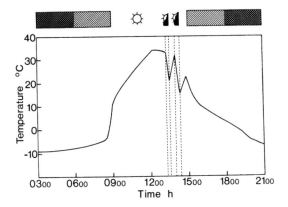

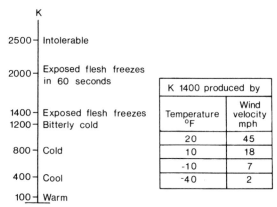

2.2 *Effect of direct sunlight on the 'exposed-black-bulb temperature' at 4880 m on the Ripimu Glacier in eastern Nepal as measured by Swan (1961). The hours indicated by cross-hatched blocks are those of darkness, while those shown by hatching are dawn to dusk. Note that a temporary obscuring of the sun by cloud induces an immediate and significant fall in temperature. (After Swan (1961).)*

2.3 *Relation between ascending values of the wind-chill factor (K) to various bodily sensations. Also shown are various combinations of temperature and wind velocity that produce a value for K of 1400 at which exposed flesh freezes. (After Unsworth (1977).)*

creasing altitude there is less atmospheric absorption of transmitted radiant energy and less effective cloudiness. Swan (1961) refers to Marmet and Schmidt who climbed Mt Everest in 1956 and removed their down-filled clothing because of the heat at 8530 m. Such conditions occur only in sunshine and with a low wind velocity. In view of all these variations it is impossible to make definitive statements concerning altitude and temperature, and average values have to be assumed. The pathological changes in the tissues induced by exposure to severe cold and the nature of man's immediate response and long-term acclimatization to cold are described in Chapter 24.

Exposure to wind is a factor that has to be considered closely in association with cold at high altitude, for with increasing wind velocity the effective skin temperature drops. In essence the insulating layer of warm air around the skin is blown away. This is known as the wind-chill factor (Ward 1975) and we shall refer to it further in Chapter 24. Unsworth (1977) relates ascending levels of the wind-chill factor (K) to various body sensations, ranging from warmth to freezing of exposed flesh in 60 seconds (Fig 2.3). At a value of 1400 for K, exposed flesh freezes, and Unsworth gives examples of how this value may be reached by various combinations of temperature and wind velocity (Fig. 2.3).

HUMIDITY

The cold air of the mountain environment has a reduced water vapour pressure. This is proportionate to the progressive fall of temperature with increasing altitude. Absolute humidity is extremely low at extreme altitude and Ward *et al.* (1989) refer to the fact that at $+20°C$ water vapour pressure is 17 mmHg whereas at $-20°C$, a temperature likely to be faced on the summits of very high mountains, it is only 1 mmHg. This has important physiological effects for in this dry air there is much insensible water loss caused by ventilation, which is increased at high altitude. Water loss through sweating is increased during work. In many mountainous areas, such as the western slopes of the Andes or in the Karakorams, these effects of high altitude are bolstered by the aridity of the terrain. The combination of low temperature and low relative humidity can be subjectively very unpleasant. Sensitive areas such as the lips can dry and crack in a matter of hours due to the dehydration caused by dry air and increased water loss consequent upon ventilation and sweating. The dehydration at extreme altitudes may assume significance in predisposing to thrombosis (Chapter 9).

SOLAR RADIATION

The electromagnetic radiation emitted from the photosphere of the sun incorporates a wide spectrum of wavelength ranging from 20 000 nm down to extreme ultraviolet radiation below 140 nm

(McCullough 1970). The much thinner atmosphere absorbs less of this solar radiation, especially that of lower wavelength. Furthermore, the dryness of the air at high altitude denies the customary protection afforded by absorption of radiation by water vapour. According to Ward (1975), at sea level the average amount of solar radiation absorbed is 963 kJ/m^2 per hour. On the other hand, at 5790 m in clear weather, Pugh (1963) found that the solar heat absorbed by the surface of the clothed human body was 1465 kJ/m^2. The solar heat absorbed by the body depends on several factors not attributable to the environment such as the clothing, with dark garments absorbing more than light, and the position of the individual. However, there are environmental factors that increase the amount of solar radiation at high altitude. One is the clear air of mountainous areas, which facilitates the passage of the radiation to the earth's surface. Another is reflection from snow. In Western Europe, the altitude of the permanent snowline varies from one mountain range to another. On the northern slopes of the Pyrenees it is at 2750 m, whereas on Mont Blanc it is at 2990 m. Permanent snow reflects solar radiation so that the effect is enhanced. Such reflectivity of solar radiation, known as the *albedo*, is less than 25% if there is no snow, but rises to a range of 75–90 % in its presence. The factor is greatest at high altitude in polar regions.

ULTRAVIOLET RADIATION

Radiation of very short wavelength is associated with sunspot activity and accounts for a negligible proportion of the total energy of solar radiation. The segment that is of far greater physiological significance is ultraviolet (uv) radiation. This part of the electromagnetic spectrum extends from 200 to 400 nm. It is often considered in three ranges: uv-A (400–315 nm); uv-B (315–280 nm); uv-C (280–200 nm).

When direct radiation from the sun streams in towards the earth, it passes through an ozone layer at 24 000 m and there is considerable absorption of ultraviolet radiation. At present there is concern about holes that have appeared in the ozone layer above both poles. These have been growing for some years. It is commonly held that this is due to the increasing use in aerosols and refrigerators of chlorofluorocarbons that escape into the atmosphere and then into the stratosphere and ozone layer where they release free chlorine. This removes an oxygen atom from ozone to produce chlorine monoxide and molecular oxygen. The monoxide is

unstable, reacting with atomic oxygen to produce molecular oxygen and free chlorine able to destroy yet more ozone. Chlorofluorocarbons are inert in the lower atmosphere but may exert their serious effects in the stratosphere for decades. Should the holes in the ozone layer continue to enlarge, the effects of ultraviolet radiation at the earth's surface and particularly at high altitude could assume increasing severity. In passing to the earth's surface, further absorption by the atmosphere takes place. Hence *direct* solar ultraviolet intensity increases with altitude, because the radiation has passed through a thinner layer of absorbing atmosphere. Factors other than altitude influence the amount of direct radiation reaching the earth's surface, since tangential entry of the radiation will increase the thickness of atmosphere through which it passes. The air mass traversed will thus depend on several additional factors such as time of day, time of year, and latitude.

In addition to direct radiation from the sun there is much so-called 'sky radiation' (McCullough 1970). This is produced by scattering of the ultraviolet radiation. This may be at the molecular level where the scattering particles, such as oxygen or nitrogen, are small compared with the wavelength of the radiation. Large-particle scattering is caused by clouds, dust, and aerosols where the particles have a diameter comparable to the wavelength of the radiation. Hence sky radiation *decreases* with increasing altitude, because the lower, more turbid atmosphere is responsible for most of the scattering.

Measurement of the *direct* solar radiation of wavelengths less than 313 nm showed that the intensity on the San Francisco Peaks (3200 m) was about 35% higher than that at the Lowell Observatory (2200 m) (Koller 1952). On the other hand, *the combined direct and sky radiation* on a horizontal surface in the Alps showed the effects of decreasing sky radiation with increasing elevation, so that the overall increase was only 15% per 1000 m (Koller 1952). The effect of elevation above sea level on intensity of ultraviolet radiation of wavelength 295 nm for different values of solar altitude is shown in Fig. 2.4.

The significantly increased ultraviolet radiation at high altitude has disproportionately serious physiological effects. This is because of the predominance in the blue and ultraviolet end of the spectrum of the shorter wavelengths, which are most easily scattered and thus make a disproportionate contribution to sky radiation. Thomas (see Heath and Williams 1981) estimates from data in Tousey (1966) and Elterman (1964) that at 4000 m the intensity of ul-

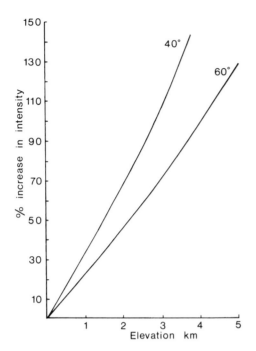

2.4 *Effect of elevation on direct solar intensity of ultraviolet radiation of wavelength 295 nm for two values of solar altitude. (After Koller (1952).)*

traviolet radiation of wavelength 400 nm is increased by 147%, whereas that of wavelength 300 nm is increased by 250%. The scattering of this radiation of short wavelength produces the blue colour of the sky. If light from the sun reached the earth in a straight line with no scattering, the sky would appear black (Mason 1967). The increased ultraviolet radiation of high altitude is of medical importance and we shall consider its effect on the skin and eyes in Chapters 25 and 27, respectively.

COSMIC RADIATION

Another physical factor characteristic of high altitudes is the increased intensity of cosmic radiation compared to that at sea level. Charged particles of very high kinetic energy continually bombard the earth. Almost all of them are positively charged protons. They constitute the primary cosmic radiation. When these particles enter the earth's atmosphere, they repeatedly collide with nitrogen or oxygen atoms. These collisions are of two types. They make a grazing contact with the electronic structure of the atom or, on the other hand, the protons of extraterrestrial origin may smash into the nucleus. On emerging from this collision the ex-

traterrestrial proton, still preserving half its energy, may go on to bring about repeated further collisions. A simultaneous result of this collision is the liberation of protons and neutrons from the target nucleus, collectively termed 'nucleons'. At the same time there is a liberation of a series of intermediate particles of very short life, termed 'mesons'. The π type of mesons, called pions, decay to form muons, neutrinos, and gamma radiation. The muons themselves then decay to form charged electrons and neutrinos. Hence the primary extraterrestrial cosmic radiation, consisting of protons, brings about an intense secondary cosmic radiation, comprising a wide variety of charged particles and electromagnetic radiation, through its contact with the high atmosphere of the earth (Fig. 2.5). The level of cosmic radiation reaches a plateau at 30 000 m (Wilson 1976), for above this altitude there is only the primary cosmic radiation. Below this elevation it is accentuated by the increased levels of secondary cosmic radiation brought about by the impact of galactic particles on the earth's high atmosphere.

At altitudes of the magnitude dealt with in this book, there is a significant increase in the levels of radiation. Thus, at 3000 m there is a threefold increase in the sea-level value of radiation of approximately 24 mrad per year (Baikie 1970). A rad is the dose of radiation equalling an absorption of 100 ergs per gram of substance irradiated. The radiation level

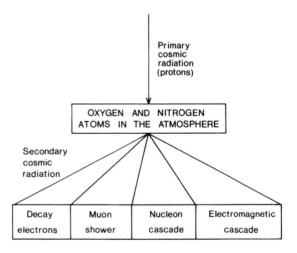

2.5 *Components of the secondary cosmic radiation produced by the collision of primary cosmic radiation with oxygen and nitrogen atoms in the upper atmosphere (see text).*

derived from cosmic radiation, as expressed in μrad/hour, in Denver (1600 m) was 5.9–6.3, and in New York, Conway (New Hampshire), and Burlington (Vermont) at low altitude was 3.6 (Lowder and Condon 1965; Beck *et al.* 1966; Shapiro 1972). These diminished levels at low altitude reflect the fact that at sea level galactic radiation contributes only about 4 μrad/hour to the environmental ionizing radiation of 10–15 μrad/hour, which is in fact largely due to gamma radiation from radioactive trace minerals in the ground (Schaefer 1971). The recognition that there is a high level of cosmic radiation at high altitude is evidenced by the building of the Cosmic Ray Observatory on the slopes of Mt Chacaltaya (5220 m) in the Bolivian Andes. This provides the highest permanent facility in the world for investigation of cosmic radiation.

HYPOXIA AND IONIZING RADIATION

The potentially damaging effects of increased ionizing radiation at high altitude may be ameliorated by the hypobaric hypoxia of that environment. The mechanism by which ionizing radiation affects cells is not clearly understood. Formerly, it was considered that most of its effects were due to direct action on the intracellular organelles causing either ionization or excitation of molecules. It is now thought that such direct action is less important that the indirect effects mediated by the cell water (Baikie 1970). The main radiochemical effect on tissues appears to be the formation of 'hot radicals' such as HO_2 and H_2O_2. Tissue oxygen tension appears to have an important influence on the formation of such radicals. Normally, an increased oxygen tension increases radiosensitivity, whereas a decrease in oxygen tension, such as occurs at high altitude, reduces the effects of radiation. Some reducing substances that produce tissue hypoxia give a degree of protection against the biological effects of radiation. They include cyanides, nitrites, 5-hydroxytryptamine, adrenaline, and derivatives of cysteine. On the other hand, ascorbic acid, which is a reducing agent, has little protective effect. These protective chemicals may compete for the free radicals referred to above. As HO_2, a powerful oxidizing agent, is found only in the presence of oxygen, this would explain why hypoxia and chemical protection are related. Oxygen has the ability to combine freshly severed ends of molecular structures, thus preventing them from rejoining, which they commonly do if the opportunity presents itself. Thus it interferes with a natural recovery process and causes

a given dose of radiation to be much more damaging than it would be in hypoxic conditions (Orr 1985).

There do not appear to have been any reports of disease at high altitude associated with increased levels of cosmic radiation. The levels of radiation in mountainous areas have to be put into perspective by comparing them with the levels of background radiation at sea level. This depends on radioactive elements in soil, rocks, and some building materials, notably granite. Because of this latter factor, the houses built of this material in Aberdeen produce a mean dose rate of 85 mrad per year (i.e. 10 μrad/hour). In addition, populations are increasingly exposed to higher levels of radiation resulting from such factors as routine medical radiography and the use of radioisotopes. Exceptionally, there are incidents such as the leak of radioactive materials from the Chernobyl Atomic Energy Plant in the former USSR.

INFLUENCES OF PARTICULAR MOUNTAINOUS AREAS OF THE WORLD ON HIGH-ALTITUDE MEDICINE

Areas at high altitude are scattered throughout the world (Fig. 2.6) and demonstrate that many factors in addition to elevation have to be taken into account in assessing the health problems the various mountain ranges present. Such factors may be geographical, climatic, economic, and even historical.

The Andes

The Andes extend the whole length of the western side of the South American continent from Ecuador to the Argentine (Fig. 2.7). They consist of three principal ranges or cordillera, running approximately from north-west to south-east in parallel with the coast and separated one from the other by high plateaux forming the altiplano (Marett 1969). The western range runs in a continuous chain along the whole continent, but the central and eastern cordillera, although well defined in the north and to a lesser extent in the south, become merged and lost in great knots of transverse mountain ranges (Marett 1969).

The western slopes of the Andes are as dry as dust, these desert-like conditions being the result of the Humboldt current in the Pacific (Fig. 2.7). This current runs along the whole length of the Peruvian coast, cooling the air above the sea and reducing its capacity to retain the moisture, which in normal circumstances would have fallen on the land as rain. Moreover, once the air passes over the land, it is warmed up again, increasing its capacity to retain

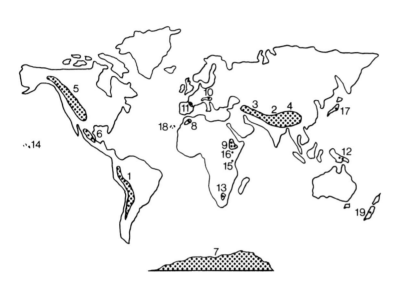

2.6 *World distribution of areas of high altitude exceeding 3000 m. 1, Andes; 2, Himalaya; 3, mountain ranges of Eastern Turkey, Persia, Afghanistan and Pakistan; 4, Tibetan plateau and southern China; 5, Rocky Mountains; 6, Sierra Madre; 7, Antarctica, 8, Atlas Mountains; 9, high plains of Ethiopia; 10, Alps. 11, Pyrenees; 12, highlands of New Guinea; 13, Basutoland; 14, Mauna Kea and Mauna Loa, volcanoes on Hawaii; 15, Kilimanjaro, volcano in East Africa; 16, Mt Kenya, volcano in East Africa; 17, Mt Fuji, volcano in Japan; 18, Mt Teide, volcano on Tenerife; 19, Mt Cook, New Zealand.*

moisture and making precipitation impossible. Such climatic factors turn the coastal strip of Peru into desert and indeed it is commonly said that 'it never rains in Lima'. On the ascent up the western aspects of the Andes everything is dust, and cacti and eucalyptus trees abound. This brings about a very low relative humidity with all its attendant medical problems as outlined above. Only a few high mountain ranges such as that including Huascarán (6765 m) (Table 2.1) are snow-covered. On the other hand, the eastern slopes of the Andes descend into the Amazon jungle and are progressively more humid and tree-covered.

Studies in the Andes have probably yielded more data on high-altitude medicine and pathology than any other area in the world. At first glance at Table 2.1 this seems unlikely, for the heights of the highest Andean peaks are well below those of the Himalayan ranges. However, the Quechua and Aymara Indians of the Andes live permanently at much higher altitudes than do the Sherpas of Nepal and the Ladakhis of the Karakorams. This permanent residence at 4300 m and above predisposes to the development of chronic mountain sickness

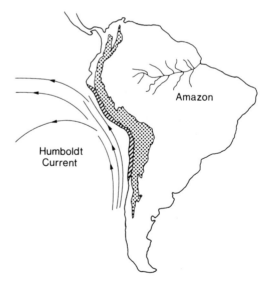

2.7 *Path of the cold Humboldt current, which cools the overlying air, reducing its capacity to hold moisture, and thus ensuring the aridity of the coastal strip of Peru and Chile (hatched area) and the western slopes of the Andes (stippled area).*

Table 2.1 Heights of selected mountains (to nearest 5 m)

Peak	Height (m)	Situation
Mt Everest (Chomolungma, Tibetan Goddess Mother of the Earth)*	8850	Everest range, Tibet/Nepal
K2 (Godwin-Austen)	8610	Karakorams
Kangchenjunga ('Five Treasures of the Eternal Snows')	8600	Everest range, Sikkim
Lhotse	8500	Everest range, Tibet/Nepal
Makalu	8470	Everest range, Nepal
Dhaulagiri	8170	Everest range, Nepal
Cho Oyu	8155	Tibet/Nepal border
Nanga Parbat ('Naked Mountain')	8125	Karakorams, Kashmir
Manaslu	8125	Everest range, Nepal
Annapurna I and II ('Giver of Life')	8080	Everest range, Nepal
Gasherbrum II and IV	8070	Karakorams†
Hidden peak	8065	Karakorams, Kashmir
Broad peak	8045	Karakorams†
Aconcagua	6960	Andes
Huascarán	6765	Andes
Chimborazo	6310	Ecuador
Mt McKinley	6195	Alaska
Kilimanjaro	5895	Tanzania
Mt Kenya	5200	Kenya
Mont Blanc	4810	France
Monte Rosa	4635	Switzerland
Weisshorn	4505	Switzerland
Matterhorn	4480	Swiss/Italian border
Mt Rainier	4400	Washington, USA
Pike's Peak	4300	Colorado, USA
Mauna Kea	4210	Hawaii
Mt Fuji	3775	Japan
Mt Cook	3765	New Zealand

*In 1865 Sir Andrew Waugh, Director of the Indian Survey, suggested the highest mountain should be named after Sir George Everest, Surveyor-General of India from 1830 to 1843.
†Disputed area between Sinkian and Kashmir.

(Monge's disease), and most of the studies of the clinical and pathological features of this condition (Chapter 15) have been carried out in the Andes.

The South American mountain ranges are quite heavily populated, and some routes of major economic importance joining Lima and the Peruvian coast to the Amazon ascend to penetrate the mountains via the Ticlio pass (4850 m). On these routes one finds processions of ancient buses and *collectivos* (communal taxis). The roads, if not wide and modern, allow rapid ascent from the coast to altitudes exceeding 4000 m in 1–6 hours. This easy accessibility to the mountains for lowlanders, tourists, and highlanders returning to their homes enhances the risk of developing acute mountain sickness (Chapter 12) and high-altitude pulmonary oedema (Chapter 13). It is no coincidence that much important work on high-altitude pulmonary oedema has been carried out in the hospital of La Oroya, situated by the side of the road just emerging from the Ticlio pass. This mining centre is also the area in which one finds the classic infectious disease of high altitude, Oroya fever, due to *Bartonella bacilliformis* (Chapter 26).

In South America, considerable mining activity goes on at Cerro de Pasco (4330 m), Potosi (4070 m), and Oruro (3760 m). This relative ease of access to the Andean heights has influenced the history of the region. The empire of the Incas extended throughout the Andes and had its capital at Cuzco (3400 m). This highland race built for itself at 2440 m a fortress at Majchu Picchu on the edge of the Amazon, to prevent the fierce jungle tribes penetrating the deep gorges to reach the sacred city of Cuzco. At this altitude the Inca people built a town with incredible terracing and lived on these precipitous mountainsides. At Sacsayhuaman (3580 m), remains of fortresses and temples still exist as testimony that in the past large communities have existed at high altitude just as they do today. Finally, the Andes have their high-altitude camelids to offer for the study of genetic adaptation, as contrasted to acclimatization to the mountain environment (Chapter 35). With the wealth of human and veterinary material it is not surprising that Peruvian physicians and pathologists have played a leading role in the study of high-altitude medicine and pathology.

The Himalaya

'The Himalaya' is a singular noun from the Sanskrit meaning 'the abode of snow' and throughout this book we shall use this instead of the commonly employed but incorrect plural form. The Himalayan range extends across the base of the Indian subcontinent for about 2740 km (1700 miles) from Assam in the south-east to Afghanistan in the west, and it is up to 240 km (150 miles) wide. This range comes under the influence of the monsoon that originates in the Indian Ocean (Fig. 2.8). Water-laden air flows from east to west across India, ascending the mountain slopes and cooling as it does so. Eventually the water vapour condenses and rain pours in torrents between April and October over the eastern part of the Himalayan range. However, as the monsoon passes to the west, it becomes progressively depleted of its content of water vapour. As a result the eastern Himalaya is drenched and the western Himalaya is arid. At Darjeeling, on the border of Sikkim, the rainfall is 123 in (3.1 m) a year. At Simla, north of Delhi, in the central

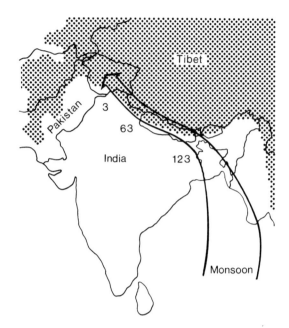

2.8 *As the monsoon sweeps inland from the Indian Ocean, heavy with moisture, it gives rise to an annual downpour of 123 in (3.1 m) a year at Darjeeling, with heavy snowfalls in the Nepal Himalaya. As it crosses the subcontinent it becomes drier, so that the annual rainfall at Simla in the central Himalaya is 63 in (1.6 m). By the time the wind reaches the western extremities of the Himalayan range in Kashmir it is dry and the rainfall is merely 3 in (76 mm) a year. Hence, the Karakorams are arid in contrast to the Nepal Himalaya. Areas of high altitude are indicated by stippling.*

Himalayan range it is 63 in (1.6 m). In contrast, the mountains of the western extremity of the Himalaya in Leh, the capital of Ladakh, have an annual rainfall of only 3 in (76 mm) (Nicolson 1975; see also Fig. 2.8). The Karakorams, derived from Turki words giving the meaning 'black and crumbling rock', dividing Pakistan from China in the west, are arid. Indeed, one of the highest mountains in this range is called 'the naked mountain' (Nanga Parbat) because it is not permanently covered by snow. The other dry western extremity of the Himalaya is represented by the Hindu Kush ('Hindu killer') which is 965 km (600 miles) long and rises to 7620 m. It is situated mainly in Afghanistan.

Much of the Tibetan plateau, at an altitude of between 4600 and 4900 m, is also arid with a low rainfall. It is the largest and highest plateau in the world and has an area of some half a million square miles. It extends from the Himalaya and high Himalayan valleys in the south to the Kun Lun range in the north that separates it from Xinjiang (Chinese Turkestan). To the west it is bordered by the northward curve of the Himalaya that continues into Kashmir to Gilgit and into the Karakorams. Eastwards lie the Quinghai lake, the valleys of Sikiang province, and the gorges of south-east Tibet.

Silicosis in arid Ladakh

For some years local doctors have been concerned at the frequency of chest disease in some villages of the Indus valley in Ladakh, a high-altitude region of the Himalaya in north-west India. Norboo and his colleagues (1991*a*) surveyed the villages of Chucot Shamma (3200 m) and Stok (3500 m) because silicosis had been suspected from the radiographs of some of the inhabitants. These villages are agricultural, and Chucot is exposed to frequent dust storms. In spring dust storms occur in most parts of Ladakh. During these storms the affected villages are covered by a thick blanket of fine dust, and inhabitants are exposed to considerable amounts of the dust for several days (Saiyed *et al.* 1991). Chest radiographs of villagers aged 50–62 years were examined. In Chucot five of seven men and all of the nine women examined showed varying grades of silicosis, compared with three of 13 men and seven of 11 women in Stock (3500 m), which is exposed to fewer dust storms. The women are more heavily exposed to dust because they do most of the farming work and they sweep the dusty houses and carry baskets of earth for the traditional toilets. The houses are often smoky owing to the lack of an effective chimney. There is no occupational exposure to dust.

The difference in prevalence of silicosis between the two villages was significant, as was the difference between men and women. Three patients from the village adjoining Chucot were later found to have radiological evidence of progressive massive fibrosis (Fig. 2.9).

Lung slices showed numerous black nodules, 1–2 mm in diameter. Histological examination of the lungs and a lymph node showed heavy deposition of black dust, which in the lung was aggregated focally as centriacinar collections. Polarizing microscopy revealed many birefringent particles among the black dust. The lymph node was largely replaced by whorled hyaline collagenous nodules. Inorganic dust accounted for 141.7 mg/g of dry lung. Chemical analysis of the inorganic dust in the lung

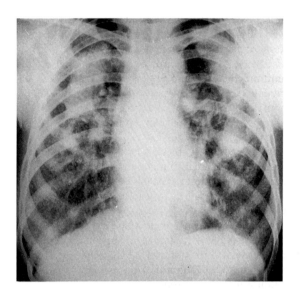

2.9 *Chest radiograph from a Ladakhi resident in the village of Chucot Shamma (3200 m) in the Indus valley. It shows progressive massive fibrosis with egg-shell calcification of hilar lymph nodes.*

showed that 54.4% was elemental silicon. This was similar to the silicon content of dust samples collected from houses in Chucot, which included particles of respirable size. X-ray microanalysis showed that quartz formed 16–21% of the inorganic lung dust. The study of Norboo *et al.* (1991*a*) indicates that silicosis is common among the older inhabitants of these Himalayan villages. The dust exposure is clearly environmental and not industrial. Non-industrial deposition of silica in the lung has been reported in other arid environments in the world such as the Sahara desert (Policard and Collet 1952).

Studies of non-occupational pneumoconiosis at high-altitude villages in central Ladakh were carried out by Saiyed *et al.* (1991) in three communities. In the first dust storms were rare, in the second they were moderate, and in the third they were severe. The prevalance of pneumoconiosis in these three villages was 2.0%, 20.1%, and 45.3%, respectively.

In the same area summer and winter surveys were carried out to examine the relation between respiratory illness and domestic pollution (Norboo *et al.* 1991*b*). The prevalence of productive chronic bronchitis rose steeply with age and was greater among women than men. Lung function was significantly worse in those with chronic cough, independently of age and sex. Carbon monoxide measurements were used to assess domestic pollution from fires. Heating and cooking in the home is provided by fires burning wood from a local bush called 'malchung' and the dung of yaks, cows, horses, and donkeys (Saiyed *et al.* 1991). Many of these fires have no chimney or emit much smoke and fumes into the living accommodation. Due to severe cold, the ventilation in the houses is usually kept at a minimum. The wood is not allowed to burn quickly but is kept smouldering to prolong its slow heating effect. The dwellers are thus exposed to high concentrations of soot. Amongst the small minority of smokers (all men) carbon monoxide in exhaled air was higher than in non-smoking men. In non-smoking men and women, levels of exhaled carbon monoxide were very significantly higher in winter than in summer, as were the levels of carbon monoxide measured in the houses. Norboo *et al.* (1991*b*) concluded that it was domestic pollution that was the important contributor to chronic bronchitis in these villagers of the Himalaya.

The ice-kingdom of the eastern Himalaya

The aridity of Ladakh and Tibet is in sharp contrast to the environment in the eastern mountain ranges of Nepal. Here above an altitude of 5000 m one enters what Nicolson (1975) has aptly described as 'the ice kingdom'. Ice and show predominate and the terrain becomes one of the glaciers, ice walls, and crevasses. Winds up to hurricane force and temperatures as low as $-40°C$ have to be contended with. The health hazards in this region for high-altitude climbers attempting to conquer the highest peaks are unique. They comprises frostbite and other manifestations of cold (Chapter 24) and the dangers inherent in the ice kingdom, namely avalanches, blizzards, and the physical dangers of crevasses.

Himalayan inaccessibility

In contrast to the Andes, the Himalayan mountains are very inaccessible. High-altitude climbers journeying to climb a peak commonly have to trek by foot through high mountain passes for 2–3 weeks to reach the mountains elected for assault. Such inaccessibility means that climbers arriving at high altitude in Nepal or Tibet are acclimatized. In recent years, however, the increasing numbers of trekkers in the region frequently fly to a high altitude to start their trek and thereby constitute a growing problem of cases of acute mountain sickness and high-altitude pulmonary oedema. This inaccessibility can be disastrous when the transport of large numbers of people to high altitude in the Himalaya has to be un-

dertaken as an emergency by air, as a suitable system of roads is not available. This occurred when large numbers of Indian troops were flown to the airstrip at Leh (3500 m) in Ladakh to face the infiltration of Chinese soldiers across the Tibetan border. It produced the explosive creation of the largest series of cases of acute mountain sickness ever reported (Chapter 12).

We have already pointed out that highlanders in these mountain ranges live permanently at altitudes considerably lower than those occupied by the Amerindians of Peru and Bolivia. Tibet and the Himalaya are largely empty above 4570 m. There are gold mines at Tok Dschalung at 4880 m at the headwaters of the Indus, but such settlements are exceptional.

The Ethiopian highlands

These areas attain a moderate altitude of 2400 m–3700 m in their northern parts known as the Amhara highlands and the highest peak in the country is Ras Dashau (4620 m). However, much of the population lives above 2000 m. The region is intersected by a number of rift valley-systems connecting the African Rift Valley to the south and the Red Sea to the north (Ward *et al.* 1989). It is thus divided into the Western highlands, the Rift valley, and the Eastern highlands. As we note in Chapter 3, studies in the Ethiopian highlanders have revealed that children living there are taller and heavier and mature earlier than their genetically similar counterparts living at low altitudes.

Alaska

The mountains of Alaska are at high latitude in the Arctic and this brings problems of exaggerated hypoxia and cold for climbers. Their geographical situation also leads to exposure to rapidly changing adverse weather conditions (Hackett 1988). Mt McKinley, situated in central Alaska, is the highest geological point (6195 m) in North America (Table 2.1). It is situated at 63°N just south of the Arctic circle at 66° 6′ N. Locally the mountain is called in Athabascan 'Denali' meaning 'the great one'.

Its situation at high latitude means that the barometric pressure on the mountain is lower for any given altitude. As noted earlier in this chapter, there is compression of the atmosphere near the poles and expansion toward the equator. The barometric pressure at the summit of Mt McKinley is equivalent to that of altitudes 200–800 m higher in the Himalaya situated at 27°N. It depends on the time of the year being highest (350 mmHg) in July and lowest (326 mmHg) in January. In July the barometric pressure at an equivalent altitude on the equator is 365 mmHg (Hackett 1988). Thus the climbers on Mt McKinley are exposed to a greater degree of hypoxia.

The high latitude of Mt McKinley makes it a much colder mountain than Mt Everest. Only the highest peaks of the Antarctic are comparable in this respect. According to Hackett (1988) the lowest temperature on Mt Everest ever measured at 8000 m was −27°C in October 1981. In contrast to this the minimum temperature at 4300 m on Mt McKinley for the first 2 weeks of May 1985 and May 1986 was −40°C. Assuming a fall-off of 6.5°C per 1000 m, the temperature at the summit of Mt McKinley would have been −53°C.

Mt McKinley and its sister Mt Foraker, situated in the Alaska range and rising abruptly from sea level, create their own microclimate and catch the frequent storm systems moving across Alaska. As a consequence changes in weather and barometric pressure are rapid and severe. Hackett (1988) refers to a drop in barometric pressure of 10 mmHg in one night, the effect of which is to make a climber wake up '152 m higher' in the morning. The lethal combination of diminished barometric pressure, extreme cold, and sudden storms led to eight deaths and 14 helicopter rescues in 1980 and led to the setting up of a rescue post and research laboratory on the mountain.

The Alps

The Swiss Alps are very moderate in altitude compared to other mountainous areas considered in this book but they deserve mention here because they form one of the major tourist centres of Western Europe. Most holiday-makers will gain their experience of mountains through the Alps. So far as mountain medicine is concerned, this mountainous area presents very characteristic features. The levels of altitude encountered are moderate. Thus the summits of the highest peaks in the Alps such as the Matterhorn (4480 m), which are reached only by alpine climbers, are only roughly of the same elevation as the streets of thriving mining towns like Cerro de Pasco (4330 m), inhabited by thousands of Peruvians occupied in the daily round of their lives. In the Alps, accessibility for the majority of holiday-makers is available only to moderate altitudes barely exceeding 3000 m.

However, the profusion of cable-cars and mountain railways means that one can ascent to the borderline of significant high altitude very rapidly

indeed. In little more than an hour it is possible to ascend by mountain railway from Zermatt (1620 m) to Gornergrat station (3130 m) and thence to the Stockhorn station (3405 m) by cable-car. Such rapidity of ascent precludes any chance of acclimatization and the Swiss are either fortunate of far-seeing in that their cable-cars end just at the altitude above which physiological troubles would be expected. Not only are the altitudes too low to present any real risk of acute mountain sickness, but the stay at these high cable-car stations is far too brief for the development of symptoms (Chapter 12). In any event, retreat from high altitude can be achieved as rapidly as entry into it, by cable-car. Nevertheless, it has to be kept in mind that this group of newcomers to high altitude is peculiarly vulnerable, often including small children and the family dog.

References

Baikie, A.G. (1970). *A Companion to Medical Studies*, Vol. 2, Chapter 33. Oxford; Blackwell Scientific

Beck, H.L., Lowder, W.M., and Bennett, B.G. (1966). *Further studies of external environmental radiation*, Report HASL 170. U.S. Atomic Energy Commission

Brunt, D. (1952). In *Physical and Dynamical Meteorology*, 2nd edn. Cambridge; Cambridge University Press, p. 379

Elterman, L. (1964). *Atmospheric attenuation model, 1964, in the ultraviolet, visible and infra-red regions for altitudes to 50 km*, Environmental Research Paper No. 46, AFCRL-64-70. U.S. Air Force Cambridge Research Laboratories

Frisancho, A.R. (1975). Functional adaptation to high altitude hypoxia. *Science*, **187**, 313

Habeler, P. (1979). *Everest: Impossible Victory*. London; Arlington Books

Hackett, P.H. (1988). Medical research on Mount McKinley. *Annals of Sports Medicine*, **4**, 232

Heath, D. and Williams, D.R. (1981). Physical factors at high altitude. In *Man at High Altitude*, 2nd edn. Edinburgh; Churchill Livingstone, p. 9

International Civil Aviation Organization (1968). *Manual of the ICAO Standard Atmosphere*, 2nd edn. Montreal; International Civil Aviation Organization

Koller, L.R. (1952). *Ultraviolet Radiation*. New York; John Wiley/London; Chapman and Hall

Lowder, W.M. and Condon, W.J. (1965). Measurement of the exposure of human populations to environmental radiation. *Nature (London)*, **206**, 658

McCullough, E.C. (1970). Qualitative and quantitative features of the clear day terrestrial solar ultraviolet radiation environment. *Physics in Medicine and Biology*, **15**, 723

Marett, R. (1969). The setting. In *Peru*. London; Ernest Benn, p. 25

Mason, G.W. (1967). Altitude effects on the human body. Ultraviolet, cold and low pressure. *Northwest Medicine*, **66**, 917

Messner, R. (1979). The mountain. In *Everest: Expedition to the Ultimate*. London; Kaye and Ward

Nicolson, N. (1975). *The Himalayas. The World's Wild Places*. Amsterdam; Time-Life Books

Norboo, T., Angchuk, P.T., Yahya, M., Kamat, S.R., Pooley, F.D., Corrin, B., Kerr, I.H., Bruce, N., and Ball, K.P. (1991*a*). Silicosis in a Himalayan village population: role of environmental dust. *Thorax*, **46**, 341

Norboo, T., Yahya, M., Bruce, N.G., Heady, J.A., and Ball, K.P. (1991*b*). Domestic pollution and respiratory illness in a Himalayan village. *International Journal of Epidemiology*, **20**, 749

Norton, E.F. (1925). Norton and Somervell's attempt. In *The Fight for Everest*. London; Edward Arnold

Orr, J.S. (1985). Cell damage in ionising radiation. In *Muir's Textbook of Pathology* (J.R. Anderson, Ed.). London; Edward Arnold, p. 326

Policard, A. and Collet, A. (1952). Deposition of silicosis dust in the lungs of the inhabitants of the Sahara regions. *Archives of Industrial Hygiene and Occupational Medicine*, **5**, 527

Pugh, L.G.C.E. (1957). Resting ventilation and alveolar air on Mount Everest: with remarks on the relation of barometric pressure to altitude in mountains. *Journal of Physiology, London*, **135**, 590

Pugh, L.G.C.E. (1963). Tolerance to extreme cold at altitudes in a Nepalese pilgrim. *Journal of Applied Physiology*, **18**, 1234

Saiyed, H.N., Sharma, Y.K., Sadhu, H.G., Norboo, T., Patel, P.D., Venkaiah, K., and Kashyap, S.K. (1991). Non-occupational pneumoconiosis at high altitude villages in central Ladakh. *British Journal of Industrial Medicine*, **48**, 825

Schaefer, H.J. (1971). Radiation exposure in air travel. *Science*, **173**, 780

Shapiro, J. (1972). Ionizing radiation and public health. In *Radiation Protection. A Guide for Scientists and Physicians*. Cambridge, Mass; Harvard University Press, p. 278

Swan, L.W. (1961). The ecology of the high Himalayas. *Scientific American*, **205**, 68

Tousey, R. (1966). The radiation from the sun. In *The Middle Ultraviolet: Its Science and Technology* (A.E.S. Green, Ed.). New York; Wiley

Unsworth, W. (1977). *Encyclopaedia of Mountaineering*. Harmondsworth; Penguin Books, p. 369

Ward, M. (1975). Temperature regulation, ch. 14; Insulation, ch. 15. In *Mountain Medicine. A Clinical Study of Cold and High Altitude*. London; Crosby Lockwood Staples, pp. 191–2; 209–10

Ward, M.P., Milledge, J.S., and West, J.B. (1989). 'The atmosphere' In *High Altitude Medicine and Physiology*, London Chapman and Hall Medical, p. 27

West, J.B. (1984). Man on the summit of Mount Everest. In *High Altitude and Man* (J.B. West and S. Lahiri, Ed.). Bethesda, Maryland; American Physiological Society, p. 5

West, J.B., Lahiri, S., Maret, K.H., Peters, R.M. Jr, and Pizzo, C.J. (1983). Barometric pressures at extreme altitudes on Mt. Everest: physiological significance. *Journal of Applied Physiology: Respiratory, Environmental and Exercise Physiology*, **54**, 1188

West, J.B. and Wagner, P.D. (1980). Predicted gas exchange on the summit of Mt. Everest. *Respiration Physiology*, **42**, 1

Wilson, J.G. (1976). *Cosmic Rays*. London; Wykeham Publications

3

The native highlander

Throughout the world there are populations of people who are native to high altitudes. Large numbers of Quechua and Aymara Indians live in sizeable mining towns and communities of the Andes, predominantly in Peru and Bolivia. Most Tibetans live on the high plateau of their country and this population merges with the people of the Karakorams of Ladakh. The high-altitude Sherpas live in the Himalayan ranges of Nepal. There are also other smaller groups of native highlanders who are to be found in areas other than South America and Central Asia. They include the people of the Ethiopian highlands and the natives of the mountains of New Guinea. At first sight it would seem an easy matter to determine anthropometric characteristics of such native highlanders manifesting their adjustment to the high-altitude environment. This would establish the bodily features of a 'high-altitude man' whose physique fits him specifically for life at great heights. The problem in fact proves to be complex, for the various peoples referred to above have very different ethnic origins and their physique may be determined by a variety of factors in addition to the hypobaric hypoxia of high altitude. These include genetic background, diet, and chronic infection (Fig. 3.1).

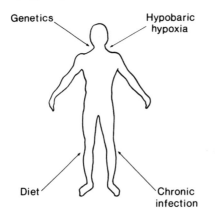

3.1 *Genetic and environmental factors that influence body build in various mountain ranges in the world.*

ANDEAN INDIANS

These peoples were the subjects for the classic early study of the physical anthropology of mountain people by Alberto Hurtado in 1932. His findings and his subsequent views came to have an authoritative influence on the popular image of 'high-altitude man'. This has been unfortunate in the sense that the features he described in Quechuas living at very high altitudes in the Andes have come to be regarded by many, erroneously, as applying to all native highlanders throughout the world. The Quechuas and Aymaras are of Mongoloid stock, and it is generally accepted that their remote ancestors emigrated from Asia by way of the Bering Strait in late glacial times. Proof of their subsequent prolonged undisturbed residence in the mountain habitat is provided by the finding of traces of man at Lauricocha in Peru, with a radiocarbon date of about 7500 BC (Marett 1969).

Facially, these Andean Indians are mongoloid in type (Figs 3.2 and 3.3(a)). The eyes are almond-shaped with thick epicanthic folds (Fig. 3.3(b)). The skin is pigmented and of a dark olive hue and forms a striking contrast to the russet-red colouration of the mucous membranes, the lips, and the lobes of the ears, which is an expression of the high level of haemoglobin described in Chapter 5. Superimposed on this dark red colour is associated central cyanosis consequent upon the systemic arterial oxygen unsaturation due to hypobaric hypoxia. Cyanosis is usually detected when the systemic arterial oxygen saturation falls below 80% and the arterial oxygen tension has fallen to 50 mmHg or less (Cumming and Semple 1973). Such conditions are readily met at high altitude and cyanosis becomes apparent because of the elevated haematocrit in the Quechua Indian. Some 4–5 g of deoxyhaemoglobin need to be present per decilitre of blood for cyanosis to be detected and, since the normal level of haemoglobin in the Andean Indians living at altitudes above 4000 m is in the region of 20 g/dl (Chapter 5), the necessary conditions are readily met. The combination of erythraemia and cyanosis also produces suffusion of the

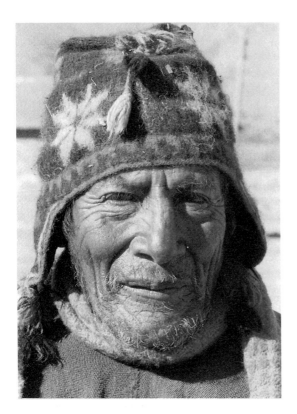

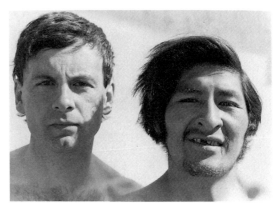

(a)

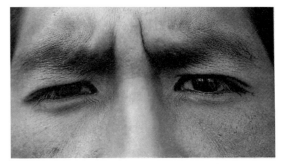

(b)

3.2 *Facial features of a Quechua, 66 years of age, from La Raya (4200 m) in the Peruvian Andes. The skin is pigmented (see Chapter 25) and the lips are of a deep russet-red colour due to the high haematocrit (see Chapter 5).*

3.3 *(a) The facial features of a Quechua Indian (right), 23 years of age, from Cerro de Pasco (4330 m) compared with those of one of the authors (D.R.W.); (b) the Indian's eyes, showing thick epicanthic folds.*

conjunctival vessels, which are both tortuous and prominent. The conjunctiva has a creamy-yellow appearance, rather than the clear white opaque appearance seen in the lowlander in good health. The lips tend to be bulbous and the nose straight. The hair is straight and black.

Hurtado (1932) came to the conclusion that the reduced systemic arterial oxygen saturation of life at high altitude leads to widespread clubbing of the fingers in the native Peruvian highlanders. He made a clinical study of 950 males between the ages of 4 and 75 years and concluded that clubbing is to be found in 59% of Quechua children between 4 and 9 years of age and in 94% of adults. Its degree was said to vary widely between individuals and was frequently limited to the thumb, index, and little fingers. Our personal observations in the Andes lead us to believe that clubbing of the fingers in the healthy Indian population is far less common than

this. It seems to us that the fingers are commonly what British clinicians would term 'beaked' rather than 'clubbed' (Fig. 3.4). In our opinion, true clubbing or the fingers is more likely to be encountered in patients with Monge's disease (see Fig. 15.2), in whom the degree of systemic arterial oxygen unsaturation and cyanosis are greater.

Small haemorrhages within the fingernails are common in the Indian population (see Fig. 25.10) and they are probably related to repeated minor trauma to the nails just as they are at sea level (Chapter 25). Nail haemorrhages are commoner and of more generalized distribution in patients with Monge's disease (Chapter 15). In this condition they are related to a much elevated level of haematocrit, as in patients with cyanotic congenital heart disease

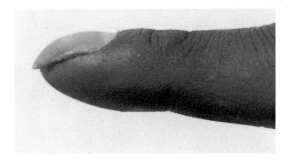

3.4 *A finger of the young Quechua Indian shown in Fig. 3.3. It shows 'beaking' in contrast to the clubbing of the fingers in cases of Monge's disease illustrated in Fig. 15.2(d).*

with secondary polycythaemia in whom they also occur.

The Quechua is shorter than the Caucasian or the mestizo from the coast. In the Andes of 1932, Hurtado found that the average height of young adult Quechua Indians was 159 cm compared with 168 cm in Caucasian students of the same age living at sea level. The shortness in stature was associated with a correspondingly low body weight. In 1932 the average body weight in Quechua Indians was 55.4 kg in the age range 20–34 years, 56.8 kg in those between 35 and 49 years, and 55.2 kg in those between 50 and 75 years. Obesity is a rarity in native highlanders of the Andes.

The bodily feature that attracted most attention from Hurtado (1932) was the thoracic cage. This is not surprising since this is where one might anticipate finding the greatest structural adaptation to provide an increased ventilatory reserve compatible with a healthy and active life at high altitude. He stated: 'Since early childhood there is a definite appearance of a prominent and large chest as proportionally compared with the rest of the body dimensions, and at this age it is often continuous in front with a prominent abdomen. Later in adolescence this outstanding appearance of the chest is more evident on account of the thin lower extremities. This is particularly true in adult life. The native at this time, in the vast majority of cases, gives the impression that practically all the body mass lies on the chest.' This overstates the case and commonly the differences between the configuration of the chest of the native highlander and that of sea-level man are more subtle and require for their demonstration different methods of measurement that, over

the years, have varied considerably in their complexity and validity with different observers.

It is of historical interest that in his classic study of 1932 Hurtado attempted to calculate the so-called 'chest volume' in his cases in the field from the somewhat crude physical measurements of 'chest width, depth and height'. He defined 'width' as the distance between the mid-axillary lines at the level of the sixth ribs. 'Depth' was the distance from the middle of the sternum to the vertebral column at the level at which width was determined. 'Height' was the distance between the upper level of the sternum and its lower tip. He found that in men between 20 and 34 years of age the chest volume was greater in Andean highlanders than in non-native residents at high altitudes, or in white Peruvian students, in spite of the much taller stature of the latter two groups. The so-called 'chest index' is derived from such data as (depth/width) × 100 and gives some idea of the shape of the thorax. In the child at sea level the value of the index falls so that the chest changes from being rounded to ellipsoidal. In the Andes the chest in childhood maintains a more rounded shape. There is a widening of the costal angle. Monge and Monge (1966) compared physical measurements of the chest in 120 subjects from Lima (150 m) and in 53 subjects from altitudes of between 3500 and 4500 m in Bolivia. The average anteroposterior diameter in the highlanders was 213 mm compared with 203 mm in the lowlanders, while the average transverse diameter was 283 mm. As a result of this the chest was rounded rather than ellipsoidal, as described above. The height of the sternum in the Andean Indians was also increased to 199 mm from 183 mm in sea-level subjects, so that the chest as a whole was more voluminous.

In our experience there is considerable variation in the size and shape of the chest in native highlanders of the Andes (Fig. 3.5 (a)–(d)). In Fig 3.5 (a) and (b) is shown the massive chest of a young Aymara Indian resident in the city of La Paz (3800 m). His appearance appeared to confirm the classic views on the voluminous chest of the native highlanders, but close questioning revealed that his spare time was devoted to the hobby of weightlifting and body-building! In contrast, Fig. 3.5 (c) and (d) reveals that other Aymara natives of the Bolivian capital have a small flat chest. Personal observation thus demonstrates that, even in the High Andes, not all the native highlanders manifest the features of a 'high-altitude man' with a voluminous chest and pronounced erythraemia and cyanosis.

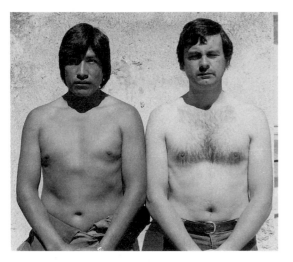

(a)

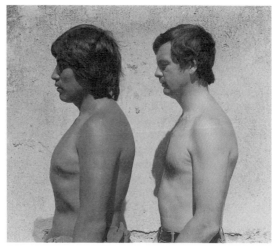

(b)

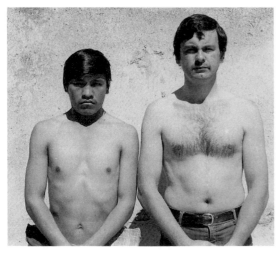

(c)

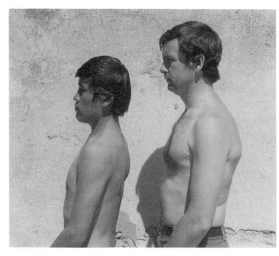

(d)

3.5 *(a) Front view of chest in a young Indian native of La Paz, Bolivia (3800 m) (left) compared with that of one of the authors (D.R.W.). The chest of this highlander is very prominent and well developed and this appearance could be held to be consistent with the classic view that 'high-altitude man' has a barrel-shaped chest. (b) Side view of chest in the same two subjects. The barrel-shaped configuration of the highlander's chest appears even more obvious from this angle. The apparent confirmation of the big chest of the highlander is, however, cast into doubt when questioning reveals that the Indian is an enthusiastic weight-lifter in his spare time! (c) Front view of the chest in another young native of La Paz (left) compared with that of D.R.W. This photograph indicates that the Andean highlanders are usually shorter than Caucasians, but it also shows that the chest of many of them is anything but prominent and hardly confirms the classic view referred to in the text. (d) Side view of chest in the same two subjects. It shows how flat is the thorax in some highlanders. It will be readily appreciated from parts (a)–(d) that with such variation in chest size and shape it is hazardous to make any generalization as to the internal surface area of the lung in native highlanders.*

Internal surface area of the lung and vital capacity

It has not been established that the rounded chest of the Andean highlander demonstrated by anthropometry is associated with an increased internal surface area of the lung. Reliable macroscopic and histological methods of tissue morphometry are available for the determination of the internal surface area of the lung and of the number of alveolar spaces it contains. We have employed these methods extensively in the study of the emphysematous lung (Hicken *et al.* 1966), and their application to the lung of high-altitude man is long overdue. It would clearly be of great interest to ascertain how the internal surface area of the lung is related to the rounding of the chest.

Vital capacity is increased in native highlanders of the Andes (Fig. 3.6). The mean body surface area (BSA) in 612 Quechua Indians between the ages of 20 and 75 years was found to be 1.56 m² (Hurtado 1932). The mean vital capacity in 478 Indians in the age group 20–34 years was 2.72 l/m² BSA. This compared to 2.61 l/m² BSA in non-native residents at high altitude, and 2.46 l/m² BSA in sea-level Caucasian Peruvian students. Vital capacity depends on age as well as body surface area and in high-altitude natives it fell from a mean value of 2.72 l/m² BSA in 478 Quechuas between 20 and 34 years of age, to a mean value of 2.37 l/m² BSA in 29 Indians between 50 and 75 years of age.

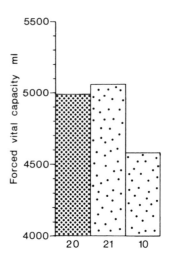

3.7 *Forced vital capacity, adjusted for age, weight, and height in subjects tested at 3400 m. The heavily stippled column is the mean value for 20 high-altitude natives. The lightly stippled columns refer first to 21 sea-level subjects acclimatized during growth, and secondly to 10 Caucasian subjects from the USA acclimatized as adults. (After Frisancho (1975).)*

The vital capacity in subjects living at high altitude depends on the time of life when acclimatization takes place (Frisancho 1975). The forced vital capacity (the maximum amount of air expired after maximum inspiration) was measured by Frisancho *et al.* (1973*a*,*b*) in high-altitude natives at 3400 m, in sea-level subjects acclimatized during growth, and in American subjects acclimatized as adults. Frisancho and his colleagues found that the lowland natives who were acclimatized to high altitude during growth, when adjusted for variations in body size, attained the same values of forced vital capacity as the native highlanders (Fig. 3.7). In contrast, lowlanders, both of Peruvian and American extraction, who had acclimatized as adults had a significantly lower vital capacity than native highlanders (Fig. 3.7). Frisancho (1975) postulates that the enlarged lung volume of the native highlander in the Andes is the result of changes occurring during growth and development and we shall consider this problem now.

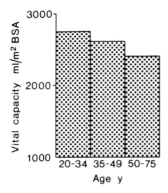

3.6 *Vital capacity (ml/m² body surface area) in three different age groups of high-altitude natives of Morococha (4540 m). The mean values for the three age groups shown are based respectively on data from 478, 105, and 29 Quechua Indians, the smallest group being composed of the eldest subjects. (From data of Hurtado (1932).)*

CHEST DIMENSIONS OF EUROPEAN AND AMERINDIAN CHILDREN AT HIGH ALTITUDE

In an attempt to separate genetic and environmental factors in producing the big chest of the highlander,

Stinson (1985) compared the chest dimensions of European children raised at high altitude with those of Andean natives. The children of European extraction comprised 216 pupils between eight and 14 years of age who attended a private French school in La Paz, Bolivia (3200–4000 m). All of them were born at an altitude over 2400 m and lived all their lives at elevations between 3200 and 3600 m. Although there was some Indian admixture, they were primarily of Spanish ancestry and were genetically closer to Europeans than the indigenous Indian population. The Andean natives were 253 Aymara children from the rural canton of Ancoraimes near Lake Titicaca in Bolivia, at altitudes between 3800 and 4000 m. The standard anthropometric techniques used were measurements of chest width, depth, and shape, and the relation of chest width and depth to stature.

In general, Stinson (1985) found chest width and depth to be larger in the 'European' children, but this was due to their much larger overall body size. From the ages of 8 to 14 years they were 13 cm taller and 6 kg heavier than the Aymaras. This difference in overall size was almost certainly the result of superior diet and other advantages of a higher socio-economic status. However, the Aymara children had larger chest dimensions relative to body stature throughout the age range studied. The reason for this may rest in the fact that in La Paz, built on a steep incline from 3200 m to the altiplano exceeding 4000 m, the native Indian population tends to live at the higher altitudes. In this respect Frisancho and Baker (1970) found that Quechuas living at elevations above 4500 m had significantly larger chest circumferences than those living at 4000 m. A most interesting finding from this study was that the children of European and Indian extraction showed a similar ratio of chest width to depth. Thus the European children raised at high altitude are similar to the Indians in having a round chest, although not the large relative chest dimensions characteristic of native populations. Thus exposure to the hypobaric hypoxia of high altitude during growth may affect the relation of chest width and depth more than it affects relative chest size, which may be of genetic basis. It has been suggested that the effects of hypoxia on growth are greater during adolescence than during childhood (Beall *et al.* 1977), so that it is possible that the trends noted by Stinson progress into adolescence and adulthood. Later in the chapter we consider experimental work on the effects of hypoxia on the developing lung and theo-

retical consideration of the nature of enlargement of the lung at high altitude.

In summary, the Quechua and Aymara highlanders of the Andes have increased chest circumference, although not to the extent suggested in the early descriptions by Hurtado (1932). This is associated with an increased vital capacity. These larger chest dimensions relative to general body build are characteristic of the developing child of the Andean Indian, but an increased ratio of chest depth:width is also found in children of European ancestry living and growing at high altitude (Stinson 1985). We shall see later in the chapter that hypoxia brings about enlargement of the lung of the developing rat. All of these data point to a relation between increased chest circumference, with enhanced lung size and vital capacity, and development size.

TIBETAN AND HAN RESIDENTS OF LHASA

The policy of the Chinese government in introducing large numbers of immigrants of Han origin to mingle with the native Tibetan highlanders in large centres of population like Lhasa (3600 m) has led to an intriguing biological situation where the non-acclimatized and acclimatized (and perhaps partly genetically adapted) have been thrown together at high altitude. In Chapter 17 we allude to this fascinating scenario in connection with infantile subacute mountain sickness but here we may consider it with regard to the physical anthropology of native highlanders in Tibet (Fig. 3.8). Droma *et al.* (1991) set out to determine if native Tibetan highlanders had large lung volumes like the Quechuas of the Andes compared to the Chinese newcomers from low altitude. They studied 38 Tibetan and 43 Han residents of Lhasa matched for age, height, weight, and smoking history. The native highlanders had larger chest measurements and lung volumes (Table 3.1). The total lung capacity and vital capacity of the Tibetans in relation to body size were similar to values reported earlier in this chapter for native highlanders in the Andes. These larger lung volumes may be important in raising lung diffusing capacity by increasing internal surface area and thus improving arterial oxygen saturation during exercise.

SHERPAS

Anthropometric studies on the Sherpas of the Nepalese Himalaya led Gupta *et al.* (1985) to rather different conclusions. Sherpas live in the eastern Himalaya and their name is in fact derived from the Tibetan language meaning inhabitants (*pa*) of the

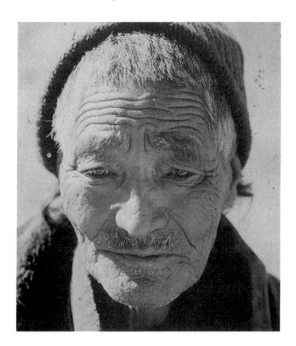

3.8 *Facial features of a native highlander of the Himalayan village Sakti (4500 m) in Ladakh in the Karakoram range on the Tibetan border. They differ from the features of the Andean Indian illustrated in Figs 3.2 and 3.3. The body build of native highlanders from various mountain ranges throughout the world depends on genetic factors as well as on the hypobaric hypoxia of high altitude.*

east (*shar*). They represent an offshoot of the people of Tibet, continuing to speak the dialect of that country and following one of its sects of Buddhism (Gupta *et al.* 1985). the original homeland of the Sherpas was in Kham province, Salmo Gang, some

2000 km away from their present home in the Solu and Khumbu regions of Nepal (Gupta *et al.* 1985). High-altitude Sherpas in the main live in villages such as Namche Bazar, Khumjung, Khunde, and Thamichok, situated at heights of between 3500 and 4050 m. These elevations are comparable to but, it should be noted, distinctly lower than those of the communities of the Andean altiplano. It is possible that the Sherpas emerged as a distinct group only after settling in the Khumbu region (Pawson 1974). There are also low-altitude Sherpas who emigrated directly into the Kalimpong area around Darjeeling (Sikkim) about 200 years ago (Gupta 1980). They live in the villages of the hill districts of Darjeeling at altitudes between 1200 and 1500 m. Also living in the low-altitude areas of the eastern Himalaya are the Lepchas who are the original inhabitants of the region.

Gupta *et al.* (1985) compared the anthropometric characteristics of high- and low-altitude Sherpas and found little difference between them thus confirming previous findings by Beall (1982). They extended their study to compare the body build of Sherpas domiciled at similar altitudes but living in different socio-economic circumstances. Multivariate statistical analysis confirmed that anthropological analysis of people in mountainous areas must include economic and cultural factors as well as environmental ones such as hypobaric hypoxia (Majunder *et al.* 1986). Genetic factors must also be kept in mind. The study of Gupta *et al.* (1985) confirmed that lifestyle is important in determining body build. As a general example we may note that, in the past, the fact that adult Sherpas were leaner than lowland Tibetans was almost certainly related to their poorer economic conditions. In recent times there has been a considerable influx of mountaineers and trekkers requiring Sherpa guides and porters, and this has led

Table 3.1 Chest circumference and lung volumes in Tibetan and Han residents of Lhasa* (after Droma *et al.* 1991)

Parameter	Tibetans	Han Chinese	*p* value
n	38	43	
Total lung capacity (l)	6.80 ± 0.19	6.24 ± 0.18	<0.05
Vital capacity (l)	5.00 ± 0.08	4.51 ± 0.10	<0.05
Residual volume (l)	1.86 ± 0.12	1.56 ± 0.09	<0.06
Chest circumference (cm)	85 ± 1	82 ± 1	<0.05

*Matched for age, height, weight, and smoking history.

to a change in the economic structure from yak-breeding and the growing of potatoes and yams to a more affluent labour for wages (Pawson 1974). Such social and economic changes may well lead in the future to a blurring of the differences in body build between Sherpas and lowland Tibetans. In the same way, differences between low-altitude Sherpas and Lepchas may largely be due to the better nutrition of the latter.

GROWTH AND DEVELOPMENT

Child-growth surveys in Peru, Ethiopia, and Nepal illustrate the pitfalls of such comparative studies in different areas at high altitude. Patterns of growth appear to be population-specific for the reasons we have just outlined and it is not possible to extrapolate the effects of environmental stress from one population to another (*Lancet* Annotation 1975). Studies in Peru showed that children born and raised at altitudes above 3500 m tended to have lower birth weights (Chapter 23), slower growth rate, a longer overall period of growth, a poorly defined adolescent growth spurt, and delayed onset of certain aspects of psychomotor development (Pawson 1976). In an early study of 21 native highlanders, 10 years of age, born and living at Morococha (4540 m), the average height was 122.2 cm, this being some 8.5% less than a comparable low-altitude group in North America (Hurtado 1932).

Subsequent studies in Ethiopia showed that children living at high altitude were taller and heavier, and matured earlier, than their genetically similar counterparts living at low altitude (Clegg *et al.* 1972). The situation of the two communities studies, Adi Arkai (1500 m) and Debarek (3000 m), was unusual in that a high degree of genetic homogeneity has been established for two adjacent populations subject to diverse environmental conditions, notably differences in altitude and temperature and the presence of infectious disease (Pawson 1976). Hence the effects of environmental differences could be assessed by investigation of persons from the two villages. Although the main difference between the two villages was that of altitude, the comparative difference in body measurement between children of the two villages did not conform to the pattern of altitude effects on growth predicted on the basis of work carried out in Peru (Frisancho and Baker 1970). In the Amerindians, growth retardation appears to be proportional to the degree of hypoxia along the altitude gradient, making it seem likely that hypoxia is the main agent responsible. The

work of Stinson (1985), quoted earlier in this chapter, suggests that in children growing in the Andean environment both genetic and environmental factors are of importance, involving respectively the size of the chest relative to general stature, and the ratio of chest depth to width. It is, however, difficult to draw valid comparisons between the work from Ethiopia and that from the Andes. Thus the degree of hypoxic stress encountered in the highland communities of Ethiopia at 3000 m may not be great enough to affect growth adversely. Socio-economic influences including diet may be of considerable importance. Another factor predisposing to retarded growth in Ethiopian lowlanders may be the greater prevalence among them of malaria and intestinal parasitism. It is apparent that growth and development in high-altitude populations are influenced in a complex fashion by genetics, factors related to the mountain environment such as hypobaric hypoxia, socio-economic influences including diet, and complicating disease such as malaria, parasitism, and other infectious disease (see Fig. 3.1).

In order to clarify the effects of genetic and environmental influences on growth among high-altitude populations, a study was made by Pawson (1976) of the growth characteristics of peoples of Tibetan origin living in Nepal (Figs 3.9 and 3.10). The individuals studied were Sherpas living in several villages in the Everest region at altitudes

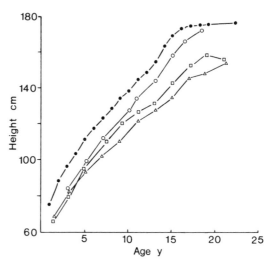

3.9 *Height (in cm) of white American children at low altitude (filled circle) in comparison with that of children at high altitude in Ethiopia (open circle), of Quechua children in the Andes (square), and of Sherpa children in Nepal (triangle). (After Pawson (1976).)*

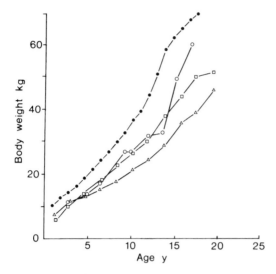

3.10 *Body weight (in kg) of white American children at low altitude (filled circle) in comparison with that of children at high altitude in Ethiopia (open circle), of Quechua children in the Andes (square), and of Sherpa children in Nepal (triangle). (After Pawson (1976).)*

between 3500 and 4050 m. This people had migrated from the Tibetan plateau, where they had existed for several thousand years, to their present habitat a few hundred years ago and were thus comparable to the Quechuas and Aymaras of the Andes. The other group studied was composed of refugee Tibetan children living near Kathmandu (1000 m); they lived in better social conditions than the Sherpa villagers at high altitude.

Overall somatic growth in the Sherpa and Tibetan children was compared with that of children in the Andes, the Ethiopian highlands, and in the USA (Figs 3.9 and 3.10). The American children were consistently taller than any of the highland populations. The Ethiopians were the tallest of the highlanders (Fig. 3.9). The Quechuas were taller than the Sherpas. The Sherpas were shortest (Fig. 3.9) and most closely resembled the Tibetans. A small sample of adult Tibetans was more similar in height to adult Ethiopians, suggesting that the period of growth of Sherpa and Tibetan children may extend past the age at which other high-altitude populations have stopped growing.

All the children from the three highland groups were lighter than the children from the USA (Fig. 3.10). The Ethiopians were the heaviest of the young highlanders. The high-altitude Sherpas were

the lightest of the three mountain groups (Fig. 3.10). However, eventually Sherpa and Tibetan populations attain body weights that are equal to or greater than those of Quechua or Ethiopian populations. As with height, there is evidence that body weight continues to increase in Tibetan and Sherpa populations well into the third decade of life.

Earlier in this chapter we referred to the classic 'barrel-shaped' chest of the Andean highlander as described by Hurtado (1932). Pawson (1976) compared chest circumference and its relation to height in the three groups of high-altitude natives referred to above. He found that Quechua children have the largest chest circumferences up to the age of 13 years when they are surpassed by Ethiopians. On the other hand, the chest dimensions of Sherpa and Tibetan children are generally less than those of the other populations, especially after the age of 13 years. Quechua boys do not appear to be developing unusually large chest dimensions for their height at least up to the age of 13 years. After that time, Quechua and Sherpa boys resemble each other in their individual chest circumference:height ratios. Any enlargement of chest dimensions in native Andean highlanders must be part of a prolonged process of growth in chest circumference that extends well into the third decade.

Skinfold thicknesses showed that Sherpa children have a greater amount of body fat than Quechua children when young, but that this decreases progressively as they become older. Ethiopian children have less body fat than Tibetan or Sherpa children. Bone development in the hand is consistently retarded over much of the period of growth in highlanders, particularly among Sherpas and Tibetans (Pawson 1976).

It is clear that comparative studies of growth among various high-altitude populations are beset by great difficulties. Specific effects seen in one population may not occur in another. In the Ethiopian highlander, the major factor causing him to be heavier and taller is the healthier environment with less prevalent malaria and intestinal parasitism. Genetic factors seem to be important, since there is genetic homogeneity with persons living at lower altitude in the region. The degree of hypoxia encountered in the Ethiopian highlands is inadequate to influence chest and lung development. In the Andes there seems to be growth retardation induced by increasing levels of hypoxia along the altitude gradient. Here the increased chest dimensions may reflect structural adaptations of the chest wall to hypoxia during the period of growth. In the Himalaya the effects of altitude on the chest are not so demonstrable as in the Amerindian. Here genetic influences seem to be predominant and 'the growth characteristics of Himalayan peoples may reflect the presence of an extremely ancient Tibetan gene pool' (Pawson 1976). One of the most conspicuous features of both Tibetan and Sherpa children is their remarkably slow growth in size and rate of skeletal maturation, despite differences in the conditions under which they live.

HYPOXIA AND THE DEVELOPING LUNG IN RATS

There is experimental evidence to suggest that the structure of the growing lung is influenced by the partial pressure of oxygen in the atmosphere. Burri and Weibel (1971) subjected three groups of rats to hypoxic, normoxic, and hyperoxic atmospheres from the 23rd to the 44th day of postnatal development. The hypoxic group was exposed to a simulated altitude of 3450 m and a Po_2 of 100 mmHg. The normal group was kept at normal barometric pressure with a Po_2 of 150 mmHg. The hyperoxic group was kept in an atmosphere of 40% oxygen and 60% nitrogen at a mean pressure of 730 mmHg and a Po_2 of 290 mmHg. A fourth group of rats of the same age and stock was killed on the 23rd day of postnatal development in order to provide control data.

The absolute lung volume measured by water displacement, on the 23rd day, was 2.5 ml. On the 44th day this rose to 6.34 ml in the control group, 6.84 ml in the hypoxic group, and 5.51 ml in the hyperoxic group. The animals in the hypoxic group weighed less than the other groups so that lung volume per 100 g body weight is more relevant. The control group had a value of 4.5 ml/100 g compared with 5.5 ml/100 g in the hypoxic animals and 3.9 ml/100 g in the hyperoxic animals. This means that the lung volume per 100 g body weight in the hypoxic animals was some 20% more than in the controls (Fig. 3.11). Light and electron microscopy showed no significant quantitative changes in the relative composition of the lung. Hence the increase in lung volume could be attributed to increases in alveolar capillary and tissue volumes.

The importance of relating lung volume to body weight can be seen from the above results. Cook *et al.* (1970) exposed young rats to a barometric pressure of 390 mmHg for 21–91 days. They found that the growth rate of the lung was normal, although the increase in body weight was reduced when compared with the controls. Hence the lung volume per 100 g body weight in their hypoxic animals was

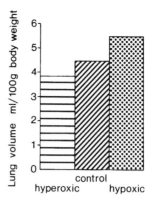

3.11 *Lung volumes (expressed as ml/100 g body weight) in three groups of rats exposed to hyperoxic, normal, and hypoxic atmospheres from the 23rd to the 44th day of postnatal development. The Po_2 to which the groups were exposed was 290, 150, and 100 mmHg, respectively. (From data of Burri and Weibel (1971).)*

considerably increased. After a return to normal barometric pressure the animals gained weight and after 1 month the lung weights and body weights were normal. However, Bartlett (1970) conducted a similar experiment to that of Burri and Weibel (1971) when he exposed 1-month-old rats to differing oxygen concentrations of 10.4, 18.3, and 45.8% at sea-level barometric pressure. His findings as to body weight were similar to those of Burri and Weibel (1971), but he found that lung development was not affected relative to body weight in the group exposed to a low oxygen concentration, whereas in the group exposed to a high oxygen concentration body weight increased more rapidly than in controls and the lung growth was inhibited. Although at first the results of Bartlett (1970) with the group exposed to a low oxygen concentration appear to be in conflict with those of Burri and Weibel (1971), there are two important differences in his method. The rats used were 1 month old as opposed to 23 days and at such an early stage of postnatal life such a difference may be significant. Also it cannot be said with certainty that a low oxygen concentration at normal barometric pressure is the same stimulus as normal oxygen concentration at a low barometric pressure.

NATURE OF ENLARGEMENT OF THE LUNG AT HIGH ALTITUDE

Brody *et al.* (1977) studied the nature of enlargement of the lung at high altitude. They were able to confirm from determination of forced vital capacity in Peruvian mountain dwellers between 17 and 20 years of age that the lung volume of highlanders is 30–35% greater than that of lowlanders similar in race, age, and body size. Vital capacities of Peruvian lowlanders were only 84% of values found in Caucasians, confirming that there are genetic differences in lung size between Aymara and Caucasian populations. Aymaras living in the mountains, however, had a vital capacity some 116% of that of Caucasian values. Lung elastic recoil in highlanders and lowlanders is similar to that of Caucasian subjects of similar age, suggesting that neither increased muscle strength nor alterations in connective tissue properties of the lung are primarily responsible for the larger forced vital capacities in highlanders. However, in spite of the larger lungs of high-altitude natives, absolute flow rates are not greater and, when expressed as a function of lung volume, are actually less in highlanders (Brody *et al.* 1977). Such a difference in flow rate may be an expression of the manner in which hypoxia stimulates the growth of the lung.

The growth of lung associated with genetic or early fetal adaptation would be likely to be brought about by increasing the size and/or number of both airways and alveolar spaces (Fig. 3.12). Hence the volume of airways matches the increase in alveolar mass, as occurs in the lungs of people of different sizes. On the other hand, the postnatal effects of environmental hypoxia on lung growth would not involve the airways (Fig. 3.12). Hence one would have the combination of the bronchial tree of a lowlander and increased alveolar numbers of a highlander (Fig. 3.12). In this situation, the cross-sectional area or volume of the airways would be the same in highlanders and lowlanders but would have to coexist with increased lung volume in highlanders. In summary, the hypoxia of high altitude appears to bring about enlargement of the alveolar spaces but not of the airways.

BLOOD GROUPS

The difference in the blood groups in the two major peoples living at high altitudes supports the importance of genetic factors in determining their characteristic features. Of particular interest is the remarkable predominance of blood group O among the Indian population of the Andes. Although studies of the ABO blood groups in Liverpool show that only half of the population is of blood group O (Mourant *et al.* 1958), in the Andes of Northern Peru 100% of the population are of this group (Arce

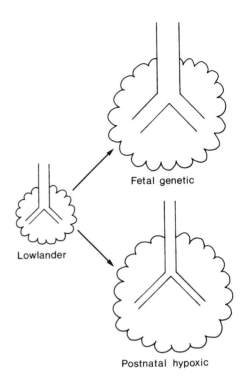

3.12 *Nature of the enlargement of the lung at high altitude. In an enlargement of fetal genetic basis both airways and alveolar lung tissue would be enlarged together. In fact, in the highlander the bronchial tree is not enlarged but only the alveolar spaces, suggesting that the enlargement is due to postnatal effects of environmental hypoxia on lung growth.*

Larreta 1930; see Fig. 3.13). Intermediate incidence of the group is found in the mestizos of Lima, where intermarriage of Spanish stock and Andean Indians is commonplace (Escajadillo 1948; see Fig. 3.13). A high proportion of the population with blood group O is also found in the Andean town of Junin (San Martin 1951; see Fig. 3.13). Blood group O has also been reported in 95% of Bolivian Indians (Quilici 1968), in 85% of Quechuas in Milpo and Colquijirca in Peru (4000 m) (Ruiz and Peñaloza 1970), and in 93% of the Aymaras of the Andean altiplano (Durand 1971). Arias-Stella (1971) studied a native group called the Lamistas in a province of Peru near the jungle and found that 100% of them were of blood group O.

In contrast, in Nepal only 33% of subjects are of blood group O (Macfarlane 1937; Mourant *et al.* 1958) and in Tibet the incidence of blood group O is only 42% of the population (Büchi 1952). Hence it is clear that blood group O is not common to all

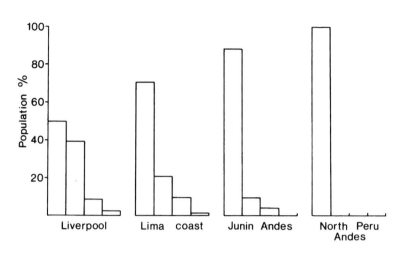

3.13 *Distribution of the ABO blood groups at Liverpool, in the mestizo population of Lima, and in the largely Quechua communities of the Andes. In each instance the first column represents group O, the second column group A, the third group B, and the fourth group AB. Note the predominance of blood group O in the Indian population at high altitude. (From data of Mourant et al. (1958).)*

highlanders and, in general, blood group appears to be related to the origin of the race rather than to any adaptation to life at high altitude. However, this view is not universally accepted. In particular Peñaloza (1971) believes that the present predominance of group O in the indigenous race of the High Andes is the result of a genetic mutation occurring as an adaptive phenomenon over the centuries. Such a belief arises from the study of the blood groups in Peruvian mummies.

Blood groups in Peruvian mummies
Peñaloza (1971) referred to the fact that studies of blood stains found in five South American mummies from the pre-Columbian period revealed blood group A in three cases (Gilbey and Lubran 1952). In the study of Boyd and Boyd (1937), six mummies were found to be of group B and two of group AB. These findings, in face of the predominance of blood group O in most present-day Andean highlanders, has led some to believe that the finding of A, B, or AB groups is artefactual and perhaps due to contamination of mummy tissues by bacteria (Hübener–Thomsen–Friedenreich phenomenon).

This view is not shared by Allison *et al.* (1976) who believe that ABO group antigens have palaeoserological value since they are not restricted to red cells but are distributed throughout the body to include white cells. Thus bone and hair can be used to determined ABO groups and Allison *et al.* (1976) have studied material from dry muscle of forearm or calf, apex of heart, and abdominal skin. They determined the blood groups of Peruvian

mummies of known origin by agglutination–inhibition, induction of antibody production, and mixed cell agglutination. Their results indicate unequivocally the presence of A, B, and AB blood groups in America prior to known European contact.

It seems likely that group B has been eliminated from the Andes by natural selection. Thus, in the province of Pisco in the most northerly area of Peru, the incidence of blood group O in mummies is only 53.1% (Table 3.2). As one moves south to Arequipa (Table 3.2), groups B and AB disappear and Boyd (1959) suggests that the B group may have been eliminated by natural selection. In the Ica culture (Table 3.3), group O was present in 57.1% but in the Incas it rose to 92.4% (Allison *et al.* 1976). The Murga colonial people had three times as many A individuals as the Incas, but the group B of the Ica culture had gone (Table 3.3). One must be careful before ascribing too readily blood group O to mummies, in the realization that A and B antigens may simply have been destroyed by time so that α and β agglutinins are not absorbed.

LONGEVITY
The question is frequently posed whether or not the high-altitude native has a life expectancy similar to that of sea-level subjects. The answer is that the great majority of highlanders achieve a high level of natural acclimatization to the hypobaric hypoxia of high altitude, so that its effects on the body do not shorten life. Most spend long lives in an occupation demanding hard physical work such as mining and

Table 3.2 ABO blood group distribution of Peruvian mummies, based on geographical location of cemetery where mummies were found. The provinces listed are progressively more southerly situated (after Allison *et al.* 1976)

	Blood group (%)			
Province	**A**	**B**	**AB**	**O**
Pisco and Ica	28.6	6.1	12.2	53.1
Nazca	16.6	0	11.2	72.2
Arequipa and Tarapaca	7.2	0	0	92.8

Table 3.3 Cultural groups and carbon 14 dating of Peruvian mummies: agglutination–inhibition technique (after Allison *et al.* 1976)

		ABO blood group distribution (%)			
Culture	**Carbon 14 dating**	**A**	**B**	**AB**	**O**
Paracas	265–85 BC	28.5	7.1	21.4	43.0
Nazca	95 BC–700 AD	0	0	40.0	60.0
Huari	890–1235	26.7	0	20.0	53.3
Ica	1350–1550	32.2	7.1	3.6	57.1
Inca	1245–1650	7.6	0	0	92.4
Tarapaca colonial	1550–1600	10.0	0	0	90.0
Murga colonial	1580–1700	23.6	0	3.7	72.7
Total		22.9	2.2	7.8	67.1

are symptom-free. Only a small minority living at very high altitude in the Andes develop chronic mountain sickness (Monge's disease) with increasing age and are forced to leave their mountain home for the coast or else risk an early death. At the same time it has to be kept in mind that in such areas there are many other potential causes of an early death. Thus in the Andes tuberculosis, infectious hepatitis, malnutrition, and typhus are all common.

In contrast, there are remote mountainous areas in the world where people are alleged to live much longer and remain more vigorous in old age than in most modern societies. To investigate these claims Leaf (1973) visited the Andean village of Vilcabamba (the 'Sacred Valley' according to Davies 1975) in Ecuador at an altitude of 2250 m. He also visited the area inhabited by the Hunza in the Karakoram range of Kashmir (Fig. 3.14) and the Abkhazia region of the Caucasian mountains of Georgia in the former USSR rising to 2000 m (Fig.

3.14). Claims of longevity in such regions are hard to confirm because of the difficulty of establishing unequivocally the age of the subjects. In the absence of birth certificates, church baptismal records are sometimes useful in supporting the age claimed. A census in 1971 suggested that in Vilcabamba no fewer than nine of the population of 819 were centenarians (Leaf 1973). Asadov and Berdyshev (1986) studied longevity in 138 men and 178 women between the ages of 80 and 100 years in Azerbaydzhan (Fig. 3.14). They found that the ages had been exaggerated in a quarter of the subjects studied. Nevertheless, in 1970 the area had 48.4 centenarians per 100 000 of the population, the highest rate in the former USSR. In the Hunza people (Fig. 3.14) the confirmation of the date of birth is difficult, since in the high valleys between China and Afghanistan the language, Burushaski, bears no relationship to other tongues and there is no written form (Leaf 1973). American investigators

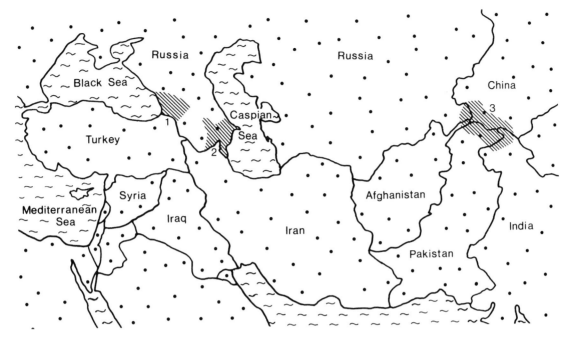

3.14 *The areas of Abkhazia (1) and Azerbaydzhan (2), and those populated by the Hunza in the Karakoram range of Kashmir (3), all famed for the longevity of their inhabitants.*

visiting Vilcabamba in 1978 concluded that the old people of the region 'lie outrageously about their age and have been doing so for years' (Ball 1978). They found that a claim to great age enhanced their prestige in the community. Many claimed their father's baptismal records as their own.

Not only is it extremely difficult to substantiate the claims of longevity of these highlanders in remote areas because of the lack of authenticated birth certificates, it is also impossible to unearth the factors in the way of life of these mountain folk that bestow long life. Indeed, one can imagine the interest that would be aroused throughout the world, in both medical and non-medical quarters, should such a factor ever emerge. Diet has, of course, been investigated as a factor. Davies (1975) dwells momentarily on the exotic possibility of trace elements in the soil, water, and diet, since considerable quantities of gold, iron, magnesium, and cadmium are said to be found in Vilcabamba. Not surprisingly, Leaf (1973) found the daily calorie (energy) intake in these old people from poor mountain societies in both Ecuador and the Karakorams to be low. In 55 men in the Hunza population there was an average intake of less than 2000 cal (8.4 kJ), with 50 g protein, 36 g fat, and 354 g carbohydrate, and a low consumption of meat and dairy products.

In Vilcabamba the average daily diet provided but 1200 cal (5.0 kJ), with 35g protein, 12–19 g fat, and 200–260 g carbohydrate. Under these circumstances it is not surprising that Leaf found that there were no obese subjects in these communities and it has long been appreciated that the life expectation of the obese is less than that of the thin.

However, any views Leaf may have formed on the relation between low calorie intake and longevity received a rude shock when he visited the Caucasus. There he found that everyone, including the aged, consumed a diet high in calories and rich in dairy and meat products. As a result many of the population were fat. One obese woman, said to be 107 years old, remarked: 'I became fat when I stopped having children. For 60 years I have been fat as a barrel and all my children are like me.'

Furthermore, many enjoyed intemperate habits. Leaf (1973) was impressed by the heavy alcohol intake of some of the centenarians at a meal he attended in Georgia. Davies (1975) also commented on the heavy alcohol intake of natives of Vilcabamba. One woman, believed to be 130 years old, had smoked a packet of cigarettes a day for 62 years. It is noteworthy that all highlanders undertake much hard physical labour from childhood onwards.

Simply traversing the mountainous terrain each day sustains a high level of fitness.

It is difficult to be certain of the importance of genetic factors. Probably they have an influence and Leaf (1973) notes that almost all the supposed centenarians had at least one parent or sibling who had enjoyed the same longevity. However, one should not think of these areas claimed to favour longevity as isolated, genetically pure communities. In the Caucasus there are many different ethnic groups such as Georgians, Azerbaydzhanis, Russians, Jews, and Armenians. Davies (1975) also points out that La Thoma in Ecuador, famed for its centenarians, is a hotchpotch of humanity on the way to Peru.

One factor that must not be overlooked is the sociological structure of these communities, in which the family unit is still of great importance. Not only that, but the aged still have an important role in the family group, a condition no longer applying in the so-called developed countries of the West. A feeling of being wanted and needed must be an incentive to survive, but present evidence suggests that the prime need is to prove that the centenarians of these high-altitude areas actually exist before finding reasons for the supposed longevity.

References

Allison, M.J., Hossaini, A.A., Castro, N., Munizaga, J., and Pezzia, A. (1976). ABO blood groups in Peruvian mummies. I. An evaluation of techniques. *American Journal of Physical Anthropology*, **44**, 55

Arce Larreta, J. (1930). *Anales del Hospital de Lima*, **3**, 74 (Quoted by Mourant *et al.* (1958)

Arias-Stella, J. (1971). In *High Altitude Physiology: Cardiac and Respiratory Aspects*,. Ciba Symposium (R. Porter and J. Knight, Ed.). Edinburgh; Churchill Livingstone, p. 12

Asadov, S.A. and Berdyshev, G.D. (1986). Familial longevity in the Azerbaijan SSR. *Journal of Clinical and Experimental Gerontology*, **8**, 75

Ball, I. (1978). Lies explode Andean claims for long life. *Daily Telegraph*, London 18 March, p. 20

Bartlett, D. (1970). Postnatal growth of the mammalian lung: influence of low and high oxygen tensions. *Respiration Physiology*, **9**, 58

Beall, C.M. (1982). A comparison of chest morphology in high altitude Asian and Andean populations. *Human Biology*, **54**, 145

Beall, C.M., Baker, P.T., Baker, T.S., and Haas, J.D. (1977). The effects of high altitude on adolescent growth in southern Peruvian Amerindians. *Human Biology*, **49**, 109

Boyd, W.C. (1959). A possible example of the action of selection in human blood groups. *Journal of Medical Education*, **34**, 398

Boyd, W.C. and Boyd, L.G. (1937). Blood grouping tests on 300 mummies. *Journal of Immunology*, **32**, 307

Brody, J.S., Lahiri, S., Simpser, M., Motoyama, E.K., and Velasquez, T. (1977). Lung elasticity and airway dynamics in Peruvians native to high altitude. *American Journal of Physiology: Respiratory, Environmental and Exercise Physiology*, **42**, 245

Büchi, E.C. (1952). *Bulletin of the Department of Anthropology, India*, **1**, 71 (Quoted by Mourant *et al.* 1958)

Burri, P.H. and Weibel, E.R. (1971). Environmental oxygen tension and lung growth. *Respiration Physiology*, **11**, 247

Clegg, E.J., Pawson, I.G., Ashton, E.H., and Flynn, R.M. (1972). The growth of children at different altitudes in Ethiopia. *Philosophical Transactions of the Royal Society of London*, **B264**, 403

Cook, C., Barer, G.R., Shaw, J.W., and Clegg, H.S. (1970). Growth of the heart and lungs in normal and hypoxic rodents. *Journal of Anatomy*, **107**, 384

Cumming, G. and Semple, S.J. (1973). *Disorders of the Respiratory System*. Oxford; Blackwell Scientific, pp. 171 and 199

Davies, D. (1975). *The Centenarians of the Andes*. London; Barrie and Jenkins, p. 113

Droma, T., McCullough, R.G., McCullough, R.E., Zhuang, J., Cymerman, A., Sun, S., Sutton, J.R., and Moore, L.G. (1991). Increased vital and total lung capacities in Tibetan compared to Han residents of Lhasa (3,658 m). *American Journal of Physical Anthropology*, **86**, 341

Durand, J. (1971). In *High Altitude Physiology: Cardiac and Respiratory Aspects*, Ciba Symposium (R. Porter and J. Knight, Ed.). Edinburgh; Churchill Livingstone, p. 12

Escajadillo, I. (1948). *2° Curso sudamer, de transfus, y hematol*. Santiago-Chile (1946), p. 58. (Quoted by Mourant *et al.* 1958)

Frisancho, A.R. (1975). Functional adaptation to high altitude hypoxia. *Science*, **187**, 313

Frisancho, A.R. and Baker, P.T. (1970). Altitude and growth: a study of the patterns of physical growth of a high altitude Peruvian Quechua population. *American Journal of Physical Anthropology,* **32**, 279

Frisancho, A.R., Martinez, C., Velásquez, T., Sanchez, J., and Montoye, H. (1973a). Influence of developmental adaptation on aerobic capacity at high altitude. *Journal of Applied Physiology,* **34**, 176

Frisancho, A.R., Velásquez, T., and Sanchez, J. (1973b). Influence of developmental adaptation on lung function at high altitude. *Human Biology,* **45**, 583

Gilbey, B.E. and Lubran, M. (1952). Blood groups in South American Indian mummies. *Man,* **52**, 115

Gupta, R. (1980). Altitude and demography among the Sherpas. *Journal of Biosocial Science,* **12**, 103

Gupta, R., Basu, A., Pawson, I.G., Bharati, P., Mukhopadhyay, B., Roy, S.K., Mukhopadhyay, S., Majumder, P.P., Bhattacharyo, S.K., and Bhattacharya, K.K. (1985). *Is high altitude a specialised environment in the human case? Analyses of some Eastern Himalayan data.* Indian Statistical Institute Technical Report No. Anthropology/2

Hicken, P., Brewer, D., and Heath, D. (1966). The relationship between the weight of the right ventricle of the heart and the internal surface area and number of alveoli in the human lung in emphysema. *Journal of Pathology and Bacteriology,* **92**, 529

Hurtado, A. (1932). Respiratory adaptations in the Indian natives of the Peruvian Andes. *American Journal of Physical Anthropology,* **17**, 137

Lancet Annotation (1975). High living in Ethiopia. *Lancet,* **ii**, 17

Leaf, A. (1973). Every day is a gift when you are over 100. *National Geographic Magazine,* **143**, 93

Macfarlane, E.W.E. (1937). East Himalayan blood groups. *Man,* **37**, 127

Majunder, P.P., Gupta, R., Mukhopadhyay, B., Bharati, P., Roy, S.K., Masali, M., Sloan, A.W.,

and Basu, A. (1986). Effects of altitude, ethnicity–religion, geographical distance, and occupation on adult anthropometric characters on eastern Himalayan populations. *American Journal of Physical Anthropology,* **70**, 377

Marett, R. (1969). *Peru,* London; Ernest Benn, p. 33

Monge-M,C. and Monge-C, C. (1966). The high-altitude native. In *High-Altitude Diseases. Mechanism and Management.* Springfield, Illinois; Charles C. Thomas, p. 14

Mourant, A.E., Kopéc A.C., and Domaniewska-Sobczak, K. (1958). *The ABO Blood Groups, Comprehensive Tables and Maps of World Distribution.* Oxford; Blackwell Scientific, pp. 88 and 207

Pawson, I.G. (1974). The growth and development of high altitude children with special emphasis on populations of Tibetan origin in Nepal. Unpublished D.Phil. thesis, Pennsylvania State University, USA

Pawson, I.G. (1976). Growth and development in high altitude populations: a review of Ethiopian, Peruvian, and Nepalese studies. *Proceedings of the Royal Society of London,* **B194**, 83

Peñaloza, D. (1971). In *High Altitude Physiology: Cardiac and Respiratory Aspects,* Ciba Symposium (R. Porter and J. Knight, Ed.), Edinburgh; Churchill Livingstone, p.13

Quilici, J.K. (1968). Les altiplanides du corridor Andin. In *Étude hemotypologique.* Toulouse; Centre d'Hemotypologie

Ruiz, L. and Peñaloza, D. (1970). *Altitude and Cardiovascular Diseases,* Progress Report on World Health Organisation, pp. 1–48

San Martin, M. (1951). *Anales de la Facultad de medicina Casilla 529,* Lima, **34**, 276 (Quoted by Mourant *et al.* 1958)

Stinson, S. (1985). Chest dimensions of European and Aymara children at high altitude. *Annals of Human Biology,* **12**, 333

4

Ventilation and pulmonary diffusion

At rest, the quantity of oxygen consumed by the tissues of the body each minute is 220–260 ml (standard temperature and pressure on a dry gas, STPD) (Harris and Heath 1977). There is an inexhaustible reservoir of oxygen in the ambient air and the problem of providing an adequate supply of the gas to the mitochondria where it will be used lies in the complex nature of the route in the body along which the oxygen must travel to reach the cells. This flow of oxygen can be analysed in terms of the *resistances* met on the route or as *conductances*, which are the reciprocal to resistances and describe the facilitating processes that make the journey of the oxygen easier (Denison 1986).

STAGES OF RESPIRATION

Respiration entails four distinct stages of conduction of oxygen from the atmosphere to the cells. In *ventilation*, air flows through the trachea and bronchial tree to the alveolar spaces of the lung. *Pulmonary diffusion* is the stage by which oxygen in the alveoli comes into contact with the alveolar-capillary walls and passes through them to reach the blood. The gas is then carried by *blood transport* from the capillaries of the lung to those of the tissues. Finally, in the fourth stage of *tissue diffusion*, oxygen passes from the systemic capillaries to the respiratory enzymes of the intracellular mitochondria where it will be utilized.

OXYGEN GRADIENTS

Respiration thus entails a complex combination of transport mechanisms and, even at sea level, various diseases may interfere with one or more of these stages, impairing the conduction of oxygen to the tissues. However, in healthy man living at sea level the operation of transporting the oxygen to the mitochondria functions efficiently because the difference between the partial pressure of oxygen in the atmosphere and that required in the mitochondria is so great. Thus, as we have already seen in Chapter 2, the partial pressure of oxygen in ambient air at sea level is 159 mmHg, whereas the critical P_{O_2} at the

mitochondrial site for oxidative phosphorylation is less than 3 mmHg (Mithoefer 1966). At each of the four stages of respiration there is a fall in oxygen tension. The magnitudes of these changes at sea level, at high altitude, and at extreme altitude are shown in Fig. 4.1. The succeeding falls in P_{O_2} at each stage of respiration are referred to as 'the oxygen cascade'. At high altitude the barometric pressure is diminished and with it the pressure difference of oxygen available to transport the gas to the mitochondria. This is the central problem of respiration at high altitude.

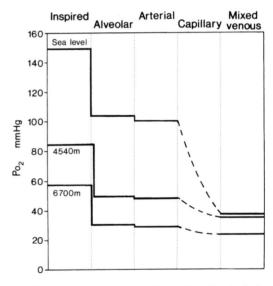

4.1 *Mean oxygen pressure gradients from inspired air to mixed venous blood in lowlanders at sea level, in native highlanders at 4540 m, and in climbers at the extreme altitude of 6700 m. The 'oxygen cascade' in subjects at high altitude is seen to be much less steep than in sea-level residents. Thus, although the partial pressure of oxygen in the ambient air at high altitude is much less than at sea level, the final partial pressure of oxygen achieved in the mixed venous blood of subjects at high altitude is not greatly diminished. (Based on data from Hurtado (1964a) and Luft (1972).)*

The oxygen cascade and acclimatization

There are two ways in which the shortfall in the P_{O_2} of ambient air could be compensated. The first is the modification of tissue metabolism, so that metabolic demands are satisfied in spite of reduced availability of oxygen (Luft 1972). The second is the adjustment by various means of the oxygen transport system so that the impact of the loss of oxygen pressure in the atmosphere is minimized for the tissues and particularly for the mitochondria (Luft 1972). Most features of acclimatization fall within the second category and Fig. 4.1 reveals how adjustments in the transport mechanisms for oxygen render 'the oxygen cascade' much less steep than would be anticipated if such adjustments did not take place. Thus, in mountaineers climbing at 6700 m there is a diminution of 92 mmHg in the partial pressure of oxygen of inspired air, but that of mixed venous blood is only 13 mmHg less than at sea level.

In this and succeeding chapters we shall consider some of the processes of acclimatization that bring about this remarkable alteration in the steepness of 'the oxygen cascade'. In the present chapter we shall deal with changes in ventilation and pulmonary diffusion. In the next chapter we describe the changes in the blood that occur at high altitude to facilitate oxygen transport and release to the tissues. In Chapter 6 we shall consider alterations in tissue diffusion. Changes of acclimatization in the systemic circulation are considered in Chapter 18.

Partial pressure of oxygen of ambient, inspired, and alveolar air

At sea level the partial pressure of oxygen in ambient air is 20.93% of 760 mmHg which is 159 mmHg. As inspired air passes through the bronchial tree to the alveolar spaces it is humidified. The partial pressure of water vapour in fully saturated air at body temperature is 47 mmHg. Hence the partial pressure of oxygen in inspired air is 20.93% of (760 – 47) mmHg which is 149 mmHg. Once in the alveolar spaces, oxygen diffuses through the alveolar walls to the pulmonary capillaries, whereas carbon dioxide diffuses out from the blood into the alveoli. Hence the partial pressure of oxygen in the alveolar spaces at sea level approximates to 100 mmHg and already one-third of the oxygen gradient transporting the gas to the mitochondria has been lost (see Fig. 4.1). At each breath only some 15% of the alveolar air is replaced by fresh ambient air. This slow replacement of alveolar air is important in preventing sudden changes in gas concentrations in the blood and stabilizes the control of respiration and helps to prevent sudden and excessive changes in tissue oxygenation.

VENTILATION AT HIGH ALTITUDE

Ventilation is increased at high altitude due to the response to the hypobaric hypoxia and this represents a most important component of the process of acclimatization to the mountain environment. As the partial pressure of oxygen in inspired air is reduced, there is little increase in ventilation at first and then ventilation increases exponentially. This non-linear relationship has meant that different workers have used different ways of expressing hypoxic ventilatory response (Milledge 1987). The fall of P_{O_2} from inspired to alveolar air is less in subjects at high altitude. This is because they maximize the flow of oxygen into the alveoli by increasing alveolar ventilation. Hurtado (1964a) found that the mean total ventilation for 103 persons at sea level was 7.77 l/min (SD 1.24), but for 80 highlanders at 4540 m was 9.49 l/min (SD 1.77). Expressed per square metre of body surface area the figures were respectively 4.56 and 6.19 l/min. In general, the native highlander hyperventilates some 25–35% above the value for sea-level man. In the newcomer to high altitude, hyperventilation occurs within a few hours of arrival and increases rapidly during the first week. It comes to exceed that of native highlanders by some 20% (Lenfant and Sullivan 1971). With increasing duration of residence at high altitude this difference between the sojourner and the native diminishes. However, even this smaller difference in ventilation response keeps the partial pressure of oxygen in the alveolar spaces and blood elevated in the sojourner compared with the native highlander.

Such hyperventilation maintains an adequate oxygen tension in the alveolar spaces in the face of a low partial pressure of oxygen in the ambient air. Thus, at Morococha (4540 m) in the Peruvian Andes, where ambient P_{O_2} is 84 mmHg, if the normal oxygen pressure differential from atmosphere to alveolar space of 50 mmHg found at sea level were operative, the resulting partial pressure of oxygen in the alveoli would be a critical 34 mmHg. In fact, hyperventilation at this altitude leads to an oxygen pressure of 50 mmHg, the gradient from ambient to alveolar air having been improved by some 16 mmHg (see Fig. 4.1).

The increase in ventilation varies greatly in different subjects and does not usually begin until the partial pressure of oxygen in inspired air is reduced to about 100 mmHg (Ward *et al.* 1989), corresponding to an alveolar oxygen tension of just over

50 mmHg. This corresponds to an altitude of 4000 m. In our experience the hyperventilation that occurs on acute exposure to high altitude is due to an increase in tidal volume rather than in respiratory rate. This view is not accepted by everyone. Burki (1984) studied six young men, of mean age 19.5 years, at an altitude of 518 m and subsequently on the first 4 days in Kaghan (3940 m) in the Karakorams. He wished to study the relative alterations in the components of ventilation that led to the well-documented hyperventilation at high altitude. He was able to confirm the expected increase in resting expired minute ventilation from a control mean of 9.9 ± 1.78 l/min to 14.25 ± 2.67 l/min on the third day of exposure to high altitude. However, he found no significant change in tidal volume, which was 0.60 ± 0.21 litres at sea level and 0.61 ± 0.12 litres on the third day of exposure to high altitude. In contrast he found that there was a sharp, significant rise in respiratory rate from 15.6 ± 3.5 to 23.8 ± 6.2 breaths/min on the third day of exposure. This led him to believe that acute exposure to high altitude in normal lowlanders causes the well-known increase in resting expired minute ventilation primarily by an alteration in central breath timing with no change in respiratory drive. We find these conclusions surprising, for on visits to the Andes and the Himalaya we have been impressed by the singular lack of increase of respiratory rate at rest.

Ward (1975) is also of the opinion that on exposure to high altitude the initial change in ventilation appears to be an increase in tidal volume rather than in rate. He reports that minute volume increases above 3660 m, but respiratory rate at rest does not increase significantly until an altitude exceeding 6000 m is reached. We are inclined to believe that psychological factors, perhaps apprehension on acute exposure to high altitude, led to the high respiratory rates in the six teenagers studied by Burki (1984). He quotes the remarkably high mean figure of 27.6 ± 5.8 breaths/min for his subjects on the second day of exposure to high altitude. In our opinion such a high rate at rest, if not due to psychological factors, is likely to indicate incipient high-altitude pulmonary oedema (Chapter 12).

At sea level, once alveolar Po_2 exceeds about 100 mmHg, there is normally little further benefit to be derived from hyperventilation because pulmonary capillary blood becomes saturated with oxygen (Denison 1986). At first sight it would seem that increasing alveolar ventilation would be worthwhile whenever pulmonary end-capillary Po_2 fell below 100 mmHg, but this is not so. Increasing alveolar ventilation above metabolic need dilutes alveolar carbon dioxide excessively. This disturbs arterial pH and eventually cerebral pH, leading to protective constriction of cerebral vessels and a paradoxical reduction in the provision of oxygen to cerebral tissue, where many critical oxygen-dependent reactions occur (Denison 1986).

Initial hyperventilation and peripheral arterial chemoreceptors

On ascent to high altitude the initial hyperventilation is due to stimulation of the peripheral arterial chemoreceptors, namely, the carotid and aortic bodies. Moderate elevation will not bring about such stimulation immediately (Rahn and Otis 1949). In hypoxia induced acutely it is necessary to lower arterial oxygen tension to about 55 mmHg before hyperventilation occurs (Cumming and Semple 1973). However, once acclimatization has taken place, hyperventilation will be provoked by an arterial oxygen tension as high as 90 mmHg. The hypoxic drive from the peripheral arterial chemoreceptors is maintained in the newly acclimatized for many weeks on exposure to high altitude (Michel and Milledge 1963; Tenney *et al.* 1964). Lowlanders who live for years at high altitude do not lose their hypoxic drive due to the sensitivity of their peripheral arterial chemoreception to a diminished arterial oxygen tension. There has been just one study of lowlanders resident at high altitude for decades that suggested that blunting of the hypoxic ventilatory response did eventually take place slowly (Weil *et al.* 1971). This could be explained by the gradual proliferation of sustentacular cells relative to chief cells which is a feature of the ageing of the carotid body at high and low altitudes (Chapter 7). In striking contrast, native highlanders, and indeed anyone exposed to severe hypoxia during the first few years of his life, do not show that same degree of sensitivity to hypoxia. The role of the carotid bodies in the respiratory adjustments to the hypobaric hypoxia of high altitude is considered in Chapter 7. It will be apparent that there is a controversy here as to whether a brisk ventilatory response to hypoxia, as seen in the newcomer to the mountains, or a blunted response, as seen in the native highlander, offers the greatest benefit for life at high altitude. This problem is considered at length in Chapter 32, where it is considered especially in relation to high-altitude climbing.

Respiratory alkalosis and acid–base balance

The hyperventilation resulting from stimulation of the carotid bodies by the hypoxaemia brought about by the hypobaric hypoxia of high altitude results in increased exhalation of carbon dioxide. As a result the arterial carbon dioxide tension falls and arterial pH rises. This respiratory alkalosis is gradually corrected by the renal excretion of excess bicarbonate restoring blood H^+ concentration towards normal. This metabolic compensation for the alkalosis may be complete with the arterial pH returning to normal or incomplete with a pH that exceeds 7.4 and remains stabilized at that level.

There have been several studies of arterial pH when healthy lowlanders are taken rapidly to high altitude (Severinghaus *et al*. 1963; Lenfant *et al*. 1971; Dempsey *et al*. 1978). In one typical study with ascent to 4500 m in less than 5 hours arterial pH initially rose to a mean of 7.47 within a day and then very slowly declined but was still about 7.45 at the end of 4 days. On return to sea level the pH fell gradually to return to a normal value of 7.40 after 2 days (Lenfant *et al*. 1971). In the study of Severinghaus *et al*. (1963) in which four normal subjects were taken rapidly to an altitude of 3800 m for 8 days, the arterial pH rose rapidly from a mean of 7.42 at sea level to 7.48 after 2 days and remained at this level at the end of 8 days.

Metabolic compensation is slow. We found that on acute exposure to high altitude in the Andes the pH of the urine may show little or no change during the first 2 or 3 weeks. In fact, on further ascent from 3000 to 4300 m we found the urine to become even more acid. During an expedition at high altitude in Colombia, Waterlow and Bunjé (1966) found the urine to be alkaline on only three occasions during the testing of 500 specimens. Ward (1975) refers to this apparent paradox and believes it may be accounted for by the fact that many visitors to high altitude suffer from acute mountain sickness with anorexia and loss of weight. Acetone bodies may occur in the urine, masking the sluggish renal compensation.

After this early compensatory process the subject is left with an arterial carbon dioxide that is lower than normal and a reduced blood bicarbonate concentration (Monge and Monge 1966; Mithoefer 1966). Typical values for their reduced levels at an altitude of 4540 m are shown in Fig. 4.2. Thus native highlanders show a fully compensated respiratory alkalosis with arterial pH values close to 7.40. Typical values reported are 7.36 at 4300 m (Aste-Salazar and Hurtado 1944), 7.37 at 4500 m (Hurtado *et al*. 1956), 7.40 at 4510 m (Chiodi 1957), 7.43 at 4300 m (Monge *et al*. 1964), 7.40 at 4880 m (Lahiri *et al*. 1967), 7.40 at 4500 m

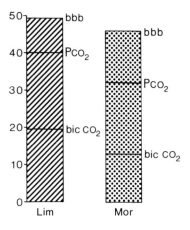

4.2 *Partial pressure of carbon dioxide and blood buffer base in systemic arterial blood in native residents of Lima (Lim) at 150 m (hatched column) and Morococha (Mor) at 4540 m (stippled column). In both columns the top line (bbb) represents blood buffer base in mmol/l. The middle line P_{CO_2} represents partial pressure of carbon dioxide in mmHg. The bottom line (bic CO_2) represents bicarbonate CO_2 in mmol/l. (Based on data from Hurtado (1964a).)*

(Torrance *et al*. 1970–71), and 7.40 at 4300 m (Rennie *et al*. 1971).

There has been one controversial report by Winslow *et al*. (1981) to the effect that the mean plasma pH in 46 Quechua Indians (4540 m) was 7.44. Their blood was thus slightly on the alkaline side of normal and the respiratory alkalosis did not appear to be fully compensated. There was some concern that the elevated haematocrit had had an effect on the glass electrode for measuring pH, a problem that had been considered by one of the authors some years before (Whittembury *et al*. 1968). In spite of this possible reservation about their data, Ward *et al*. (1989) point out that no other workers in this field had made a correction for this effect on the electrode and they conclude that the mild alkalinity representing an incompletely compensated respiratory alkalosis was genuine.

Ward *et al*. (1989) note that, when sufficient time is allowed for acclimatization in lowlanders to high altitude, the arterial pH returns close to the normal value of 7.4 up to an altitude of 3000 m. Above this altitude the blood becomes somewhat alkaline. As long ago as 1937 Dill *et al*. found mean arterial pH to be 7.45 at 5340 m. West *et al*. (1962) reported values in the range of 7.41 and 7.46 at 5800 m. Winslow *et al*. (1984) made extensive measurements of arterial pH during the 1981 American Medical Research Expedition to Everest. The mean arterial pH of acclimatized lowlanders living at 6300 m was 7.47. The mean arterial pH of two climbers on 8050 m was 7.55 and in one subject one the summit of Mt Everest the calculated arterial pH was over 7.7. These climbers were at these extreme altitudes for very short periods and were in no sense acclimatized. Ward *et al.* (1989) point out that metabolic compensation for respiratory alkalosis appears to be extremely slow.

Cerebrospinal fluid and ventilation

Within the medulla there is a receptor to levels of carbon dioxide that responds rapidly to an increased H^+ concentration in the cerebrospinal fluid (CSF). Respiration is stimulated and the hyperventilation reduces the partial pressure of carbon dioxide, thereby returning the pH of the CSF to normal. On initial exposure to high altitude there is stimulation of the carotid bodies and peripheral arterial chemoreceptors which thereby reduces the partial pressure of carbon dioxide in the CSF. This brings about a relative alkalinity of the fluid as part of the general respiratory alkalosis described above and tends to inhibit respiration by its action on the medullary H^+ receptors.

Some years ago Severinghaus *et al.* (1963) and Severinghaus and Mitchell (1964) presented physiological evidence to suggest that this cerebrospinal alkalosis does not occur, due to active transport of bicarbonate ions out of the CSF, which brings about a relative increase in its acidity that stimulates ventilation and thus aids acclimatization. This concept of the role of the pH of the CSF as a homeostatic mechanism was soon challenged. Dempsey *et al.* (1974) and Forster *et al.* (1975) found that the pH of the lumbar CSF were more alkaline than at sea level in men stopping at 3100 m for 3–4 weeks and at 4300 m for only 5–10 days. Weiskopf *et al.* (1976) also found that, in six healthy men subject to a simulated altitude of 4300 m for 5 days, both lumbar and intracranial CSF were significantly more alkaline than at sea level. It would appear that the strong hypoxic peripheral chemoreceptor drive is in fact partly offset by alkaline inhibition of the medullary chemoreceptors.

Sustained hyperventilation

At low altitude ventilation is largely controlled by the level of carbon dioxide, the sensor being a paired region beneath the surface of the fourth ventricle in the medulla. The response of ventilation to the gas is influenced by the prevailing partial pressure of oxygen, so that with increasing hypoxia the line of the response curve of ventilation to carbon dioxide steepens (Milledge 1975). Hence, using various levels of arterial oxygen tension, a 'fan of curves' may be produced (Fig. 4.3). On ascent to high altitude the 'fan of curves' moves to the left, so that at an extreme altitude of 5800 m its origin moves from 38 to 23 mmHg. Hence the respiratory centre now responds to a level of carbon dioxide reduced by almost half. Furthermore, having started to respond, the respiratory centre responds more briskly to any increment in carbon dioxide. The influence of hypoxia on the response to carbon dioxide remains in principle the same as at sea level, so that a fall in the partial pressure of oxygen still increases the response to carbon dioxide (Fig. 4.3). Hence in highlanders the sensitivity to carbon dioxide remains high, but that to hypoxia is blunted. Indeed, some authorities believe that a heightened sensitivity to carbon dioxide is an important factor in sustaining hyperventilation. Thus, Hurtado (1964*b*) reported an increased ventilatory response to carbon dioxide inhaled at high altitude as compared with sea level, although Chiodi (1957) found no such response in two high-altitude natives at 4520 m. Once this increased sensitivity has been induced in the acclimatized lowlander, he will show only an insignificant fall in ventilation even when breathing oxygen, which raises his arterial oxygen tension to equal or exceed that which was found at sea level (Cumming and Semple 1973).

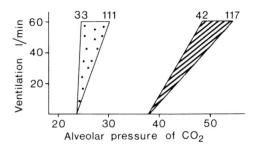

4.3 *Ventilatory response at sea level and at 5800 m. The numbers at the upper ends of the lines indicate the P_{O_2} value of that response line. At high altitude (stippled triangle) the respiratory centre responds to a level of carbon dioxide that is only half of sea-level values (hatched triangle). Furthermore, the response is brisker to any increment in carbon dioxide. (From data of Milledge (1975).)*

The respiratory sensitivity to carbon dioxide starts to increase after only some 15 hours at high altitude and it continues to increase to the eighth day when no further changes occur. The magnitude of the increase in sensitivity is roughly proportional to the degree of altitude. After this early stage there is a slow decrease in ventilation that starts after a few weeks and continues over years. As we have seen, newcomers on ascent sustain a higher ventilation than native highlanders whose resting ventilation, however, still exceeds that of sea-level man. As a result of this, at any given altitude, the resident highlander has a lower arterial oxygen tension and a higher arterial carbon dioxide tension than the acclimatized lowlander.

Carbon dioxide transport at high altitude

Carbon dioxide transport is modified in those living at high altitude. This is because the partial pressure of the gas in the alveolar spaces is abnormally low and because the haemoglobin content of the blood is increased (Chapter 5). Carbon dioxide is carried in the blood in a variety of ways. In both plasma and cells small amounts are in solution, but larger quantities are combined with base. At sea level, the partial pressure of carbon dioxide of systemic arterial blood reaching the tissues is about 40 mmHg, whereas that of resting tissues is some 46 mmHg. Hence there is a diffusion of carbon dioxide into the blood. At high altitude the diminished barometric pressure of the ambient air and the hyperventilation responding to it both lead to a diminished partial pressure of carbon dioxide in the alveolar spaces. This leads to a fall in arterial carbon dioxide tension. Hurtado (1964*a*) found its mean value to fall from 40.1 mmHg in 80 subjects living at sea level to 33.0 mmHg in 40 subjects living at 4540 m (see Fig. 4.2). The fall in arterial carbon dioxide tension is compensated for by a proportional decrease in plasma bicarbonate (Fig. 4.2), so that blood pH is maintained within normal limits as we have already seen. In the subjects referred to above, the plasma pH was found to be 7.41 at sea level and 7.39 at 4540 m.

The increased number of red cells in the blood occurring during acclimatization participate in carbon dioxide transport, modifying the process. Carbon dioxide combines with haemoglobin to form carbaminohaemoglobin, which may be expressed as Hb NH COOH. Reduced haemoglobin has a much greater power of forming carbaminohaemoglobin at any given level of P_{CO_2} than has oxyhaemoglobin. Carbon dioxide is taken up in the tissues and released in the lungs very rapidly on account of carbonic anhy-

drase activity in the erythrocytes. This catalyses the formation of carbonic acid from carbon dioxide and water, and the reverse reaction. As carbon dioxide from the tissues diffuses into the red cells to form carbaminohaemoglobin, oxygen leaves them. This reduces the affinity of haemoglobin for base because the isoelectric point of reduced haemoglobin is on the alkaline side of that of oxyhaemoglobin. At the same time carbon dioxide diffusing into the red cells under the action of carbonic anhydrase becomes carbonic acid. This acid acquires the base no longer so firmly held by the haemoglobin. Some of the carbonic acid diffuses from the erythrocytes into the plasma where it combines with base and is transported in the blood. In addition there is a reciprocal chloride shift into the red cells. In this way plasma base plays an important role in carbon dioxide transport.

In the pulmonary capillaries the reverse processes occur. Carbon dioxide dissociates from the carbamino compound and leaves the blood to enter the alveolar air. Oxygen enters the blood to form oxyhaemoglobin, which combines more readily with base. The bicarbonate liberated splits into carbon dioxide and water, which are lost to the alveoli. Bicarbonate passes from plasma to erythrocytes and chloride in the reverse direction.

The reduced levels of partial pressure of carbon dioxide, blood bicarbonate concentration, and blood buffer base at high altitude are shown in Fig. 4.2. The various components of the transport of carbon dioxide in the blood in subjects at low and high altitude are shown in Fig. 4.4. They include estimations of the total carbon dioxide and those portions free in the plasma and transported as bicarbonate and carbamino compound. It will be seen that in high-altitude subjects, although there is a reduction in total and free carbon dioxide and that bound as bicarbonate, the level of carbamino compound rises (Fig. 4.4). A normal balance between concentrations of anions and cations is maintained. The mean values of plasma sodium, potassium, and calcium are the same at high and low altitudes, so that the decrease in bicarbonate is quantitatively compensated for by an increase in chloride. The buffering power for carbon dioxide is greater at high altitude than at sea level (see Fig. 4.2) and this is because of the increase in haemoglobin concentration that is considered in the next chapter.

Suprapontine influences on hypoxic ventilatory control

The hypoxic ventilatory response is attenuated by sleep and by prolonged residence at high altitude.

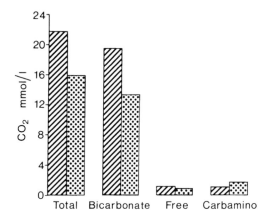

4.4 *Arterial carbon dioxide levels in 80 subjects at sea level (hatched columns) and in 40 highlanders at 4540 m (stippled columns). In the high-altitude residents total arterial carbon dioxide levels are decreased; this is true of free carbon dioxide and of that in the form of bicarbonate. In highlanders, however, carbamino-bound carbon dioxide is elevated compared with sea-level subjects. (After Hurtado (1964a).)*

The basis for this may be a failure of the peripheral arterial chemoreceptor, as discussed in Chapter 7, but Tenney *et al.* (1971) thought it possible that chronic hypoxia modifies a central mechanism influencing the respiratory centres in the pons and the medulla. On the basis of experimental studies in cats exposed to simulated high altitude, they postulated that there is a cortical influence that is inhibitory and that can be removed to release an underlying facilitatory influence originating in the diencephalon. They thought it possible that early in acclimatization arousal by the reticular activating system accounts for the hyperresponsiveness and is the origin of symptoms such as insomnia and irritability that are common on exposure to high altitude. The cortical inhibitory influence is presumed to develop more slowly, but eventually it overrides the diencephalic facilitatory influence and then the blunted hypoxic drive becomes apparent. Tenney *et al.* (1971) regard the orbital region of the frontal lobes, Walker's area 13, as the likely region of the cortex from which the inhibitory stimuli arise.

PULMONARY DIFFUSION

In the lung the oxygen tension in the alveolar spaces is higher than in the arterial blood. Raine and Bishop (1963) found this 'A–a difference' to average 6 mmHg in normals under the age of 40 years and

17 mmHg in normals over that age. This is brought about by an anatomical diffusion barrier in the form of the alveolar-capillary wall, and two physiological shunts that tend to reduce the oxygenation of the arterial blood. The first of these is an anatomical shunt of venous blood from bronchial and Thebesian veins or through pulmonary vessels that have no contact with alveoli. The second is the effective shunt caused by uneven ventilation–perfusion. The addition of the two represents the 'physiological shunt' or 'venous admixture' (Harris and Heath 1986). Clearly, diffusion of oxygen across the alveolar-capillary membrane is enhanced by a higher partial pressure of oxygen in the alveolar spaces. An increased internal surface area of the lung will also increase the capacity for pulmonary diffusion. The rate of transfer of a gas through a sheet of tissue is also proportional to a diffusion constant that depends on the properties of the tissue and the gas concerned (Ward *et al.* 1989). This means that carbon dioxide diffuses about 20 times more rapidly than oxygen through tissue sheets since its solubility is about 24 times greater at 37°C (Ward *et al.* 1989). At sea level the A–a difference is relatively unimportant, since the quantity of oxygen carried by the blood does not fall substantially. However, at high altitude the A–a difference, were it maintained at sea-level magnitude, would assume significance, as the fall in arterial oxygen tension on the steep slope of the oxygen–haemoglobin dissociation curve would cause a pronounced fall in the quantity of oxygen carried by the haemoglobin.

Alveolar-capillary wall

Oxygen in the alveolar spaces has to diffuse through the alveolar-capillary wall to reach the blood in the pulmonary capillaries. The capillary vessels lie on supporting connective tissue elements, so that one side of the alveolar-capillary wall is thin whereas the other is thick (Fig. 4.5). It is the thin side that is concerned with the exchange of respiratory gases. Its alveolar aspect is composed of the delicate cytoplasmic extensions of the membranous (type I) pneumonocytes (Fig. 4.6). This is covered by surfactant material derived from the granular (type II) pneumonocytes found in the corners of alveolar spaces (Fig. 4.7). The membranous pneumonocytes lie on a 'fused basement membrane' that is common to it and the underlying endothelial cells of the pulmonary capillaries (Fig. 4.6). Thus oxygen must diffuse through alveolar epithelial cells and their covering of surfactant, fused basement membrane, and endothelial cells to

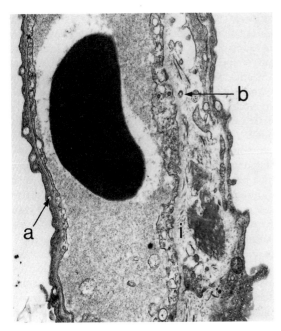

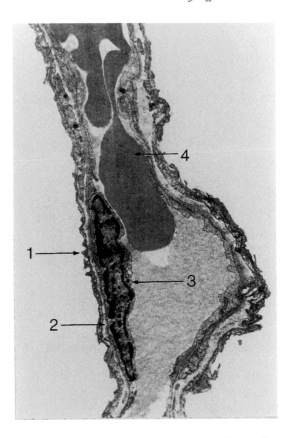

4.5 *Electron micrograph of lung from a Wistar albino rat. It shows the two aspects of a pulmonary capillary. The thin wall of the capillary (arrow a) is concerned with the exchange of respiratory gases. From the alveolar space inwards it consists of the attenuated cytoplasm of the membranous pneumonocytes, the fused basement membrane of the alveolar capillary wall, and the thinned cytoplasm of the pulmonary endothelial cells. The thick wall of the capillary (arrow b) is concerned with the movement of interstitial fluid in the lungs. It comprises interstitial tissue (i), which includes collagen fibres embedded in ground substance. This is bounded internally by the pulmonary endothelium with its basement membrane, and externally by the attenuated cytoplasm of the membranous pneumonocytes and their basement membrane. The J receptors are thought to lie in the interstitial layer.* × 12 500.

4.6 *Electron micrograph of the alveolar-capillary wall in a mestizo male aged 22 years who was born and resided all his life at La Paz, Bolivia (3800 m). The thin side of the wall, concerned with the exchange of respiratory gases, is composed of the delicate membranous extensions of the membranous pneumonocytes (arrow 1), the fused basement membrane (arrow 2), and the endothelial cells of the pulmonary capillaries (arrow 3). Oxygen diffusing through this wall reaches erythrocytes (arrow 4).* × 6000.

reach the plasma and erythrocytes in the pulmonary capillaries (Fig. 4.6).

The thick wall of the alveolar-capillary membrane shows a layer of interstitial connective tissue between the separated basement membranes of the alveolar epithelial cells and the pulmonary endothelial cells (Fig. 4.5). The interstitial tissue is concerned with the transport of tissue fluid and is the site of J receptors. We shall consider this aspect of the alveolar-capillary wall and these receptors in relation to high-altitude pulmonary oedema in Chapter 13.

Measurement of the thickness of the alveolar-capillary wall is a time-consuming business that requires the application of morphometric methods to large numbers of electron micrographs. Even then the results obtained by different workers may be conflicting and this depends to a large extent on the morphometric technique employed. One may calculate the so-called 'arithmetic' or 'harmonic mean thickness' of the alveolar-capillary wall. Put simply, arithmetic mean thickness is estimated by determining, by complex morphometric techniques on electron micrographs, the volume and surface density of

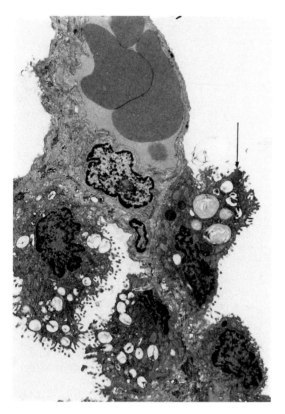

4.7 *Electron micrograph of the corner of an alveolar space in a mestizo girl aged 4 years who was born and resided all her life at La Paz, Bolivia (3800 m). There are many granular pneumonocytes (arrow), which contain within their cytoplasm numerous lamellar bodies. These form the surfactant that covers the cytoplasmic extensions of membranous pneumonocytes shown in Fig. 4.6. × 3700.*

the alveolar-capillary wall and by then dividing the former by the latter. Harmonic mean thickness is determined by direct measurement of the thickness of the air–blood barrier as defined on an electron micrograph (Weibel and Knight 1964).

We studied the thickness of the alveolar-capillary wall in 14 guinea-pigs (*Cavia porcellus*) (Hogan *et al.* 1986*a*) by both methods. Seven were laboratory bred from sea level and seven were wild guinea-pigs collected from the countryside around La Raya in the Andes at an elevation of 4200 m. In absolute terms we found by direct measurement on the electron micrograph that the harmonic mean thickness of the alveolar-capillary wall of the sea-level guinea-pig was 0.45 μm (SD 0.061), whereas in the

Peruvian animals it was 0.29 μm (SD 0.035). This represents a statistically significant thinning of the air–blood barrier at high altitude ($p<0.05$). Forrest and Weibel (1975) found a comparable harmonic mean thickness of 0.42 μm in sea-level guinea-pigs.

There is less agreement on the thickness of the air–blood barrier employing the estimation of arithmetic mean thickness. Forrest and Weibel (1975) found a much higher value of 1.59 μm using this technique and the reason for this is that they included the large amounts of connective tissue in the thick parts of the alveolar wall that is characteristic of this species. They recognized how high this value was and pointed out that it was calculated by this technique to be of the same order of magnitude as that found in dogs of a body weight 26 times greater than that of the guinea-pig. We modified the technique to include only those areas of connective tissue around alveolar capillaries and arrived at the much lower figure of 0.70 μm for the arithmetic mean thickness of the alveolar-capillary wall in guinea-pigs (Hogan *et al.* 1986*a*); the value fell to 0.51 μm for the high-altitude guinea-pigs. In spite of the discrepancy in the value of the alveolar-capillary wall found by the two morphometric technique, it is clear that at high altitude there is thinning of the air–blood barrier of the wild Andean guinea-pig. In assessing the significance of this finding it has to be kept in mind that these animals are indigenous to the area and over countless generations have probably become adapted rather than acclimatized to the hypobaric hypoxia of high altitude (Chapter 35). It is of interest that the villous membrane of the placenta has been shown to be thinned in Aymara women in Bolivia (Mayhew 1986; Chapter 23, this volume). Like the alveolar-capillary wall, the placental villous membrane represents a resistance to the conduction of oxygen in the tissues.

Burri and Weibel (1971) found that the pulmonary diffusion capacity, calculated from morphometric data, was increased in hypoxia in rats and decreased in hyperoxia and concluded that this was due to a greater surface area of the alveolar-capillary membrane rather than to any decrease in the thickness. They exposed three groups of developing rats to hypoxic, normoxic, and hyperoxic atmospheres from the 23rd to 44th day of their life, the respective partial pressures of oxygen being 100, 150, and 290 mmHg. Under hypoxic conditions the lung volumes were increased by 20% above those of controls, in contrast to hyperoxia where volumes fell by 16%. The proportions of alveolar space, pulmonary capillaries, and lung tissue all took part equally in the growth, so that the greater size of the lung was thought to arise from an increase in the number of respiratory units rather than by any appreciable alteration in structure. Pearson and Pearson (1976), from a stereological analysis of the ultrastructural composition of the alveolar-capillary wall of mice (*Phyllotis darwini*) living at sea level compared with that of the same species adapted to natural high altitude at 4660 m in Peru, were unable to detect any difference in its thickness.

We have also measured the harmonic mean thickness of the alveolar-capillary wall in man from both low and high altitudes (Hogan *et al.* 1986*b*). This ultrastructural study of lung biopsy specimens from an adult mestizo highlander from La Paz (3800 m) and three patients undergoing resection of lung tissue from London (Table 4.1) showed no significant difference in the thickness of the alveolar-capillary wall, the thickness in the highlander being 0.65 μm and the range in the lowlanders being 0.57–0.69 μm. The thickness of the blood–air barrier in a 4-year-old mestizo girl born and living in La Paz was 0.47 μm. It is a rarity to be able to obtain fresh lung biopsy specimens at high altitude fixed in a suitable manner for subsequent electron microscopy, but even so it is impossible to base generalization on such a small number of specimens. Nevertheless, the above data are suggestive that the alveolar-capillary wall in the acclimatized non-Indian highlander does not differ in thickness from that in the lowlander. This contrasts with the findings in the native high-altitude guinea-pigs referred to above that indicated that the air–blood barrier is thinner in such indigenous mountain species that are probably adapted genetically rather than acclimatized to hypobaric hypoxia.

Another shortcoming in our study is the difference in age of the patients between the low- and high-altitude groups. It is well known that the blood–air barrier in the normal human lung increases after the age of 20–30 years, largely due to interposition of collagen and fibrocyte processes between the basement membranes of the thin portion of the alveolar-capillary wall. We were unable to obtain lung biopsy specimens from patients of equivalent age to those collected in La Paz. For the purposes of comparison, the fact that the three adult patients from sea level were older than the adult highlander would tend to make the blood–air barrier appear thinner in the mestizo. We have no information on the thickness of the alveolar-capillary wall in native Quechua or Aymara highlanders. It would certainly be of interest to study them to see if in fact they have unusually thin alveolar-capillary walls to aid diffusion of oxygen into the blood like the adapted guinea-pigs. So far as we are aware, although the numbers in whom our laboratory has studied the ultrastructural morphometry are small, they represent the only such measurements carried out so far in man.

Pulmonary diffusing capacity at high altitude

There are no pronounced changes in pulmonary diffusing capacity in lowlanders shortly after their ascent to high altitude (Kreuzer and Van Lookeren Compagne 1965; De Graff *et al.* 1970; Guleria *et al.* 1971). During exercise there is a slight increase in diffusing capacity, but it does not exceed that which would be expected under similar conditions of work at sea level. Hence exercise on arrival at high altitude leads to a pronounced fall in arterial oxygen saturation, despite any elevation in the partial

Table 4.1 Age, sex, diagnosis, and harmonic mean thickness of alveolar-capillary wall in two patients from La Paz and three from London

Sex	Age (years)	Domicile	Altitude (m)	Diagnosis	Harmonic mean thickness (μm) (SD)
F	4	La Paz	3800	Lung abscess	0.47 (0.04)
M	22	La Paz	3800	Bronchiectasis	0.65 (0.1)
M	51	London	0	Bronchial carcinoma	0.61 (0.12)
M	52	London	0	Thoracotomy for oesophageal polyp	0.57 (0.15)
M	51	London	0	Bronchial carcinoma	0.69 (0.13)

pressure of oxygen in the alveolar spaces brought about by hyperventilation.

Indeed the A–a difference in newcomers to mountainous areas may be a limiting factor on exercise. It is considered by some authorities that this represents the major significance of pulmonary diffusion at high altitude (Ward *et al.* 1989). These authors refer to the classic studies of Barcroft and his party (1923) at Cerro de Pasco (4330 m) who concluded from their measurements of pulmonary diffusing capacity for carbon monoxide that equilibration of arterial oxygen tension between alveolar gas and the blood at the end of the pulmonary capillary could not be achieved, especially on exercise. West *et al.* (1962) reported that, during the Himalayan Scientific and Mountaineering Expedition of 1960–61, measurements of arterial oxygen saturation by ear oximetry were made on five subjects who lived for 4 months at an altitude of 5800 m. The average arterial oxygen saturation at rest was 67% and at a work level of 900 kg/min this fell to 56%. The A–a difference was found to be 26 mmHg. Some 20 years later confirmation of these results was obtained during the American Medical Research Expedition to Everest in 1981. Fifteen subjects spent up to a month at an altitude of 6300 m. There was a progressive fall in arterial oxygen saturation as the work level was raised from rest to 1200 kg/min and A–a difference rose to 21 mmHg (West *et al.* 1983).

In striking contrast the pulmonary diffusing capacity of native highlanders is increased. We have already pointed out earlier in this chapter that at sea level the A–a difference averages 6 mmHg in normal subjects under the age of 40 years but may climb to 17 mmHg with the advance of age (Raine and Bishop 1963). Native highlanders living at 4270 m were found to have an A–a difference of only 2 mmHg (Houston and Riley 1947). Hurtado (1964*b*) found the A–a difference in Quechua Indians at Morococha (4540 m) to be only 1 mmHg. Later work confirms that the pulmonary diffusing capacity is some 20–50% higher than in residents at sea level. Remmers and Mithoefer (1969) found this both at rest and during exercise in Quechua Indians at 3700 m and De Graff *et al.* (1970) confirmed it in Caucasians domiciled at 3100 m. The rate of diffusion of a gas through a sheet of tissue is inversely proportional to the thickness of the tissue. As noted above, we have been able to confirm by morphometric techniques that there is indeed a difference in the thickness of the alveolar-capillary membrane in native guinea-pigs of the Andes compared with members of the same species from a sea-level

habitat, suggesting some genetic adaptation to high altitude. On the other hand, we have been unable up to present to demonstrate a similar difference between the lungs of lowlanders and highlanders, but this may be because we have gained access for such study to the lungs of only two natives of La Paz (3600 m) one being a child (see Table 4.1). It is likely, however, that the diminished A–a difference in the native highlander is associated with a thinning of the alveolar-capillary wall compared with man at sea level.

The rate of gas transfer through a sheet of tissue is also proportional to its area. Thus an increased internal area of lung may be a significant factor in increasing the pulmonary diffusing capacity of native highlanders. Hurtado (1964*a*) regarded a barrel-shaped chest as characteristic of the physique of the Quechua Indians, as discussed in Chapter 3. He found that the native highlander of the Andes shows an increase in the volume of some compartments of the lung. This applies to the volume of gas remaining in the lung at the end of a normal expiration (functional residual capacity) and that remaining after a forced expiration (residual volume) (Fig. 4.8). (For definitions of the various functional lung compartments the reader is referred to Fig. 31.4.) The lungs are thus held in a position of increased inflation in native highlanders and the same change can be detected in newcomers to high altitude during initial acclimatization (Tenney *et al.* 1953). It is possible that this hyperinflation of the lungs increases their internal surface area, aiding the diffusion of oxygen. The effect of such hyperinflation on the pulmonary blood flow or the distribution of ventilation and perfusion is not yet clear.

It has not been determined if this sustained hyperinflation in highlanders is associated with the development of an increased internal surface area. Certainly rats reared from birth in a hypoxic environment develop lungs with an abnormally large internal surface area. Methods of tissue morphometry to determine the internal surface area of the lungs, and the number and size of alveoli, such as we have employed in the study of pulmonary emphysema (Hicken *et al.* 1966), have not been applied to high-altitude lungs. Such morphometric study of the lungs of highlanders would seem to be a fruitful area for research.

Another factor that may operate in improving the pulmonary diffusing capacity at high altitude is the moderate degree of pulmonary hypertension that occurs in subjects at such elevations (Chapter 10).

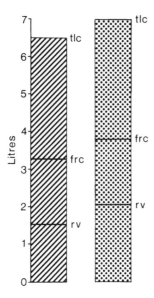

4.8 *Compartments of the total lung capacity (in litres) in 60 men, average age 23 years, at sea level (hatched column) and in 38 men, average age 23.3 years, at 4540 m (stippled column). In both columns the top line (tlc) represents total lung capacity, the middle line (frc) represents functional residual capacity, and the bottom line (rv) represents residual volume. (Based on data from Hurtado (1964a).) For definitions of the various functional lung compartments the reader is referred to Fig. 31.4.*

The elevation of pulmonary arterial pressure is possibly associated with a more uniform perfusion of the lung, especially of the upper zone that is underperfused at sea level. At high altitude there is an increase in total blood volume and this hypervolaemia associated with the mild pulmonary hypertension referred to above may distend patent capillaries and perhaps perfuse those unopened at sea level. This would enhance pulmonary diffusing capacity. In the final analysis the efficiency of pulmonary diffusing capacity depends on the perfect matching of ventilation and perfusion or, in the case of the lung at high altitude, the matching of hyperventilation and pulmonary hypertension.

Clara cells

These are non-ciliated cells found in the terminal portions of the bronchial tree. They have mushroom-shaped caps that project into the lumen and are attached to the basal, nucleated portion of the cell by only a long narrow isthmus. The apices are

extruded into the bronchiolar lumen, but the nature and function of this apocrine secretion are not known. We have found an increased activity of Clara cells in llamas living at 4720 m compared with that in those born and living in a zoo at sea level (Heath *et al.* 1976, 1980; see Fig. 4.9). Ultrastructural study of the extruded apices revealed a paler and looser cytoplasm and dilatation of the endoplasmic reticulum (Fig. 4.10), with globules of cytoplasm discharged into the bronchiolar lumen. Such electron microscopical appearances are consistent with increased synthesis, storage, and apocrine secretion of some product into the bronchiolar lumen and alveolar space. The autoradiographical studies of Etherton *et al.* (1973) suggest that the extensive smooth endoplasmic reticulum of the Clara cell may contain accumulations of a phospholipid, dipalmitoyl lecithin. This is a known pulmonary surfactant and its presence offers one possible explanation for the activity

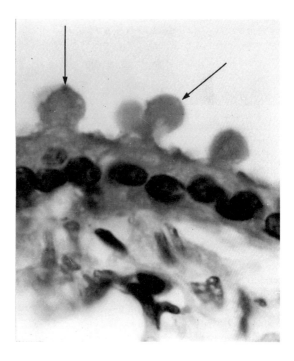

4.9 *Clara cells in a terminal bronchiole from a 2-year-old llama born and bred at Rancas (4720 m) in the Peruvian Andes. The apical caps of these cells (arrows) project into the lumen of the bronchiole. Subsequently they are extruded with liberation of their intracytoplasmic chemical substance, the function of which in the bronchial tree is unknown. The nuclei appear darkly stained in the basal portions of the cells. HE, × 1500.*

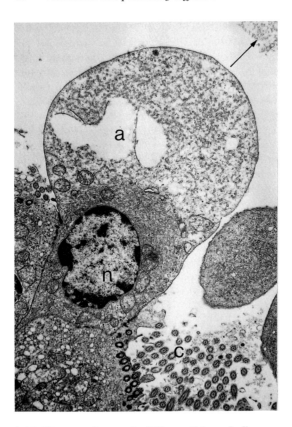

4.10 *Electron micrograph of Clara cell from the llama referred to in Fig. 4.9. The apical portion of the cell (a) forms a mushroom-shaped cap that is extruded into the bronchiolar lumen (arrow). The basal portion of the cell with its nucleus (n) remains in situ. The cilia of the surrounding respiratory epithelium (c) are seen.* × 7000.

of Clara cells in hypobaric hypoxia. If there were a tendency to increased surface tension in the lung at high altitude, there would be a need for a constant and perhaps enhanced supply of surfactant and hence the activity of the Clara cells.

In this connection there was a claim by Castillo and Johnson (1969) that there was an increase in surface tension of lung extracts of mice after their acute exposure to a simulated altitude of 4270 m for 45 minutes. However, the technique of sonication employed in this study has been criticized on the grounds that it would liberate so much cellular lipid that it would swamp the surfactant lipids which would account for only 5–10 % of the total. Thus, the surface tension–area loops revealed in the paper are predictable from knowledge of the extraction

procedure and are not specific to lung surfactant. Furthermore, blood plasma contains substances that can inhibit lung surfactant, so that mincing and sonication of lung tissue may itself be responsible for the observed increase in surface tension. It is clear that, before the suggestion that high altitude increases alveolar surface tension can be accepted, confirmation of the work of Castillo and Johnson (1969) must be forthcoming from other workers using techniques not open to the objections alluded to above.

Pulmonary endocrine cells

Scattered throughout the bronchial tree and alveolar-capillary walls are cells that contain dense-core vesicles in their cytoplasm and thus resemble the chief cells of the carotid body described in Chapter 7. They appear to represent part of a diffuse endocrine system originally described by Feyrter (1938). They occur both singly (Fig. 4.11) and in intramucosal clusters termed 'neuroepithelial bodies'. Pulmonary endocrine cells are part of the APUD system (i.e. cells capable of Amine Precursor Uptake and Decarboxylation) and the central osmiophilic cores of their dense-core vesicles contain the peptides calcitonin, bombesin, and leucine-enkephalin (Cutz, *et al.* 1981), whereas the surrounding clear halo contains the biogenic amine serotonin (Gould *et al.* 1983). It is commonly believed that neuroepithelial bodies with their sensory innervation represent chemoreceptors in the airways, sensitive to hypoxia.

Against this background it might be anticipated that pulmonary endocrine cells would show ultrastructural and histological changes on exposure to the hypobaric hypoxia of high altitude. Early studies on animals seemed to confirm this. In neonatal rats the dense-core vesicles of the pulmonary endocrine cells showed broadening of the peripheral haloes into microvacuoles and pallor, shrinking, and movement of the peptide cores into an excentric position (Moosavi *et al.* 1973). Taylor (1977) studied the argyrophilic pulmonary endocrine cells of rabbits by the Grimelius technique. He found that they were greater in number in rabbits that had been born and lived all their lives in Cerro de Pasco at an altitude of 4330 m in the Andes. There were more in both airways and lung parenchyma when compared with an age-matched sea-level control group. The increase in neuroepithelial bodies was confined to the airways, whereas solitary cells were significantly increased within the parenchyma. Since pulmonary endocrine cells are derived from the neural crest and

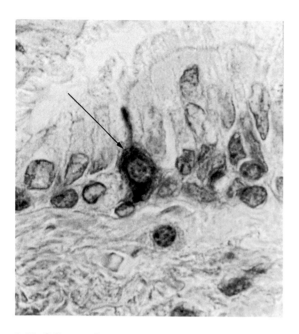

4.11 *Solitary pulmonary endocrine cell (arrow) in the bronchial wall of a sea-level man. The peptide in this cell was immunoreactive for calcitonin. Peroxidase–antiperoxidase method, × 1500.*

thus incapable of division it seems likely that their prominence in hypoxia was due to increased numbers of peptide-containing dense-core vesicles in pre-existing endocrine cells. A similar study on Bolivian highlanders by Memoli *et al.* (1983) confirmed this increase in pulmonary endocrine cells. We were unable to confirm the findings of Taylor (1977) when we studied by neurone-specific enolase the pulmonary endocrine cells in various breeds of sheep and goats from Srinagar (1500 m) in Kashmir and from Sakti (4500 m) in Ladakh (Gosney *et al.* 1988). On the same expedition we studied the pulmonary endocrine cells in the lungs of a yak, two dzos, and two stols (Chapter 35) from Sakti. We found no relation to the altitude at which the animals were living and thus to the level of hypobaric hypoxia. Rather we found that the morphology, distribution, and numbers of the pulmonary endocrine cells were species-specific. The cells were numerous and usually solitary in the bronchial tree of sheep, being especially common in merinos, irrespective of their origin or domicile at low or high altitude (Gosney *et al.* 1988). In contrast, pulmonary endocrine cells were far less obvious and largely restricted to clusters in the alve-olar-capillary wall in the goats and the interbreeds of yaks and cattle (Gosney *et al.* 1988).

Subsequently, we found no increase in the numbers of pulmonary endocrine cells immunoreactive for gastrin-releasing peptide (the human analogue of bombesin in amphibian skin) and calcitonin in three Aymara Indians and three mestizos born and living in La Paz (3600 m) compared to four White lowlanders from sea level (Williams *et al.* 1993; see Fig. 4.12). In the highlanders the number of cells containing gastrin-releasing peptide was in the range of 3.3 to 4.4 per cm^2 of lung section, compared to a range of 6.5 to 15.6 per cm^2 in the normoxic controls. In the highlanders the number of endocrine cells containing calcitonin was in the range of 0.1 to 0.3 per cm^2 of lung section, compared to a range of 0.2 to 4.5 per cm^2 in the lowlanders. We relate this lack of increase of pulmonary endocrine cells in highlanders to the nature of the pulmonary vascular remodelling that is found in them (Chapter 10). In highlanders there is but limited migration of pulmonary vascular smooth muscle cells from media to intima (Heath and Williams 1991; see Fig. 10.9). This is in striking contrast to the free migration of electron-dense smooth muscle cells from intima to vascular lumen that occurs in plexogenic pulmonary arteriopathy (Heath *et al.* 1988). In this disease there are large increases in the number of bombesin-rich pulmonary endocrine cells in the lung (Heath *et al.* 1990). In other words the pulmonary endocrine cells in man do not appear to be prominent at high altitude and seem to be related more to events in the pulmonary arterial walls than to the hypobaric hypoxia of high altitude. Sissons (1986) found an increase in the number of pulmonary endocrine cells containing calcitonin in patients with chronic bronchitis and emphysema. This could be attributed to hypoxia, although other factors such as infection are involved.

ENVIRONMENTAL AND GENETIC FACTORS IN VENTILATORY ADJUSTMENT TO HIGH ALTITUDE

Lahiri *et al.* (1976) have assessed the relative roles of environmental and genetic factors in ventilatory adjustment to high altitude. They studied the control of ventilation and the magnitude of lung volumes in different age groups from the neonatal period to adulthood, both at high altitude and sea level. Their results suggest strongly that such adjustments at high altitude are acquired and determined by environmental rather than genetic factors. The relative changes in the ventilatory response to acute hypoxia

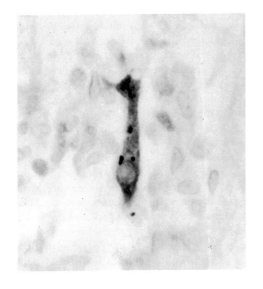

(a)

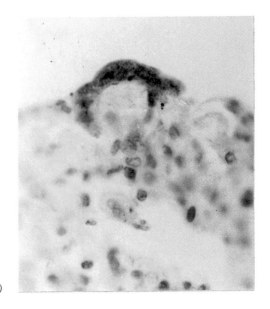

(b)

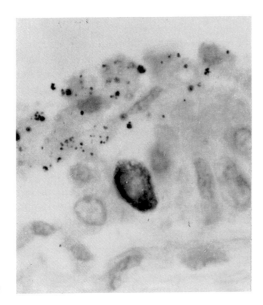

(c)

4.12 *Pulmonary endocrine cells from Aymara Indians born and living in La Paz (3600 m). (a) Solitary cell showing the characteristic shape that was immunoreactive for gastrin-releasing peptide. (b) A cluster of endocrine cells immunoreactive for gastrin-releasing peptide. (c) Solitary cell immunore active for calcitonin. All stained by avidin–biotin complex method. (a) × 1500, anti-bombesin; (b) × 1000, anti-bombesin; (c) × 1500, anti-calcitonin*

and in the increased vital capacity from predicted sea-level volume are shown in Fig. 4.13. The normal hypoxic ventilatory drive was developed in the native highlander up to the age of 8 years before it was substantially lost during adult life.

Vital capacity was the same in neonates and young children at sea level and at high altitude, but after the age of about 9 years vital capacity in the

highlander began to outpace that of sea-level children (121 ± 13.7%). Accelerated lung growth then persisted in young adult native highlanders, 18–21 years of age (145 ± 16.7%). Thus the ventilatory response to hypoxia and vital capacity are similar in neonates and infants at sea level and at high altitudes, suggesting that no genetic or intrauterine changes of acclimatization occur in these physio-

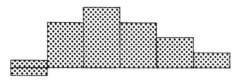

Ventilatory response to acute hypoxia

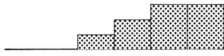

Increased vital capacity from predicted
sea-level values

birth
to
|1 week| 2-6 m |5-8 y |8-12 y |12-20y|20-25y|

4.13 *Ventilatory acclimatization to high altitude from birth to the age of 25 years. Normal hypoxic ventilatory drive develops in the native highlander up to the age of 8 years before becoming substantially lost during adult life. Vital capacity tends to increase throughout the teenage period. After data of Lahiri* et al. *(1976).)*

logical parameters in preparation for life at high altitude. Vital capacity tends to increase in the postnatal period and continues to do so through the teenage period. The blunted hypoxic response, however, only begins to manifest itself in teenage life, becoming universal in adults. A genetic trait tends to be excluded on the grounds that offspring of lowlanders born and bred at high altitude showed the same phenomena as native highlanders.

References

Aste-Salazar, H. and Hurtado, A. (1944). The affinity of haemoglobin for oxygen at sea level and at high altitudes. *American Journal of Physiology*, **142**, 733

Barcroft, J., Binger, C.A., Bock, A.V., Doggart, J.H., Forbes, H.S., Harrop, G., Meakins, J.C., and Redfield, A.C. (1923). Observations upon the effect of high altitude on the physiological processes of the human body, carried out in the Peruvian Andes, chiefly at Cerro de Pasco. *Philosophical Transactions of the Royal Society*, **B211**, 351

Burki, N.K. (1984). Effects of acute exposure to high altitude on ventilatory drive and respiratory pattern. *Journal of Applied Physiology: Respiratory, Environmental and Exercise Physiology*, **56**, 1027

Burri, P.H. and Weibel, E.R. (1971). Morphometric estimation of pulmonary diffusion capacity. II. Effect of Po_2 on the growing lung. Adaptation of the growing rat lung to hypoxia and hyperoxia. *Respiration Physiology*, **II**, 247

Castillo, Y. and Johnson, F.B. (1969). Pulmonary surfactant in acutely hypoxic mice. *Laboratory Investigation*, **21**, 61

Chiodi, H. (1957). Respiratory adaptations to chronic high altitude hypoxia. *Journal of Applied Physiology*, **10**, 81

Cumming, G. and Semple, S.J. (1973). The effects of hypoxia and hypercapnia. In *Disorders of the Respiratory System*. Oxford; Blackwell Scientific, p. 236

Cutz, E., Chan, W., and Track, N.S. (1981). Bombesin, calcitonin, and leu-enkephalin immunoreactivity in endocrine cells of human lung. *Experientia*, **37**, 765

De Graff A.C. Jr, Grover, R.F., Johnson, R.L., Hammond, J.W., and Miller, J.M. (1970). Diffusing capacity of the lung in Caucasians native to 3,100 m. *Journal of Applied Physiology*, **29**, 71

Dempsey, J.A., Forster, H.V., Chosy, L.W., Hanson, P.G., and Reddan, W.G. (1978). Regulation of CSF (HCO_3) during long-term hypoxic hypocapnia in man. *Journal of Applied Physiology*, **44**, 175

Dempsey, J.A., Forster, H.V., and DoPico, G.A. (1974). Ventilatory acclimatization to moderate hypoxemia in man. *Journal of Clinical Investigation*, **53**, 1091

Denison, D. (1986). Where and how hypoxia works. In *Aspects of Hypoxia* (D. Heath, Ed.). Liverpool; Liverpool University Press

Dill, D.B., Talbott, J.H., and Consolazio, W.V. (1937). Blood as a physiochemical system. XI. Man at high altitudes. *Journal of Biological Chemistry*, **118**, 649

Etherton, J.E., Conning, D.M., and Corrin, B. (1973). Autoradiographical and morphological evidence for apocrine secretion of dipalmitoyl lecithin in the terminal bronchiole of mouse lung. *American Journal of Anatomy*, **138**, 11

Feyrter, F. (1938). *Über diffuse endokrine epitheliale Organe*. Leipzig; J.A. Barth

Forrest, J.B. and Weibel, E.R. (1975). Morphometric estimation of pulmonary diffusion capacity. VII. The normal guinea pig lung. *Respiration Physiology*, **24**, 191

Forster, H.V., Dempsey, J.A., and Chosey, L.W. (1975). Incomplete compensation of CSF (H+) in man during acclimatization to high altitude (4,300 m). *Journal of Applied Physiology*, **38**, 1067

Gosney, J., Heath, D., Williams, D., Deen, M., Harris, P., Anand, I., and Ferrari, R. (1988). Pulmonary endocrine cells in different animal species in the Himalaya. *Journal of Comparative Pathology*, **99**, 93

Gould, V.E., Linnoila, R.I., Memoli, V.A., and Warren, W.H. (1983). Biology of disease. Neuroendocrine components of the bronchopulmonary tract: hyperplasias, dysplasias and neoplasms. *Laboratory Investigation*, **49**, 519

Guleria, J.S., Pande, J.N., Sethi, P.K., and Roy, S.B. (1971). Pulmonary diffusing capacity at high altitude. *Journal of Applied Physiology*, **31**, 536

Harris, P. and Heath, D. (1977). The relation between ventilation and perfusion. In *The Human Pulmonary Circulation. Its Form and Function in Health and Disease*, 2nd edn. Edinburgh; Churchill Livingstone, p. 567

Harris, P. and Heath, D. (1986). *The Human Pulmonary Circulation. Its Form and Function in Health and Disease*, 3rd edn. Edinburgh; Churchill Livingstone

Heath, D. and Williams, D. (1991). Pulmonary vascular remodelling in a high-altitude Aymara Indian. *International Journal of Biometeorology*, **35**, 203

Heath, D., Smith, P., and Harris, P. (1976). Clara cells in the llama. *Experimental Cell Biology*, **44**, 73

Heath, D., Smith, P., and Biggar, R. (1980). Clara cells in llamas born and living at high and low altitudes. *British Journal of Diseases of the Chest*, **74**, 75

Heath, D., Smith, P., and Gosney, J. (1988). Ultrastructure of early plexogenic pulmonary arteriopathy. *Histopathology*, **12**, 41

Heath, D., Yacoub, M., Gosney, J.R., Madden, B., Caslin, A.W., and Smith, P. (1990). Pulmonary endocrine cells in hypertensive pulmonary vascular disease. *Histopathology*, **16**, 21

Hicken, P., Brewer, D., and Heath, D. (1966). The relation between the weight of the right ventricle of the heart and the internal surface area and number of alveoli in the human lung in emphysema. *Journal of Pathology and Bacteriology*, **92**, 529

Hogan, J., Smith, P., Heath, D., and Harris, P. (1986*a*). The thickness of the alveolar capillary wall in guinea-pigs at high and low altitude. *Journal of Comparative Pathology*, **96**, 217

Hogan, J., Smith, P., Heath, D., and Harris, P. (1986*b*). The thickness of the alveolar capillary wall in the human lung at high and low altitude. *British Journal of Diseases of the Chest*, **80**, 13

Houston, C.S. and Riley, R.L. (1947). Respiratory and circulation changes during acclimatization to high altitude. *American Journal of Physiology*, **149**, 565

Hurtado, A. (1964*a*). Some physiologic and clinical aspects of life at high altitudes. In *Aging of the Lung* (L. Cander and J.H. Moyer, Ed.). New York; Grune and Stratton, p. 257

Hurtado, A. (1964*b*). Animals in high altitudes: resident man. In *Handbook of Physiology*, Section 4, Adaptation to Environment. Washington; American Physiological Society, p. 843

Hurtado, A., Velásquez, T., Reynafarje, C., Lozano, R., Chavez, R., Aste-Salazar, H., Reynafarje, B., Sánchez, S., and Munoz, J. (1956). Mechanisms of natural acclimatization. Studies on the native resident of Morochocha, Peru, at an altitude of 14,900 feet. Report 56.1 to the Air University, School of Aviation Medicine, USAF, Randolph AFB, Texas, p. 57

Kreuzer, F. and Van Lookeren Compagne, P. (1965). Resting pulmonary diffusing capacity for CO and O_2 at high altitude. *Journal of Applied Physiology*, **20**, 519

Lahiri, S. Milledge, J.S., Chattopadhyay, G.P., Bhattacharyya, A.K., and Sinha, A.K. (1967). Respiration and heart rate of Sherpa highlanders during exercise. *Journal of Applied Physiology*, **23**, 545

Lahiri, S., Delaney, R.G., Brody, J.S., Simpeer, M., Velasquez, T., Motoyama, E.K., and Polgar, C. (1976). Relative role of environmental and genetic factors in respiratory adaptation to high altitude. *Nature (London)*, **261**, 133

Lenfant, C. and Sullivan, K. (1971). Adaptation to high altitude. *New England Journal of Medicine*, **284**, 1298

Lenfant, C., Torrance, J.D., and Reynafarje, C. (1971). Shift of the O_2–Hb dissociation curve at altitude: mechanism and effect. *Journal of Applied Physiology*, **30**, 625

Luft, U.C. (1972). Principles of adaptations to altitude. In *Physiological Adaptations. Desert and Mountain* (M.K. Yousef, S.M. Horvath, and R.W. Bullard, Ed.). New York and London; Academic Press, p. 145

Mayhew, T. (1986). Morphometric diffusing capacity for oxygen of the human term placenta at high altitude. In *Aspects of Hypoxia* (D. Heath, Ed.). Liverpool; Liverpool University Press, p. 186

Memoli, V.A., Linnoila, I., Warren, W.H., Rios-Dalenz, J., and Gould, V.E. (1983). Hyperplasia of pulmonary neuroendocrine cells and neuroepithelial bodies. *Laboratory Investigation*, **48**, 57A

Michel, C.C. and Milledge, J.S. (1963). Respiratory regulation in man during acclimatization to high altitude. *Journal of Physiology*, **168**, 631

Milledge, J.S. (1975). Physiological effects of hypoxia. In *Mountain Medicine and Physiology* (C. Clarke, M. Ward, and E. Williams, Ed.). London; Alpine Club, p. 73

Milledge, J.S. (1987). The ventilatory response to hypoxia: how much is good for a mountaineer? *Postgraduate Medical Journal*, **63**, 169

Mithoefer, J.C. (1966). Physiological patterns; the respiration of Andean natives. In *Life at High Altitude*, Scientific Publication No. 140. Washington, DC; Pan American Health Organization, p. 21

Monge-C, C., Lozano, R., and Carcelén, A. (1964). Renal excretion of bicarbonate in high altitude natives and in natives with chronic mountain sickness. *Journal of Clinical Investigation*, **43**, 2303

Monge-M, C. and Monge-C, C. (1966). *High-Altitude Diseases. Mechanisms and Management*. Springfield, Illinois; Charles C. Thomas

Moosavi, H., Smith, P., and Heath, D. (1973). The Feyrter cell in hypoxia. *Thorax*, **28**, 729

Pearson, O.P. and Pearson, A.K. (1976). A stereological analysis of the ultrastructure of the lungs of wild mice living at low and high altitude. *Journal of Morphology*, **150**, 359

Rahn, H. and Otis, A.B. (1949). Man's respiratory response during and after acclimatization to high altitude. *American Journal of Physiology*, **157**, 445

Raine, J.M. and Bishop, J.M. (1963). A–a difference in O_2 tension and physiological dead space in normal man. *Journal of Applied Physiology*, **18**, 284

Remmers, J.C. and Mithoefer, J.C. (1969). The carbon monoxide diffusing capacity in permanent residents at high altitudes. *Respiration Physiology*, **6**, 233

Rennie, I.D.B, Lozano, R., Monge-C, C., Sime, F., and Whittembury, J. (1971). Renal oxygenation in male Peruvian natives living permanently at high altitude. *Journal of Applied Physiology*, **30**, 450

Severinghaus, J.A. and Mitchell, R.A. (1964). The role of cerebrospinal fluid in the respiratory acclimatization to high altitude in man. In *The Physiological Effects of High Altitude* (W.H. Weihe, Ed.) Oxford; Pergamon Press, p. 273

Severinghaus, J.W., Mitchell, R.A., Richardson, B.W., and Singer, M.M. (1963). Respiratory control at high altitude suggesting active transport regulation of cerebrospinal fluid pH. *Journal of Applied Physiology*, **18**, 1155

Sissons, M. (1986). Pulmonary endocrine cells in hypoxia. In *Aspects of Hypoxia* (D. Heath, Ed.). Liverpool; Liverpool University Press

Taylor, W. (1977). Pulmonary argyrophilic cells at high altitude. *Journal of Pathology*, **122**, 137

Tenney, S.M., Rahn, H., Stroud, R.C., and Mithoefer, J.C. (1953). Adaptation to high altitude: changes in lung volume during the first seven days at Mount Evans, Colorado. *Journal of Applied Physiology*, **5**, 607

Tenney, S.M., Remmers, J.E., and Mithoefer, J.C. (1964). Hypoxic–hypercapnic interaction at high altitude. In *The Physiological Effects of High Altitude* (W.H. Weihe, Ed.). Oxford; Pergamon Press, p. 263

Tenney, S.M., Scotto, P., Ou, L.C., Bartlett, D., and Remmers, J.E. (1971). Suprapontine influences on hypoxic ventilatory control. In *High Altitude Physiology, Cardiac and Respiratory Aspects* (R. Porter and J. Knight, Eds). Edinburgh; Churchill Livingstone, p. 89

Torrance, J.D., Lenfant, C., Cruz, J., and Marticorena, E. (1970–71). Oxygen transport mechanisms at high altitude. *Respiration Physiology*, **11**, 1

Ward, M. (1975). *Mountain Medicine. A Clinical Study of Cold and High Altitude*. London; Crosby Lockwood Staples

Ward, M.P., Milledge, J.S., and West, J.B. (1989). In *High Altitude Medicine and Physiology*. London; Chapman and Hall Medical, p. 195

Waterlow, J.C. and Bunjé, H.W. (1966). Observations on mountain sickness in the Colombian Andes. *Lancet*, **ii**, 655

Weibel, E.R. and Knight, B.W. (1964). A morphometric study on the thickness of the pulmonary air–blood barrier. *Journal of Cell Biology*, **21**, 367

Weil, J.V., Byrne-Quinn, E., Sodal, I.E., Filley, G.F., and Grover, R.F. (1971). Acquired attenuation of chemoreceptor function in chronically hypoxic man at high altitude. *Journal of Clinical Investigation*, **50**, 186

Weiskopf, R.B., Gabel, R.A., and Fencl, V. (1976). Alkaline shift in lumbar and intracranial CSF in man after five days at high altitude. *Journal of Applied Physiology*, **41**, 93

West, J.B., Lahiri, S., Gill, M.B., Milledge, J.S., Pugh, L.G.C.E., and Ward, M.P. (1962). Arterial oxygen saturation during exercise at high altitude. *Journal of Applied Physiology*, **17**, 617

West, J.B., Boyer, S.J., Graber, D.J., Hackett, P.H., Maret, K.H., Milledge, J.S., Peters, R.M., Jr., Pizzo, C.J., Samaja, M., Sarnquist, F.H., Schoene, R.B., and Winslow, R.M. (1983). Maximal exercise at extreme altitudes on Mount Everest. *Journal of Applied Physiology*, **55**, 688

Whittembury, J., Lozano, R., and Monge, C.C. (1968). Influence of cell concentration in the electrometric determination of blood pH. *Acta Physiologica Latino Americana*, **18**, 263

Williams, D., Heath, D., Gosney, J., and Rios-Dalenz, J. (1993). Pulmonary endocrine cells of Aymara Indians from the Bolivian Andes. *Thorax*, **48**, 52

Winslow, R.M., Monge, C.C., Statham, N.J., Gibson, C.G., Charache, S., Whittembury, J., Moran, O., and Berger R.L. (1981). Variability of oxygen affinity of blood: human subjects native to high altitude. *Journal of Applied Physiology*, **51**, 1411

Winslow, R.M., Samaja, M., and West, J.B. (1984). Red cell function at extreme altitude on Mount Everest. *Journal of Applied Physiology: Respiratory, Environmental, and Exercise Physiology*, **56**, 109

5

Transport and release of oxygen to the tissues

At rest the tissues of the body need some 220–260 ml of oxygen per minute, but on exercise this requirement may increase 10-fold or even more (Thomas *et al.* 1974). The amount of oxygen transported per minute from the lungs to the rest of the body is a function of the cardiac output, the quantity of oxygen in systemic arterial blood, and the affinity of haemoglobin for oxygen, which influences the ease with which the gas is passed to the tissues. Increased requirements of oxygen in the early stages of acclimatization can be met to some extent by an increase in cardiac output up to four times its normal level of 5 litres per minute (Chapter 18).

In this chapter we shall be concerned with the quantity of oxygen carried in the blood and with the ability of haemoglobin to release it to the tissues. The oxygen content of blood depends on the efficiency of ventilation and pulmonary diffusion (Chapter 4) and on the concentration of haemoglobin in the blood according to the following formula:

Oxygen supply (ml/min) = Cardiac output (1/min)
× Haemoglobin concentration × 1.34 (g/l)
× % oxygen saturation of arterial blood (ml O_2/ g Hb)

At sea level, haemoglobin leaving the lungs is 97% saturated and in venous blood in the tissues this saturation has fallen to 70%. The oxygen content of 100 ml blood leaving the lungs is 19.4 ml and that of blood leaving the capillaries of the tissues is 14.4 ml. Thus, at sea level this volume of blood delivers 5 ml of the gas to the tissues. At high altitude the diminished partial pressure of oxygen in the alveolar spaces consequent upon the diminished barometric pressure might be thought to demand a significantly raised haemoglobin concentration in all native highlanders, to provide a maximum level of transport for such oxygen as is available. This is not the case. The level of haemoglobin manifested depends on the severity of the altitude and on the constancy of exposure to it. The ethnic background of the native highlander and individual variation may also have an influence.

HAEMOGLOBIN CONCENTRATION

Haemoglobin concentration depends on the ratio of red cell mass to plasma volume. As Ward *et al.* (1989) point out, these two variables are regulated by different mechanisms. Red cell mass is determined by the rate of erythropoiesis and the rate of loss of red cells. At high altitude the normal sea-level life span of erythrocytes is maintained at 120 days. Plasma volume is considered below and in Chapter 18. Central control of plasma volume is through distention of the right atrium which induces release of atrial natriuretic peptide which causes the kidney to excrete sodium and water thus reducing plasma volume.

The increase in haemoglobin concentration in some individuals at high altitude was first demonstrated by Viault (1891) not in man but in animals living in the vicinity of the Andean settlement Morococha (4540 m). This is rather strange since the level of haemoglobin in adapted indigenous mountain species, such as the Andean llama, is low compared with that of man (Chapter 35). The large number of small ellipsoidal erythrocytes in this species noted by Viault (1891) is a characteristic of the camel family, including the Andean camelids such as the llama (Chapter 35).

In man the hypobaric hypoxia at high altitude may induce an increased haemoglobin concentration, but this is by no means universal. It depends on the magnitude of the elevation and the constancy of exposure to it. After only 5 days at an altitude of 4200 m at the summit of the Hawaiian volcano Mauna Kea, 32 astronomers manning the UK infrared telescope showed a small but significant increase in the haemoglobin concentration (15.9 ± 1.1 g/dl to 16.6 ± 1.0 g/dl; $p < 0.001$) (Forster 1983). At the same time there were small but significant increases in haematocrit (46.1 ± 3.3% to 47.9 ± 3.4%; $p < 0.001$), and in red cell count (5.09 ± 0.41 10^{12}/l to 5.29 ± 0.46 10^{12}/l; $p < 0.001$). After the same brief period there were no changes observed in red cell indices such as mean corpuscular haemoglobin and mean corpuscular haemoglobin concentration (Forster

1983). Within 20 days of the return to sea level the red cell count and haemoglobin concentration had returned to pre-ascent levels. Mairbäurl (1988) found that during a 2-week stay at moderate altitude there was a significant increase of reticulocytes, more pronounced in active than sedentary subjects, but haemoglobin, haematocrit, and red cell count did not change.

When lowlanders ascend to remain for a longer period at high altitude, the increases in haemoglobin concentration are greater. In India, Chohan and Singh (1979) studied 66 lowlanders at sea level, 45 lowlanders ascending to reside at 3690 m for 2 years, and 24 highlanders native to that altitude in the Himalaya. Haemoglobin level in g/dl was 14.11 (11.5–16.5) in the lowlanders, 16.03 (13.4–19.0) in temporary residents, and 13.66 (12.5–15.5) in native highlanders. Percentage haematocrit levels were 43.5 (34–59) in the lowlanders, 53 (43–64) in temporary residents, and 47 (42–56) in native highlanders. Winslow *et al.* (1984) found a range of 17.8 to 20.6 g/dl for haemoglobin concentrations in climbers at extreme altitudes between 5350 and 6300 m. There was no correlation between altitude and haemoglobin concentration. Several interesting features emerged from these data. First, lowlanders ascending to reside at high altitude for a period of 2 years show a significant elevation of haemoglobin concentration and haematocrit, although there is much variation from person to person. Second, the levels of haemoglobin in the Indian subjects in the lowlands is lower than in the astronomers from the Royal Observatory, so that there are nutritional aspects to this problem. Third is the fact that Chohan and Singh (1979) found that the haemoglobin concentration and haematocrit levels were not raised in the sample of native highlanders from Ladakh that they studied.

This latter finding was confirmed by Beall and Reichsman (1984). In a sample of 270 healthy Tibetan adults, 20–79 years of age, resident at 3250–3560 m in Upper Chumik, Nepal, the mean haemoglobin concentration was found to be 16.1 ± 1.2 g/dl among 126 adult males, 14.4 ± 1.4 g/dl among 100 pre-menopausal women, and 15.0 ± 1.1 g/dl among 44 post-menopausal women. No less than 98% of the men, 96% of the pre-menopausal women, and 82% of the post-menopausal women had haemoglobin concentrations within two standard deviations ('the normal range') of sea-level men. It is clear that a healthy population may reside at high altitude in the Himalaya without a significant elevation in haemoglobin.

In this context, it is of historical interest that Hurtado (1932), one of the first and most distinguished workers in the field of high-altitude medicine, also found the elevation in haemoglobin in Andean highlanders to be often modest in extent. As later pointed out by Winslow and Monge (1987), Hurtado used only a simple optical device for his estimations of haemoglobin levels and this may have yielded artificially low results. However, at the time he found this, and the individual variation, so disturbing that it led him to doubt the importance of an increase in haemoglobin as a factor in acclimatization. In his early study, no fewer than 26% of the highlanders examined had a red cell count below 6×10^{12}/l and in 11% it was even lower than the average at sea level. There was pronounced individual variation from 4.8 to 10.4×10^{12}/l. The average haemoglobin level in 100 highlanders was 15.93 g/dl, a value only slightly higher than the normal at sea level. He concluded that a normal sea-level count was not incompatible with health in such high regions, a view restated half a century later by Beall and Reichsman (1984). He said: 'If we know that the native lives at high altitudes with a lower saturation of his arterial blood and with less circulating oxygen, as compared with the recent arrival, and yet is much more physically efficient than the latter, we have great difficulty in accepting the assumption that an increase of haemoglobin is of great importance.' This view also received support many years later from Winslow and Monge (1987).

Different individuals may reach an equilibrium with a haematocrit that may be anywhere in the range of 50–70%. One factor that may operate is whether the subject obtains relief from the chronic exposure to hypoxia by descending to lower altitude from time to time. On one visit to Cerro de Pasco (4330 m) in Peru we worked closely with two highlanders at the High Altitude Research Laboratory. One was a man in late middle age who had worked there as a miner for 30 years, but had made frequent visits to Lima on the coast; his haematocrit was only moderately elevated. The other was a young man of 23 years who had never left his mountain home; he had a haematocrit that was so high as to give concern that he was likely to develop chronic mountain sickness (Chapter 15).

Some 30 years later, further haematological studies were carried out by Hurtado (1964a) on 83 Quechua Indians from a higher altitude of 4540 m at Morococha and on 250 sea-level residents from Lima. In this series he used more sophisticated photoelectric equipment and the haemoglobin and haematocrit levels reported were much higher. The mean value for the haematocrit was 46.6% at sea level and 59.5% at high altitude. The haemoglobin levels were 15.6 and 20.1 g/dl respectively. The mean red cell count in the sea-level dwellers was 5.1, but was $6.4 \times 10^{12}/l$ in the native highlanders. The reticulocyte counts were, respectively, 17.9 and $45.5 \times 10^9/l$. These data for residents of Morococha were confirmed by Reynafarje (1966) who found that in 50 members of the settlement the average haemoglobin level was 20 g/dl and the average haematocrit was 60%. Monge and Monge (1966) gave somewhat lower values for natives of Huancayo (3260 m) who went to Morococha (4540 m) for 15 days. They found the average haemoglobin level of these visitors to the settlement to be 17.98 g/dl. The number of erythrocytes was $6.05 \times 10^{12}/l$ and the haematocrit level was 54.3%. In native highlanders in the Andes the red cell mass may rise to be up to 83% greater than that of lowlanders (Sanchez *et al.* 1970).

These very high figures derived from the work of Hurtado and his Peruvian colleagues have come to be regarded as classical manifestations of acclimatization to hypobaric hypoxia, but it has to be kept in mind that the Quechuas from whom these data were obtained were residents at particularly high altitudes. Indeed at Morococha (4540 m) some investigators have found haematological values on the very edge of those that would be regarded as criteria for the diagnosis of chronic mountain sickness (Chapter 15). Thus, Merino (1950) found the average haematocrit in the highlanders there to be 66.7%. The average haemoglobin level was stated by him to be 22.6 g/dl, a figure very close to 23 g/dl which is a diagnostic criterion for Monge's disease (Chapter 15). Merino (1950) also gives a high average value for the red cell count, namely, $7.88 \times 10^{12}/l$. It is clear that, even allowing for individual variation, haematological values are closely related to the elevation of permanent residence. Whittembury and Monge (1972) also showed that there is a relation between haematocrit and the age of permanent residents at different altitudes. They collected data from healthy volunteers at Morococha (4540 m), Cerro de Pasco (4330 m), and Puno (3800 m). They found that a haematocrit of 75% is accompanied by symptoms of chronic mountain sickness. This level is predictable at an age of 30 years of Morococha but at 63 years at Cerro de Pasco.

Theoretically, women at high altitude could lose important haematological components of acclimatization by anaemia brought about by poor socio-economic conditions, and blood loss due to menstruation and parturition. However, Moreno-Black *et al.* (1984) found iron-deficiency anaemia in only 11% of 152 non-pregnant healthy women under the age of 45 years in La Paz (3800 m). The mean haemoglobin level was 16.3 g/dl (SD 1.8).

Optimum haemoglobin concentration

The increase in haemoglobin concentration with high altitude compensates for a reduction in systemic arterial oxygen saturation. At altitudes up to 5300 m this compensation results in arterial oxygen content approximately equal to that at sea level in acclimatized men (Ward *et al.* 1989). There is clearly an optimum haemoglobin level below which oxygen-carrying capacity is reduced. Higher concentrations induce increased viscosity with its attendant problems of inadequate blood flow. However, as we discuss below, the relation between higher haemoglobin levels and increased viscosity is complex. Winslow *et al.* (1985a) found that in native highlanders in the Andes reduction of packed cell volume from 62 to 42% resulted in increased cardiac output and elevation of mixed venous oxygen tension.

Comparison of haemoglobin concentrations in native highlanders of the Andes and the Himalaya

Beall and Reichsman (1984) compared the published data on mean haemoglobin concentrations in adult Himalayan and Andean highlanders residing permanently between 3200 and 4100 m (Table 5.1). This comparison reveals quite clearly that mean levels of haemoglobin in the native highlanders from the Himalaya are lower, being only a modest 5% greater than those of a reference population at sea level. These differences are largely explained by the fact that the Tibetans and Sherpas live permanently at considerably lower altitudes than do the Quechuas and Aymaras. An alternative explanation, favoured by Adams and Strang (1975), is that, like the llama, Sherpas may rely more on greater oxygen saturation than on an increased partial pressure of oxygen in the blood. Doubt has been cast by recent investigators on the validity of supposed differences in the position of the oxygen–haemoglobin dissociation curve between Sherpas and Quechuas, as discussed later. The lower haemoglobin levels among the highlanders of Ladakh and Nepal are not explained by deficiencies of vitamin B_{12}, folate, iron, or thyroid hormone (Adams and Strang 1975), although hookworm infestation may sometimes be

Table 5.1 Comparison of haemoglobin concentrations among Himalayan and Andean samples of native highlanders living permanently at altitudes between 3200 and 4100 m (from Beall and Reichsman 1984, by courtesy of Alan R. Liss Inc, Publishers)

Mean Hb concentration (g/dl)	Standard deviation	No.	Altitude (m)	Age (years)	Ethnic group	Reference
Native highlanders, men, samples of 30 or more						
Himalayan						
16.1	1.2	126	3400	20–79	Tibetan	Beall and Reichsman (1984)
Andean						
17.5	1.5	38	4000	20–56	Quechua	Garruto (1976)
18.2	1.1	85	3600	22±3	Aymara	Arnaud *et al.* (1979)
18.8	1.5	40	3700	19–48	Indian	Hurtado *et al.* (1945)
Native highlanders, adolescents and men (samples of less than 30)						
Himalayan						
17.0	1.9	13	3900	14–50	Sherpa	Samaja *et al.* (1979)
Andean						
17.4	1.4	18	3700	18–36	Indian	Moret *et al.* (1972)
High-altitude residents (length of residence unknown), adolescents and men						
Himalayan						
14.7	1.3	25	3700	18–28	Ladakhi	Guleria *et al.* (1971)
16.8	1.4	?	3650	'Adult'	Tibetan	Adams and Shrestha (1974)
17.0	1.3	28	4000	15–57	Sherpa	Adams and Strang (1975)
Andean						
19.0	1.7	529	3600	29 ± 11	Indian Mestizo	Tufts (1982)
Native highlanders, women (samples of 30 or more)						
Himalayan						
14.4	1.4	100	3400	20–49	Tibetan	Beall and Reichsman (1984)
Andean						
16.3	1.8	152	3600	18–45	Indian Mestizo	Moreno-Black *et al.*, (1984)
High-altitude residents (length of residence unknown), adolescent girls and women						
Himalayan						
14.5	0.7	?	3650	'Adult'	Tibetan	Adams and Shrestha (1974)
15.3	0.8	23	4000	15–51	Sherpa	Adams and Strang (1975)

responsible (Beall and Reichsman 1984). In conclusion, in contrasting haemoglobin levels in natives of the Himalaya and the Andes it has to be kept in mind that the values from South America, which have come to be accepted as some of the classic criteria of acclimatization to hypobaric hypoxia, are based on residents at extremely high settlements.

When interpreting comparisons between haematological data collected by different or even the same workers at different times and in different areas, due consideration must be given to the techniques employed. Thus, as we have seen, Hurtado (1932) initially reported that increases in haemoglobin concentration in native highlanders of the Andes were modest but in this investigation he used only a simple optical device to estimate the haemoglobin levels. In a later study when Hurtado *et al.* (1945) employed a more sophisticated photoelectric instrument, they found haemoglobin concentrations to be higher. The lower haemoglobin levels found in native highlanders of Nepal by Beall and Reichsman (1984) were arrived at by finger-stick and measurements using a simple optical comparator method. The use of oxalate will artificially reduce observed levels of haematocrit. It is obvious that environmental factors such as silicosis in Andean miners or non-occupational silicosis in Ladakh (Chapter 2) will influence haemoglobin levels. Thus, for many reasons the determination of haemoglobin concentrations in high-altitude populations is not without its pitfalls.

BLOOD RHEOLOGY

A pronounced rise in haematocrit at high altitude might be thought to pose problems by increasing blood viscosity to dangerous levels thus compromising blood flow and oxygen delivery to the tissues. The equation that relates pressure, flow, dimensions of the tube, and viscosity of the liquid under streamline is that of Poiseuille, an early nineteenth century French physician,

$$\Delta P = \frac{8 \eta l \dot{Q}}{\pi r^4}$$

where ΔP is expressed in $N \cdot m^{-2}$, l is the length of the tube in m, r is the radius in cm; $\dot{Q}$ is the flow in $m^3 \cdot s^{-1}$; and η is the coefficient of viscosity of the liquid in $N \cdot s \cdot m^{-2}$ (Harris and Heath 1986). Thus the fluidity of blood is a complex function of the haematocrit, the composition of the plasma, the diameter of the vessel through which the blood flows, and the driving pressure of the cardiac ventricle

(Schmid-Schönbein 1982). The raised haematocrit of some highlanders does not have the anticipated deleterious effect on the flow of blood, for the viscosity of rapidly flowing polycythaemic blood is lower than expected. Thus, while most suspensions and emulsions exhibit an extremely high viscosity at volume fractions above 0.4, mammalian blood remains fluid, even at a haematocrit above 0.9 when it has a viscosity comparable to that of olive oil (Schmid-Schönbein 1982).

The explanation is that the non-nucleated red cells assume flow properties similar to those of fluid droplets. The normal disc-shaped erythrocytes have a favourable ratio of surface area to volume so that they can be deformed without straining the membrane. The flexible membrane and fluid cytoplasm of red cells allow them to squeeze through very narrow blood vessels without being sequestered and phagocytosed. In doing so they become elongated and the cell membrane is driven with rotation around the cell contents, the so-called 'tank-treading' in small capillaries. The cells rapidly migrate to the axial core surrounded by a marginal lubricating layer of plasma of low viscosity and as a result the fluidity of cells is increased in narrow capillaries.

Due to this squeezing, rapid and highly effective intracellular mixing is induced. The motion of the membrane brings about complex, intracellular laminar flow of haemoglobin, oxyhaemoglobin, and dissolved oxygen (Zander and Schmid-Schönbein 1973). Consequently, the diffusive transport of oxygen in and out of the red cells is augmented by a convective motion in moving cells. The blood capillaries of man and other mammals are much smaller than those of species with nucleated red cells. Consequently, the exchange area for any given capillary volume is much higher and the diffusion distance of oxygen to the wall of the capillary is smaller.

This unusually high fluidity of blood in capillaries is dependent on an adequate flow. When flow diminishes to low levels, a sharp transition to a very viscous suspension occurs. This is brought abut by aggregation of red cells into rouleaux, which then form larger elastic networks, the density and stability of which increase with progressive elevation of haematocrit. When rouleaux straddle bifurcations or impact into the lumens of capillaries, the fluidity of the blood may be sharply diminished or even abolished. Under such conditions of low flow, a haematocrit exceeding 55% may prove to be very serious. The degree of aggregation is influenced by the concentration of plasma proteins of high molecular weight such as fibrinogen, α_2 macroglobulins and IgM (Schmid-Schönbein 1982). These creeping masses of red cells constitute what is termed 'sludging'. Such masses are deoxygenated long before they leave the capillaries. They impede the further supply of fresh oxygenated blood and, hence, a condition of stagnation hypoxia is brought about. In general, the consequences of a loss of blood fluidity are very dependent on local factors such as flow, driving pressure, and geometry of blood vessels. Hence, the effects are likely to vary in different organs.

Sarnquist *et al.* (1986) studied the effects of acute, isovolaemic haemodilution on the exercise ability and mental function of four polycythaemic mountain climbers at 5400 m. About 15% of their blood volume was removed and replaced with an equal volume of 5% human albumin solution. Thus the original haematocrit of 58 ± 1.25% fell to 50.5 ± 1.5%. The oxygen-carrying ability of the blood was reduced by 13%. However, maximum work level, oxygen uptake, minute ventilation, and blood oxygen saturation did not change. There was a small but significant improvement in psychological tests. It was concluded that a haematocrit of greater than 50% conferred no advantage for exercise.

Pentoxifylline

In spite of the demonstration that the viscosity of rapidly flowing polycythaemic blood is lower that expected (Schmid-Schönbein 1982) some workers believe that exercise performance at high altitude may be worsened by increased blood viscosity (Mairbäurl *et al.* 1986; Wood and Appenzeller 1988*a*). In their experience blood is made less viscous and thus able to flow more easily at high altitude by the drug pentoxifylline (Trental ®) which is a theobromine derivative of methylxanthine introduced in 1972 as a vasodilator. When given orally, it does not have such an effect and does not influence heart rate, arterial blood pressure, or systemic vascular resistance (Weisse *et al.* 1975). Subsequently, the drug was found to reduce the viscosity and improve the flow properties of blood thus improving blood flow and tissue oxygenation in peripheral vascular disease (Accetto 1982). The drug helped prevent thrombus formation in patients with polycythaemia vera, who are prone to cerebrovascular accidents (Sedova *et al.* 1984).

Pentoxifylline appears to act by increasing the deformability of erythrocytes through the spectrin–actin meshwork of their cell membranes. The state of the membrane is dependent on intra-cellular concentrations of calcium and adenosine triphosphate (ATP), a fall in the latter causing an increase in blood viscosity (Nakao *et al.* 1960). In the severe hypoxaemia of high altitude the increased amounts of deoxyhaemoglobin bind with ATP thus leading to a stiffening of red cells (Wood and Appenzeller 1988*b*). Pentoxifylline may reverse this effect of hypoxaemia by increasing intracellular ATP by enhancing glucose uptake or by increasing the rate of glycolysis. The increased ATP chelates free calcium, reducing calcium-dependent membrane stiffness.

Palareti *et al.* (1984) found that pentoxiphylline prevented increased blood viscosity and fibrinogen and decreased red-cell deformability immediately after return from high altitude (7500 m) in the Himalaya. Wood and Appenzeller (1988*a*) made a similar study in Tibet and Nepal and reported results consistent with decreased deformability of red cells. Appenzeller and Wood (1988) also demonstrated that pentoxifylline affects neurogenic vasomotor function and they postulate that this drug may be useful in the prevention of frostbite (Chapter 24).

RED CELL MORPHOLOGY AT HIGH ALTITUDE

Observations on the morphology of red cells in venous blood samples from four climbers ascending to 7200 m over a period of 5 weeks were made by Rowles and Williams (1983). The erythrocytes were studied by scanning electron microscopy and categorized on the criteria of Brecher and Bessis (1972). They found that even a mild degree of hypoxia (3555 m) for a short period of 2 days brought about an increase in the proportion of morphologically abnormal red cells. As longer time was spent at high altitude, so the proportion of abnormal cells rose. Thus, the authors found 88.5% of red cells to be morphologically normal discocytes at sea level, but this had fallen to 24.7% after 39 days above 4600 m with quick ascents to 6200 and 7200 m. Multiple irregularities or gross distortion of shape, including echinocytes, rose from 0.6 to 12.7% over the same period.

This study led Reinhart and Bärtsch (1986) to investigate by light microscopy blood from five men and five women ascending to 3400 m in a cable-car. After a night's rest at 3600 m, they reached by foot, the next day, an altitude of 4560 m, virtually the same altitude of the study of Rowles and Williams (1983). They found that about 90% of the cells were discocytes both at 1190 and 4560 m and there was no difference in morphology at the two altitudes. Hence they found nothing to suggest that short-term exposure to high altitude influences red cell morphology. They suggested that such changes in erythrocytes may take place only after brief ascents to extreme altitude (6200 and 7200 m) or after a longer time of exposure to high altitude. The significance of these possible alterations in red cell morphology is as yet unclear, although such abnormal shapes, especially echinocytes, can increase blood viscosity (Meiselman 1978).

BLOOD VOLUME

During the first 1 or 2 weeks at high altitude there is an initial decrease of 15–20% in plasma volume that results in an increase in circulating haemoglobin of 1–2 g/dl (Surks *et al.* 1966). It has to be kept in mind that this haemoconcentration accounts for at least part of the initial rise in haemoglobin levels found in those acutely ascending into high altitude, such as the astronomers on Mauna Kea described above. Mairbäurl (1988) accepts that the early elevation of haemoglobin on ascent to high altitude is in part due to dehydration. Once polycythaemia is underway, it leads to an increase in the red cell volume and this in turn results in an increase in total blood volume (see Fig. 18.2), in spite of the plasma volume being reduced.

ERYTHROKINETICS AT HIGH ALTITUDE

Initially, it was reported that there was an elevation of erythropoietin in the first 24 to 48 hours after exposure to high altitude (Siri *et al.* 1966; Albrecht and Littell 1972). However, the work of Reynafarje (1966) suggested that increased activity occurs within as little as 2 hours. More sensitive modern techniques have confirmed that serum immunoreactive erythropoietin concentration rises within 3 hours of exposure to hypobaric hypoxia and reaches a maximum after 24–48 hours. Thereafter, it declines to reach after 3 weeks values not measurably different from those at sea level (Milledge and Coates 1985). The kidney is the main site of erythropoietin production in adult animals and man, probably in the juxtaglomerular apparatus (Fisher and Langston 1967). It is uncertain whether the kidney produces erythropoietin directly or a proerythropoietin that then reacts with a serum factor to produce erythropoietin (Wickramasinghe and Weatherall 1982). Later reports suggested that 10–15% of erythropoietin is produced in the liver (Erslev 1987). Erythropoietin is a glycoprotein which in man has a molecular weight of 39 000. Ward *et al.* (1989) note

that the two major stimuli for erythropoietin production are hypoxia and blood loss. They believe it likely that the latter is of greater evolutionary significance for survival. It is of interest that the hypoxia of anaemia stimulates the rate of synthesis of erythropoietin, which is regulated by the rate of oxygen delivered to the renal cells producing it. This is in contrast to the stimulation of the carotid bodies by the level of arterial oxygen tension (Chapter 7). Erythropoietin stimulates responsive cells in the bone marrow derived from haemopoietic cells into proerythroblasts. These develop through various stages into reticulocytes. After a period in the marrow they enter the circulation where they mature into erythrocytes. The degree of stimulation of erythropoietin production is proportional to the severity of the hypobaric hypoxia within certain limits. Thus up to an elevation of 3660 m the haemoglobin level increases in a linear relation to altitude. Above this height the haemoglobin concentration rises more rapidly with altitude than previously. However, in conditions of extreme hypoxia, such as occur around 6000 m, a limit is reached and there begins a decrease in the formation of erythrocytes and haemoglobin (Hurtado *et al.* 1945). Erythropoietic hyperactivity falls away when the systemic arterial oxygen saturation falls to 60%. The initial rise in plasma and urinary erythropoetin that occurs within hours of the first ascent to high altitude falls in a few days to a value intermediate between the initial pronounced response and that at sea level (Siri *et al.* 1966; Faura *et al.* 1969). This secondary fall in the level of erythropoietin is related to the gradual rise in arterial oxygen tension that follows hyperventilation and the other mechanisms of acclimatization described elsewhere in this book. Mairbäurl (1988) found that, initially on exposure to high altitude, serum-immunoreactive erythropoietin was increased fourfold but transiently, subsequently returning almost to prealtitude values. Serum iron and ferritin decreased but the utilization of injected ^{59}Fe was higher in subjects at high altitude. The reticulocyte count increased about threefold in 5 days at 4559 m but haemoglobin, haematocrit, and red cell count remained unchanged. The duration of the stay was too short to induce a significant change in these parameters.

Reynafarje *et al.* (1964) had earlier presented experimental evidence to confirm this falling away of initial erythropoietin production. To detect evidence of erythropoiesis, they injected rats with plasma obtained from natives of Morococha (4540 m), from sea-level subjects, and from newcomers to this Andean town 1, 3 and 10 days after their arrival from sea level. They found erythropoietic activity in plasma from newcomers only 1 day after their arrival. Erythropoietin was not found in plasma taken from newcomers 3 or 10 days after their arrival. The increase in red cell mass is slow but it continues to rise for a long time so that after 6 months at altitudes over 4000 m it has increased by a mean of 50%. Earlier work on the measurement of erythropoietin in blood was by bioassay and indirect indices of erythropoietin activity such as intestinal iron absorption or reticulocyte counts. Newer methods using radioimmunoassay are more sensitive.

The hyperactivity of erythropoietin gives rise to an increase in the iron turnover rate. Within 2 hours of exposure to high altitude the iron turnover rate (in mg/day per kg body weight) increased on average from 0.37 to 0.54 in eight lowlanders taken to 4540 m (Reynafarje 1964). The iron turnover rate rises to a maximum of 0.91 in 1 to 2 weeks, so that erythropoietic activity is about three times higher than at sea level. Thereafter, the iron turnover rate falls, but even after 6 months it is still elevated. Even after a year's residence at high altitude the erythropoietic balance is still not achieved, for while the red cell mass increases the total blood volume is higher (Reynafarje 1964).

There is a consequent stimulation of the intestinal absorption of iron to three or four times sea-level values during early exposure to high-altitude hypoxia. The maximal absorption of iron is reached after 1 week (Reynafarje and Ramos 1961). Permanent residents at high altitude do not have an iron absorption significantly different from that of people born and living at sea level. The stimulus for iron absorption was considered by Reynafarje and Ramos (1961) to be the demand of the bone marrow for the production of more red cells so that native highlanders who remain hypoxaemic but who are not forming excess erythrocytes do not show a significant elevation of iron absorption. In newcomers to high altitude actively becoming more polycythaemic, the effect of erythropoietin on the bone marrow is limited by available iron.

The bone marrow of the newcomer to high altitude undergoing active acclimatization shows a hyperplasia of the erythroid elements, whereas the megakaryocytes remain normal in number and maturation (Merino and Reynafarje 1949; Huff *et al.* 1951). The erythroid hyperplasia, with increase in red cells with normal white cells, differentiates this condition of high-altitude polycythaemia from polycythaemia vera. We consider the peripheral and dif-

ferential white cell count in Chapter 26 and the platelet count in Chapter 9. The increased activity of the bone marrow leads to a daily red cell production some 30% higher than that of lowlanders at sea level (Reynafarje 1964). The life span of erythrocytes in both native highlanders and in lowlanders acclimatized to high altitude is said to be within the normal limit of 120 days (Berlin *et al.* 1954). The change in red cell mass is slow and the rise in haemoglobin levels constitutes one of the slower components of acclimatization.

BILIRUBINAEMIA

Bilirubinaemia occurs in man at high altitude. This may be due to the greatly increased number of erythrocytes, so that a normal rate of destruction will lead to increased levels of bilirubin. An inability of the liver to handle increased levels of serum bilirubin may be another factor. The serum bilirubin concentration of permanent residents at 4540 m in Peru was found to range from 1.27 to 1.56 mg/ 100 ml compared with 0.76 mg/100 ml for men at sea level (Hurtado *et al.* 1945; Merino 1950; Berendsohn 1962). The elevation was due almost entirely to indirect bilirubin. A study was made by Altland and Parker (1977) of the serum bilirubin concentration and the extent of intravascular haemolysis in rats during acclimatization to a simulated altitude of 5500 m. During both continuous and intermittent exposure of 4 hours per day the serum bilirubin was significantly elevated at the end of 4–6 weeks. The rises occurred only after the development of severe polycythaemia, with a haematocrit of 68% and a haemoglobin level of 21.6 g/dl. An increase in intravascular haemolysis was found after 2 weeks' intermittent exposure and after 4 weeks' continuous exposure to 5500 m. There was no alteration of erythrocyte fragility to account for increased intravascular haemolysis. No liver pathology was observed in the rats exposed to simulated high altitude.

EFFECTS OF DESCENT TO SEA LEVEL

There is a progressive decrease in red cell iron turnover rate in high-altitude natives when they are brought down to sea level, reaching its lowest value from the third to the fifth week (Reynafarje *et al.* 1959). It is then only one-third of its initial value, indicating great depression of red cell production. Three months after descent to sea level the red cell volume reaches a value lower than normal, indicating a true anaemia. At the same time, there is an increase in plasma bilirubin and in faecal urobilinogen, and this has been considered to be consistent with increased red cell destruction as well as inhibition of erythropoietic activity (Merino 1950). However, Reynafarje (1964) found the red cell life span to be normal, as was also the rate of sequestration in the spleen and liver of autogenous red cells labelled with ^{51}Cr. Hence there is unlikely to be an accelerated destruction of circulating red cells. On descent to sea level, erythropoietin becomes undetectable. There is a progressive decrease in the activity of the bone marrow. The mobilization and utilization of iron decreases progressively, reaching a minimum after 2 to 3 weeks. The red cell mass diminishes slowly and after 2 months is even lower than that of sea-level subjects (Chapter 33). Reynafarje (1966) reported that filtrates of plasma from polycythaemic subjects from the Andes brought to sea level produced a statistically significant depression of erythropoiesis in rats previously exposed to high altitude to make them sensitive to such a depression factor. This suggests that an inhibitory humoral factor exists in the plasma of high-altitude natives brought down to sea level.

OXYGEN RELEASE TO THE TISSUES

So far in this chapter we have been concerned with the increase in the *quantity* of haemoglobin in man living at high altitude, which enables a greater supply of oxygen to be transported to the tissues. The properties of haemoglobin itself must now be considered, for they present a seeming paradox. Acclimatization to the hypoxia of high altitude might appear to be better served by an *enhanced affinity* of haemoglobin for oxygen, which will facilitate carriage of more of the gas to the tissues. On the other hand, it could be considered that acclimatization is better effected by a *decreased affinity* of haemoglobin for oxygen, so that it readily yields oxygen to the tissues maintaining an adequate oxygen tension for transport to the mitochondria. The answer to this question is complex and depends to some extent on the level of altitude and consequent degree of hypoxia being considered. We shall first consider this problem in relation to man living at high but not extreme altitude (Chapter 32). Central to this matter is the oxygen– haemoglobin dissociation curve.

Oxygen–haemoglobin dissociation curve

As 97% of the oxygen is carried in the erythrocyte and only 3% in the plasma, the increased concentration of haemoglobin in the blood at high altitude means that it transports an increased amount of oxygen to the tissues. However, its availability there

depends on the ease with which it is liberated from haemoglobin. Such affinity is expressed as the familiar oxygen–haemoglobin dissociation curve which was found by Bohr (1904) to have a sigmoid shape (Fig. 5.1). This shape has considerable physiological significance even at sea level because, over the flat portion of the curve, fluctuations in alveolar oxygen tension do not interfere with the arterial oxygen content. On the other hand, on the steep slope of the curve, minimal changes in oxygen tension at the peripheral capillaries allow considerable unloading of oxygen.

The peculiar sigmoid shape is due to changes in the conformation of the haemoglobin molecule (Finch and Lenfant 1972). Crystallographic techniques show that oxyhaemoglobin has a slightly different configuration than that of deoxyhaemoglobin in that in the former the pair of α chains and the pair of β chains are slightly closer together (Muirhead *et al.* 1967). The combination of an oxygen molecule with a haem group alters the position of the ferrous ion in the haem ring, changing in turn the position of certain amino acids and changing the affinity for oxygen of the haem group in the neighbouring subunit chain. Hence, in effect, the uptake of each oxygen molecule in turn enhances the uptake of more (Perutz 1970). There is a suggestion that, upon oxygenation of the third haem, the quarternary structure of the haemoglobin changes from the structure of deoxyhaemoglobin to that of oxyhaemo-

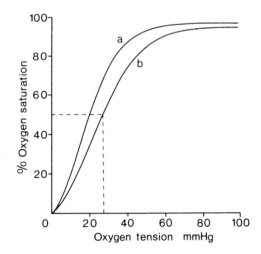

5.1 *Oxygen–haemoglobin dissociation curves of blood on different hydrogen ion (H⁺) concentrations. Curve a, normal arterial blood at sea level; curve b, normal venous blood at sea level. The value for* P_{50} *is shown to be 26.6 mmHg.*

globin. These molecular events account for the changing of the oxygen affinity of haemoglobin with oxygenation causing the oxygen dissociation curve to have a sigmoid shape.

Position of the oxygen dissociation curve at high altitude

The position of the curve is given by the partial pressure of oxygen in plasma associated with 50% oxygen saturation of blood (that is, when half the total haem groups are combined with oxygen) at 37°C and pH 7.4. This particular partial pressure is known as the P_{50}. It is of historical interest that Barcroft *et al.* (1923) suggested that an increased affinity of haemoglobin for oxygen might be an important factor in acclimatization. They found that fetal blood was superior to adult blood in its affinity for oxygen, facilitating the intrauterine transfer of oxygen. The normal value of P_{50} for adult whole blood at a P_{CO_2} of 40 mmHg, pH 7.4, and temperature 37°C is 26–27 mmHg. Human fetal blood has a P_{50} of 19 mmHg. Following an expedition to Peru, Barcroft (1925) came to the conclusion that there was a tendency for the dissociation curve to shift to the left. Later studies by Dill *et al.* (1931) in Colorado and by Keys *et al.* (1936) in Chile did not confirm this. They thought there was a slight decrease in the affinity of haemoglobin for oxygen at high altitude. This increase in P_{50} and the shift of the oxygen – haemoglobin dissociation curve to the right are favourable in maintaining an adequate level of oxygen diffusion in the tissues. They maintain a relatively high arterial oxygen tension with freer removal of oxygen from haemoglobin during passage through a systemic capillary. The amount of oxygen per minute that will diffuse from the blood to the mitochondria of tissue cells varies directly with the difference in P_{O_2} between these two regions. Since the mitochondrial P_{O_2} is probably below 1 mmHg (Chapter 6), it is the partial pressure of oxygen in the capillary that determines the rate of diffusion of the gas. A shift of the oxygen–haemoglobin dissociation curve to the right gives a higher P_{O_2} for every value of saturation and thereby provides a requisite partial pressure of oxygen further along the capillary.

This favourable effect of maintaining a higher P_{O_2} for tissue diffusion of oxygen was recognized by Aste-Salazar and Hurtado (1944). These studies were subsequently extended to a total of 40 subjects in Lima and 30 in Morococha (4540 m) (Hurtado 1964*b*). The mean value of P_{50} at pH 7.4 was 24.7 mmHg at sea level and 26.9 mmHg at high altitude.

Lenfant and Sullivan (1971) point out that the advantages of such a shift depend on the altitude. Below an elevation of 3500 m there is a substantial advantage, but at higher altitudes the advantage is very small. The reason for this is clearly that the partial pressure of oxygen in the alveolar spaces decreases greatly, so that oxygen loading of the blood in the lungs is impaired. Hence the beneficial effects of increased unloading of oxygen in the tissues are counterbalanced by the decreased oxygen loading in the lungs. In the newcomer to high altitude, the hyperventilation that occurs increases the partial pressure of oxygen in his alveolar spaces, enhancing the advantage gained by the progressive shift of the oxygen–haemoglobin dissociation curve to the right.

A cautionary note was sounded by Winslow *et al.* (1981) who studied oxygen dissociation curves on 46 highlanders in Morococha (4540 m) and confirmed that at pH 7.4 the P_{50} was significantly higher in highlanders than in lowlanders. The values were 31.2 as opposed to 29.2 mmHg. However, the highlanders showed a partially compensated respiratory alkalosis with a mean plasma pH of 7.44. When the P_{50} values were corrected to the subjects' actual plasma pH, the mean value of 30.1 mmHg could no longer be distinguished from that of the sea-level controls. They concluded that the small increase in P_{50} resulting from the increased concentration of 2,3-diphosphoglycerate in the red cells (see below) was offset by the mild degree of respiratory alkalosis. In other words the position of the oxygen dissociation curve was the same as that in sea-level controls. Mairbäurl (1988) also confirmed that the oxygen dissociation curve is shifted to the right at high altitude only when the measurements are made under standard acid–base conditions.

2,3-Diphosphoglycerate

Events within the haemoglobin molecule determine the shape of the oxygen–haemoglobin dissociation curve. Certain conditions stabilize the deoxy shape of the haemoglobin molecule favouring oxygen release (Finch and Lenfant 1972). These include hydrogen ions, carbon dioxide, and 2,3-diphosphoglycerate (2,3-DPG). Although this organic phosphate was described in red cells over half a century ago (Greenwald 1925), it is only since 1967 that its role in regulating the oxygen affinity of haemoglobin has been recognized (Benesch and Benesch 1967; Chanutin and Curnish 1967). It is generated by the anaerobic glycolytic pathway in erythrocytes and blood contains some 15 μmol per g of haemoglobin. An increase of 2,3-DPG within the red cell increases the P_{50} by about 0.5 mmHg per mole of 2,3-DPG (Ward *et al.* 1989). Glucose is converted in cells to glucose-6-phosphate through the action of hexokinase. In erythrocytes the enzyme diphosphoglycerate mutase catalyses much of the 1,3-diphosphoglycerate arising from glucose- 6-phosphate into 2,3-diphosphoglycerate. It is able to enter the core of the haemoglobin molecule, when it is in the deoxy form, between the β chains and binding itself to each (Finch and Lenfant 1972). This stabilization of the deoxy form favours oxygen release, so it means in effect that each red cell has its own mechanism for reacting to hypoxia. When de-oxyhaemoglobin increases, there is an increase in red cell glycolysis leading to an increase in 2,3-DPG and oxygen availability (Hamasaki *et al.* 1970). Levels of 2,3-DPG are increased in diseases associated with chronic hypoxia such as chronic lung disease (Oski *et al.* 1969) and cyanotic heart disease (Woodson *et al.* 1970). High levels have been found in various forms of anaemia. It seems likely that in these con-ditions the increased amounts of 2,3-DPG may have some role in making more oxygen available to the tissues.

2,3-DPG levels rise in people living at high alti-tudes (Lenfant *et al.* 1968; Torrance *et al.* 1970*a,b*), as in the residents in Leadville and Climax in Colorado (Eaton *et al.* 1969). About half of the change in P_{50} and 2,3-DPG occurs within 15 hours of exposure to high altitude (Lenfant *et al.* 1971). Mulhausen *et al.* (1968) demonstrated a change in the P_{50} from 26.7 to 30.6 mmHg within 1 day of ascent to 3500 m. The intraerythrocytic organic phosphates appear to affect the affinity of haemoglo-bin for oxygen by the direct binding action described above and by lowering the intracellular pH (Bohr effect, see below).

There is experimental evidence to suggest that the production of 2,3-DPG falls off with age. Thus, in the study of Martin *et al.* (1975), young rats aged 2, 12, and 24 months showed significant increases of respectively 21, 14, and 22% of erythrocyte 2,3-DPG following exposure for 4 weeks to a simulated altitude of 7010 m. However, rats aged 40 months were not capable of the same exaggerated degree of erythropoiesis and the increase in 2,3-DPG in ery-throcytes was much less.

Effect of alkalosis
Lenfant *et al.* (1971) studied the oxygen dissociation curve and oxygen transport parameters in four normal subjects and in two subjects made acidotic with acetazolamide before, during, and after a stay

of 4 days at an altitude of 4500 m. In the normal subjects on ascent the oxygen dissociation curve shifted rapidly to the right and appeared to be brought about by an increase of 2,3-DPG that was related to an increase in plasma pH above sea-level values. In the acidotic subjects there was no rise in plasma pH, no increase in 2,3-DPG, and no shift in the oxygen dissociation curve. Gerlach *et al.* (1970) found an increased erythrocytic level of 2,3-DPG in rats following exposure to 11% oxygen. However, the addition of 5% carbon dioxide to the inspired gas prevented alkalosis and the expected changes in 2,3-DPG. Such data are consistent with the view that the altitude-induced increase in 2,3-DPG is the result of alkalosis accompanying expo-sure (Klocke 1972). In other words, the primary cause of the increase in 2,3-DPG is the increase in plasma pH above that at sea level brought about as a result of respiratory alkalosis, as part of acclimatiza-tion. Respiratory alkalosis at high altitude activates red cell glycolysis and inhibits 2,3-DPG phos-phatase, the enzyme responsible for the breakdown of 2,3-DPG. This leads to an accumulation of this substance in the erythrocyte (Brewer and Eaton 1971; Duhm and Gerlach 1971).

Thus it comes about that there is a significant re-lation between the degree of altitude, the extent of respiratory alkalosis, and the level of 2,3-DPG. At moderate altitudes a slight elevation of 2,3-DPG re-sulting from respiratory alkalosis occurs within the first few hours after ascent (Mairbäurl 1988). Then alkalosis is compensated and plasma and red cell pH values become normal. At moderate altitudes the ar-terial oxygen saturation falls only by a few per cent. A change in blood pH occurs rapidly and there is a slow increase in 2,3-DPG. The increase in 2,3-DPG is more pronounced in subjects who are physically active rather than in sedentary ones. At altitudes of above 4500 m the compensation for respiratory alka-losis is almost complete after 10 days and arterial oxygen saturation falls significantly (Mairbäurl 1988). Hence alkalosis and deoxygenation of the haemoglobin contribute to the enhanced formation of 2,3-DPG.

The change in oxygen affinity under *in vivo* acid–base conditions deviates considerably from that under standard conditions. A few hours at moderate altitude leaves oxygen affinity virtually unchanged because within this period respiratory alkalosis is not yet fully compensated for and balances the effect of an increase in 2,3-DPG. A prolonged stay at a mod-erate altitude, however, results in a decrease in oxygen affinity as respiratory alkalosis is then compensated for, allowing pH-independent factors such as 2,3-DPG to rise. At 4559 m oxygen affinity is comparable to that at sea level. Here respiratory alkalosis and the decrease in arterial P_{CO_2} neutralize the effect of 2,3-DPG on oxygen binding by haemoglobin. At altitudes above that, an altitude-related increase in oxygen affinity results from an increased degree of alkalinization that overrides the 2,3-DPG increase. Winslow *et al.* (1984) calculated that *in vivo* P_{50} values should decrease far below normal at the summit of Mt Everest (8848 m) because of a plasma pH of about 7.7 and a very low arterial carbon dioxide tension.

Increased Bohr effect in Quechuas

Morpurgo *et al.* (1970) confirmed the 'shift to the right' of the oxygen–haemoglobin dissociation curve, to which we have referred above, in acclimatized Quechuas of the Peruvian Andes. They claimed that another feature of acclimatization in these native highlanders of the Andes was an increased Bohr effect, that is, a greater decrease in affinity of haemoglobin for oxygen at lower tissue pH. They determined the oxygen–haemoglobin dissociation curves at pH 7.4 and 6.7 for haemolysates from 26 native highlanders in the Andes and from eight subjects of European origin living for different periods at high altitude. In addition, the dissociation curves were determined on 18 Europeans living at sea level in Rome. The typical 'shift to the right' was noted at pH 7.4 and 6.7. However, in the latter case the mean P_{50} and P_{80} values (the partial pressure of oxygen required for 50 and 80% saturation of haemoglobin, respectively) of Europeans at high altitude were found by them to be lower than those of native Andean highlanders (Fig. 5.2; Table 5.2). In other words, Morpurgo *et al.* (1970) claimed to have demonstrated an increased Bohr effect in the Amerindians, which would in theory facilitate the supply of oxygen to the tissues. The magnitude of the Bohr effect is usually given in terms of the increase in log P_{50} per pH unit. The normal value for human blood is 0.4 at constant P_{CO_2} (Ward *et al.* 1989). This phenomenon might arise from a modification of the haemoglobin molecule, but no such abnormality could be detected. In a later publication, the same group (Battaglia *et al.* 1971) showed that the effect was not due to 2,3-DPG.

Subsequently, Winslow *et al.* (1985*b*) were unable to substantiate these findings. They measured whole blood oxygen affinity by an automatic technique that allowed recording of oxygen saturation continuously over a range of P_{O_2} of 1–150 mmHg at constant pH

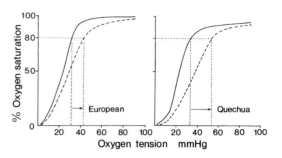

5.2 *Compared with Europeans, Quechua Indians seem to show an increased Bohr effect, so that there is a greater decrease in affinity of haemoglobin for O_2 at the lower tissue pH of 6.7 (-----) compared with a pH of 7.4 (———). Note the greater increase in the value for P_{80}, with the fall in pH in the case of the Quechuas. This would imply that in the hypoxic conditions of life at high altitude there is a higher P_{O_2} available for use by the tissues where the pH is lower. However, see text for contradictory findings. (Based on data from Morpurgo et al. (1970).)*

and P_{CO_2}, on fresh samples of blood obtained from five native highlanders from Morococha (4540 m) in the Peruvian Andes. The results were not significantly different from those obtained with controls living at sea level, so that their findings do not support the earlier concept that native highlanders from the Peruvian Andes have an increased Bohr effect.

Effects at extreme altitude

At extreme attitude (Chapter 32) a shift of the oxygen–haemoglobin dissociation curve to the right would exacerbate the dangerous degree of arterial desaturation and introduce the possibility of severe hypoxaemia and death. Such considerations reactivate the classical controversy in the early part of the century when Barcroft *et al.* (1923) suggested that an *increased* affinity of haemoglobin and a shift of the oxygen-dissociation curve to the left for oxygen might be an important factor in acclimatization.

Eaton *et al.* (1974) sought to establish whether or not artificially increased oxygen–haemoglobin affinity would protect rats when they were subsequently acutely exposed to very low environmental oxygen pressures. Fourteen Sprague–Dawley rats were given drinking water containing 0.5% sodium cyanate, which irreversibly carbamoylates haemoglobin amino groups, thereby increasing oxygen–haemoglobin affinity. Two weeks later 80% of the

Table 5.2 Comparison of partial oxygen pressures required for 50% (P_{50}) and 80% (P_{80}) saturation of haemoglobin in haemolysates diluted in 0.1 mol/l phosphate buffer, at pH 7.4 and pH 6.7, from Europeans and Quechua Indians (with standard deviations of the mean). The Bohr effect is calculated as the difference between the values obtained at pH 6.7 and 7.4. (From the data of Morpurgo *et al.* 1970)

Subjects	No. of individuals	P_{50}			P_{80}		
		pH 7.4	pH 6.7	Bohr effect	pH 7.4	pH 6.7	Bohr effect
Europeans at sea level	18	19.5 ± 1.30	26.4 ± 1.48	6.9	27.0 ± 1.91	37.9 ± 2.80	10.9
Europeans above 3500 m	8	24.8 ± 2.23	31.3 ± 3.21	6.5	35.1 ± 2.86	46.3 ± 4.14	11.2
Quechuas above 3500 m	26	25.0 ± 2.80	33.7 ± 2.94	8.7	35.5 ± 4.83	52.7 ± 5.98	17.2

reactive haemoglobin amino groups had been carbamoylated and the P_{50} of the test animals had been reduced from 37.3 to 21 mmHg. The concentration of 2,3-DPG in the erythrocytes had fallen. The control and test rats were then exposed to a simulated altitude of 9180 m. Eight of the 10 control animals died, but all the test rats, with their artificially induced 'shift to the left', survived. Such experimental evidence supports the view that *increased affinity* of haemoglobin for oxygen has survival value at *extreme* altitude. It suggests that the characteristic 'shift to the right' of the oxygen–haemoglobin dissociation curve in the highlander and in the newcomer to the mountains is of little value and potentially dangerous at extreme altitude. On the steep portion of the oxygen–haemoglobin dissociation curve, any increase in oxygen delivery to the tissues by decreased affinity of haemoglobin for the gas will be accompanied by an almost equal loss of Pa_{O_2}.

The relative merits of polycythaemia and increased or decreased affinity of haemoglobin for oxygen were also studied by Penney and Thomas (1975). They tested the survival over 90 minutes of acute decompression (228 mmHg) of three groups of rats that had been treated in various ways to bring about changes in the level of 2,3-DPG and the value of P_{50} (Fig. 5.3). The first group was exposed to a simulated altitude of 4570 m for up to 9 weeks to give rise to progressive polycythaemia and to elevate 2,3-DPG levels and raise P_{50} values. A second group was exposed to carbon monoxide for 9 weeks, bringing no change in 2,3-DPG but a fall in P_{50} (Fig. 5.3). A third group was treated for 10 days with

sodium cyanate to produce big decreases in 2,3-DPG and P_{50}. Cyanate reacts irreversibly by carbamoylating the α-amino groups of both the α and β chains of haemoglobin, increasing its affinity for oxygen. When exposed to the acute hypoxia, only 5% of the control animals survived (Fig. 5.3). Some 44% of the polycythaemic rats with a raised P_{50} survived.

More of the animals in the other two groups where P_{50} had been artificially diminished lived through the acute hypoxia. No fewer than 75% of the cyanate-treated animals with big falls in 2,3-DPG levels and P_{50} values survived (Fig. 5.3). Clearly, such experimental results indicate that survival at extreme altitude is better aided by *increased* oxygen haemoglobin affinity and a shift of the oxygen–haemoglobin dissociation curve *to the left*. Once the level of arterial oxygen tension falls below the 'shoulder' of the curve, saturation declines rapidly, thereby decreasing total oxygen transport. If the affinity of haemoglobin for oxygen increased, its oxygen saturation is moved back from the mid-portion of the sigmoid to the shoulder. Oxygen unloading becomes more difficult, but oxygen transport is increased by the higher oxygen saturation of the haemoglobin.

During the American Medical Research Expedition to Mount Everest in 1981, Winslow *et al.* (1984) studied acclimatized lowlanders at an altitude of 6300 m. They also studied two subjects at the summit (8850 m). The venous blood samples taken at 8850 m were studied the morning after the summit climb. There was an increase in 2,3-DPG and this was associated with a slightly increased P_{50} value when expressed at pH 7.4. However, the

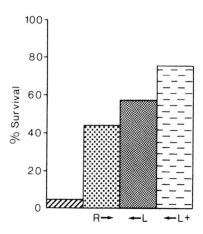

5.3 *Percentage survival in four groups of rats exposed to a simulated altitude of 8840 m for 90 min. The hatched column represents control animals; the stippled column represents rats previously acclimatized to an altitude of 4570 m for 9 weeks. After such acclimatization there is a rise in P_{50} indicating a fall in the systemic arterial saturation, but there is a rise in 2,3-DPG suggesting an increased release of oxygen to the tissues. The wavy line column represents rats exposed to carbon monoxide for 9 weeks bringing no change in 2,3-DPG but a fall in P_{50}, indicating increased oxygen saturation of the blood. The dashed column represents rats treated with sodium cyanate for 10 days to bring about big falls in P_{50} and 2,3-DPG, indicating increased arterial oxygen saturation but decreased release of oxygen to the tissues. The rise in P_{50} is indicated in the diagram by a shift to the right of the oxygen dissociation curve, whereas a fall in P_{50} is indicated by a shift of the curve to the left. (Based on data from Penney and Thomas (1975).)*

respiratory alkalosis was not fully compensated so that at the summit the subject's *in vivo* P_{50} was as low as 19.4 mmHg in one subject. Their data showed that at extreme altitude the oxygen-dissociation curve shifted progressively leftwards primarily because of the respiratory alkalosis. This effect completely overwhelmed the relatively small tendency for the curve to shift to the right because of the increased in red-cell 2,3-DPG.

Oxygen–haemoglobin dissociation curve in animals indigenous to high altitude

Monge and Whittembury (1974) contrast the 'shift to the right' of the oxygen–haemoglobin dissociation curve of man at high altitude with the 'shift to the left' of indigenous high-altitude animals (Chapter

35). Such highland animals include camelids such as the alpaca, vicuña, and llama, rodents such as the mountain-viscacha, ruminants such as the yak, and birds such as the hualiata. All of these indigenous high-altitude animals have a higher haemoglobin–oxygen affinity than their sea-level relatives, such as the camel, rabbit, and ox, and a variety of sea-level birds.

Biological significance of shifts in the oxygen–haemoglobin dissociation curve

In summary, a shift of the oxygen–haemoglobin dissociation curve to the right implies a lowered affinity of haemoglobin for oxygen with elevated levels of 2,3-DPG. This means that oxygen unloading at the tissues is facilitated, maintaining an elevated Po_2 in association with some loss of oxygen saturation of the haemoglobin. This system is characteristic of *acclimatization* (Chapter 36), allowing high survival at high altitude, but it is not advantageous under conditions of extreme hypoxia (Table 5.3). It is typical of man at high but not extreme altitude and is best developed in the native highlander.

On the other hand, a shift of the curve to the left implies increased affinity of haemoglobin for oxygen, so that oxygen transport and haemoglobin saturation are enhanced at the expense of oxygen unloading at the tissues (Table 5.3). Such a system is found in indigenous high-altitude animals and is characteristic of *genetic adaptation* in contrast to acclimatization (Fig. 5.4). It may also be induced artificially in labo-

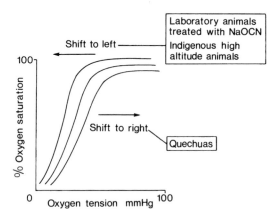

5.4 *In the acclimatized Quechua there is a shift to the right of the oxygen–haemoglobin dissociation curve. However, in adapted indigenous high-altitude animals the curve shifts to the left. A leftward shift may also be induced experimentally by treatment with sodium cyanate.*

Table 5.3 Biological significance of shifts of the oxygen–haemoglobin dissociation curve at high altitude

Shift of dissociation curve	To the right	To the left
P_{50}	Raised	Lowered
2,3-DPG	Raised	Lowered or weak interaction between haemoglobin and intraerythrocytic phosphates
Affinity of Hb for O_2	Lowered	Raised
Survival at high altitude (3000–5800 m)	High	Raised
Survival at extreme altitude (>5800 m)	High compared with sea-level subjects	Higher still
Groups showing features	Quechua Indians of the Peruvian Andes and to less extent newcomers to high altitude	Indigenous high-altitude animals; rats artificially treated with NaOCN
Typical biological status	Acclimatization	Genetic adaptation

ratory animals, as we have already seen (Fig. 5.4). A shift of the oxygen–haemoglobin dissociation curve to the left favours survival at extreme altitudes. Hebbel *et al.* (1978) reported a family with two members (termed 'human llamas'!) who had a haemoglobin with a very high affinity (Hb Andrew–Minneapolis, P_{50} 17.1 mmHg). The two members performed noticeably better on exercise at an altitude of 3100 m than two siblings with normal blood.

References

Accetto, B. (1982). Beneficial hemorrheologic therapy of chronic peripheral arterial disorders with pentoxifylline; results of a double-blind study versus vasodilator nylidrin. *American Heart Journal.* **103**, 864

Adams, W.H. and Shrestha, S.M. (1974). Hemoglobin levels, vitamin B$_{12}$ and folate status in a Himalayan village. *American Journal of Clinical Nutrition*, **27**, 217

Adams, W.H. and Strang, L.J. (1975). Hemoglobin levels in persons of Tibetan ancestry living at high altitude. *Proceedings of the Society for Experimental Biology and Medicine*, **149**, 1036

Albrecht, P.H. and Littell J.K. (1972). Plasma erythropoietin in men and mice during acclimatization to different altitudes. *Journal of Applied Physiology*, **32**, 54

Altland, P.D. and Parker, M.G. (1977). Bilirubinaemia and intravascular haemolysis during acclimatization to high altitude. *International Journal of Biometeorology*, **21**, 165

Appenzeller, O. and Wood, S.C. (1988). Pentoxifylline: thermoregulatory and vasomotor effects at high altitudes. *Annals of Sports Medicine*, **4**, 279

Arnaud, J., Quilici, J.C., Gutierrez, N., Beard, J., and Vergnes, H. (1979). Methaemoglobin and erythrocyte reducing systems in high-altitude natives. *Annals of Human Biology*, **6**, 585

Aste-Salazar, H. and Hurtado, A. (1944). The affinity of hemoglobin for oxygen at sea level and at high altitudes. *American Journal of Physiology*, **142**, 733

Barcroft, J. (1925). *Respiratory Function of the Blood.* Part 1, Lessons from High Altitude. London and New York; Cambridge University Press

Barcroft, J., Binger, C.A., Bock, A.V., Doggart, J.H., Forbes, H.S., Harrop, G., Meakins, J.C., and Redfield, A.C. (1923). Observations upon the effect of high altitude on the physiological processes of the human body carried out in the Peruvian Andes chiefly at Cerro de Pasco. *Philosophical Transactions of the Royal Society of London*, B**211**, 351

Battaglia, P., Morpurgo, G., and Passi, S. (1971). Variability of the Bohr effect in man. *Experientia*, **27**, 321

Beall, C.M. and Reichsman, A.B. (1984). Hemoglobin levels in a Himalayan high altitude population. *American Journal of Physical Anthropology*, **63**, 301

Benesch, R. and Benesch, R.E. (1967). The effect of organic phosphates from the human erythrocyte on the allosteric properties of haemoglobin. *Biochemical and Biophysical Research Communications*, **26**, 162

Berendsohn, S. (1962). Hepatic function at high altitude. *Archives of Internal Medicine*, **109**, 256

Berlin, N.H., Reynafarje, C., and Lawrence, J.H. (1954). Red cell life span in the polycythaemia of high altitude. *Journal of Applied Physiology*, 7, 271

Bohr, C. (1904). Theoretische Behandlung der Quantitativen Verhältnisse bei der Sauerstoffaufnahme des Hamoglobins. *Zentralblatt für Physiologie*, **17**, 682

Brecher, G. and Bessis, M. (1972). Present status of spiculed red cells and their relationship to discocyte–echinocyte transformation: a critical review. *Blood*, **40**, 333

Brewer, G.J. and Eaton J.W. (1971). Erythrocyte metabolism: interaction with oxygen transport. *Science*, **171**, 1205

Chanutin, A. and Curnish, R.R. (1967). Effect of organic and inorganic phosphates on the oxygen equilibrium of human erythrocytes. *Archives of Biochemistry and Biophysics*, **121**, 96

Chohan, I.S. and Singh, I. (1979). Cell mediated immunity at high altitude. *International Journal of Biometeorology*, **23**, 21

Dill, D.B., Edwards, H.T., Folling, A., Oberg, S.A., Pappenheimer, A.M., and Talbott, J.H. (1931). Adaptations of the organism to change in oxygen pressure. *Journal of Physiology (London)*, **71**, 47

Duhm, J. and Gerlach, E. (1971) On the mechanism of the hypoxia-induced increase of 2-3 diphosphoglycerate in erythrocytes. *Pflügers Archiv*, **326**, 254

Eaton, J.W., Brewer, G.J., and Grover, R.F. (1969). Role of red cell 2,3 diphosphoglycerate in the adaptation of man to altitude. *Journal of Laboratory and Clinical Medicine*, **73**, 603

Eaton, J.W., Skelton, T.D., and Berger, E. (1974). Survival at extreme altitude; protective effect of increased hemoglobin–oxygen affinity. *Science*, **183**, 743

Erslev, A. (1987). Erythropoietin coming of age. *New England Journal of Medicine*, **316**, 101

Faura, J., Ramos, J., Reynafarje, C., English, E., Finne, P., and Finch, C.A. (1969). Effect of altitude on erythropoiesis. *Blood*, **33**, 668

Finch, C.A. and Lenfant, C. (1972). Oxygen transport in man. *New England Journal of Medicine*, **286**, 407

Fisher, J.W. and Langston, J.W. (1967). The influence of hypoxia and cobalt on erythropoietin production in the isolated perfused dog kidney. *Blood*, **29**, 114

Forster, P.J.G. (1983). *Work at High Altitude. A Clinical and Physiological Study at the United Kingdom Infrared Telescope, Mauna Kea, Hawaii.* Edinburgh; Royal Observatory

Garruto, R.M. (1976). Hematology. In *Man in the Andes: A Multidisciplinary Study of High-Altitude Quechua* (P.T. Baker and M.A. Little, Eds). US/IBP Synthesis Series, no. 1, Stroudsburg, Pennsylvania; Dowden, Hutchinson and Ross, p. 261

Gerlach, E., Duhm, J., and Deuticke, B. (1970). Metabolism of 2,3-diphosphoglycerate in red blood cells under various experimental conditions. In *Red Cell Metabolism and Function* (G.J. Brewer, Ed.). New York; Plenum Press

Greenwald, I. (1925). A new type of phosphoric acid compound isolated from blood with some remarks on the effect of substitution and the rotation of L-glyceric acid. *Journal of Biological Chemistry*, **63**, 339

Guleria, J.S., Pande, J.N., Sethi, P.K., and Roy, A.B. (1971). Pulmonary diffusing capacity at high altitude. *Journal of Applied Physiology*, **31**, 536

Hamasaki, N., Asakura, T., and Minakami, S. (1970). Effect of oxygen tension in glycolysis in human erythrocytes. *Journal of Biochemistry*, **68**, 157

Harris, D. and Heath, D. (1986). In *The Human Pulmonary Circulation*. Edinburgh; Churchill-Livingstone, p. 123

Hebbel, R.P., Eaton, J.W., Kronenberg, R.S., Zanjani, E.D., Moore, L.G., and Berger, E.M. (1978). Human llamas: adaptation to altitude in subjects with high haemoglobin oxygen affinity. *Journal of Clinical Investigation*, **62**, 593

Huff, R.L., Lawrence, J.H., Siri, W.E., Wasserman, L.R., and Henessy, T.G. (1951). Effects of changes in altitude on haematopoietic activity. *Medicine*, **30**, 197

Hurtado, A. (1932). Studies at high altitude. Blood observations on the Indian natives of the Peruvian Andes. *American Journal of Physiology*, **100**, 487

Hurtado, A. (1964a). Some physiologic and clinical aspects of life at high altitude. In *Aging of the Lung*, 10th Hahnemann Symposium (L. Cander and J.H. Moyer, Ed.). New York; Grune and Stratton, p. 257

Hurtado, A. (1964b). Animals in high altitudes: resident man. In *Handbook of Physiology. Adaptation to the Environment* (D.B. Dill, Ed.). Washington, DC; American Physiological Society

Hurtado, A., Merino, C., and Delgado, E. (1945). Influence of anoxaemia on the hemopoietic activity. *Archives of Internal Medicine*, **75**, 284

Keys, A., Hall, F.G., and Guzman-Barron, E.S. (1936). The position of the oxygen dissociation curve of human blood at high altitude. *American Journal of Physiology*, **115**, 292

Klocke, R.A. (1972). Oxygen transport and 2,3-diphosphoglycerate (DPG). *Chest*, **62**, 795

Lenfant, C. and Sullivan, K. (1971). Adaptation to high altitude. *New England Journal of Medicine*, **284**, 1298

Lenfant, C., Torrance, J., English, E., Finch, C.A., Reynafarje, C., Ramos, J., and Faura, J. (1968). Effect of altitude on oxygen binding by hemoglobin and on organic phosphate levels. *Journal of Clinical Investigation*, **47**, 2652

Lenfant, C., Torrance, J.D., and Reynafarje, C. (1971). Shift of the O_2–Hb dissociation curve at altitude: mechanisms and effect. *Journal of Applied Physiology*, **30**, 625

Mairbäurl H. (1988). Red blood cell function at high altitudes. *Annals of Sports Medicine*, **4**, 189

Mairbäurl, H., Schobersberger, W., Humpeler, E., Hasibeder, W., Fischer, W., and Raas, E. (1986). Beneficial effects of exercising at moderate altitude on red cell oxygen transport and on exercise performance. *Pflügers Archiv*, **406**, 594

Martin, L.G., Connors, J.M., McGrath, J.J., and Freeman, J. (1975). Altitude-induced erythrocytic 2,3-DPG and haemoglobin changes in rats of various ages. *Journal of Applied Physiology*, **39**, 258

Meiselman, H.J. (1978). Rheology of shape-transformed human red cells. *Biorheology*, **15**, 225

Merino, C. (1950). Studies on blood formation and destruction in the polycythaemia of high altitudes. *Blood*, **5**, 1

Merino, C. and Reynafarje, C. (1949). Bone marrow studies in the polycythaemia of high altitude. *Journal of Laboratory and Clinical Medicine*, **34**, 637

Milledge, J.S. and Coates, P.M. (1985). Serum erythropoietin in humans at high altitude and its relation to plasma renin. *Journal of Applied Physiology*, **59**, 360

Monge-C, C. and Whittembury, J. (1974). Increased hemoglobin–oxygen affinity at extremely high altitudes. *Science*, **186**, 843

Monge-M, C. and Monge-C, C. (1966). *High Altitude Diseases: Mechanism and Management*, Springfield, Illinois; Charles C. Thomas, pp. 58 and 59

Moreno-Black, G., Quinn, V., Haas, J., Franklin, J., and Berard, J. (1984). The distribution of haemoglobin concentration in a sample of native high-altitude women. *Annals of Human Biology*, **11**, 317

Moret, P., Cobarrubias, E., Coudert, J., and Duchosal, F. (1972). Cardiocirculatory adaptation to chronic hypoxia: III. Comparative study of cardiac output, pulmonary and systemic circulation between sea level and high altitude residents. *Acta Cardiologica*, **27**, 596

Morpurgo, G., Battaglia, P., Bernini, L., Paolucci, A.M., and Modiano, G. (1970). Higher Bohr effect in Indian natives of Peruvian Highlands as compared with Europeans. *Nature (London)*, **227**, 387

Muirhead, H., Cox, J.M., Mazzarella, L., and Perutz, M.F. (1967). Structure and function of haemoglobin. III. A three-dimensional former synthesis of human deoxyhaemoglobin at 5.5Å resolution. *Journal of Molecular Biology*, **28**, 117

Mulhausen, R.O., Astrup, P., and Mellemgaard, K. (1968). Oxygen affinity and acid–base status of human blood during exposure to hypoxia and carbon monoxide. *Scandinavian Journal of Clinical Laboratory Investigation*, Suppl. 103, p. 9

Nakao, M., Nakao, T., and Yamazoe, S. (1960). Adenosine triphosphate and maintenance of shape of the human red cells. *Nature*, **187**, 945

Oski, F.A.A, Gottlieb, A.J., Delivoria-Papadopoulos, M., and Miller, W.W. (1969). Red cell 2,3 diphosphoglycerate levels in subjects with chronic hypoxaemia. *New England Journal of Medicine*, **280**, 1165

Palareti, G., Coccheri, S., Poggi, M., Tricarico, M.G., Magelli, M., and Cavazzuti, F. (1984). Changes in the rheologic properties of blood after a high altitude expedition. *Angiology*, **35**, 451

Penney, D. and Thomas, M. (1975). Hematological alterations and response to acute hypobaric stress. *Journal of Applied Physiology*, **39**, 1034

Perutz, M.F. (1970). Stereochemistry of co-operative effect in haemoglobin. *Nature (London)*, **228**, 726

Reinhart, W.H. and Bärtsch, P. (1986). Red cell morphology at high altitude. *Nature (London)*, **228**, 309

Reynafarje, C. (1964). Hematologic changes during rest and physical activity in man at high altitude. In *The Physiological Effects of High Altitude* (W.H. Weihe, Ed.). Oxford; Pergamon Press, p. 73

Reynafarje, C. (1966). Physiological patterns: hematological aspects. In *Life at High Altitudes*, Scientific Publication No. 140. Washington, DC; Pan American Health Organization, p. 32

Reynafarje, C. and Ramos, J. (1961). The influence of altitude changes on intestinal iron absorption. *Journal of Laboratory and Clinical Medicine*, **57**, 848

Reynafarje, C., Lozano, R., and Valdivieso, J. (1959). The polycythemia of high altitude. Iron metabolism and related aspects. *Blood*, **14**, 433

Reynafarje, C., Ramos, J., Faura, J., and Villavicencio, D. (1964). Humoral control of erythropoietic activity in man during and after altitude exposure. *Proceedings of the Society for Experimental Biology and Medicine*, **116**, 649

Rowles, P.M. and Williams, E.S. (1983). Abnormal red cell morphology in venous blood of men climbing at high altitude. *British Medical Journal*, **286**, 1396

Samaja, M., Veicsteinas, A., and Cerretelli, P. (1979). Oxygen affinity of blood in altitude Sherpas. *Journal of Applied Physiology*, **47**, 337

Sanchez, C., Merino, C., and Figallo, M. (1970). Simultaneous measurement of plasma volume and cell mass in polycythemia of high altitude. *Journal of Applied Physiology*, **28**, 775

Sarnquist, F.H., Schoene, R.B., Hackett, P.H., and Townes, B.D. (1986). Hemodilution of polycythemic mountaineers; effects of exercise and mental function. *Aviation, Space and Environmental Medicine*, **57**, 313

Schmid-Schönbein, H. (1982). Blood rheology in hemoconcentration. In *High Altitude Physiology and Medicine* (W. Brendel and R.A. Zink, Ed.). New York; Springer Verlag, p. 109

Sedova, G.T., Krasiukova, L.I., Kovaleva, L.G., Malykhina, L.S., and Ermil'chenko, G.V. (1984). Use of Trental as an agent for preventing thrombus formation in patients with polycythemia vera. *Gematologiia I Transfuziologiia*, **29**, 19

Siri, W.E., Van Dyke, D.C., Winchell, H.S., Pollycove, M., Parker, H.G., and Cleveland, A.S. (1966). Early erythropoietin, blood and physiological responses to severe hypoxia in man. *Journal of Applied Physiology*, **21**, 73

Surks, M.I., Chinn, K.S.K., and Matoush, L.O. (1966). Alterations in body composition in man after acute exposure to high altitude. *Journal of Applied Physiology*, **21**, 1741

Thomas, J.M., Lefrak, S.S., Irwin, R.S., Fritts, H.W., and Caldwell, P.R.B. (1974). The oxyhemoglobin dissociation curve in health and disease. *American Journal of Medicine*, **57**, 331

Torrance, J.D., Jacobs, P., Restrepo, A., Eschbach, J.W., Lenfant, C., and Finch, C.A. (1970*a*). Intraerythrocytic adaptation to anemia. *New England Journal of Medicine*, **283**, 165

Torrance, J.D., Lenfant, C., Cruz, J., and Marticorena, E. (1970*b*). Oxygen transport mechanisms in residents at high altitudes. *Respiration Physiology*, **11**, 1

Tufts, D. (1982). Hemoglobin and work capacity in Bolivian males living at high altitude. Unpublished, Cornell University, USA

Viault, F. (1891) Sur la quantité d'oxygene contenue dans la sang des animaux des hauts plateaux de l'Amérique du Sud. *Compte Rendus Hebdomadaires des Séances de l'Académie des Sciences, Paris*, **112**, 295

Ward, M.P., Milledge, J.S., and West J.B. (1989). Haematological changes and plasma volume. In *High-Altitude Medicine and Physiology*. London; Chapman and Hall Medical, p. 161

Weisse, A.B., Moschos, C.B., Martin, F.J., Levinson, G.E., Cannilla, J.E., and Regan, T.J. (1975). Hemodynamic effects of staged hematocrit reduction in patients with stable cor pulmonale and severely elevated hematocrit levels. *American Journal of Medicine*, **58**, 92

Whittembury, J. and Monge-C., C. (1972). High altitude, haematocrit and age. *Nature (London)*, **238**, 278

Wickramasinghe, S.N. and Weatherall, D.J. (1982). The pathophysiology of erythropoiesis. In *Blood and Its Disorders*, 2nd edn (R.M. Hardisty and D.J. Weatherall, Ed.). Oxford; Blackwell Scientific, p. 101

Winslow, R.M and Monge-C., C. (1987). *Hypoxia, Polycythemia and Chronic Mountain Sickness.* Baltimore and London; Johns Hopkins University Press, p. 37

Winslow, R.M, Monge-C., C., Statham, N.J., Gibson, C.G., Charache, S., Whittembury, J., Moran, O., and Berger, R.L. (1981). Variability of oxygen affinity of blood: human subjects native to high altitude. *Journal of Applied Physiology*, **51**, 1411

Winslow, R.M., Samaja, M., and West, J.B. (1984). Red cell function at extreme altitude on Mount Everest. *Journal of Applied Physiology (Respiratory Environmental and Exercise Physiology)*, **56**, 109

Winslow, R.M., Monge-C., C., Brown, E.G., Klein, H.G., Sarnquist, F., Winslow, N.J., and McKneally, S.S. (1985a). Effects of hemodilution on O_2 transport in high-altitude polycythemia. *Journal of Applied Physiology*, **59**, 1495

Winslow, R.M., Monge-C., C., Winslow, N.J., Gibson, C.G., and Whittembury, J. (1985b). Normal whole blood Bohr effect in Peruvian natives of high altitude. *Respiration Physiology*, **61**, 197

Wood, S.C. and Appenzeller, O. (1988a). Effects of pentoxifylline on blood rheological properties and exercise performance of endurance-trained athletes at high altitudes. *Annals of Sports Medicine*, **4**, 263

Wood, S.C. and Appenzeller, O. (1988b). Physiology and pharmacology of a rheologically active drug pentoxifylline. *Annals of Sports Medicine*, **4**, 260

Woodson, R.D., Torrance, J.D., Shapell, S.D., and Lenfant, C. (1970). The effect of cardiac disease on hemoglobin–oxygen binding. *Journal of Clinical Investigation*, **49**, 1349

Zander, R. and Schmid-Schönbein, H. (1973). Intracellular mechanisms of oxygen transport in flowing blood. *Respiration Physiology*, **19**, 279

6

Tissue diffusion

The components of acclimatization considered in the preceding chapters maintain oxygen tension in the blood capillaries as high as possible to preserve the most advantageous driving power for the gas through the tissues to the mitochondria of the cells, where it is ultimately required. At sea level this diffusing pressure from the venous end of the capillary to the mitochondria is in the region of 30 mmHg (Luft 1972). At high altitude it seems likely that oxygen tension in capillaries must be considerably lower and a fall of 10–15 mmHg at the venous end of the capillary would be expected to have serious effects in providing adequate oxygen for the mitochondria. In fact, the critical Po_2 for the functioning of mitochondria is extremely low and of the order of 1–3 mmHg (Chance *et al.*1964; Lübbers and Kessler 1968; Luft 1972). Tenney and Ou (1969) give an even lower figure of 0.5 mmHg. Nevertheless, further factors appear to operate at the level of tissue diffusion to complete the process of acclimatization. Increased capillary density seems to diminish the distance over which oxygen has to diffuse in the tissues. An increased amount of myoglobin in the cells constitutes a reservoir of oxygen in them and aids its translation to the mitochondria.

CAPILLARY DENSITY

One possible microanatomical adjustment to the hypoxaemia resulting from life at high altitude would be a reduction of the distance over which oxygen has to diffuse from blood capillaries to reach the cells. The distance between open capillaries in resting muscle is of the order of 50 μm and is much greater than the distance of 0.5 μm over which oxygen has to diffuse to cross the alveolar-capillary membrane of the lung (Chapter 4). Early studies of capillary density suggested that in acclimatized animals there is an increased number of capillaries per unit of tissue in the cerebral cortex (Diemer and Henn 1965), skeletal muscle (Valdivia 1958) and myocardium (Cassin *et al.* 1966). Detailed histological morphometric studies on the sternothyroid muscle were carried out by Banchero (1975) on three

adult mongrel dogs native to Denver (1600 m) before and after exposure for 3 weeks to a simulated altitude of 4880 m. Subsequently, these studies were extended to include five mongrel dogs native to the Andes (4350 m) (Eby and Banchero 1976). The sternothyroid was chosen in order to minimize the possible effects of exercise on the skeletal muscle. The mean capillary density in cross-sections of the muscle (Fig. 6.1(a)) and the relative surface area of

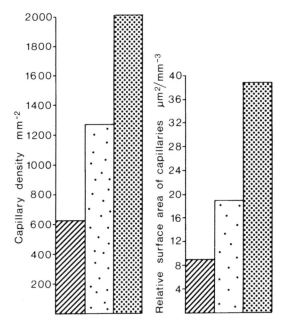

6.1 *Results of histological morphometric studies on blood capillaries in striated muscle by Banchero (1975) and Eby and Banchero (1976) on the sternothyroid muscle of three adult dogs native to Denver (1600 m) (hatched column), the same three dogs after residence for 3 weeks at a simulated altitude of 4880 m (lightly stippled column), and of five dogs native to the Andes (4350 m) (stippled column). (a) Capillary density in sternothyroid muscle; (b) relative surface area of capillaries. (For explanation see text.)*

capillaries per unit volume of tissue (Fig.6.1 (b)) both rose after 3 weeks at 4880 m, but did not reach the levels found in native highland dogs.

However, some recent reports suggest that ambient hypoxia *per se* is not a sufficient stimulus for the development of new capillaries (Turek *et al.* 1972; Appell 1978; Banchero 1982). Snyder *et al.*(1985) believe that the negative results in these studies might be explained by the fact that they were carried out on systemic skeletal muscle in caged animals subjected to forced lack of activity. To test this hypothesis they compared the effects of ambient hypoxia in laboratory rats on gastrocnemius, a systemic muscle that may be relatively non-functional in caged animals, versus diaphragm, a muscle that is thought to experience approximately the same work load during normoxia and hypoxia. In fact, their study showed no differences in capillary density. Newly hatched goslings subjected to hypoxia as embryos have a higher ratio of blood capillaries to muscle fibres (Snyder *et al.* 1984) and this suggests that increased capillary density may be restricted to the very early stages of maturation and that hypoxia *per se* is not an adequate stimulus on its own. High capillary density counts may indicate capillary recruitment during exercise rather than the development of new capillaries.

MUSCLE FIBRE SIZE

A further microanatomical component of acclimatization in muscle is a decrease in size of muscle fibres which, in association with the increased capillary density, diminishes the distance over which oxygen has to diffuse to reach mitochondria. In the studies of dogs by Banchero (1975) and Eby and Banchero (1976) referred to above the average diameter of the muscle fibres fell (Fig. 6.2(a)) and the relative surface area of muscle fibres increased (Fig. 6.2(b)). This occurred after the animals from 1600 m had been at 4880 m for 3 weeks but even then the levels did not reach those seen in dogs native to high altitude (Fig. 6.2(b)).

The same pattern has been described in acclimatized man. Cerretelli *et al.* (1984) took muscle biopsy specimens on climbers immediately after they had spent several weeks attempting to climb Lhotse Shar (8400 m). They found that, although the capillary density was somewhat raised, it could be wholly accounted for by a reduction of muscle fibre size. Boutellier *et al.* (1983) are of the same opinion. (Ward *et al.* 1989) reported that a similar result was found in Operation Everest II in which eight volunteers were gradually decompressed to the simulated

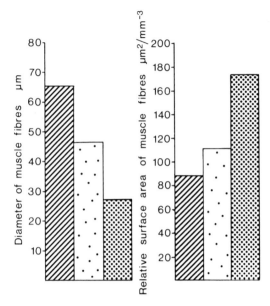

6.2 *Results of histological morphometric studies on muscle fibres in the investigation described in Fig. 6.1. (a) Diameter of muscle fibres in sternothyroid; (b) relative surface area of muscle fibres. (For explanation see text.)*

altitude of Mt Everest over a period of 40 days. Capillary density increased by a mean of 18% in the vicinity of type I fibres and by 9% for type II fibres. The corresponding muscle fibre area was reduced by 21% for type I and 7% for type II. Thus, again the changes in capillary density reflected atrophy of muscle and not an increased number of capillaries *per se*.

Muscle fibre size and capillary density in Sherpas

The ultrastructure of the vastus lateralis muscle of five male Sherpas from Nepal was studied and compared with that of sedentary lowlanders and of Caucasian climbers before and after exposure to high altitude by Kayser *et al.* (1991). The mean cross-sectional area of the muscle fibres was found to be similar to that of Caucasian elite high-altitude climbers and a group of climbers after 6 to 8 weeks' stay at 5000–8000 m but was slightly, but not significantly, smaller than that of sedentary lowlanders (Table 6.1). The number of capillaries per mm² of muscle cross-section was similar to that found in the high-altitude climbers but was significantly greater than that of sedentary lowlanders (Table 6.1). Hence the trend towards increased capillary

Table 6.1 Muscle (vastus lateralis) fibre size and capillary density in different groups in the Himalaya. (Investigations carried out in the same laboratory with identical techniques)

Group	Average muscle fibre cross-sectional area (μm^2)	Capillary density (no./mm^2)	Reference
Sherpas	3186 ± 521	467 ± 22	Kayser *et al.* (1991)
Elite climbers	3108 ± 303 (NS)	542 ± 127 (NS)	Oelz *et al.* (1986)
Climbers after Himalayan expedition	3360 ± 580 (NS)	538 ± 89 (NS)	Hoppeler *et al.* (1990)
Sedentary subjects of comparable age	3640 ± 260 (NS)	387 ± 25†	Hoppeler *et al.* (1973)

NS, Not statistically significant difference from Sherpas.
† p <0.05.

density and smaller muscle fibres in muscles found experimentally in animals compared to subjects from low altitude has been confirmed in man.

It was also found by Kayser *et al.* (1991) that in Sherpas at high altitude the volume density of mitochondria was 3.96 ± 0.54% which was significantly ($p < 0.05$) less than the values found for any other group investigated, including sedentary subjects at sea level (4.74 ± 0.30%). Studies of maximal oxygen consumption in the Sherpas showed that its ratio to mitochondrial volume was higher than in lowlanders despite the reduced mitochondrial volume density. This may be related to increased oxygen conductance in the tissues associated with a shorter diffusion path due to increased capillary density and reduced muscle fibre size. Other factors may be increased myoglobin concentration and an increased activity of mitochondrial enzymes controlling oxidative phosphorylation such as we describe later in this chapter. All these features are found in elite and acclimatized Caucasian climbers as well as in Sherpas and thus cannot be held to be the ultrastructural basis for the endurance capacity at high altitude for which the Sherpa is renowned.

The decrease in the size of muscle fibres at high altitude has been associated by some with the lack of physical activity that often characterizes lowlanders struggling to achieve acclimatization to the hypobaric hypoxia, but this could hardly be said to apply to Sherpas or high-altitude climbers. As we shall see in Chapter 21, sustained sojourn at altitudes exceeding 5500 m is associated with progressive loss of body weight due to catabolism of muscle protein. On acute exposure to hypobaric hypoxia high

capillary counts could indicate capillary recruitment in the general congestion that takes place, rather than the development of new capillaries (Fig. 6.3).

THE KROGH MODEL

Findings on capillary density and muscle fibre size have often been considered in relation to a traditional but rather artificial model for oxygen diffusion in tissues, the so-called Krogh model. An orderly tissue like skeletal muscle, with parallel capillaries, was taken as its basis. It was conceived that each capillary would serve a column of tissue, somewhat hexagonal in cross-section. The distribution of oxygen to the tissues was assessed by dividing the

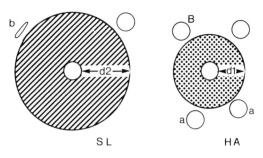

6.3 *Contributory factors in acclimatization in tissue diffusion. Compared to sea level (SL), at high altitude (HA) there is an increased number of new blood capillaries (a) and opening (B) of hitherto closed capillaries (b). The diameter of striated muscle fibres at high altitude (d1) is smaller than at sea level (d2).*

cylinder into a sequence of discs, each of which was radially symmetrical and could be considered independently (Denison 1986). The concept was one of a gradual, almost even, loss of oxygen along the capillary, with the final disc being the least well served, and its outer rim, the so-called 'lethal corner', being the most vulnerable of all. This Krogh model of diffusion of oxygen in the tissues has been widely used in assessing the significance of the reported combination of increased capillary density and diminution in muscle fibre size at high altitude.

The way in which the Krogh model has been used to calculate the effectiveness of a combination of increased capillary density and decreased muscle diameter is illustrated by the studies of Eby and Banchero (1976) and Banchero *et al.* (1976). They estimated that, at an atmospheric pressure of 635 mmHg, the oxygen tension at the remotest extremity of the tissue cylinder at the venous end of a capillary (the 'lethal corner' referred to above) was 25 mmHg. They postulate that at an increased altitude of 4350 m, with a barometric pressure of 435 mmHg, the corresponding oxygen tension would be only 16 mmHg in the absence of tissue factors of acclimatization. In fact they estimate the oxygen tension in the 'lethal corner' to be 31 mmHg and attribute this to the effectiveness of the modifications in capillary density and muscle fibre size.

Such assumptions and assessments have attracted considerable reserve for in most tissues capillaries are not orderly but arranged in a complex and seemingly haphazard way, about which it is very difficult to think analytically. Denison (1986) notes that the traditional Krogh model ignores the ease with which oxygen can flow through the large flat surfaces of the model, from one disc to the next, down the blood column of tissue, parallel to the capillary. Recent studies by computer suggest that most oxygen leaves blood in the first 10–20% of capillary length, with little change thereafter. A small cone of tissue at the arteriolar end of the capillary will have a high oxygen tension. The remainder of the tissue column will have an oxygen tension that falls away slowly radially, but varies little down the long axis parallel to the capillary. Tissue near the capillary will share something very close to end-capillary oxygen tension. Denison (1986) concludes that the prime determinant of oxygen tension in the tissues is local venous oxygen tension; the shorter the intercapillary distance the less its radial fall.

It is clear from these considerations that there are three ways in which mechanisms of acclimatization can operate in the tissue to elevate oxygen tension. The blood flow may increase to elevate local venous oxygen tension. The capillary density may increase to diminish the distance over which oxygen has to diffuse to reach the cells. Finally, the transfer of oxygen to reach the mitochondria may be eased by increasing the amounts of myoglobin in the cells.

MYOGLOBIN

In spite of the fact that an increased number of capillaries is able to bring the supply of oxygen closer to the cells, in the final analysis the gas must pass from those vessels to the mitochondria by the slow process of diffusion. Its rate appears to be enhanced by increased amounts of tissue myoglobin. This is a protein found within cells, which has a molecular weight of about 17 500 and consists of a single chain of 152 amino acid residues and one iron-containing haem group. It has relevance to high-altitude studies because it has the property of combining loosely and reversibly with oxygen. Hence, from the time of the early studies of Millikan (1939), the general view has been that myoglobin takes up oxygen rapidly at low oxygen tissue tensions and acts as a reserve store of oxygen which is available during periods of cellular activity. The dissociation curve for myoglobin is a rectangular hyperbola, in contrast to the classical sigmoid shape of the curve for haemoglobin. Thus at a Po_2 of 40 mmHg, haemoglobin is 75% saturated, whereas myoglobin is 95% saturated. At a Po_2 of 10 mmHg, haemoglobin is only 10% saturated, whereas myoglobin is 70% saturated (Ward 1975). In this way the protein retains oxygen in loose combination at an oxygen tension at which haemoglobin readily gives it up. This allows oxygen to be carried in relatively large quantities at a low oxygen tension across the cytoplasm to the surface of the mitochondria where it is released.

The chemical basis for the combination of myoglobin with oxygen probably lies in the fact that one of the coordination sites of the iron atom situated on one aspect of the tetrapyrrole structure is occupied by a water molecule and it is this that is presumably displaced by oxygen when myoglobin is converted to its oxygenated form (Mahler and Cordes 1966). A survey of aqueous extracts of 8000 samples of human skeletal muscle by Boulton and Huntsman (1972) revealed five variants of myoglobin. These resulted from single amino acid substitution. Boulton (1973) examined human psoas muscle and found a myoglobin content of about 4.5 mg/g of muscle. If one assumes this to be a representative skeletal muscle, 0.4–0.5 g (that is, 10–12%) of the total body iron of a 70-kg man is present as myoglobin.

Striated muscle fibres exist in two main forms, white and red. In man, all skeletal muscles are a mixture of white and red fibres. White fibres contain little myoglobin and few mitochondria and their supply of cellular energy comes predominantly from glycolysis. Functionally they are adapted to rapid, brief activities. In contrast, red fibres contain a high concentration of myoglobin and many mitochondria. Their supply of energy comes mainly from oxidative phosphorylation, and free fatty acid is utilized in preference to glucose. Muscles that are functionally required to maintain tension for postural purposes or a rhythmic contraction, as in the heart, tend to be red. High concentrations of myoglobin are found in the mammalian myocardium.

In many animal species whole individual muscles may be recognizably pale or dark. In chicken, the leg muscles, which walk and engage in the periodic heavy work of scratching for food, are red and contain much myoglobin, but the pectoral muscles, which are used very intermittently for feeble attempts at flying, are white (Wittenberg 1966). On the other hand, the well-developed pectoral muscles of flying birds, which are constantly used, are red. Although the sustained slow swimming muscles of fish are red, the mass of body musculature used for sudden spurts of activity is white (Wittenberg 1966). The amount of myoglobin in muscle depends on how hard it works. Thus the myoglobin content of rats, pigs, and racehorses is increased by habitual exercise (Lawrie 1950, 1953a). Myoglobin increases in muscle with age, and this has been ascribed to the need to aid diffusion as the tissue elements increase in bulk (Lawrie 1950, 1953a). The myoglobin content of cells is closely related to their capacity for oxygen uptake, as indicated by the activities of the cytochrome oxidase and succinate dehydrogenase system (Lawrie 1953b,c). A cautionary note is sounded by Harris (1971) as to the function of myoglobin as a reserve store of oxygen in the tissues. He points out that, while myoglobin combines reversibly with oxygen, it gives it up slowly.

Increased amounts of myoglobin are present in the tissues of man and animals at high altitude. An enhanced content of this protein in skeletal muscle at high altitude has been reported in dogs (Hurtado et al. 1937), guinea-pigs (Tappan and Reynafarje 1957), and rats (Anthony et al. 1959). An increase

in myoglobin as part of acclimatization to hypobaric hypoxia has also been reported in hamster heart muscle by Clark et al. (1952) and in rat heart and diaphragm. Reynafarje (1962) found that in the sartorius muscle the mean level of myoglobin (in mg/g fresh tissue) was 6.07 in nine healthy young men of average age 28.8 years at sea level, but was 7.03 in nine healthy young highlanders of average age 24.3 years at 4330 m. An absolute increase in the quantity of myoglobin in heart muscle has been found in rats exposed continuously to a simulated altitude of 5490 m (Anthony et al. 1959) and in rats subjected intermittently to a simulated altitude of 7620 m.

An alternative function for this increased amount of myoglobin at high altitude rather than as a reserve store of oxygen is that it facilitates diffusion of the gas (Biörck 1949). This is a physiochemical phenomenon discovered independently by Wittenberg (1959) and Scholander (1960). Haemoglobin molecules must move to facilitate the diffusion of oxygen; those of earthworms have a molecular weight of 3 000 000 and do not fulfil this function. Proteins of lower molecular weight, such as myoglobin, are capable of facilitating diffusion of the gas. Since haemoglobin molecules are closely packed in an orderly lattice (Wittenberg 1966), translational movements of the molecules are very limited. It is more likely that facilitation of diffusion of oxygen is mediated by rotation of molecules, particularly if they are in an environment of concentrated proteins. Wittenberg (1966) is of the opinion that oxygen molecules diffuse from the capillaries to the mitochondria by random movement interspersed with larger advances of translational and rotational movements of myoglobin molecules. There is evidence that the myoglobin-facilitated oxygen flux is about six times as great as the ordinary diffusive flux and accounts for most of the oxygen reaching the mitochondria. When a high-altitude animal such as the alpaca is brought down to sea level, it shows a progressive diminution in the content of myoglobin in its skeletal muscles (Reynafarje et al. 1975; see Fig. 6.4).

MITOCHONDRIA

Mitochondria are the organelles where oxygen transported from the atmosphere is finally combined in a biologically controlled manner with hydrogen ions derived from the respiratory chain, whereby phosphate combines with adenosine diphosphate (ADP) to form the energy-rich ATP and thus provide cellular energy. Oxidative phosphorylation can proceed

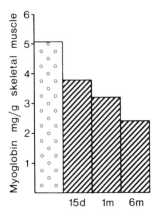

6.4 *Myoglobin content of skeletal muscle in six alpacas at 4540 m (open circles column) and 15 days, 1 month, and 6 months after removal to sea level (hatched columns). (From data of Reynafarje et al. (1975).)*

in cardiac mitochondria with a Po_2 at the remarkably low level of 0.5 mmHg (Tenney and Ou 1969). Theoretically it might be conceived that an increase in the number of mitochondria would increase the probability of an oxygen molecule finding an enzyme site in a short time and would thus have an apparent effect of increasing intracellular diffusion capacity (Ou and Tenney 1970). On the other hand, the small intracellular dimensions involved, and the diffusion speed of oxygen in tissues, must imply that the time delay for the diffusion process is so short that no major advantage would be likely to be gained by an increase in the number of mitochondria. Ou and Tenney (1970) felt that, while such objections were valid with the subject at rest, such an increase in mitochondria could assume significance at exercise with increased metabolism. They have described an increase in the numbers of mitochondria in the myocardium of eight cattle born and raised at 4250 m, compared with sea-level cattle. The sites of ventricular sampling were not specified. The method employed was one of differential centrifugation and counting of mitochondria from hearts stored in dry ice for 5 days. They found a 40% increase in the number of mitochondria in the animals at high altitude, although the size of the organelles remained the same. In this study, the technique in essence comprised the counting of granules in tissue homogeneates and the authors themselves were well aware of the possibility that not all the granulates counted were mitochondria, but could have been other types of organelle such as the lysosome.

Kearney (1973), working in our laboratory, was unable to confirm this increase in mitochondria by stereological analysis of random electron micrographs of the myocardium of rabbits and guinea-pigs from Cerro de Pasco (4330 m) and from sea level. He found no quantitative differences in the myocardial mitochondria using the methods introduced by Weibel and colleagues (Weibel 1969; Weibel et al. 1966, 1969). Mitochondrial volume, expressed as a percentage of cytoplasmic volume, was the same in rabbits and guinea-pigs from sea level and high altitude (Fig. 6.5). The numbers of mitochondria per millilitre of cytoplasm were the same in the same species at low and high altitude (Fig. 6.6). There was no significant difference between the control and high-altitude animals so far as the surface areas of outer and inner mitochondrial membranes, expressed per millimetre of cytoplasm, were concerned (Figs 6.7 and 6.8). A study of muscle biopsy specimens of seven climbers returning from the Swiss 1986 Everest Expedition revealed a decrease of mitochondrial volume of 26%, associated with a decrease of 10% in muscle mass, and a fall of 15% in muscle fibre diameter (Ward et al. 1989).

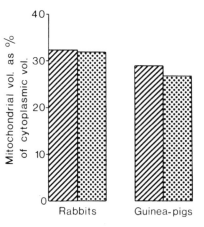

6.5 *Mitochondrial volume expressed as a percentage of cytoplasmic volume in three rabbits and three guinea-pigs born and bred at sea level (hatched columns) and the same numbers of the two species born and bred at Cerro de Pasco (4330 m) (stippled columns). There is no significant difference between the mitochondrial volume in high- and low-altitude representatives of these species). (Figs 6.5–6.8 are based on data from Kearney (1973).)*

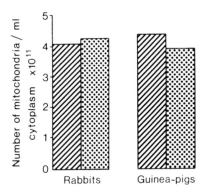

6.6 *Numbers of mitochondria per millilitre of cytoplasm in the animals listed in Fig. 6.5. Identification of groups as in that figure. There is no significant difference between the numbers of mitochondria in high- and low-altitude representatives of these species.*

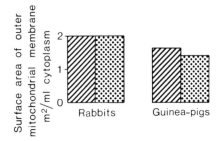

6.7 *Surface area of the outer mitochondrial membrane in m²/ml cytoplasm in the animals listed in Fig. 6.5. Identification of groups as in that figure. There is no significant difference between the surface area of the outer mitochondrial membrane in high- and low-altitude representatives of these species.*

Oxidative phosphorylation in the mitochondria

Finally, by the processes of acclimatization and adaptation described in the preceding chapters and in Chapter 35, oxygen reaches the mitochondria at an adequate partial pressure. Here it is reduced to water in a biologically controlled fashion by hydrogen ions and electrons accepted from the respiratory chain (Fig. 6.9). Phosphate is utilized to combine with adenosine diphosphate (ADP) to give rise to the energy-rich triphosphate, ATP. Thus by this process of oxidative phosphorylation in the mitochondria, the ultimate function of the provision of cellular energy is achieved.

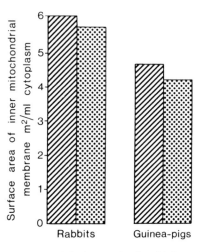

6.8 *Surface area of the inner mitochondrial membrane in m2/ml cytoplasm in the animals listed in Fig. 6.5. Identification of groups as in that figure. There is no significant difference between the surface area of the inner mitochondrial membrane in high- and low-altitude representatives of these species.*

The mitochondrial respiratory chain is itself driven by hydrogen ions and electrons from the Krebs cycle (Figs 6.9 and 6.10). This cycle of tricarboxylic acids also liberates to the blood carbon dioxide, the transport of which we considered in Chapter 4.

Acetyl coenzyme A which enters this cycle (Fig. 6.11) is produced either from glucose through the process of glycolysis or from fatty acids through the process of lipolysis with the formation of the intermediary fatty acyl coenzyme A (Fig. 6.11). In the process of glycolysis with the formation of pyruvate there is liberation into the bloodstream of lactate (Chapters 19 and 32). Each molecule of glucose passes through the glycolytic pathway (Fig. 6.11), then the Krebs cycle (Fig. 6.10) and finally the respiratory chain (Fig. 6.9) to liberate 38 mol of ATP. This is the ultimate biochemical significance of the delivery of oxygen at adequate partial pressure by the processes of acclimatization: to allow the formation of energy-rich chemical bonds that are available for the vital functions of the cell and for conversion into physical energy in such phenomena as muscle contraction.

INTRACELLULAR ENZYMES

There are differences in the activity in intracellular enzymes in the three stages of energy metabolism

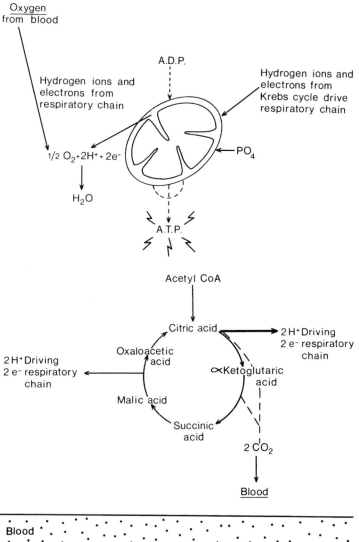

Oxygen
from blood

A.D.P.

Hydrogen ions and
electrons from
respiratory chain

Hydrogen ions and
electrons from
Krebs cycle drive
respiratory chain

$1/2\ O_2 + 2H^+ + 2e^-$

PO$_4$

H$_2$O

A.T.P.

6.9 *Final destination of oxygen delivered by the process of acclimatization. Oxygen from the blood diffuses through the tissues to the vicinity of mitochondria, where it combines with hydrogen from the respiratory chain to form water. Hydrogen and electrons from the Krebs cycle drive the respiratory chain, and phosphate combines with ADP to form the energy-rich ATP.*

Acetyl CoA

Citric acid

2 H$^+$ Driving
2 e$^-$ respiratory
chain

Oxaloacetic
acid

∝Ketoglutaric
acid

2 H$^+$ Driving
2 e$^-$ respiratory
chain

Malic acid

Succinic
acid

2 CO$_2$

Blood

6.10 *Source of hydrogen driving the respiratory chain and of the carbon dioxide diffusing into the blood in the tricarboxylic acid cycle.*

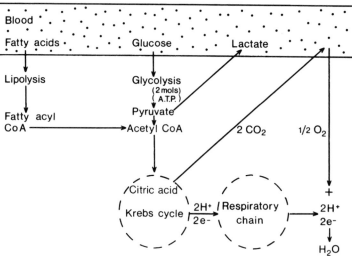

Blood

Fatty acids

Glucose

Lactate

Lipolysis

Glycolysis
(2 mols)
(A.T.P.)

Fatty acyl
CoA

Pyruvate

Acetyl CoA

2 CO$_2$

$1/2\ O_2$

Citric acid

Krebs cycle

2H$^+$
2e$^-$

Respiratory
chain

+
2H$^+$
2e$^-$

H$_2$O

6.11 *Formation of fatty acyl coenzyme A (CoA) from fatty acids and of acetyl coenzyme A from glucose. Acetyl coenzyme A enters the Krebs cycle which donates hydrogen to drive the respiratory chain.*

illustrated in Figs 6.9 to 6.11. Glucose, amino acids, and fatty acids may be converted to acetyl coenzyme A which feeds into the Krebs cycle (Figs 6.10 and 6.11). Oxygen is not needed for the glycolytic breakdown of glucose or glycogen and so glycolysis represents an important but temporary source of energy under conditions of oxygen shortage or absence. Hence the hypobaric hypoxia of high altitude does not affect the enzymes in the glycolytic pathway. We studied the enzyme activity of myocardial homogenates from guinea-pigs, rabbits, and dogs indigenous to high altitude (4330 m) in the Andes and compared it with that of similar homogenates of the same species at sea level in London (Harris *et al.* 1970). There proved to be no significant difference in the level of lactate dehydrogenase in the groups from low and high altitudes confirming the lack of effect of hypoxia on this intracellular enzyme.

In contrast, the Krebs cycle is unable to produce energy in the absence of oxygen. Hence the hypobaric hypoxia of high altitude increases the activity of some enzymes involved in the citric acid cycle. One such enzyme is succinate dehydrogenase. In the study of myocardial homogenates just referred to (Harris *et al.* 1970) we found an increased activity of this enzyme. Ou and Tenney (1970) also found increased levels of succinate dehydrogenase. We thought a weakness of our study might lie in our comparison of inbred laboratory animals at sea level with outbred domestic animals at high altitude. When outbred guinea-pigs and rabbits at the two altitudes were subsequently studied, no difference was found in the activity of succinate dehydrogenase or in other enzymes (Barrie and Harris 1976). However, the increased activity of succinate dehydrogenase might reflect changes in emphasis of the importance of different metabolic pathways on long-standing exposure to the hypobaric hypoxia of high altitude. Careful reading of studies on intracellular enzymes at high altitude illustrates the complexity of the factors involved, such as differences between strains of species and between cardiac ventricles, and the effects of diet.

With regard to the enzymes of the respiratory, electron transport chain, Reynafarje (1962) studied the enzymatic activity of human muscle at high altitude. Biopsy specimens were taken from the Quechua Indians of Cerro de Pasco (4330 m) and compared with those from Lima at sea level. He found that enzymes of the electron transport chain, (NADH, NADPH-cytochrome C-reductase, and NAD(P)+), were significantly increased in the native highlanders. Ou and Tenney (1970) also found in-

creased levels of several enzymes of the electron transport chain including cytochrome oxidase, NADH-oxidase, and NADH-cytochrome C-reductase in high-altitude cattle.

Exposure to extreme altitudes exceeding 6000 m may cause a reduction in the activity of certain enzymes. This has been demonstrated in the study of muscle-biopsy specimens from climbers taken before and after the Swiss expedition to Lhotse Shar in 1981 (Cerretelli 1987). Results from this expedition indicate that extreme altitude reduces the activity of both Krebs cycle (succinate dehydrogenase) and glycolytic (phosphofructokinase, lactate dehydrogenase) enzymes (Cerretelli 1987).

References

Anthony, A., Ackerman, E., and Strother, G.K. (1959). Effects of altitude acclimatization on rat myoglobin; changes in myoglobin content of skeletal and cardiac muscle. *American Journal of Physiology*, **196**, 512

Appell, H.J. (1978). Capillary density and patterns in skeletal muscle. III. Changes of the capillary pattern after hypoxia. *Pflügers Archiv*, **377**, R-53

Banchero, N. (1975). Capillary density of skeletal muscle in dogs exposed to simulated altitude. *Proceedings of the Society for Experimental Biology and Medicine*, **148**, 435

Banchero, N. (1982). Long term adaptation of skeletal muscle capillarity. *Physiologist*, **25**, 385

Banchero, N., Gimenez, M., Rostami, A., and Eby, S.H. (1976). Effects of simulated altitude on O_2 transport in dogs. *Respiration Physiology*, **27**, 305

Barrie, S.E. and Harris, P. (1976). Effects of chronic hypoxia and dietary restriction on myocardial enzyme activities. *American Journal of Physiology*, **231**, 1308

Biörck, G. (1949). On myoglobin and its occurrence in man. *Acta Medica Scandinavica Supplementa*, **226**, 133

Boulton, F.E. (1973). The myoglobin content of human skeletal muscle. *British Journal of Haematology*, **25**, 271

Boulton, F.E. and Huntsman, R.G. (1972). Variants of human myoglobin: their oxygen dissociation curves. *British Journal of Haematology*, **22**, 633

Boutellier, U., Howald, H., di Prampero, P.E., Giezendanner, D., and Cerretelli, P. (1983). Human muscle adaptations to chronic hypoxia.

Progress in Clinical and Biological Research, **136**, 273

Cassin, S., Gilbert, R.D., and Johnson, E.M. (1966). Capillary development during exposure to chronic hypoxia, *Technical Report 66*. San Antonio, Texas; Brooks Air Force Base, p. 16

Cerretelli, P. (1987). Extreme hypoxia in air breathers. In *Comparative Physiology of Environmental Adaptations* (P. Dejours Ed.). Basel; Karger

Cerretelli, P., Marconi, C., Deriaz, O., and Giezendanner, D. (1984). After effects of chronic hypoxia on cardiac output and muscle blood flow at rest and exercise. *European Journal of Applied Physiology*, **53**, 92

Chance, B., Schoener, B., and Schindler, F. (1964). The intercellular oxidation reduction state. In *Oxygen in the Animal Organism*. New York; Macmillan, p. 367

Clark, R.T., Criscuolo, D., and Coulson, D.K. (1952). Effects of 20 000 feet simulated altitude on myoglobin content of animals with and without exercise. *Federation Proceedings*, **11**, 25

Denison, D. (1986). Where and how hypoxia works. In *Aspects of Hypoxia* (D. Heath, Ed.). Liverpool; Liverpool University Press p. 239

Diemer, K. and Henn, R. (1965). Kapillarvermehrung in der Himvinde der Ratte unter chronischem Sauerstoffmangel. *Die Naturwissenschaften*, **52**, 135

Eby, S.H. and Banchero, N. (1976). Capillary density of skeletal muscle in Andean dogs. *Proceedings of the Society for Experimental Biology and Medicine*, **151**, 795

Harris, P. (1971). In *High Altitude Physiology, Cardiac and Respiratory Aspects*, Ciba Foundation Symposium (R. Porter and J. Knight, Ed.). Edinburgh; Churchill Livingstone, p. 8

Harris, P., Castillo, Y., Gibson, K., Heath, D., and Arias-Stella, J. (1970). Succinic and lactic dehydrogenase activity in myocardial homogenates from animals at high and low altitudes. *Journal of Molecular and Cellular Cardiology*, **1**, 189

Hoppeler, H., Lüthi, P., Claassen, H., Weibel, E.R., and Howald, H. (1973). The ultrastructure of the normal human skeletal muscle. *Pflügers Archiv*, **344**, 217

Hoppeler, H., Kleinert, E., Schlegel, C., Claassen, H., Howald, H., Kayar, S.R., and Cerretelli, P.

(1990). Morphological adaptations of human skeletal muscle to chronic hypoxia. *International Journal of Sports Medicine*, **11** (Suppl. 1), S3

Hurtado, A., Rosta, A., Merino, C., and Pons, J. (1937). Studies of myohemoglobin at high altitude. *American Journal of the Medical Sciences*, **194**, 708

Kayser, B., Hoppeler, H., Claassen, H., and Cerretelli, P. (1991). Muscle structure and performance capacity of Himalayan Sherpas. *Journal of Applied Physiology*, **70**, 1938

Kearney, M.S. (1973). Ultrastructural changes in the heart at high altitude. *Pathologia et Microbiologia*, **39**, 258

Lawrie, R.A. (1950). Some observations on factors affecting myoglobin concentrations in muscle. *Journal of Agricultural Science*, **40**, 356

Lawrie, R.A. (1953a). Effect of enforced exercise on myoglobin concentration in muscle. *Nature (London)*, **171**, 1069

Lawrie, R.A. (1953b). The activity of the cytochrome system in muscle and its relation to myoglobin. *Biochemical Journal*, **55**, 298

Lawrie, R.A. (1953c). The relation of energy-rich phosphate in muscle in myoglobin and to cytochrome-oxidase activity. *Biochemical Journal*, **55**, 305

Lübbers, D.W. and Kessler, M. (1968). Oxygen supply and rate of tissue respiration. In *Oxygen Transport in Blood and Tissues* (D.W. Libben, Ed.). Stuttgart; Thieme, p. 90

Luft, U.C. (1972). Principles of adaptations to altitude. In *Physiological Adaptations, Desert and Mountain* (M.K. Yousef, S.M. Horvath, and R.W. Bullard, Eds). New York; Academic Press, p. 143

Mahler, H.R. and Cordes, E.H. (1966). *Biological Chemistry*. New York; Harper

Millikan, G.A. (1939). Muscle hemoglobin. *Physiological Reviews*, **19**, 503

Oelz, O., Howald, H., Di Prampero P.E., Hoppeler, H., Claassen H., Jenni, R., Bühlman, A., Ferreti, G., Brückner, J.C., Veicsteinas, A., Gussoni, M., and Cerretelli, P. (1986). Physiological profile of world-class high-altitude climbers. *Journal of Applied Physiology*, **60**, 1734

Ou, L.C. and Tenney, S.M. (1970). Properties of mitochondria from hearts of cattle acclimatized to high altitude. *Respiration Physiology*, **8**, 151

Reynafarje, B. (1962). Myoglobin content and enzymatic activity of muscle and altitude adaptation. *Journal of Applied Physiology*, **17**, 301

Reynafarje, C., Faura, J., Villavicencio, D., Curaca, A., Reynafarje, B., Oyola, L., Contreras, L., Vallenas, E., and Faura, A. (1975). Oxygen transport of hemoglobin in high-altitude animals (Camelidae). *Journal of Applied Physiology*, **38**, 806

Scholander, P.F. (1960). Oxygen transport through hemoglobin solutions. *Science*, **131**, 585

Snyder, G.K., Byers, R.L., and Kayar, S.R. (1984). Effects of hypoxia on tissue capillarity in geese. *Respiration Physiology*, **58**, 151

Snyder, G.K., Wilcox, E.E., and Burnham, E.W. (1985). Effects of hypoxia on muscle capillarity in rats. *Respiration Physiology*, **62**, 135

Tappan, D.V. and Reynafarje, B. (1957). Tissue pigment manifestations of adaptation to high altitude. *American Journal of Physiology*, **190**, 99

Tenney, S.M. and Ou, L.C. (1969). In *Biomedicine Problems of High Terrestrial Elevations* (A.H. Hegnauer, Ed.). U.S. Army Research Institute of Environmental Medicine, p. 160

Turek, S., Grandtner, M., and Kreuzer, F. (1972). Cardiac hypertrophy, capillary and muscle fibre density, muscle fibre diameter, capillary radius and diffusion distance in myocardium of growing rats and adapted to a simulated altitude of 3,500 m. *Pflügers Archiv*, **335**, 19

Valdivia, E. (1958). Total capillary bed in striated muscle of guinea pigs native to the Peruvian Mountains. *American Journal of Physiology*, **194**, 585

Ward, M. (1975). *Mountain Medicine, A Clinical Study of Cold and High Altitude*. London; Crosby Lockwood Staples

Ward, M.P., Milledge, J.S., and West, J.B. (1989). Peripheral tissues. In *High Altitude Medicine and Physiology*; London Chapman and Hall, p. 201

Weibel, E.R. (1969). Stereological principles for morphometry in electron microscopic cytology. *International Review of Cytology*, **26**, 235

Weibel, E.R., Kistler, G.S., and Scherle, W.F. (1966). Practical stereological methods for morphometric cytology. *Journal of Cell Biology*, **30**, 23

Weibel, E.R., Staubli, W., Gnagi, H.R., and Hess, F.A. (1969). I Morphometric model, stereological methods and normal morphometric data for the rat liver. *Journal of Cell Biology*, **42**, 68

Wittenberg, J.B. (1959). Oxygen transport: a new function proposed for myoglobin. *Biological Bulletin*, **117**, 402

Wittenberg, J.B. (1966). Myoglobin facilitated diffusion of oxygen. *Journal of General Physiology*, **49**, 57

7

The carotid bodies

Situated in the neck in the bifurcations of the common carotid arteries are two nodules of tissue, 3mm in diameter, that are responsive to levels of respiratory gases in the blood. These chemoreceptors respond rapidly to alterations of partial pressure of oxygen and carbon dioxide and to disturbances of blood pH. In man at sea level respiration is largely controlled by minor fluctuations in arterial carbon dioxide tension influencing the medullary respiratory centres, and the influence of stimulation of the carotid bodies by arterial oxygen tension is minor, accounting for only 15% of the overall stimulation of respiration. The predominantly afferent nature of the nerve supply of the carotid bodies of the glossopharyngeal nerves demonstrated that the carotid bodies had an important sensory function (de Castro 1928). His interpretation of the structure of the carotid bodies as being consistent with the monitoring of blood gases was soon confirmed by the physiological studies of Heymans et al. (1930). This does not exclude the possibility that the carotid bodies may have additional functions to chemoreception, perhaps of an endocrinological nature. At high altitude the situation is transformed, for the significant falls in arterial oxygen tension have a powerful effect, altering the structure of the carotid bodies.

STRUCTURE
The carotid bodies form part of what is known as the paraganglionic system, which includes nodules of tissue scattered widely throughout the body ranging from the glomus jugulare around the jugular vein to the organ of Zuckerkandl at the bifurcation of the aorta. All these widely dispersed tissues and the tumours arising from them are composed of the same basic histological unit, but it should be noted that, in spite of this, only the carotid bodies and the aortico-pulmonary bodies have been shown to be chemoreceptors.

The carotid body is a vascular, spherical nodule composed of a complex network of arteries, capillaries, and veins that is intimately associated with two distinctive types of cell designated chief and sustentacular. The Latin term for such a rolled-up body is 'glomus' and it is classically used in descriptive histology to indicate a spherical conglomeration of cells and small vessels. In the carotid body glomic tissue forms lobules embedded in connective tissue, each lobule being composed of cellular clusters some 80 μm in diameter. Running through the fibrous stroma are elastic interlobular arteries derived from the main glomic arteries, which themselves arise from the carotid bifurcation. The elastic interlobular arteries divide into muscular intralobular arteries that enter the lobules and terminate as arterioles.

Also ramifying in the stroma are myelinated radicles of the glossopharyngeal nerves carrying away afferent impulses from the cell clusters. Other nerves running in the stroma are sympathetic in nature and derived from the ganglioglomerular nerve; they appear to supply the blood vessels in the glomus.

The cells comprising the clusters are of two distinct types. The first is the chief (type 1) cell, some 13 μm in diameter, with cytoplasmic borders that are so poorly defined as to resemble a syncytium (Fig. 7.1). The large (7 μm), round or oval nucleus is very characteristic, with an open vesicular network of chromatin (Fig. 7.1). The cytoplasm is palely eosinophilic and contains small vesicles. At ultrastructural level the vesicles have a central dense osmiophilic core and a surrounding clear halo and are thus termed 'dense-core vesicles'. The dense cores contain a variety of peptides while the surrounding haloes include several biogenic amines. We found the concentration of six peptides in the human carotid body as shown in Table 7.1 by the use of radioimmunoassay (Heath et al. 1988). Immunolabelling for both methionine-and leucine-enkephalin (Met-and Leu-enkephalin) is predominantly within glomic chief cells with no labelling at all in the sustentacular cells described below. We found that substance P was present in the chief cells of man in 16 of 24 cases studied (Smith et al. 1990). Vasoactive intestinal peptide also occurs in all variants of chief cell but is absent from sustentacular cells and nerves (Smith et al. 1990). We identified

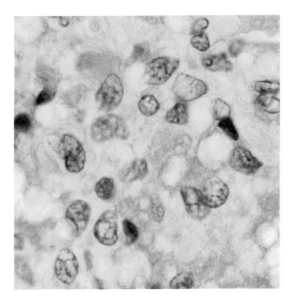

7.1 *A group of light chief cells from the core of a cluster in a lobule from a carotid body of an adult lowlander. Their nuclei are pale and vesicular with strands or fine dots of chromatin. The cytoplasm is pale, indistinct, and vacuolated. Haematoxylin and eosin (HE), × 1500.*

trations are dopamine 64%, noradrenaline 14.8%, and adrenaline 2.5%, the remaining 18.8% consisting of 5-hydroxytryptamine (Steele and Hinterberger 1972).

There are three histological variants of the chief cell. The description given above is that of the light variant, which is the commonest form and corresponds to the classic glomic cell (Heath and Smith 1992). There are two other variants, the dark and the progenitor. In the dark variant the nucleus is smaller and more compact and the heterochromatin is more densely packed together (Fig. 7.2). The cytoplasm is more basophilic and forms characteristic streamers (Fig. 7.2). There are many small cytoplasmic vesicles and many of these are prominent dense-core vesicles. The dark cell is particularly prominent in the carotid body of the infant and young adult at sea level and is probably best regarded as an active chemoreceptor cell (Hurst *et al.* 1985). The progenitor variant has a much smaller and more compact nucleus (Fig. 7.2). This cell is probably to be regarded as the forerunner of the dark variant, which itself undergoes subsequent transposition into the classic, light variant. The rich content of dense-core vesicles in the cytoplasm of the progenitor variant suggests that it too is biochemically active. In the rat the variants of chief cell have been dismissed as artefacts due to inadequate fixation (McDonald 1981) but such reservations do not apply to the human carotid body.

The second type of cell to be found in the clusters is the sustentacular (type 2) cell, which is to be found predominantly at their periphery. It is elongated and wrapped around non-myelinated nerve axons and it gradually merges into the Schwann cells embracing myelinated nerves in the interlobular fibrous stroma. The sustentacular cell has an elon-

neurotensin in only eight of 23 pairs of carotid bodies and even then the labelling was weak and involved only a few chief cells. Immunostaining for bombesin is entirely different from that of the other five peptides in that it is confined almost entirely to the glomic vasculature (Smith *et al.* 1990). Catecholamines can be demonstrated in the human carotid body by formalin-induced fluorescence (Hamburger *et al.* 1966) where their relative concen-

Table 7.1 Concentrations of six peptides in the human carotid body as determined by radioimmunoassay (after Heath *et al.* 1988)

Peptide	No. carotid bodies assayed	Concentration (pmol/g)	
		Mean	Range
Met-enkephalin	10	612	219–1267
Leu-enkephalin	10	162	53–353
Bombesin	13	73	30–124
Neurotensin	13	67	36–114
Substance P	8	16	4–25
Vasoactive intestinal peptide	13	9	4–16

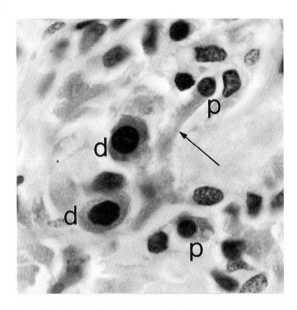

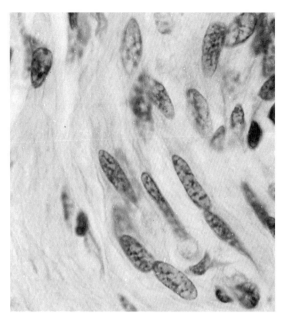

7.2 *Dark cells (d) in the carotid body contain haematoxyphilic nuclei and dark, clearly defined cytoplasm. Progenitor cells (p) have small, dark nuclei and less copious cytoplasm of a staining intensity similar to that of dark cells. A cytoplasmic streamer extends from one progenitor cell (arrow). HE, × 1500.*

7.3 *Sustentacular (type 2) cells from the normal right carotid body of a woman of 71 years. The nucleus is elongated and the spindle-shaped cytoplasm is pale and fibrillary. HE, × 1500.*

gated nucleus (13 × 4μm); its cytoplasm contains numerous filaments but virtually no organelles (Fig. 7.3). It is commonly thought to have only a supporting role for nerve axons.

ENLARGEMENT ON ACUTE EXPOSURE TO HYPOBARIC HYPOXIA

On acute exposure of the lowlander to hypobaric hypoxia on ascent to high altitude it seems likely that the carotid bodies enlarge. The nature of this enlargement can only be inferred by analogy to what occurs in rats kept in a decompression chamber. Such experiments show that the carotid bodies enlarge rapidly on acute exposure to diminished barometric pressure and just as rapidly return to normal size once the hypoxic stimulus is withdrawn (Heath *et al.* 1973; Laidler and Kay, 1975*a*, *b*). In one experiment we studied the tissue volume of the carotid body by an application of Simpson's rule to histological sections in three groups of 10 adult male Wistar albino rats (Heath *et al.* 1973). The first group was kept for 5 weeks in a hypobaric chamber exposed to a barometric pressure of 380 mmHg, equivalent to a simulated altitude of 5500 m above sea level. The second was exposed to

the same barometric pressure for 5 weeks and then allowed to recover in room air for a further period of 5 weeks. The third group acted as controls and was kept at normal barometric pressure throughout. In the control animals the mean carotid body volume (expressed in units of $\mu m^3 \times 10^6$) was 13.45, but after exposure to hypobaric hypoxia for only 5 weeks this volume rose to 47.81. After the hypoxic stimulus was withdrawn the tissue volume fell after only 5 weeks to 19.82. Similarly, when Laidler and Kay (1975*a*) exposed rats to a barometric pressure of 460 mmHg for between 25 and 96 days, the mean value of the total volume of the combined left and right carotid bodies rose from 47.16 to 187.39 $\mu m^3 \times 10^6$. Blessing and Wolff (1973) found that, when they subjected rats to a simulated high altitude of 7500 m for 3 months, the carotid bodies increased in volume from 32.8 to 194.5 $\mu m^3 \times 10^6$.

The reason for the rapid enlargement of the carotid bodies and the equally quick reversibility to almost normal levels is that the enlargement is due almost entirely to vascular engorgement, the cellular elements of the carotid body playing little or no part in it. Laidler and Kay (1975*a*) agreed with this interpretation, but were uncertain as to the functional significance of the increased vascularity. They thought it might be nothing more than a non-specific reaction designed to increase blood flow and thus oxygen transport to a hypoxic organ with increased metabolic activity. The studies of Hellström and Pequignot (1985) suggest that the vascularity of the organ in acute hypoxia is regulated through adrenergic β-receptors. They found that rats treated with propanolol adjusted more easily to hypoxia, and showed but slight enlargement of their carotid bodies in which the vascular density remained normal. The location of adrenergic β-receptors in the carotid body is not known.

CAROTID BODIES OF NATIVE HIGHLANDERS

The carotid bodies of native highlanders, born and spending their whole lives at high altitude, also show enlargement but here it is permanent and has an organic basis with changes in the histological structure of the chemoreceptors. In a verbal presentation at a scientific meeting in the United States, Arias-Stella (1969) reported that the carotid bodies of Quechua Indians born and living in the Peruvian Andes were larger than those of mestizos living on the coast. This important observation, which laid the basis for the study of the pathology of the carotid body, was subsequently extended and published by Arias-Stella and Valcarcel (1973). They described the carotid bodies in two series of necropsies, one from sea level on mestizos from Lima and one from the Peruvian mining town of Cerro de Pasco at an altitude of 4330 m on native Quechua highlanders. The cases were matched for age and sex and mostly comprised accidental deaths with no significant cardiovascular or pulmonary pathology. The cases were compared in three age groups. The carotid bodies of the highlanders were heavier (Fig. 7.4) and larger (Fig. 7.5) in each group and the differences became greater with increasing age.

Arias-Stella and Valcarcel (1976) found that the enlargement of the carotid bodies was associated with prominence of the chief cells which were so dense and so diffuse as to give the section a homogeneous appearance. The lobes and lobules were abnormally large and the intervening bands of fibrous stroma were thinner. In this study the authors attempted to measure what they termed 'the functional area' of glomic tissue in 51 lowlanders and 56 highlanders. They equated this with the area occupied by glomic tissue in sections through the centre of the carotid bodies. They found that the functional area increased in highlanders due to hy-

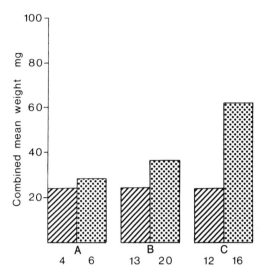

7.4 *Combined weights of the carotid bodies from two series of necropsies, one from mestizos at sea level (hatched columns) and one from native highlanders at 4330 m (stippled columns). The cases from sea level and high altitude are compared in the age groups: (A) 10–20 years; (B) 21–40 years; and (C) 41–70 years. The numbers of cases in each of the six subgroups is indicated beneath the respective columns. Note that the carotid bodies of the highlander are heavier in each group. In addition, there is a definite progressive increment in weight with age in the high-altitude series. (Data from Arias-Stella and Valcarcel (1973, 1976).)*

perplasia of chief cells, the range being 857–1171 μm² in lowlanders and 600–1800 μm² in highlanders. It was noted that the hyperplastic chief cells showed intense vacuolation. After fixation in formaldehyde vapour, the dense-core vesicles normally show a green–yellow natural fluorescence due to the biogenic amines. In the enlarged carotid bodies of highlanders such fluorescent granules were scarce or absent. Arias-Stella and Valcarcel (1976) interpreted their findings as indicating a hyperplasia of chief cells, indicating them as primary sensors of the hypoxaemia in the native highlanders brought about by the hypobaric hypoxia. The loss of formaldehyde-induced fluorescence suggested to them that there had been a discharge of biogenic amines from the chief cells.

Through the courtesy of Dr Tsering Norboo we have had the opportunity to study the carotid bodies of four native highlanders of Leh (3600 m) in the

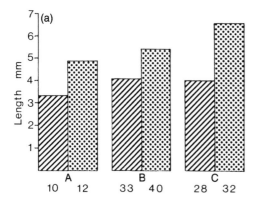

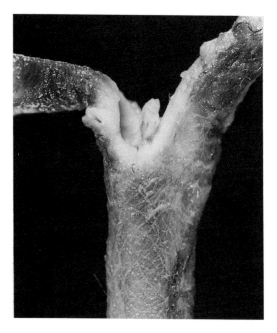

7.6 *Right carotid body from a native highlander, aged 29 years, from Chusul (4200 m). He died in an accident and was free from cardiopulmonary disease. The right carotid body weighed 8 mg and the left 10 mg. These weights are normal by sea-level standards and make it clear that the carotid bodies are not enlarged in all natives to high altitude. × 3.*

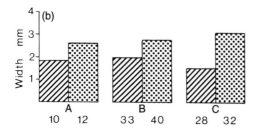

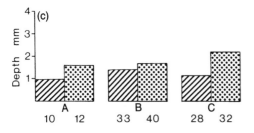

7.5 *(a) Length, (b) width, and (c) depth of the carotid bodies from the two series of necropsies referred to in Fig. 7.4, one from sea level (hatched columns) and one from 4330 m (stippled columns). As in the previous figure, the cases from sea level and high altitude are compared in the same three age groups, and the numbers of cases in each of the six subgroups are indicated beneath the respective columns. Note that the dimensions of the carotid bodies of the highlanders are greater in each group. In addition, there is a definite progressive increment in dimensions with age in the high-altitude series. (Data from Arias-Stella and Valcarcel (1976).)*

Karakorams (Fig. 7.6; Table 7.2). Our histological findings differ significantly in several respects from those of Arias-Stella and Valcarcel (1976). We studied four male Ladakhi highlanders whose ages ranged from 4 to 52 years (Table 7.2). We were able to confirm that, as with the Quechua Indians, there was a progressive increase of carotid-body-weight with age. There was an increase in size of glomic lobules but this was due to a proliferation of distinct clusters, which were smaller than those found in lowlanders (Table 7.3). Mini clusters less than 45 μm were found in abundance in contrast to the normal lobules of over 80 μm found in lowlanders (Table 7.3).

Dark cells in the carotid bodies in highlanders

A significant difference in our histological findings in the Ladakhi highlanders was an increase in the differential count of the dark variant of chief cells (Fig. 7.7; Table 7.3). Dark cells were very prominent in a boy of 4 years but even in the two older highlanders aged 35 and 52 years the incidence was

Table 7.2 Altitude of domicile and carotid body-weight in four native highlanders of Ladakh (after Khan *et al.* 1988)

Age (years)	Sex	Altitude (m) of birth place and domicile	Carotid-body weight (mg)		
			Right	Left	Total
4	M	Choglamsar 3500	3.6	3.0	6.6
29	M	Chusul 4200	8	10	18
35	M	Choglamsar 3500	25	25	50
52	M	Stok 3300	50	28	78

Table 7.3 Diameters of lobules and clusters and differential cell counts in four Ladakhi highlanders (after Khan *et al.* 1988)

Age (years)	Sex	Lobule diameter (μm)			Cluster diameter (μm)			Differential cell count (%)			
		n	Mean	CL	*n*	Mean	CL	L	D	P	S
4	M	22	314	40.4	50	76	4.6	48	23	1	28
29	M	21	355	46.8	40	75	3.6	54	17	2	27
35	M	19	495	56.3	40	44	2.6	47	14	2	37
52	M	22	518	81.4	40	45	2.6	26	14	2	58
Sea level (Smith *et al.* 1982)		57	411	154	57	82	28.0	54	5	2	39

CL, 95% confidence limits; *n*, number of samples; L, light cells; D, dark cells; P, progenitor cells; S, sustentacular cells.

14%, about three times higher than the values anticipated for adult lowlanders. The dark cells showed a striking cytological appearance. There was a pronounced increase in the size of the nuclei, which contained much more heterochromatin arranged in a denser, coarser pattern. These dark cells were much larger than those seen in the carotid bodies of normal lowlanders and the copious basophilic cytoplasm formed long streamers. The dense cytoplasm contrasted strikingly with that of the faintly staining, eosinophilic cytoplasm of the surrounding light chief cells. Its margins were sharply defined in contrast to the syncytium-like appearance of the adjacent light chief cells. The cytoplasm of the dark cells contained clear vesicles. In many cells these vesicles were small and of a bubbly appearance but in some they ap-

peared to have fused to form large vesicles that had been discharged from the cell surface (Fig. 7.7). Progenitor cells were present but not prominent and the differential count revealed no increased incidence of this type of cell. After incubation with Met-enkephalin antisera strong positive immunoreactivity was observed in the dark and progenitor variants of the chief cells (Fig. 7.8). Dark cells with streamers were particularly strongly positive for Met-enkephalin.

In conclusion, the carotid bodies of native highlanders are enlarged due to the sustained stimulation of the chemoreceptor tissue by hypobaric hypoxia. This results in the development of numerous mini clusters of chief cells that group together and lead to an increase in size of lobules. There is a

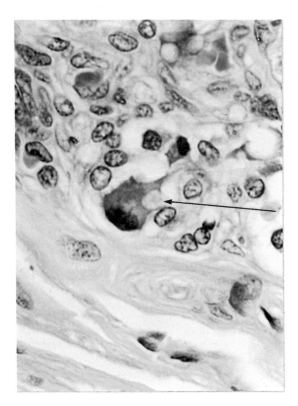

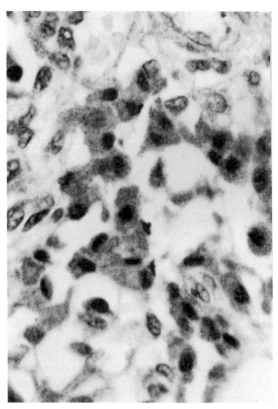

7.7 *Dark variant of chief cell of carotid body from a male Ladakhi highlander of 35 years (Table 7.2). The cell has a large dense nucleus and voluminous cytoplasm containing vesicles some of which appear to have fused to form large vesicles that have discharged from the cell surface (arrow). HE, × 1250.*

7.8 *A group of dark cells from the same case as in the previous figure containing Met-enkephalin. Peroxidase–antiperoxidase, anti-Met-enkephalin, × 1250.*

loss of formaldehyde-induced fluorescence, which suggests discharge of biogenic amines from the chief cells. There is a prominence of the dark variant of chief cells, which contain much Met-enkephalin in vesicles that accumulate to form larger intracytoplasmic cysts that then seem to be discharged from the cell. It is likely that the discharge of both the biogenic amines and peptides are associated functionally in some way with the chemoreceptor response to sustained hypobaric hypoxia.

The same response to hypoxia is produced by reversal of an intracardiac shunt in a ventricular septal defect (Smith *et al.* 1986b) or by an exacerbation of alveolar hypoxia in chronic obstructive lung disease (Heath *et al.* 1984). They are found in the carotid bodies of cattle in transit through the Andes where they became exposed to subacute

hypoxia (Heath *et al.* 1985). We have examined the numbers and ultrastructure of dark cells in rabbits kept in a hypoxic chamber for 3 and 6 months, respectively (Smith *et al.* 1986a). In the rabbits exposed to hypoxia for the shorter period there was a striking response but in those kept hypoxic for 6 months the dark cell prominence had disappeared to be replaced by the light variant of chief cells. Such experimental data suggest that the initial cellular reaction to hypobaric hypoxia is by the dark cell while the stable situation is characterized by light cells. Dark cells are rich in a variety of peptides and biogenic amines but the functional significance of the early response by these cells is unknown. The relation of the three variants of chief cell appears to be that the progenitor cell gives rise to the dark cell that in turn is transformed into the light cell, which, in fact; may develop the ageing pigment of lipofuscin.

DIFFERENCES IN THE REACTION OF THE CAROTID BODIES IN CHRONIC OBSTRUCTIVE LUNG DISEASE

The histological changes reported in the carotid bodies of Quechua Indians (Arias-Stella and Valcarcel 1976) and of Ladakhi highlanders (Khan *et al.* 1988) differ significantly from those to be found in patients with chronic bronchitis and emphysema (Heath *et al.* 1982; Smith *et al.* 1982). In patients with pulmonary emphysema there is prominent sustentacular cell hyperplasia with whorls of type 2 cells and Schwann cells, whereas as we have seen in native highlanders the enlargement is produced by numerous mini clusters of chief cells surrounded by thin rims of sustentacular cells as in the normal carotid body. To distinguish the two appearances it has been suggested that the condition be termed 'chief cell hyperplasia' in native highlanders and 'sustentacular cell hyperplasia' in patients with chronic obstructive lung disease (Heath and Smith 1992). Chief cell hyperplasia is also found in children and young adults with hypoxaemia secondary to congenital heart disease or cystic fibrosis of the lung. It may be that chief cell hyperplasia is an early stage of carotid body hyperplasia and that with the passage of time, sustentacular cells with their axons (Fitch *et al.* 1985) continue to proliferate at the expense of chief cells to produce the histological picture of sustentacular cell hyperplasia. An alternative view is that the two forms of carotid body hyperplasia are distinct entities and that their initiation depends at least upon the age of the individual at the time of commencement of the hypoxaemic stimulus. Finally, it has to be kept in mind that the hypobaric hypoxia of the native highlander is associated with hypocarbia, whereas the hypoxia of the subject with chronic obstructive airways disease is associated with hypercarbia. This may influence the nature of the histological changes in the glomic tissue.

ULTRASTRUCTURAL CHANGES

Ultrastructural changes occur in the carotid bodies of animals living at high altitude but there is scant information on the ultrastructure of either the normal or abnormal human glomera, with the exception of studies on the chemodectoma. Previously, fresh specimens of glomic tissue were resected during therapeutic glomectomy for bronchial asthma, allowing studies on the ultrastructure of normal glomic tissue (Grimley and Glenner 1968), but now that this operation is discontinued in most countries the electron microscopist must rely on tissues obtained from necropsy, with all the attendant problems of autolysis and its associated artefacts. As a consequence of this, much of what we know about the ultrastructural responses of the carotid body to hypoxia, and particularly hypobaric hypoxia, is derived from animals exposed to natural or simulated high altitude. Although this provides us with some information and insights, it is prudent to keep in mind the dangers of applying to man too readily data derived from experimental animals in decompression chambers.

Thus, electron microscopic changes have been described in the chief cells, and particularly their dense-core vesicles, in animals acutely exposed to hypoxia, but the validity of these observations is questionable. In one of the early attempts to demonstrate the effects of acute hypoxia on chief cells, rats were subjected for up to 20 min to very severe deprivation of oxygen so that it comprised only 2.5% of the inspired air (Blümcke *et al.* 1967). This reduced the number of dense-core vesicles with their apparent discharge from the surface of cells, but it also damaged both nuclei and mitochondria so it should be regarded as a pathological response to unduly severe hypoxia. Subsequent studies on cats and hamsters by, respectively;, Al-Lami and Murray (1968) and Chen *et al.* (1969) have failed to demonstrate exocytosis of dense-core vesicles in response to hypoxia. The fact that acute hypoxia does not cause dense-core vesicles to discharge their contents opposes the idea that these vesicles function as catecholamine-containing neurotransmitters to mediate chemoreception. When the potent catecholamine-releasing drug reserpine is administered to hamsters (Chen *et al.* 1969) there is no vacuolation in the granules of the chief cells of carotid bodies fixed for electron microscopy by glutaraldehyde with post-fixation in osmium. Since this is a fixative for protein, it may be that the dense-core vesicles are largely proteinaceous in composition, thus explaining their lack of response to an agent that causes depletion of biogenic amines. This lack of response, coupled with the failure of acute hypoxia to cause exocytosis of the vesicles, suggests that they may play an entirely different role. They may, for example, be concerned with secretion of a peptide hormone and this possibility has to be kept in mind when we consider the ultrastructural changes in the carotid bodies of animals exposed chronically to natural or simulated high altitude.

In contrast to acute hypoxia, chronic exposure to natural high altitude appears to induce characteristic ultrastructural changes in the chief cells and, in view of what has just been said, these features raise the distinct possibility that they represent secretion of a hormone rather than a sustained chemoreception to persistent hypoxia. We found that, in the carotid bodies of guinea-pigs born and bred in Cerro de Pasco (4330 m) in the Peruvian Andes, the chief cells showed a pronounced increase in size and vacuolation of the dense-core vesicles (Edwards *et al.* 1972). In sea-level guinea-pigs the average diameter of the bodies ranges from 100 to 150 nm. The vesicles consist of a central dense osmiophilic core with a very narrow clear halo subjacent to an outer limiting membrane (Fig. 7.9). In the high-altitude animals there was a striking increase in the diameter and vacuolation of the dense-core vesicles (Fig. 7.10). The central proteinaceous core was often reduced in size and density and was situated excentrically within the enlarged vesicle. In some the core was virtually absent, producing vacuoles up to 350 nm in diameter. Other workers were unable to confirm the existence of this vacuolation in the dense-core vesicles in rabbits living on the Bolivian altiplano at a comparable altitude (Møller *et al.* 1974) and in rats exposed to the prolonged hypoxia of a simulated altitude of 7000 m (Blessing and Kaldeweide 1975). The same vacuolation of dense-core vesicles was, however, found by Laidler and Kay (1978*a*), who subjected rats to a simulated altitude of 4300 m for 4–5 weeks.

Quantitative ultrastructural techniques were also used to assess changes in the population density of dense-core vesicles (Laidler and Kay 1978*b*). A striking reduction in the number of vesicles per unit area was found, but was associated with a proportionately large increase in area of the whole cell. Thus the absolute number of vesicles per cell was unchanged. The problem was investigated further by Smith *et al.* (1986*a*) who examined the carotid bodies of rabbits that were born at Cerro de Pasco (4330 m) in the Andes, and rabbits that were subjected to a comparable simulated high altitude for periods of either 3 or 6 months. Vacuolation of dense-core vesicles was seen in all three groups of rabbits, but was confined almost exclusively to the smaller type of granule. The vacuolation was most pronounced in the Peruvian rabbits involving about half of the vesicles, and fewer vacuoles were found in the rabbits exposed to simulated high altitude for 6 months. Vacuolation was, however, rare in the rabbits exposed to hypoxia for only 3 months. It is thus clear that the development of vacuolation of dense-core vesicles is related to the duration of the exposure to hypoxia.

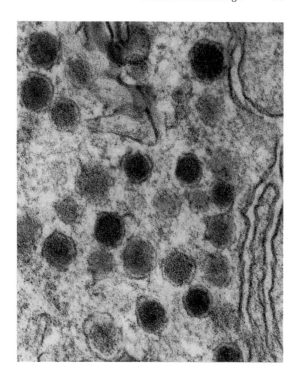

7.9 *Electron micrograph of carotid body from a low-altitude guinea-pig. It shows membrane-bound granules in the cytoplasm of a chief cell. In many granules there is a central dense osmiophilic core with a very narrow clear halo subjacent to an outer limiting membrane. In others there is no limiting membrane and the contents appear to merge into the surrounding cytoplasm. × 52 500.*

The functional significance of vacuolation of dense-core vesicles is not known, but certain observations and speculations can be made (Smith 1986). It is unlikely to represent discharge of catecholamines in response to hypoxia, since in the rabbit the change takes some 6 months to develop and is not seen on acute exposure to hypoxia. Conceivably, the change may represent storage of catecholamines consistent with the increased levels of dopamine that have been demonstrated in the chief cells of hypoxic animals. The change could represent secretion of a soluble peptide, the diminution in size of the core indicating loss of proteinaceous substance, and the distension of the surrounding 'halo' may be due to inhibition of fluid following an increase in osmotic pressure of the granule contents. The enlarged carotid bodies of spontaneously hypertensive rats do not show vacuolation of the vesicles (Smith *et al.* 1984), indicating that carotid body hyperplasia *per se* is not the factor

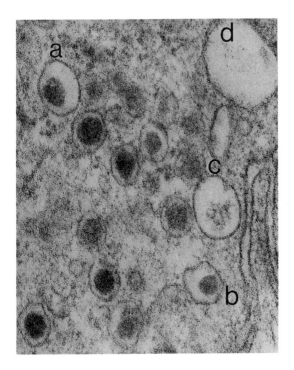

7.10 *Electron micrograph of carotid body from a high-altitude guinea-pig. It shows that some of the dense-core vesicles are distended by widening of the clear halo, which leaves the hitherto central osmiophilic core in an excentric position (a). In others the core is much less dense than normal (b) or is represented by only faint remains (c). In some granules the core has been lost and the appearances are those of a microvacuole (d). × 52 500.*

responsible for its genesis. Clearly, this ultrastructural change is in some way an effect of hypoxia, perhaps indirectly produced. It is not known if these changes occur in the carotid body of man living at high altitude.

BLUNTED VENTILATORY RESPONSE OF THE CAROTID BODIES OF THE HIGHLANDER TO HYPOXIA

The enlarged carotid bodies of the native highlander show a blunted ventilatory response to the hypobaric hypoxia of high altitude. The lowlander hyperventilates vigorously early on exposure to altitude. While the native highlander hyperventilates compared to the lowlander, he still hypoventilates compared to the newcomer to the mountains. This relative hypoventilation is unlikely to be based on genetic factors (Lahiri 1971) for it is found in natives of both the Andes and the Himalaya (Chiodi 1957; Lahiri and Milledge 1965; Pugh *et al.* 1964; Severinghaus *et al.* 1966; Sørensen and Severinghaus 1968a; Lefrançois *et al.* 1968). Both the Quechua people of the Andes and the Sherpas of the Himalaya are mongoloid, but genetically unrelated Caucasians living permanently in Kashmir at 3500 m (Ramaswamy 1962) and in Colorado at 3100 m (Forster *et al.* 1969) also show a blunted ventilatory response to hypoxia.

It seems more likely that the blunted response is acquired. Two factors seem to be of importance in the loss of sensitivity to hypoxaemia: the age of the subject at the time of exposure to hypoxia and the duration of the exposure. It appears to develop after about 12 years' residence, manifesting itself in teenagers and becoming universal in adults. Some children, however, who spend only 2 or 3 years at high altitude fail to achieve normal sensitivity to hypoxia even after prolonged residence at sea level (Sørensen and Severinghaus 1968b; Lahiri *et al.* 1969). On the other hand, the offspring of native highlanders born at sea level show the same ventilatory response as lowlanders. All these features suggest that the reduced sensitivity of the carotid bodies of native highlanders is associated with the development of miniclusters of glomic chief cells as described earlier in the chapter.

The resetting of the carotid bodies to different levels of arterial oxygen tension is one of their characteristic features at both low and high altitudes at different periods of life. The carotid body is active as chemoreceptor in fetal life. Cross and Malcolm (1952) found positive chemoreceptor and baroreceptor activity in kittens, a rabbit, lambs, and a monkey. Dawes *et al.* (1969) confirmed that, in fetal lambs delivered by Caesarean section, injection of sodium cyanide into both common carotid arteries simultaneously caused a substantial cardiovascular response and often a respiratory effort. Hertzberg *et al.* (1990) found that the peripheral arterial chemoreceptors of the carotid body are active and responsive in the fetal rat. Hanson *et al.* (1987) found that the peripheral chemoreceptors in the carotid body were spontaneously active and responsive in the exteriorized fetal lamb at the lower arterial oxygen tension prevalent during pregnancy. Cross and Oppé (1952) studied the effects of high and low concentrations of oxygen on the respiration of premature and full-term human infants and concluded that there was an active chemoreceptor reflex at these ages. All of these data confirm that the carotid bodies in the hypoxia of late fetal life show a spontaneously active and responsive chemoreceptor activity.

However, at birth when the newborn child is exposed to much elevated arterial oxygen tension, the carotid bodies show a dramatic resetting. As early as 1955 Miller and Smull proposed, as a result of experiments in which newborn infants inhaled hypoxic gas mixtures, that the peripheral chemoreceptors were not active at birth but only mature in the subsequent days or weeks. These observations were confirmed by Blanco *et al.* (1984) who found that in the sheep the arterial chemoreceptors are active and responsive in the fetus, but quiescent in the lamb on the day of birth when arterial oxygen tension has risen. Thus, in spite of the completed innervation of the carotid body in late fetal life, chemoreceptor function alters so that hypoxic sensitivity of the glomic tissue is reset of necessity on the first day of birth when arterial oxygen tension rises abruptly.

It is important to understand the functional basis of the resetting of the carotid body at birth because a comparable process operating in the reverse direction explains the resetting of glomic tissue leading to diminished sensitivity of the carotid bodies to hypobaric hypoxia at high altitude. Hertzberg *et al.* (1990) studied the strength of the chemoreflex in newborn rats and correlated this in particular with the content of dopamine of the carotid bodies of newborn pups and near-term fetuses. They found that the chemoreceptor reflex is silenced at birth but re-emerges after about 1 day in the newborn rat. The development of this reflex is preceded by a decrease in dopamine turnover in the carotid body suggesting a lifting of the inhibition of the chemosensory mechanism. This biogenic amine is produced by the glomic chief cells and exerts an inhibitory influence on impulses travelling up the carotid sinus nerve. On the first day of extrauterine life the fetal levels of dopamine are sufficient to block the diminished nerve impulses arising in response to the heightened levels of arterial oxygen tension. The fall of dopamine levels at birth allows chemoreflex activity to be renewed by lifting of the inhibition of nerve impulses travelling up the carotid sinus, now reset to be commensurate with the heightened arterial oxygen tension. Hence the complete innervation of the carotid body demonstrated by silver staining of nerve fibrils and boutons can be associated with vigorous chemosensory activity in late fetal life, with silence on the first day of life, and with re-emergence of chemosensory activity in the first few days of extrauterine life. The activity of the

nerve fibrils is clearly greatly influenced by the biochemical environment, particularly the level of dopamine.

In the same way there may be a resetting of chemoreceptor activity in native highlanders once there is hyperplasia of chief cells to form miniclusters (Khan *et al.* 1988; Heath and Smith 1992). The ability to synthesize and release dopamine in response to hypoxia is an intrinsic property of chief cells since this process occurs even when they are dissociated in tissue culture (Fishman *et al.* 1985). Hence the resetting of the chemosensory response at high altitude and in chronic lung disease so that the carotid body becomes less responsive to alveolar hypoxia appears to be the result of chief cell hyperplasia and the resultant secretion of increased amounts of dopamine.

Attenuation of the ventilatory response occurs during prolonged residence at high altitude (Severinghaus *et al.* 1966; Sørensen and Severinghaus 1968c). The reduction in sensitivity to hypoxaemia is often accompanied by a decrease in sensitivity to carbon dioxide (Chiodi 1957). A characteristic feature of this blunted ventilatory response to the hypoxia of high altitude is its irreversibility. It is not restored even after prolonged residence at sea level. There are important clinical applications of diminished ventilatory response in the face of prolonged hypoxia. Thus a blunted sensitivity also occurs in chronic respiratory disease complicated by hypoxia (Flenley and Millar 1967; Richards *et al.* 1968). Such patients also show an insensitivity to carbon dioxide. Blunted ventilatory responses also occur in cyanotic congenital heart disease (Sørensen and Severinghaus 1968c; Edelman *et al.* 1970), but in these patients there is no decrease in sensitivity to carbon dioxide.

Arias-Stella and Valcarcel (1976) related the augmented carotid body size and weight with increasing age of highlanders to progressive insensitivity of those chemoreceptors. They refer to the studies of Sime (1973) who was able to demonstrate that there is a progressive fall in pulmonary ventilation with age at high altitude. He submitted highlanders at 4330 m to a steady-state exposure to various levels of arterial oxygen tension ranging from hyperoxia to hypoxia, and in isocapnic as well as in hypercapnic conditions. Subjects sleeping naturally were also studied. His studies showed that highlanders progress irreversibly with age from hyperventilation to hypoventilation irrespective of whether they are tested under basal, or acute hypoxic or hyperoxic conditions. The progressive hypoventilation with age in native highlanders may be related to the progressive proliferation of sustentacular cells around cores of chief cells as an ageing phenomenon (Hurst *et al.* 1985). Earlier in this chapter we referred to this process occurring in a middle-aged highlander from Ladakh.

ATRIAL NATRIURETIC PEPTIDE

Recent immunocytochemical studies have demonstrated that atrial natriuretic peptide-like (ANP) activity is present in the chief (type 1) cells in the carotid body of the cat (Wang *et al.* 1991). These authors found that the biologically active ANP fragment atriopeptin III is a potent inhibitor of carotid sinus nerve activity evoked by hypoxia. Thus atrionatriuretic peptide in the carotid body may be a further factor in modulating and depressing chemosensory activity at high altitude.

CAROTID BODIES OF ANIMALS AT HIGH ALTITUDE

We have compared the size of the carotid bodies of groups of guinea-pigs, rabbits, and dogs from high and low altitudes and found those from high altitudes to be significantly larger (Edwards *et al.* 1971*b*; see Fig. 7.11). In guinea-pigs and dogs the enlargement is associated with the appearance of large numbers of chief cells of the light variety.

The carotid bodies of the llama and alpaca are small and show a quiescent histology of large chief cells and elongated sustentacular cells (Fig. 7.12; Heath *et al.* 1985).

In cattle Arias-Stella and Bustos (1976) reported a proliferation of light chief cells such as they have seen in native highlanders. In contrast, we have found focal collections of the dark variant of chief cells in the carotid bodies of cattle from Cerro de Pasco (4330 m) (Heath *et al.* 1985; Fig. 7.13).

No state comparable to a 'blunted' ventilatory response to hypoxia has been found in animals living at high altitude. A normal ventilatory response has been reported in cattle (Lahiri 1971), in the dog (Lefrançois *et al.* 1968), and in the llama (Brooks and Tenney 1968). Lahiri (1971) found that yaks, sheep, and goats born and raised at high altitude in the Himalaya showed hypoxic responses comparable to those of sea-level man and unlike those of the native highlander. All of these animals, like the Andean camelids, may be regarded as indigenous mountain animals and adapted genetically to the environment (Chapter 35). Occasionally, cattle may show some depression of ventilation with time during exposure to hypoxia. Attempts to produce

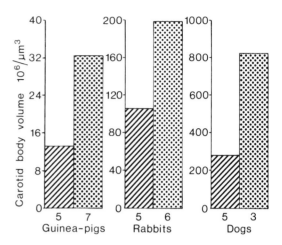

7.11 *Mean size of the left carotid body (in 10^6 μm^3) in guinea-pigs, rabbits, and dogs born and bred at low and high altitude, respectively. The low-altitude animals are represented by hatched columns and the high-altitude animals by stippled columns. The numbers of animals studied in each of the six groups are indicated beneath the columns. The size of the carotid body is larger at high altitude in each of the three species. Data from Edwards* et al. *(1971b).)*

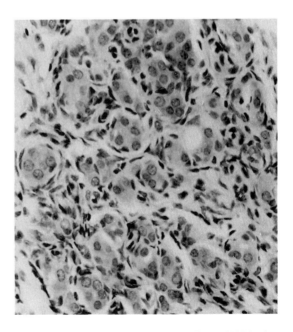

7.12 *Carotid body of alpaca from La Raya (4200 m) in the Peruvian Andes showing clusters of chief cells, with round prominent nuclei, separated by intervening sustentacular cells with elongated nuclei. HE, × 375*

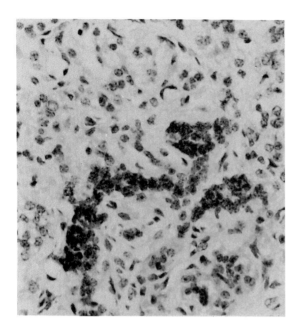

7.13 *Carotid body of cow from Cerro de Pasco (4330 m) in the Peruvian Andes. Large groups of the dark variants of chief cells are seen. This may represent an early cellular response to hypobaric hypoxia during their transit through the mountains. HE, × 375.*

hypoxic blunting in the laboratory have had limited success (Barer *et al.* 1986). Temporary blunting that persists for a few days only on return to normoxia has been produced in rats (Barer *et al.* 1976) and cats (Tenney and Ou 1977). In contrast, highlanders who return to sea level retain their poor response to hypoxia and it is disputed as to whether there is a changed response in patients whose congenital cardiac defects have been corrected by surgery. Some athletes are also said to have a blunted ventilatory response to hypoxia (Barer *et al.* 1986). We have found that at moderate altitude (3370 m) the earliest histological response to hypobaric hypoxia of rabbits occurred in the carotid bodies. This altitude failed to induce muscularization of the pulmonary arterioles in these animals. The change in the chemoreceptor took the form of an increase in the number of the dark variant of chief cells after 3 months that returned to normal after 6 months (Smith *et al.* 1993).

CHEMODECTOMAS AT HIGH ALTITUDE

An increased incidence of chemodectoma at altitude has been reported many times. Morfit *et al.* (1953) reported a series of 12 patients with carotid body tumours seen over a period of 14 years in a tumour clinic of the University of Colorado, but they did not associate this prevalence with the high altitude of the city (1610 m). However, 20 years later Saldaña *et al.* (1973) reported a series of cases of chemodectoma in 25 Peruvian adults, all but two of whom had been born and lived at altitudes between 2105 and 4350 m above sea level, whereas only 38% of the Peruvian population of 13.5 million at that time had lived at or about an altitude of 3000 m according to the Peruvian census of 1966. These authors believed that carotid body tumours are 10 times more frequent at high altitude than at sea level. In their series they found that females predominated over males by about six to one and left-sided tumours were three times more prevalent.

Histologically the tumour cells were arranged in classic 'Zellballen' of chief cells but it is of special interest that Saldaña *et al.* (1973) reported a predominance of dark cells. As we have noted, the dark variant of the chief cell is known to become prominent in diseases and environmental conditions predisposing to chronic hypoxaemia. When the effects of hypobaric hypoxia inherent in life at high altitude are buttressed by alveolar hypoxia, brought about by lung disease, the hypoxic stimulus thought to be responsible for carotid body hyperplasia and perhaps subsequent development of chemodectoma is likely to be enhanced. In this respect Saldaña and his colleagues (1973) reported the occurrence of bilateral carotid body tumours in a 29-year-old Quechua Indian who had worked at an altitude of 3870 m as a miner in the Andes, where he developed silicosis. Perhaps stimulated by the proposed association of increased numbers of carotid body tumours at high altitude, Gaylis and Mieny (1977) subsequently reported that no fewer than 27 chemodectomas were encountered in 25 patients seen in a surgical unit in Johannesburg Hospital at an altitude of 1800 m. This is a moderate degree of altitude which is lower than that considered by Saldaña and his associates to be of significance. Rodriguez-Cuevas *et al.* (1986) reported that, over a period of 21 years at an oncology head and neck clinic in Mexico City (2380 m), 40 patients were diagnosed as having paragangliomas, 87% of them being carotid body tumours. All of them were residents of Mexico City or neighbouring communities on a plateau with a mean altitude of 2000 to 2500 m above sea level. They noted that no fewer than 38 (95%) of their patients were women who accounted for only 52% of the patients attending the clinic. This propensity of the tumour for women is reminiscent of similar findings by

Saldaña *et al.* (1973). Rodriguez-Cuevas and his colleagues (1986) noted that, in the reported series of patients at high altitude with paragangliomas, no malignant tumours had been reported. They were of the opinion that at high altitude carotid body tumours appeared later in life and they thought it likely that they might represent carotid body hyperplasia rather than neoplasia. Pachecho-Ojeda *et al.* (1988) reported a high prevalence of carotid body tumours at high altitude in Ecuador. The hospital from which this report came provided care to workers and to some Indian peasants, mostly from the Andean region, living at altitudes of between 2000 and 4000 m. Twenty carotid body tumours were operated on in 19 patients over a period of 5 years. The series comprised 5 men and 14 women. Nine were from Quito (2800 m) and 10 were from other Andean provinces; all of the patients lived at high altitude. It has to be kept in mind that, while the increased prevalence of chemodectomas in the Andes may be a reflection of chronic stimulation by hypobaric hypoxia, an alternative explanation may be an inherent genetic susceptibility to the tumours in Quechua and Aymara Indians.

Albores-Saavedra and Durán (1968) reported the association of chemodectoma with thyroid carcinoma in two patients in Mexico City (2380 m). In these cases the carcinomas were of papillary and follicular type, in contradistinction to the medullary carcinoma of the thyroid that occurs in association with phaeochromocytoma. The carotid body and the adrenal medulla share a common origin from neural ectoderm and a common function in secretion of catecholamines. Two of the patients from the Andes with chemodectomas, reported by Saldaña and Salem (1970) and Saldaña *et al.* 1973), died of metastasizing thyroid carcinoma.

It has been claimed that cattle as well as man show the same tendency to develop chemodectomas at high altitude. Arias-Stella and Bustos (1976) stated that as many as 40% of cattle living at an elevation of 4330 m in the vicinity of Cerro de Pasco in the Andes of Central Peru develop histological changes in their carotid bodies suggestive of chemodectomas.

CLINICAL APPLICATIONS

Just as the carotid bodies enlarge in response to hypobaric hypoxia in highlanders, so they do in response to alveolar hypoxia resulting from chronic obstructive lung disease. In a series of 44 subjects with pulmonary emphysema coming to routine necropsy (Edwards *et al.* 1971*a*), we point-counted lungs fixed in distension, so that the type and severity of the emphysema could be determined accurately. Thirteen of these cases had no 'significant' emphysema, arbitrarily taken to be 5% or more of centrilobular emphysema or 10% or more of the alveolar duct or panacinar variety, and in them the mean combined weight of the carotid bodies was 21.1 mg. Eleven of the remaining 31 subjects had significant emphysema. In four of them the right ventricular weight was normal and the mean combined carotid body weight was 32.4 mg. In seven of the emphysematous subjects there was right ventricular hypertrophy and the mean combined carotid body weight was 56.2 mg. In one case in this latter group the combined carotid body weight was 89.3 mg. In the remaining 20 subjects in this series there was systemic hypertension, which in itself has an effect on the carotid bodies, and they are accordingly not considered further here.

The lack of relation between the type and severity of the pulmonary emphysema on the one hand and the weight of the carotid bodies on the other makes it clear that the lung disease *per se* does not lead to enlargement of the glomic tissue. Rather, the increase in size occurred only in those cases with right ventricular hypertrophy that followed increased pulmonary vascular resistance associated with alveolar hypoxia. Hence the basic cause of enlargement of the carotid bodies in pulmonary emphysema is the same as that operating in man and animals at high altitude, namely hypoxaemia.

Chronic alveolar hypoxia occurring as a complication of cardiopulmonary pathology can also lead to chemodectoma formation, with or without the exaggerating hypoxia of diminished barometric pressure of high altitude. Chedid and Jao (1974) reported the occurrence of 11 chemodectomas of the carotid body and one vagal paraganglioma in six members of two consecutive generations of a family. All affected members had bilateral tumours of the carotid bodies, with a single exception. No fewer than four of these patients had associated chronic obstructive lung disease which had led to persistent hypoxaemia and hypercarbia.

The same considerations as to the cellular and pharmacological environment of the nerve network in the carotid body apply in various forms of cardiac disease just as they do in the neonatal period and in native highlanders. These relationships are illustrated in the schema comprising Fig. 7.14. Patients with congenital cardiac disease are commonly cyanotic and hypoxaemic for the whole of their lives. This occurs in such conditions as Fallot's tetralogy and after the development of a reversed in-

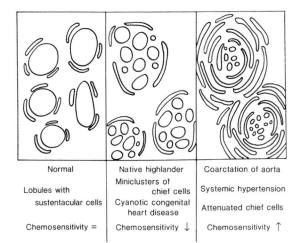

Normal	Native highlander	Coarctation of aorta
Lobules with sustentacular cells	Miniclusters of chief cells	Systemic hypertension
	Cyanotic congenital heart disease	Attenuated chief cells
Chemosensitivity =	Chemosensitivity ↓	Chemosensitivity ↑

7.14 *Schema to illustrate the relation between the level of chemosensitivity and the cellular environment of the nerve network of the carotid body. In the fetus at a late stage of gestation the carotid body, consisting of lobules of chief cells with surrounding sustentacular cells, functions vigorously in a hypoxic environment. On the day of birth fetal dopamine levels paralyse the carotid body by inhibiting the carotid sinus nerve. In the succeeding 2 or 3 days dopamine turnover in the glomus falls and chemosensitivity rises, reset to the less hypoxic environment. In the second column is the situation in the native highlander where there are numerous miniclusters of chief cells capable of producing dopamine and thus depressing chemosensitivity. The same occurs with chief cell hyperplasia in cyanotic congenital heart disease. In the third column is the situation in coarctation of the aorta where concentric rings of sustentacular cells compress remaining groups of attenuated chief cells. Under such conditions of systemic hypertension chemosensitivity has been reported to be increased.*

tracardiac shunt such as with a large ventricular septal defect and patent ductus arteriosus. Such patients show chief cell hyperplasia just as do subjects with cystic fibrosis (Lack *et al.* 1985). Such cellular changes are associated with a blunted ventilatory response to hypoxia occurring in cyanotic congenital heart disease (Sørensen and Severinghaus 1968c; Edelman *et al.* 1970; see Fig. 7.14).

The reverse appears to be the case where the fully developed nerve network of the carotid body finds itself in an environment in which the chief cell population is compressed or obliterated by a pro-

nounced proliferation of sustentacular cells. This is to be found in essential systemic hypertension and even more so in coarctation of the aorta where the sustentacular cell hyperplasia may be extreme (Heath *et al.* 1986; see Fig. 7.14). It may be that hypertension exerts a primary deleterious effect on the clusters of chief cells, the proliferation of sustentacular cells being secondary (Heath *et al.* 1986). One of the characteristic histological features in the carotid bodies in the case of coarctation that we reported was a striking dilatation of thin-walled vessels in the glomic clusters. Possibly the transmission of the elevated systemic arterial pressure into the centres of the clusters leads to destruction of the chief cells (Fig. 7.14). It is of interest that, in the face of this destruction of dopamine-producing chief cells in systemic hypertension, chemoreceptor drive to ventilation is increased (Fig. 7.14; Trzebski *et al.* 1982). It is tempting to associate the heightened ventilatory response to hypoxia with proliferation of sustentacular cells and loss of dopamine-producing chief cells.

References

Albores-Saavedra, J. and Durán, M.E (1968). Association of thyroid carcinoma and chemodectoma. *American Journal of Surgery*, **116**, 887

Al-Lami, F. and Murray, R.G. (1968). Fine structure of the carotid body of normal and anoxic rats. *Anatomical Record*, **160**, 697

Arias-Stella, J. (1969). Human carotid body at high altitudes. Item 150 in the sixty-ninth programme and abstracts of the American Association of Pathologists and Bacteriologists, San Francisco, California, USA

Arias-Stella, J. and Bustos, F. (1976). Chronic hypoxia and chemodectomas in bovines at high altitudes. *Archives of Pathology*, **100**, 636

Arias-Stella, J. and Valcarcel, J. (1973). The human carotid body at high altitudes. *Pathologia et Microbiologia*, **39**, 292

Arias-Stella, J. and Valcarcel, J. (1976). Chief cell hyperplasia in the human carotid body at high altitudes. Physiologic and pathologic significance. *Human Pathology*, 7, 361

Barer, G.R., Edwards, C.W., and Jolly, A.I. (1976). Changes in the carotid body and the ventilatory response to hypoxia in chronically hypoxic rats. *Clinical Science*, **50**, 311

Barer, G., Wach, R., Pallot, D., and Bee, D. (1986). Almitrine, hypoxia, systemic hypertension and the carotid body. In *Aspects of Hypoxia* (D. Heath, Ed.). Liverpool; Liverpool University Press, pp. 120–122

Blanco, C.E., Dawes, G.S., Hanson, M.A., and McCooke, H.B. (1984). The response to hypoxia of arterial chemoreceptors in fetal sheep and newborn lambs. *Journal of Physiology*, **351**, 25

Blessing, M.H. and Kaldeweide, J. (1975). Light and electron microscopic observations on the carotid bodies of rats following adaptation to high altitude. *Virchows Archiv B*, **18**, 315

Blessing, M.H. and Wolff, H. (1973). The carotid bodies at simulated high altitude. *Pathologia et Microbiologia*, **39**, 310

Blümcke, S., Rode, J., and Niedorf, H.R. (1967). The carotid body after oxygen deficiency. *Zeitschrift für Zellforschung und Mikroskopische Anatomie*, **80**, 52

Brooks, J.G. III and Tenney, S.M. (1968). Ventilatory response of llama to hypoxia at sea level and high altitude. *Respiration Physiology*, **5**, 269

Chedid, A. and Jao, W. (1974). Hereditary tumours of the carotid bodies and chronic obstructive pulmonary disease. *Cancer*, **33**, 1635

Chen, I.L., Yates, R.D., and Duncan, D. (1969). The effects of reserpine and hypoxia on the amine storing granules of the hamster carotid body. *Journal of Cell Biology*, **42**, 804

Chiodi, H. (1957). Respiratory adaptations to chronic high altitude hypoxia. *Journal of Applied Physiology*, **10**, 81

Cross, K.W. and Malcolm, J.L. (1952). Evidence of carotid body and sinus activity in newborn and foetal animals. *Journal of Physiology*, **118**, 10P

Cross, K.W. and Oppé, T.E. (1952). Effect of inhalation of high and low concentrations of oxygen on respiration of premature infant. *Journal of Physiology*, **117**, 38

Dawes, G.S., Duncan, S.L.B., Lewis, B.V., Merlet, C., Owen-Thomas, J.B., and Reeves, J.T. (1969). Cyanide stimulation of the systemic arterial chemoreceptors in foetal lambs. *Journal of Physiology*, **201**, 117

de Castro, F. (1928). Sur la structure et l'innervation du sinus carotidien de l'homme et des mammifères. Nouveaux faits sur l'innervation et la fonction du glomus caroticum. Études anato-miques et physiologiques. *Trabajos del Laboratorio de Investigaciones Biologicas de la Universidad de Madrid*, **25**, 330

Edelman, N.H., Lahiri, S., Braudo, I., Cherniack, N.S., and Fishman, A.P. (1970). The blunted ventilatory response to hypoxia in cyanotic congenital heart disease. *New England Journal of Medicine*, **282**, 405

Edwards, C., Heath, D., and Harris, P. (1971a). The carotid body in emphysema and left ventricular hypertrophy. *Journal of Pathology*, **104**, 1

Edwards, C., Heath, D., Harris, P., Castillo, Y., Krüger, H., and Arias-Stella, J. (1971b). The carotid body in animals at high altitude. *Journal of Pathology*, **104**, 231

Edwards, C., Heath, D., and Harris, P. (1972). Ultrastructure of the carotid body in high-altitude guinea-pigs. *Journal of Pathology*, **107**, 131

Fishman, M.C., Greene, W.L.,and Platika, D. (1985). Oxygen chemoreception by carotid body cells in culture. *Proceedings of the National Academy of Sciences, USA*, **82**, 1448

Fitch, R., Smith, P., and Heath, D. (1985). Nerve axons in carotid body hyperplasia. *Archives of Pathology and Laboratory Medicine*, **109**, 234

Flenley, D.C. and Millar, J.S. (1967). Ventilatory response in oxygen and carbon dioxide in chronic respiratory failure. *Clinical Science*, **33**, 319

Forster, H.V., Dempsey, J.A., Birnbaum, M.L., Reddan, W.G., Thoden, J.S., Grover, R.F., and Rankin, J. (1969). Comparison of ventilatory response to hypoxic and hypercapnic stimuli in altitude-sojourning lowlanders, lowlanders residing at altitude and native altitude residents. *Federation Proceedings, Federation of American Society for Experimental Biology*, **28**, 1274

Gaylis, H. and Mieny, C.J. (1977). The incidence of malignancy in carotid body tumours. *British Journal of Surgery*, **64**, 885

Grimley, P.M. and Glenner, G.G. (1968). Ultrastructure of the human carotid body. A perspective on the mode of chemoreception. *Circulation*, **37**, 648

Hamburger, B., Ritzen, M., and Wersall, J. (1966). Demonstration of catecholamines and 5-hydroxytryptamine in the human carotid body. *Journal of Pharmacology and Experimental Therapeutics*, **152**, 197

Hanson, M.A., Kumar, D., and Williams, P.A. (1987). Developmental changes in the reflex respiratory response to alterations of F_{IO_2} in the newborn kitten. *Journal of Physiology*, **394**, 69P

Heath, D. and Smith, P. (1992). Normal histology. In *Diseases of the Human Carotid Body*. Heidelberg and London; Springer-Verlag, pp. 15–24

Heath, D., Edwards, C., Winson, M., and Smith, P. (1973). Effects on the right ventricle, pulmonary vasculature, and carotid bodies of the rat on exposure to, and recovery from, simulated high altitude. *Thorax*, **28**, 24

Heath, D., Smith, P., and Jago, R. (1982). Hyperplasia of the carotid body. *Journal of Pathology*, **138**, 115

Heath, D. Smith, P., and Jago, R. (1984). Dark cell proliferation in carotid body hyperplasia. *Journal of Pathology*, **142**, 39

Heath, D., Smith, P., Fitch, R., and Harris, P. (1985). Comparative pathology of the enlarged carotid body. *Journal of Comparative Pathology*, **95**, 259

Heath, D., Smith, P., and Hurst, G. (1986). The carotid bodies in coarctation of the aorta. *British Journal of Diseases of the Chest*, **80**, 122

Heath, D., Quinzanini, M., Rodella, A., Albertini, A., Ferrari, R., and Harris, P. (1988). Immunoreactivity to various peptides in the human carotid body. *Research Communications in Chemical Pathology and Pharmacology*, **62**, 289

Hellström, S. and Pequignot, J.M. (1985). Beta-adrenergic blockade during long-term hypoxia. Effects on carotid body. A structural and biochemical study. Programme abstract in *8th International Symposium on the Peripheral Arterial Chemoreceptors*, Oeiras, Portugal

Hertzberg, T., Hellström, S., Lagercrantz, H., and Pequignot, M. (1990). Development of the arterial chemoreflex and turnover of carotid body catecholamines in the newborn rat. *Journal of Physiology*, **425**, 211

Heymans, C., Bouckaert, J.J., and Dautrebande, L. (1930). Sinus carotidien et réflexes respiratoires: influences respiratoires réflexes de l'acidose, de l'alcalose, de l'anhydride carbonique, de l'ion hydrogène et de l'anoxémie. Sinus carotidiens et échanges respiratoires dans les poumons et au dela les poumons. *Archives Internationales de Pharmacodynamie et de Thérapie*, **39**, 400

Hurst, G., Heath, D., and Smith, P. (1985). Histological changes associated with ageing of the human carotid body. *Journal of Pathology*, **147**, 181.

Khan, Q., Heath, D., Smith, P., and Norboo, T. (1988). The histology of the carotid bodies in highlanders from Ladakh. *International Journal of Biometeorology*, **32**, 254

Lack, E.E., Perez-Atayde, A.R., and Young, J.B. (1985). Carotid body hyperplasia in cystic fibrosis and cyanotic heart disease. A combined morphometric, ultrastructural, and biochemical study. *American Journal of Pathology*, **119**, 301

Lahiri, S. (1971). Genetic aspect of the blunted chemoreflex ventilatory response to hypoxia in high altitude adaptation. In *High Altitude Physiology: Cardiac and Respiratory Aspects*, Ciba Foundation Symposium (R. Porter and J. Knight, Ed.). Edinburgh; Churchill Livingstone, p. 103

Lahiri, S. and Milledge, J.S. (1965). Sherpa physiology. *Nature, London*, **207**, 610

Lahiri, S., Kao, F.F., Velasquez, T., Martinez, C., and Pezzia, W. (1969). Irreversible blunted respiratory sensitivity to hypoxia in high altitude natives. *Respiration Physiology*, **6**, 360

Laidler, P. and Kay, J.M. (1975*a*). A quantitative morphological study of the carotid bodies of rats living at a simulated altitude of 4300 m, *Journal of Pathology*, **117**, 183

Laidler, P. and Kay, J.M. (1975*b*). The effect of chronic hypoxia on the number and nuclear diameter of type I cells in the carotid bodies of rats. *American Journal of Pathology*, **79**, 311

Laidler, P. and Kay, J.M. (1978*a*). Ultrastructure of carotid body in rats living at a simulated altitude of 4300 metres. *Journal of Pathology*, **124**, 27

Laidler, P. and Kay, J.M. (1978*b*). A quantitative study of some ultrastructural features of the type I cells in the carotid bodies of rats living at a simulated altitude of 4300 metres. *Journal of Neurocytology*, **7**, 183

Lefrançois, R., Gautier, H., and Pasquis, P. (1968). Ventilatory oxygen drive in acute and chronic hypoxia. *Respiration Physiology*, **4**, 217

McDonald, D.M. (1981). Peripheral chemoreceptors. Structure function relationships of the carotid body. In *Regulation of Breathing* (T.F. Hornbein, Ed.). New York; Marcel Dekker, p. 105

Miller, H.C. and Smull, N.W. (1955). Further studies on the effects of hypoxia on the respiration of newborn infants. *Pediatrics, Springfield*, **16**, 93

Møller, M., Møllgard, K., and Sørensen, S.C. (1974). The ultrastructure of the carotid body in chronically hypoxic rats. *Journal of Physiology (London)*, **238**, 447

Morfit, H.H., Swan, H., and Taylor, E.R. (1953). Carotid body tumors. *Archives of Surgery*, **67**, 194

Pachecho-Ojeda, L., Durango, E., Rodriquez, C., and Vivar, N. (1988). Carotid body tumors at high altitudes: Quito, Ecuador, 1987. *World Journal of Surgery*, **12**, 856

Pugh, L.G.C.E., Gill, M.B., Lahiri, S., Milledge, J.S., Ward, M.P., and West, J.B. (1964). Muscular exercise at great altitudes. *Journal of Applied Physiology*, **19**, 431

Ramaswamy, S.S. (1962). In *International Symposium on Problems of High Altitude* (S.P. Bhatia, Ed.). New Delhi; Indian Armed Forces Medical Services, p. 74

Richards, D.W., Fritts, H.W. Jr, and Davis, A.L. (1968). Observations on the control of respiration in emphysema: the effects of oxygen on ventilatory response to CO_2 inhalation. *Transactions of the Association of American Physicians*, **71**, 142

Rodriguez-Cuevas, H., Lau, I., and Rodriguez, H.P. (1986). High-altitude paragangliomas: diagnostic and therapeutic considerations. *Cancer*, **57**, 672

Saldaña, M.J. and Salem, L.E. (1970). High altitude hypoxia and chemodectomas. *American Journal of Pathology*, **59**, 91a

Saldaña, M.J., Salem, L.E., and Travezan, R. (1973). High altitude hypoxia and chemodectomas. *Human Pathology*, **4**, 251

Severinghaus, J.W., Bainton, C.P., and Carcelen, A. (1966). Respiratory insensitivity to hypoxia in chronically hypoxic man. *Respiration Physiology*, **1**, 308

Sime, F. (1973). Ventilacion humana en hipoxia cronica. Etiopatogenia de la Enfermedad de Monge a desadaptacion cronica a la altura. Unpublished D.Phil. thesis, Universidad Peruana Cayetano Heredia, Lima, Peru

Smith, P. (1986). Electron microscopy of the abnormal carotid body. In *Aspects of Hypoxia* (D. Heath, Ed.). Liverpool; Liverpool University Press, p. 81

Smith, P., Jago, R., and Heath, D. (1982). Anatomical variation and quantitative histology of the normal and enlarged carotid body. *Journal of Pathology*, **137**, 287

Smith, P., Jago, R., and Heath, D. (1984). Glomic cells and blood vessels in the hyperplastic carotid bodies of spontaneously hypertensive rats. *Cardiovascular Research*, **18**, 471

Smith, P., Heath, D. Fitch, R., Hurst, G., Moore, D., and Weitzenblum, E. (1986*a*). Effects on the rabbit carotid body of stimulation by almitrine, natural high altitude, and experimental normobaric hypoxia. *Journal of Pathology*, **149**, 143

Smith, P., Hurst, G., Heath, D., and Drewe, R. (1986*b*). The carotid bodies in a case of ventricular septal defect. *Histopathology*, **10**, 831

Smith, P., Gosney, J., Heath, D., and Burnett, H. (1990). The occurrence and distribution of certain polypetides within the human carotid body. *Cell and Tissue Research*, **261**, 565

Smith, P., Heath, D., Williams, D., Bencini, C., Pulera, N., and Giuntini, C. (1993). The earliest histopathological response to hypobaric hypoxia in rabbits in the Rifugio Torino (3370 m) on Monte Bianco. *Journal of Pathology*, **170**, 485

Sørensen, S.C. and Severinghaus, J.W. (1968*a*). Irreversible respiratory insensitivity to acute hypoxia in man born at high altitude. *Journal of Applied Physiology*, **25**, 217

Sørensen, S.C. and Severinghaus, J.W. (1968*b*). Respiratory sensitivity to acute hypoxia in man born at sea level living at high altitude. *Journal of Applied Physiology*, **25**, 211

Sørensen, S.C. and Severinghaus, J.W. (1968*c*). Respiratory insensitivity to acute hypoxia persisting after correction of tetralogy of Fallot. *Journal of Applied Physiology*, **25**, 221

Steele, R.H. and Hinterberger, J. (1972). Catecholamines and 5-hydroxytryptamine in the carotid body in vascular, respiratory and other diseases. *Journal of Laboratory and Clinical Medicine*, **80**, 63

Tenney, S.M. and Ou, L.C. (1977). Hypoxic ventilatory response of cats at high altitude, and interpretation of blunting. *Respiration Physiology*, **30**, 185

Trzebski, A., Tafil, M., Zoltowski, M., and Przybylski, J. (1982). Increased sensitivity of the arterial chemoreceptor drive in young men with mild hypertension. *Cardiovascular Research*, **16**, 163

Wang, Z.Z., He, L., Stensaas, L.J., Dinger, B.G., and Fidone, S.J. (1991). Localization and in vitro actions of atrial natriuretic peptide in the cat carotid body. *Journal of Applied Physiology*, **70**, 942

8

Haemoglobins

Haemoglobin is responsible for the transport and release of oxygen to the tissues. In man at sea level two main types of haemoglobin are to be found and they predominate at different stages of life. That found during fetal life has a high affinity for oxygen, but after birth it is replaced by a type that releases the gas more readily. It is thus of considerable interest to see which of these two forms has been selected to sustain human life in the hypobaric hypoxia of high altitude. Various abnormal haemoglobins are recognized at sea level and, when they present at high altitude, they may have serious clinical and pathological consequences.

HbA AND HbF

Haemoglobin is a globular protein of molecular weight 64 000, consisting of two pairs of coiled polypeptide chains and four haem groups, one being attached to each of the four chains. The haem groups transport the oxygen, while the surrounding globin provides a suitable environment for this to be achieved. The two types of haemoglobin employed in the hypoxic fetal and eupoxic adult stages of life at sea level are determined by the amino acid sequence in the polypeptide chains. Four different chains occur normally in adults and they are termed α, β, γ, and δ. Normal haemoglobins consist of a pair of α chains and another pair of β, γ, or δ chains. Alpha chains contain 141 amino acids and the others each contain 146 (Rowan 1985). Each globin chain has a spiral configuration and the constituent amino acids are located both internally as non-polar, non-charged radicals and externally as polar, charged radicals. The internal amino acids of the polypeptides are vital for the structure and function of the chain, forming an internal scaffold that preserves the rigidity and stability of the tertiary configuration (Rowan 1985).

In the normal fetus at sea level the hypoxaemia is so profound that it would take an altitude of 7500 m to produce the same level of arterial oxygen tension in an adult. Under these physiological conditions the haemoglobin is HbF ($\alpha_2\gamma_2$) which has a high affinity

for oxygen. It is rapidly lost on the transition to the eupoxic conditions of extrauterine life. By the age of 1 year, 98% of the circulating haemoglobin has become HbA ($\alpha_2\beta_2$), with the remainder consisting of HbA$_2$ ($\alpha_2\delta_2$). HbA releases oxygen to the tissues more readily than HbF.

On exposure to the hypobaric hypoxia of high altitude the process of acclimatization in man involves an increased level of adult haemoglobin, HbA, which enhances the volume of oxygen transported to the tissues (Chapter 5). Here, increased concentrations of intraerythrocytic organic phosphates such as 2,3-DPG facilitate its release to the tissues. It should be noted that acclimatization to high altitude in man does not involve a return to fetal haemoglobin, HbF, in spite of the hypoxic conditions. Furthermore, it does not involve the advent of a new haemoglobin. Even in native highlanders the prolonged natural acclimatization is characterized by increased levels of normal adult haemoglobin rather than by the reappearance of fetal haemoglobin. Thus, it has been shown that HbA remains the predominant form in the Sherpas of the Himalaya. Adams and Strang (1975) studied the haemoglobins of 28 men (mean age 30 years) and 23 women (mean age 35 years), all of pure Tibetan ancestry. They found the prevalent haemoglobin was HbA. HbA$_2$ accounted for only $2.96 \pm 0.58\%$ and HbF for only $0.9 \pm 0.30\%$.

It would appear, however, that in contrast to acclimatized species, such as man, the indigenous mountain animals that show genetic *adaptation* to high altitude (Chapter 35) do retain a high percentage of fetal haemoglobin in their blood. Thus, Reynafarje *et al.* (1975), employing the alkali denaturation technique of Singer *et al.* (1951), found that 50% of the haemoglobin of adult alpacas was HbF. The percentage was even higher in newborn alpacas (Fig. 8.1). This retention of HbF in adapted as contrasted to acclimatized animals means that the blood in such species as the alpaca and llama has a high affinity for oxygen. The oxygen–haemoglobin dissociation curve lies to the left of that of man (Chapter 35). A high systemic arterial oxygen saturation is maintained,

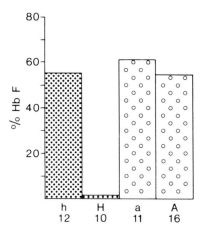

8.1 *Percentage of HbF in Quechua newborns (at 1 week of age) (h), and adults (H), newborn alpacas (at 1 week of age) (a), and adult alpacas (A). The number at the foot of each column represents the number of subjects studied in that category. (From data of Reynafarje et al. (1975).)*

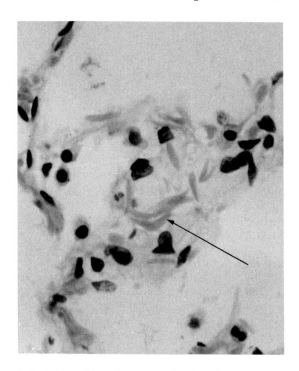

8.2 *Section of lung from a man in his early twenties who died in sickle-cell crisis associated with bronchopneumonia. Typical sickle cells are seen (arrow). In this case the crisis occurred at low altitude. HE, × 1000.*

but there is a low partial pressure of oxygen in venous blood. The extraction of oxygen by the tissues is high.

HbS

In HbS the β polypeptide differs from that of normal adult HbA by the substitution of only one amino acid. In one of the repeating eight amino acid groups, valine replaces the normally occurring glutamic acid in the sixth position (Ingram 1956). When the α chains of HbS ($\alpha_2 \beta_2^{6 \, val}$) move apart to give up oxygen, the amino acid substitution results in locking of the adjacent ends of the α chains and the abnormal β chains, and the haemoglobin molecules become stacked in rows (Rowan 1985). This causes distortion of the erythrocytes into a rigid sickle-shaped deformity in deoxygenerated blood (Fig. 8.2).

Individuals who are homozygous for HbS (HbS/S) always have the clinical manifestations of sickle-cell disease. The abnormal gene occurs among Negroes and those of negroid ancestry. The disease is characterized by chronic haemolytic anaemia, painful sickling crises, leg ulceration, and myocardial insufficiency. The crises affect especially the abdomen, bones, and joints and are brought about by occlusion of small blood vessels. One of the sites most frequently affected is the splenic artery and its branches, leading to repeated infarction with fibrous

scarring and contraction of the spleen. This presents clinically as an abdominal crisis.

Heterozygotes (HbA/S) develop symptoms only under certain circumstances and are said to have the sickle-cell trait. In particular, significant sickling with abdominal crises can occur if such individuals are subjected to severe and prolonged hypoxia such as ascent to high altitude and travel in unpressurized aircraft. Combinations of HbS with other variants are not uncommon. The most frequent, HbS/C, results in features very similar to those of sickle-cell disease in HbS/S individuals and is of particular importance with regard to air travel. The severity of haemolysis and anaemia is modified by elevation in the HbF concentration.

SICKLE-CELL TRAIT AT HIGH ALTITUDE

In sickle-cell disease, 80–100% of the haemoglobin is in the S form, the remainder being HbA (Robbins 1967), and homozygous subjects (HbS/S) have symptoms at sea level. In contrast, heterozygous subjects with the sickle-cell trait (HbA/S) have only

20–40% HbS and they are likely to be asymptomatic at sea level but susceptible to abdominal crises at high altitude. In other words, red cells with 100% HbS will sickle at normal oxygen tensions, but as the level of HbS falls there needs to be progressively lower oxygen tension to induce sickling.

In Peru many Negroes live on the coast and they are able to reach altitudes exceeding 4000 m in a few hours by car or train. Such conditions of hypobaric hypoxia are ideal for the development of deoxygenation and the abdominal crises of sickling. There is in fact a quaint Peruvian saying to the effect that 'Blackbirds do not sing well in the Andes'. Monge and Monge (1966) refer to the clinical observations of Aste-Salazar who reported that the subjects are usually in good health when setting out for destinations at high altitude. After 2 hours' travel by train or car and at altitudes between 3500 and 4500 m they often develop acute abdominal pain. When they are brought to sea level and investigated, they are found to have haemoglobins of both A and S type, indicative of the sickle-cell trait. The disease may be partly responsible for the surprisingly small Negro population inhabiting the Peruvian Andes and this despite the accessibility of the mountains and the long-established settlement of Negroes on the coast.

An illustrative example of the dangers facing heterozygous subjects with sickle-cell trait ascending into the mountains was provided by Goldberg *et al.* (1985). They report the onset of abdominal crises in two Caucasian subjects, father and son, in the moderate altitude of the south-west of the USA. There was no evidence of miscegenation by their progenitors. An 18-year-old youth travelled by bus for 36 hours from sea level to Santa Fe, New Mexico (2134 m). Two hours before the end of the journey at 2195 m he became nauseated and had a sharp pain in the left side of his abdomen that prevented his breathing deeply. Findings on examination by ultrasound were consistent with a necrotic spleen and an abdominal angiogram showed complete occlusion of the splenic artery. Quantitative haemoglobin electrophoresis showed the following pattern: HbA 51.4%; HbA₂ 2.8%; HbS 45.8%. Splenectomy was carried out and revealed an enlarged and grossly infarcted spleen. Splenic erythrocyte morphology was consistent with sickle-cell haemoglobinopathy. Eleven days after operation he was sent home by car with instructions to use oxygen at 3 litres per minute until he had descended to an altitude below 610 m to prevent further sickling.

The patient's father was 37 years old. On hearing of his son's illness, he travelled to Santa Fe by car, arriving there 24 hours later. Soon after arrival at 2134 m he also experienced abdominal pain that localized in the left upper quadrant. He became short of breath. A liver–spleen scan suggested infarction of the spleen, perhaps with rupture. Peritoneal lavage returned grossly blood-stained fluid. Quantitative haemoglobin electrophoresis showed the following pattern: HbA 55%; HbA₂ 3.4%; HbS 41%; HbCA₁ 0.6%. Splenectomy was carried out and the spleen was found to be infarcted and spontaneously ruptured. Sections of the spleen revealed grossly congested sinuses filled with abnormally shaped erythrocytes that appeared sickled. Sugarman *et al.* (1990) reported pulmonary embolism and splenic infarction in a 43-year-old Black man with sickle-cell trait documented by haemoglobin electrophoresis (39% Hb S). They presumed that the additional hypoxaemia due to the embolism created a local splenic environment which permitted infarction to occur.

O'Brien *et al.* (1972) described splenic infarction, documented by radioisotopic scan, in a 26-year-old Caucasian man of Sicilian descent while he was hiking at an altitude of only 760 m. Electrophoresis demonstrated a HbA/S pattern with 42.4% HbS and 0.5% HbF.

It has been suggested that 'autosplenectomy' early in childhood, due to repeated episodes of splenic arterial thrombosis, splenic infarction, and fibrosis, with progressive shrinkage of the organ, probably protects HbS/S patients against splenic infarction at high altitudes (Mahony and Githens 1979). Goldberg *et al.* (1985) were able to find only two reported cases of altitude-associated splenic infarction in a patient with HbS/S. One was in a 9-year-old Black boy travelling in the Colorado mountains above 2000 m (Mahony and Githens 1979). The other was in a man from Saudi Arabia travelling by commercial aircraft (Claster *et al.* 1981).

SPLENIC INFARCTION DURING AIR TRAVEL

Splenic infarction may occur in passengers with the sickle-cell trait flying in non- or inadequately pressurized aircraft. All modern aircraft have pressurized cabins, so that, irrespective of the height at which they fly, the pressure in the cabin rarely falls below that appropriate to an altitude of only 1520–1830 m, which is about the altitude of Zermatt in the Swiss Alps. Even so, Green *et al.* (1971) recommended that patients with the sickle-cell trait use oxygen continuously at standard cruising altitudes in pressurized cabins and that they should not fly at all in unpressurized aircraft.

Six Negro soldiers were reported to have developed nausea, vomiting, fever, and pain in the left upper abdomen during prolonged flights in unpressurized aircrafts at altitudes between 3050 m and 4570 m (Cooley *et al.* 1954). Previously all were in good health, with no manifestations of sickle-cell disease. Subsequently, other cases of splenic infarction were observed in military hospitals and this led Smith and Conley (1955) to obtain, for electrophoretic study, blood from 15 persons who developed splenic infarction during flight. Although 12 proved to have the sickle-cell trait (HbA/S), three had HbC in combination (HbS/C). In 11 of these subjects with splenic infarction, the amount of normal haemoglobin exceeded that of sickle haemoglobin, which is the pattern expected in the sickle-cell trait. None of the 15 persons was suspected of having sickling prior to the onset of splenic infarction. The flights leading to the abdominal crises were usually taken in unpressurized aircraft between 3050 and 4570 m, although in two instances splenic infarction occurred on commercial flights as low as between 1220 and 1830 m. Both of these subjects showed the HbS/C combination.

Since 8% of American Blacks have the sickle-cell trait it would seem that the development of splenic infarction during flight is not rare. The combination of HbS/C is, however, extremely uncommon, requiring the inheritance of both a gene for sickling and one for HbC. It has now emerged that about a quarter of persons who develop splenic infarcts at high altitudes have HbS/C disease. Air travel presents a considerable hazard to persons with this combination of abnormal haemoglobins and should disqualify them from flying. Routine tests to detect sickling are often unreliable and electrophoresis of the haemoglobin should be used to detect the susceptible.

SPLENIC SEQUESTRATION AND PSEUDOCYST

Occasionally splenic scans do not confirm the presence of splenic infarction but suggest that symptoms are due to 'splenic sequestration' of sickled cells. An acute splenic sequestration crisis is characterized by sudden trapping of the abnormal cells within the spleen, which increases in size, a drop in haemoglobin concentration, and hypovolaemia, which may cause shock and lead to death. Githens *et al.* (1977) reported five cases of the syndrome in children with HbS/C disease in association with a change in altitude. In four of them it occurred during or immediately following a trip to elevations greater than 2740 m. In the fifth child the crisis developed 10 days after travel in a pressurized aircraft from sea level to Denver (1600 m). Since 1970, only 16 cases of acute splenic sequestration crisis have been reported in patients with S/C disease who were not exposed to high altitude (Michel *et al.* 1992). Nine of these were children and adolescents aged 11 to 18 years while seven were adults aged 21 to 53 years. Michel *et al.* (1992) reported the sudden death of a 53-year-old Black woman with the syndrome at low altitude.

Rywlin and Benson (1961) reported massive necrosis of the spleen, resulting in a pseudocyst, in a White Peruvian youth aged 19 years with the sickle-cell trait, after a car trip to the Andes at an altitude of 4570 m. A sickle-cell preparation was positive. Electrophoresis revealed HbA 61.35%, HbF 0.25%, and HbS 38.40%. The patient inherited the HbS from his mother who was an Argentinian and did not manifest any negroid features. The father was born in Belgium and had HbA only. Sickle-cell haemoglobinopathy was discovered in a White Jewish family, an event never previously reported, when one of the sons was exposed at high altitude (3540 m) to strenuous physical activity precipitating massive haemorrhagic necrosis of the spleen (Shalev *et al.* 1988). The percentages of the various haemoglobins present were as follows: HbS 46.5%; HbA 50.2%; HbA_2 1.9%; HbF 1.4%.

Individuals with the sickle-cell trait who reside at moderate altitude (1600 m) do not develop impairment of splenic reticuloendothelial function as assessed qualitatively by radionuclide scanning (Nuss *et al.* 1991). The development of systemic hypertension and splenic infarction was reported by Narasimhan *et al.* (1990) in a man of 24 years with sickle-cell trait soon after travel to high altitude. The hypertension persisted for 3 days after a diagnostic laparotomy. The authors considered that sludging of red cells in the small renal blood vessels may have activated the renin–angiotensin system.

METHAEMOGLOBINAEMIA AT HIGH ALTITUDE

In methaemoglobinaemia the ferrous iron of normal haemoglobin is converted into the ferric form and as such it cannot combine with oxygen. Hypoxaemia ensues and as a result secondary polycythaemia may develop. Ferric iron combines so firmly with one atom of oxygen that the gas is not liberated even on exposure to a vacuum. Hence metHb has no oxygen-carrying capacity and during recent years it has become apparent that one of the functions of red cell metabolism is to provide reducing potential in order to protect the cell against such oxidation. In view of these considerations it is surprising that methaemoglobin has been reported as being increased at high altitude both in highlanders and indigenous animals such as the llama.

At sea level the condition is usually produced by drugs like nitrites, sulfonamides, phenacetin, acetanilide, aniline, and nitrobenzene (Walters and Israel 1974). The condition may be reversed by reducing agents such as ascorbic acid and methylene blue. Methaemoglobinaemia may also be due to congenital defects in the red cells. Thus one form of haemoglobinopathy is due to HbM, which is oxidized abnormally easily. In this type of methaemoglobinaemia, restorative agents are powerless. Clinically, there is a slate-blue cyanosis and spectroscopic examination is necessary to identify methaemoglobin and distinguish it from reduced haemoglobin.

MetHb has been found in the erythrocytes of subjects living permanently above 3500 m. Its presence does not appear to be due to ingested chemicals or drugs and the existence of HbM has been eliminated as a cause. There is no evidence of NADH-linked methaemoglobin reductase deficiency. Hence in spite of normal red cell metabolism, methaemoglobin levels are abnormally high in low oxygen tension and they return to normal on descent to low altitude. The level of methaemoglobin appears to be inversely related to the red cell count, so that it is much increased in relatively anaemic subjects. Gourdin *et al.* (1975) studied two groups of highlanders. The first consisted of 208 adult Quechuas living at 3500 m in central Peru. The mean methaemoglobin percentage was 5.3 in those with a haemoglobin level between 14 and 21 g/dl, but was 10.9 in anaemic subjects with a haemoglobin level below 14 g/dl (Fig. 8.3). The second group comprised 71 Aymaras and in them the mean methaemoglobin percentage was 2.1 in those with a haemoglobin level exceeding 21 g/dl, 3.7 in those with haemoglobin concentrations between 14 and 21 g/dl, and 9.3 in anaemic subjects with a haemoglobin level beneath 14 g/dl (Fig. 8.3). Methaemoglobin levels of 15–20% have been found in the llama, which has a low haematocrit (Chapter 35). At sea level in some areas where there are such chemicals as nitrites in the soil, the level of methaemoglobin may rise to 1.5%.

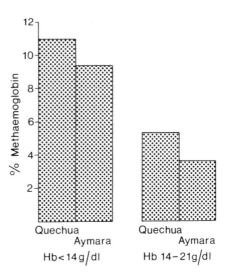

8.3 *Percentage of methaemoglobin in the blood of Quechuas and Aymaras at 3500 m, with haemoglobin levels respectively below and above 14 g/dl. (Based on data from Gourdin* et al. *(1975).)*

The presence of metHb in man and animals at high altitude is unexpected and its inverse proportion to the haemoglobin level even more so (Gourdin *et al.* 1975). As we have noted above, methaemoglobin has no oxygen-carrying capacity and its presence would appear to impose an additional disadvantage on highlanders. Gourdin and co-workers suggest that at very high altitudes the shift of the oxygen–haemoglobin dissociation curve to the right may be too great, so that there is a decrease in oxygen uptake (Chapter 5). They speculate that small amounts of methaemoglobin promote a shift of the curve to the left, thus providing some regulation. The llama has much methaemoglobin and its oxygen dissociation curve is well to the left of that of man. Smith and Ou (1975), on the contrary, believe that the phenomenon represents an adverse effect of altitude and is secondary to an increased rate of haemoglobin autoxidation that increases with decreasing oxygen tensions until it reaches a maximum at oxygen tensions corresponding to haemoglobin half-saturation. Hence at high altitude in the absence of a compensatory increase in metHb reductase activity, methaemoglobin would accumulate. Conceivably this effect might be more pronounced in anaemic than polycythaemic subjects because of the lower venous oxygen tension in the former.

CARBOXYHAEMOGLOBIN

Subjects living at high altitude who smoke cigarettes develop increased levels of haematocrit and haemoglobin compared to non-smoking native highlanders. Spielvogel *et al.* (1990) carried out a pilot study of the effects of smoking on a population at La Paz (3600 m) and published a preliminary paper on their findings at the 7th World Congress on Tobacco and Health in Perth in 1990. They investigated 33 smokers who comprised eight females of mean age 47 years, 10 young males of mean age 32 years, and 15 older males of mean age 51 years. All three groups were heavy smokers of up to 40 cigarettes a day for prolonged periods of up to 40 years or more. Spielvogel *et al.* (1990) found that haematocrit and haemoglobin levels were increased in the females by 5.2% and 3.4%, respectively. In the older males these increases were 12.8% and 8.3%, respectively; no fewer than seven smokers in this group had a haematocrit of 60% or above. The greater the number of cigarettes smoked the higher the level of carboxyhaemoglobin (COHb) saturation and the greater the worsening of hypoxaemia (Table 8.1).

These authors found that smoking at high altitude affects the respiratory more than the cardiovascular system and that females seem to be more susceptible to changes caused by smoking than males. Some of the changes found in respiratory function were the result of the high altitude *per se.* Thus all three groups of subjects studied showed a higher peak flow than that found at sea level, probably because of the lesser air density at high altitude. The expiratory flow was diminished compared to what is found at sea level due to the increased residual volume in the high altitude lung.

At sea level pregnant women who smoke have higher levels of haemoglobin and carboxyhaemoglobin than those who do not (Davies *et al.* 1979). The smokers show a greater affinity of haemoglobin for oxygen with a significantly lower P_{50} and hence a lower availability of oxygen for the tissues per gram of haemoglobin. In pregnant women who stopped smoking there was an immediate reduction in COHb and a decrease in haemoglobin–oxygen affinity, leading to a significant increase of 8% of oxygen available for the tissues within 48 hours (Davies *et al.* 1979).

Maclean (1979) felt that these studies in pregnant women could be applied to the problem of smoking and acclimatization to high altitude. As a smoker he had observed that during skiing and mountaineering he suffered less from the symptoms of acute mountain sickness than his non-smoking companions. He noted that he and several smoking mountaineers either smoked less or stopped smoking completely during these expeditions and all had suffered significantly less from altitude sickness than their non-smoking companions. Such anecdotal evidence is in keeping with a fall in carboxyhaemoglobin levels, a shift of the oxygen–haemoglobin dissociation curve to the right with an elevation of P_{50}, and an increase in the availability of oxygen to the tissues.

Endogenous COHb levels at high altitude

Endogenous carbon monoxide is produced by catabolism of haemoglobin and other haem proteins. In man this leads to an average background COHb level of 0.4–0.7%. Because of competition between oxygen and carbon monoxide for the available

Table 8.1 Effect of the number of cigarettes smoked per day on % carboxyhaemoglobin saturation and arterial oxygen tension (after Spielvogel *et al.* 1990)

Cigarettes/day	% COHb saturation	Pa_{O_2} mmHg
Males		
11.6	1.50	51
19	7.43	48
31	17.55	46.5
Females		
21	12.23	44

haemoglobin the equilibrium level of COHb in the blood depends on arterial oxygen tension as well as the level of carbon monoxide. Thus as arterial oxygen tension falls with increasing altitude the level of COHb becomes greater. McGrath (1992) measured COHb levels in laboratory rats following a 6-week exposure to clean air at simulated altitudes of 1000, 3100, and 4600 m. COHb levels at the three altitudes were 0.68 ($\pm$ 0.09), 1.16 ($\pm$ 0.28), and 1.68 ($\pm$ 0.19) %.

The effects of exogenous carbon monoxide are also greater at high altitude. When McGrath (1992) exposed rats for 6 weeks to air containing 9 ppm carbon monoxide at the same three altitudes, the COHb levels were 0.99 ($\pm$ 0.06)%, 1.77 ($\pm$0.17) %, and 2.10 ($\pm$0.08)%. The increase in erythropoiesis on ascent to high altitude increases the haemoglobin level but it also provides a greater sink for carbon monoxide, which competes against the diminished arterial oxygen tension.

HAEMOGLOBINS IN SHEEP AT HIGH ALTITUDE

The blood of healthy, adult sheep contains two types of haemoglobin, A and B. They are inherited as Mendelian traits and are present in about equal amounts in the blood in heterozygotes (Battaglia *et al.* 1969). In anaemic animals with HbA, a third type of haemoglobin, HbC, appears in large quantities in the blood (Van Vliet and Huisman 1964). This releases oxygen to the tissues more readily than HbA (Huisman and Kitchens 1968). Hence in the sheep we have the unusual situation of one species carrying haemoglobins with widely different haemoglobin–oxygen dissociation curves, with their differing influences on oxygen transport in the blood and oxygen release to the tissues. Battaglia *et al.* (1969) found that at high altitude (4340 m) sheep carrying HbA had a mean systemic arterial oxygen saturation (86.4%) significantly higher than that of HbB carriers (67.5%). The carriers of a mixture of HbA and HbB had an intermediate saturation (77.0%). P_{50} in sheep homozygote for HbA is 31 mmHg compared with that of 27 mmHg for sea-level man, whereas in sheep homozygote for HbB, P_{50} is closer to 40 mmHg. Haemoglobin B appears to be advantageous to sheep at low altitude, for here the Po_2 is sufficient to achieve 90% arterial oxygen saturation while at the same time this type of haemoglobin will ensure a plentiful release of oxygen to the tissues. On the other hand, at high altitude HbA affords an advantageous uptake of oxygen from the lung, although, of course, release of oxygen to the tissues is hindered.

Even so, as we have already noted, the P_{50} of sheep HbA is similar to that of blood from man at sea level.

HAEMOGLOBINS IN THE YAK

The yak (*Bos grunniens*) has two haemoglobins, designated 'fast' and 'slow' (Adams *et al.* 1975). *Hb slow* is unique to the yak in the genus *Bos*, but it is not yet known if it is of any importance in adaptation to high altitude with respect to its affinity for oxygen. The two yak haemoglobins share a common globin chain. Five yaks studied by these authors show the identical ratio of 38:62 of slow to fast Hb. *Hb slow* is prone to methaemoglobin formation, as described above in relation to highlanders and llamas. The erythrocytes of the yak show no tendency to sickling.

References

Adams, W.H. and Strang, L.J. (1975). Hemoglobin levels in persons of Tibetan ancestry living at high altitude. *Proceedings of the Society for Experimental Biology and Medicine*, **149**, 1036

Adams, W.H., Graves, I.L., and Pyakural, S. (1975). Hematologic observations on the yak. *Proceedings of the Society for Experimental Biology and Medicine*, **148**, 701

Battaglia, F.C., Behrman, R.E., De Lannoy, C.W., Hathaway, W., Makowski, E.L., Meschia, G., Seeds, A.E., and Schruefer, J.J.P. (1969). Exposure to high altitude of sheep with different haemoglobins. *Quarterly Journal of Experimental Physiology*, **54**, 423

Claster, S., Godwin, M.J., and Embury, S.H. (1981). Risk of altitude exposure in sickle cell disease. *Western Journal of Medicine*, **135**, 364

Cooley, J.C., Peterson, W.L., Engel, C.E., and Jernigan, J.P. (1954). Clinical triad of massive splenic infarction, sicklemia trait, and high altitude flying. *Journal of the American Medical Association*, **154**, 111

Davies, J.M., Latto, I.P., Jones, J.G., Veale, A., and Wardrop, C.A.J. (1979). Effects of stopping smoking for 48 hours on oxygen availability from the blood: a study of pregnant women. *British Medical Journal*, **ii**, 355

Githens, J.H., Gross, G.P., Eife, R.F., and Wallner, S.F. (1977). Splenic sequestration syndrome at mountain altitudes in sickle/haemoglobin C disease. *Journal of Pediatrics*, **90**, 203

Goldberg, N.M., Dorman, J.P., Riley, C.A., and Armbruster, E.J. (1985). Altitude-related splenic infarction in sickle cell trait. Case reports of a father and son. *Western Journal of Medicine*, **143**, 670

Gourdin, D., Vergnes, H., and Gutierez, N. (1975). Methaemoglobin in man living at high altitude. *British Journal of Haematology*, **29**, 243

Green, R.L., Huntsman, R.G., and Serjeant, G.R. (1971). The sickle-cell and altitude. *British Medical Journal*, **4**, 593

Huisman, T.H.J. and Kitchens, J. (1968). Oxygen equilibria studies of the hemoglobins from normal and anemic sheep and goats. *American Journal of Physiology*, **215**, 140

Ingram, V.M. (1956). A specific chemical difference between the globins of normal and human sickle haemoglobin. *Nature (London)*, **178**, 792

Maclean, N. (1979). Smoking and acclimatisation to altitude. *British Medical Journal*, **ii**, 799

Mahony, B.S. and Githens, J.H. (1979). Sickling crises and altitude. Occurrence in the Colorado patient population. *Clinical Paediatrics*, **18**, 431

McGrath, J.J. (1992). Effects of altitude on endogenous carboxyhemoglobin levels. *Journal of Toxicology and Environmental Health*, **35**, 127

Michel, J.B., Hernandez, J.A, and Buchanan, G.R. (1992). A fatal case of acute splenic sequestration in a 53-year-old woman with sickle-haemoglobin C disease. *The American Journal of Medicine*, **92**, 97

Monge-M, C. and Monge-C, C. (1966). *High Altitude Diseases. Mechanism and Management.* Springfield, Illinois; Charles C. Thomas

Narasimhan, C., George, T., George, J.T., and Pulimood, B.M. (1990). *Journal of the Association of Physicians of India*, **38**, 435

Nuss, R., Feyerabend, A.J., Lear, J.L., and Lane, P.A. (1991). Splenic function in persons with sickle cell trait at moderately high altitude. *American Journal of Hematology*, **37**, 130

O'Brien, R.T., Pearson, H.A., Godley, J.A., and Spencer, R.P. (1972). Splenic infarct and sickle-cell trait. *New England Journal of Medicine*, **287**, 720

Reynafarje, C., Faura, J., Villavicencio, D., Curaca, A., Reynafarje, B., Oyola, L., Contreras, L.,

Vallenas, E., and Faura, A. (1975). Oxygen transport of hemoglobin in high altitude animals (*Camelidae*). *Journal of Applied Physiology*, **38**, 806

Robbins, S.L. (1967). Blood and bone marrow (sickle cell anemia). In *Pathology*. Philadelphia; W.B. Saunders, p. 626

Rowan, R.M. (1985). The blood and bone marrow. In *Muir's Textbook of Pathology*, 12th edn (J.R. Anderson, Ed.) London; Edward Arnold,- p. 17.26

Rywlin, A.M. and Benson, J. (1961). Massive necrosis of the spleen, with formation of a pseudocyst. *American Journal of Clinical Pathology*, **36**, 142

Shalev, O., Boylen, A.L., Levene, C., Oppenheim, A., and Rachmilewitz, E.A. (1988). *American Journal of Hematology*, **27**, 46

Singer, K., Chernoff, A.I., and Singer, L. (1951). Studies of abnormal hemoglobin. *Blood*, **6**, 413

Smith, E.W. and Conley, C.L. (1955). Sicklemia and infarction of the spleen during aerial flight. Electrophoresis of the hemoglobin in 15 cases. *Bulletin of the Johns Hopkins Hospital*, **96**, 35

Smith, R.P. and Ou, L.C. (1975). Methaemoglobinaemia at high altitude. *British Journal of Haematology*, **31**, 411

Spielvogel, H., Aparicio, O., Bellido, D., Galarza, M., Nallar, N., Quintela, A., Peñaloza, R., Tellez, W., Vargas, E., Villena, M., and Rios Dalenz, J. (1990). The effects of smoking on a high altitude population. *Proceedings of the 7th World Congress on Tobacco and Health*. Perth, 1990

Sugarman, J., Samuelson, W.M., Wilkinson, R.H. Jr, and Rosse, W.F. (1990). Pulmonary embolism and splenic infarction in a patient with sickle cell trait. *American Journal of Hematology*, **33**, 279

Van Vliet, G. and Huisman, T.H.J. (1964). Changes in the haemoglobin types of sheep as a response to anaemia. *Biochemical Journal*, **93**, 401

Walters, J.B. and Israel, M.S. (1974). *General Pathology*, 4th edn. Edinburgh; Churchill Livingstone

9

Disorders of blood coagulation

Rapid ascent of climbers to extreme altitudes may induce in them major thrombotic episodes such as cerebral thrombosis that may bring about serious medical conditions such as hemiplegia. Pulmonary hypertension based on thrombosis in the lung vasculature at high altitude has been described in Indian soldiers in the Himalaya. It has been reported that such clinical thrombosis is related to a hypercoagulability of the blood in lowlanders during their first 2 or 3 weeks at high altitude that then reverts rapidly to sea-level values (Chohan 1984). According to this view, while this hypercoagulability is common in lowlanders, it does not reveal itself clinically in the great majority of persons and has to be demonstrated by laboratory tests. More recent studies in Europe and the United States have failed to confirm that there are significant disorders of coagulation on very early exposure to high altitude. We review these conflicting results in this chapter. There are similar disagreements as to the numbers of blood platelets on acute exposure to high altitude. There are also differences of opinion as to the time of intravascular deposition of fibrin in high-altitude pulmonary oedema and as to whether fibrin is cause or effect in this disease. In high-altitude pulmonary and cerebral oedema (Chapters 13 and 14) thrombosis may develop in pulmonary arteries or cerebral venous sinuses. It is important for the clinician to realize that these conditions are due not to oedema alone but to superimposed thrombosis, for this has important therapeutic and prognostic implications. Healthy native highlanders show no abnormalities of blood coagulation but thrombosis is a feature of the pathology of Monge's disease (Chapter 15).

PULMONARY HYPERTENSION BASED ON PULMONARY THROMBOSIS AT HIGH ALTITUDE

Acute exposure of lowlanders to high altitude may provoke widespread thrombosis in the pulmonary circulation, with the development of pulmonary hypertension. This set of circumstances has been reported in the Himalaya but not in the Andes. Singh (1973) reported this chain of events in some Indian soldiers arriving for a tour of duty in Ladakh. Clinical signs of significant pulmonary hypertension developed in the affected subjects after a stay of 5–42 months at altitudes between 3660 and 5490 m. The pathology of these cases was one of a thrombotic, occlusive hypertensive pulmonary vascular disease. Once this vascular condition has developed, periodic returns to sea level for 2 to 3 months once a year do not ameliorate it (Singh 1973). The pulmonary hypertension either persists at sea level or, if it abates, reappears within 2–3 weeks of any return to high altitude. Indeed, Singh (1973) found that, if affected soldiers were not evacuated to sea level promptly, they might not recover but die from progressive right ventricular failure. Singh and Chohan (1972a) found that such troops may also develop thrombosis in the peripheral and splenic veins and in the coronary, cerebral, and mesenteric arteries, usually when the subject had been at high altitude for several weeks or months. Singh and Chohan (1972b) believed that pulmonary thrombosis may form the organic basis for the pulmonary hypertension characteristic of all highlanders (Chapter 10).

We believe this concept to be wrong. The mild pulmonary hypertension of the healthy native Quechua and Aymara highlanders in the Andes is associated with muscularization rather than thrombosis of the most peripheral portions of the pulmonary arterial tree (Chapter 10). Thus, the raised pulmonary arterial pressure of the Andean highlander is both benign and reversible, although its complete reversibility may take many months to achieve since it requires the regression of the muscular coat around pulmonary arterioles. Singh and Chohan (1972b) did not appear to appreciate this, for they rejected the concept that the pulmonary hypertension of the native highlander is essentially muscular in nature on the grounds that administration of oxygen did not bring about total and immediate reversibility of the elevated pulmonary arterial pressure.

The clinical syndrome of pulmonary hypertension based on thrombosis that they described in Indian soldiers appears to be a much more serious and less reversible form of pulmonary hypertension than that found in the Quechua of the Andes. Furthermore, it is likely to affect the *newcomer* to high altitude on account of the hypercoagulability thought to be induced by the mountain environment (Fig.9.1). Necropsy findings in a fatal case of pulmonary hypertension induced by temporary residence at high altitude have been provided by Singh and Chohan (1972*b*). The condition was not reversed by descent to sea level, but gradually worsened during a period of 35 months at low altitude following exposure to the mountain environment. At post-mortem there was extensive occlusive thrombosis in the pulmonary

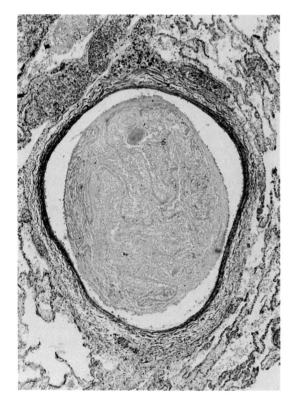

9.1 *A 54-year-old man trekked into the Solu Khumbu, Nepal, crossing the Tesi Lapcha Pass (5700 m) to climb a peak of 6300 m before descending to reach Namche Bazaar (3440 m) 4 days later. He became weak and breathless and consciousness became impaired. He died and at post-mortem the small pulmonary arteries were found to contain multiple recent ante-mortem thrombi, one of which is shown. EVG, × 60.*

trunk extending from near the pulmonary valve to the hila of the lungs (Singh *et al.* 1965*b*). It proved impossible to determine whether the widespread thrombotic occlusion of many small pulmonary arteries was autochthonous or embolic in origin. Underlying the thrombus in the pulmonary trunk the media showed patchy destruction with an inflammatory arteritis and a cellular infiltration around the vasa vasorum. In this condition there is high fibrinolytic activity, but apparently this is inadequate to counter the intensity of the coagulation process by which fibrinogen is being constantly depleted by deposition as fibrin in the pulmonary vascular bed (Chohan 1984).

MAJOR THROMBOTIC EPISODES AT EXTREME ALTITUDES

Such episodes are well recognized as a hazard facing climbers at extreme altitude. Commonly they take the form of pulmonary thromboembolism and infarction following thrombophlebitis in the calf. The thrombotic episodes reported by Ward (1975) occurred in fit young climbers between the ages of 23 and 41 years and at great heights between 5790 and 7930 m. Commonly, the climbers had spent a considerable period above 6000 m. A typical case was that reported by Genton *et al.* (1970) in a young man who developed thrombophlebitis of the calf and pulmonary thromboembolism during an attempted ascent of Mt Godwin Austen (K2)-(8610 m) in 1953. While most of these major thrombotic episodes have been in European climbers, others have occurred in Sherpas and have proven fatal.

CHRONIC THROMBOSIS OF MAJOR PULMONARY ARTERIES AT MODERATE ALTITUDE

Chronic massive thrombosis of major pulmonary arteries, usually described as occurring in 0.1% of necropsies, was found in 68 of 7753 necropsies (0.9%) in Penrose Hospital, Colorado Springs, at an altitude of 1800 m (Presti *et al.* 1990). In the same series 2.6% of the cases revealed acute massive pulmonary emboli. These data suggested to the authors that, in some unknown manner, the moderate altitude of the area was a contributory factor in the development of chronic thrombi. The frequency of acute emboli in the same hospital suggested to them that the increased incidence of chronic thrombosis at moderate altitude is not merely secondary to an overall increase in thrombogenesis but rather is due to a defect in thrombolysis.

CEREBRAL THROMBOSIS AND HEMIPLEGIA

Cerebrovascular accidents have been reported many times during the last century in men at altitudes between 4300 and 8200 m. Ward *et al.* (1989) provide an imposing list of cerebrovascular accidents reported by Roborovsky (1896), Norton (1925), Shipton (1943), Tilman (1948), Evans (1956), Ward (1968), Clarke (1983), and Asaji *et al.* (1984). Two fatal cases were in a Gurkha soldier during an expedition to Mt Everest and in a Sherpa who died on Kanchenjunga (Evans 1956). Cerebral venous thrombosis has been reported by Fujimaki *et al.* (1986). Transient ischaemic attacks and blindness have been reported in climbers by Wohns (1978). Once a person has suffered one serious thrombotic episode at high altitude it would be foolhardy for him to risk exposure to the same environmental hazards again. Ward (1975) recommends that susceptible subjects should not ascend again above 4270 m. Pugh (1962) reported that Sir Edmund Hillary became ill at 5790 m on Makalu during the Himalayan Expedition of 1960–61. He developed aphasia and right-sided facial palsy, preceded by headache. It seemed likely that he had developed a mild cerebral thrombosis. He was advised not to ascend again above 4570 m.

At such extreme altitudes it is clear that there are special factors predisposing to thrombosis. These include dehydration due to increased ventilation. Ward (1975) noted that enforced inactivity in tents on storm-bound mountainsides may also play a part. He recommended that adequate hydration and exercise should be ensured to prevent thrombosis. He believes that anticoagulants should not be administered until adequate laboratory control is available.

DISORDERS OF BLOOD COAGULATION

In view of the undoubted frequency of thrombotic episodes in European climbers and Indian soldiers at high altitude it might be anticipated that unequivocal changes would have been demonstrated and precisely defined. Such is not the case and different observers have presented conflicting results. According to Chohan (1984) there is a tendency towards hypercoagulation on immediate arrival or within a day at high altitude. He reported an increase in platelet count, and heightened levels of factors X and XII. Prothrombin and clotting times became shorter and clot retraction was impaired. This state of hypercoagulation was countered by a compensatory rise in fibrinolytic activity, evidenced by reduction of clot lysis time and levels of plasma fibrinogen (Singh and Chohan 1972*a*). Chohan (1984) found that by the end of the first week there was a progressive rise in factors X and XII and also in factors V and VIII. The platelet count and the level of platelet factor 3 also became elevated. Clotting time in glass and silicone and prothrombin time showed further shortening. However, by the end of the second week when the haematocrit had risen there was already a fall in factors V and X. Clot retraction returned to normal (Chohan 1984). Throughout the fortnight, factor XII remained high. The tendency to hypercoagulability immediately on arrival at high altitude tended to be counteracted by an increase in fibrinolytic activity (Singh and Chohan 1972*a*, *b*).

After the first week or two at high altitude the state of hypercoagulation started to regress and, with continuous stay in the mountains, this regression continued (Chohan 1984). It was indicated by a prolongation of clotting time in silicone and in prothrombin and thrombin. Platelet adhesiveness, platelet factor 3, factors V, VIII, and XII, and clot retraction were all restored to normal. However, the reduction in hypercoagulation on prolonged stay at high altitude was partly checked by a significant increase in plasma fibrinogen to which we refer below. On descent to the plains the adverse changes in blood coagulation reverted to normal. Platelet adhesiveness, clot lysis time, factors V and VIII, and thrombin clotting time all returned to normal within 1–3 weeks. Platelet factor 3, fibrinogen, thrombotest activity, and prothrombin time are all restored to baseline values (Singh and Chohan 1972*b*).

Other groups have failed to confirm this early and shortlived hypercoagulability after ascent to high altitude. There were no significant changes in blood coagulation factors in eight healthy male volunteers, 21–31 years of age, who participated in the Operation Everest II project (Andrew *et al.* 1987). During this study the participants were subjected to gradual decompression over 40 days to simulate an ascent to the summit of Mt Everest. Analysis of plasma showed no change in the activity or concentration in factors II, V, VII, VIII, and IX to XIII and a wide range of other factors in the coagulation cascade. These included prekallikrein, high-molecular-weight kininogen, fibrinogen, antithrombin III, α_2-macroglobulin, α_2-antiplasmin, C_1-esterase inhibitor, α_1-antitrypsin, and protein C. However, exercise at extreme simulated altitudes resulted in increases in the circulating concentrations of factor VIII complex, which were unequivocal but smaller than those found on exercise at sea level.

Bärtsch *et al.* (1982) also found that, in 20 subjects taken rapidly to 3700 m; there were no changes in coagulation tests 1 hour after arrival, but they too found that after strenuous exercise there was an increase in factor VIII activity, which they note is also found at sea level. This increase in levels of factor VIII was associated with a shortening of clotting time and euglobulin lysis time.

Factor VIII complex contains two proteins (Andrew *et al.* 1987). One is factor VIII procoagulant which is a cofactor for the activation of factor X and is absent in haemophilia A. The other is the von Willebrand factor which is a molecule essential for platelet adhesion to the subendothelium and is reduced or altered in von Willebrand's disease. Reductions of these proteins may lead to a severe bleeding diathesis, whereas excessive concentrations and alterations of the von Willebrand molecule are loosely associated with thrombotic states (Andrew *et al.* 1987). Exercise and exposure to acute hypoxia have been reported to produce alterations in the factor VIII complex. The effect of hypoxia on the factor VIII complex differs according to whether the exposure to hypoxia is acute or chronic.

Maher *et al.* (1976) reported alterations in the coagulation cascade, but in this study the onset of hypoxaemia was unduly rapid. The observations made during the Operation Everest II project suggest that even pronounced hypoxia does not affect the levels of the components of the coagulation system so long as the hypoxia is of gradual onset and successful acclimatization occurs. Singh and Chohan (1972*b*) reported that factor VIII precoagulant is unchanged in soldiers who have lived at and successfully acclimatized themselves to high altitudes but it is mildly increased in soldiers who have developed pulmonary hypertension at high altitude.

Plasma fibrinogen levels in long-term residents at high altitude

The coagulability and plasma fibrinogen levels of 38 soldiers who were resident at altitudes between 3690 and 5490 m for 2 years was studied by Singh and Chohan (1972*b*). Six of them were thought to have developed significant pulmonary hypertension on clinical, radiological, and electrocardiographic grounds, although this was not confirmed by cardiac catheterization. Control data were obtained from 16 men at sea level. In the healthy soldiers at high altitude there was a significant increase of plasma fibrinogen levels and fibrinolytic activity. However, in the six with clinical evidence of pulmonary hypertension, levels of plasma fibrinogen were lower sug-

gesting that it was being constantly depleted by conversion into fibrin. An abrupt fall in the plasma fibrinogen level was also reported in eight men exposed for 2 days to a simulated high altitude of 4400 m (Maher *et al.* 1976). The same fall was also demonstrated by Genton *et al.* (1970), who studied blood coagulation in calves 4–6 weeks of age at Denver (1600 m) and subsequently when the animals were taken to Mt Evans (4310 m) for 10 days prior to their return to the lower altitude. They found that plasma fibrinogen levels fell until they were about one-third below baseline values.

Lack of activation of blood coagulation in acute mountain sickness

Bärtsch *et al.* (1987) investigated blood coagulation and fibrinolysis in acute mountain sickness and high-altitude pulmonary oedema by measuring *in vivo* activity by molecular markers such as fibrinopeptide A or fibrinogen fragment E. Fibrinopeptide A is one of two polypeptides that are cleaved from fibrinogen by thrombin in the final stage of coagulation leading to fibrin monomers followed by fibrin polymerization. Elevated levels of fibrinopeptide A indicate activated coagulation with fibrin formation *in vivo*. Fragment E is a late degradation product evolving from proteolysis of fibrin and fibrinogen by plasmin (Bärtsch *et al.* 1987). It is also found elevated *in vivo* when thrombosis or intravascular coagulation is present. Bärtsch and his colleagues studied blood coagulation and fibrinolysis in 66 non-acclimatized mountaineers at 4550 m. These included 25 healthy subjects, 24 with mild acute mountain sickness, 13 with severe acute mountain sickness, and 4 with high-altitude pulmonary oedema. Coagulation times, euglobulin lysis time, and fibrin fragment E were normal in all groups without significant changes. Fibrinopeptide A was elevated in the cases of high-altitude pulmonary oedema to 4.2 ± 2.7 ng/ml compared with the other groups showing mean values between 1.6 ± 0.4 and 1.8 ± 0.7 ng/ml. This indicated activated coagulation and fibrin formation *in vivo*. Bärtsch *et al.* (1987) concluded that activation of blood coagulation is not involved in the pathogenesis of acute mountain sickness. They believe that the fibrin generation found in high-altitude pulmonary oedema is probably an epiphenomenon of oedema formation and not causative, as we discuss below. Hyers *et al.* (1979) were unable to detect any difference in the degree of coagulation activity between subjects with and without high-altitude pulmonary oedema.

BLOOD PLATELET COUNT

There is also no uniformity of opinion as to the blood platelet count in those ascending to high altitude. Chohan (1984) reported an *increase* in platelet count on exposure to a mountain environment, with increased adhesiveness and aggregation of thrombocytes with sequestration of young, adhesive platelets in the pulmonary vascular bed. On the other hand, Sharma (1986) found no significant change in the platelet count in lowlanders ascending to 3650 m. He studied 50 lowlanders at sea level and after they had travelled to high altitude, half travelling quickly by train and road and the remainder slowly over 8 days to acclimatize *en route*. No changes in platelet count were found in either group.

Thus, neither of three observers could confirm the earlier findings of Gray *et al.* (1975) that suggested that the blood platelet count *falls* on ascent to high altitude. They studied 14 men at 2990 m and found a fall of 7% in the count compared with that at sea level. After a further 2 days at 5370 m there was a reduction of 25% from control values, but after another 8 days the count recovered to a point only 7% below the baseline at sea level (Fig. 9.2). Falls of this magnitude do not amount to clinical thrombocytopenia, which is said to exist when the platelet count is less than $150 \times 10^9/l$ (Rowan 1985). Bleeding from capillaries is unusual when the count is greater than $50 \times 10^9/l$ and spontaneous haemorrhage does not usually occur with a count above $20 \times 10^9/l$ unless infection is also present. Hence any fall in platelet count of the magnitude reported by Gray *et al.* (1975) could not be held to be responsible for the bleeding from mucosal surfaces described later in this chapter.

A drop in the number of circulating thrombocytes had previously been reported in rats subjected to simulated high altitude for 22 days by exposing them to a reduced barometric pressure of 380 mmHg (De Gabriele and Penington 1967). These experimental conditions led to an unimpressive fall in platelet count from 643 to $594 \times 10^9/l$. A much more severe and persistent fall in platelet count was produced in mice exposed to the same reduction in barometric pressure (Birks *et al.* 1975). After this degree of decompression for 2 days there was an initial small rise in the platelet count, probably due to haemoconcentration. This was followed by a severe and persistent thrombocytopenia with a rapid decline in the platelet count between the fifth and ninth days of hypoxia. By the twelfth day the platelet count in the mice was only 36% of that in the control group. As we have noted above, a fall in

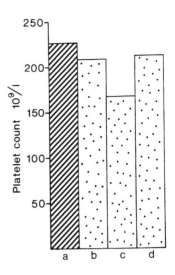

9.2 *Platelet count at various natural altitudes in 14 young men. (a) Control values at 790 m; (b) after airlift to 2990 m for 5 days; (c) in eight subjects after airlift to 5370 m for 2 days; (d) after 10 days at 5370 m. (Based on data from Gray* et al. *(1975).)*

platelet count of this magnitude is not found in man. Genton *et al.* (1970) found a similar reduction in the number of circulating platelets in calves taken to high altitude for 10 days. At the same time the number of circulating young adhesive platelets rose greatly to an average figure some 142% greater than baseline values. There was a striking decrease of 63% in platelet half-life. Platelet adhesiveness was also noted in man by Singh and Chohan (1972*b*).

Decompression *per se* may lead to a sharp fall in platelet count. Sixteen men were decompressed to simulate a rate of ascent of 1520 m/min to an altitude of 6100 m where they remained for two hours (Gray *et al.* 1975). During this period they breathed oxygen at a partial pressure of 150 mmHg, but in spite of this they showed significant fall in platelet count from control levels of 232 to $207 \times 10^9/l$, a fall of approximately 10% which persisted for 3 days. This fall in platelet count was regarded in part as being due to a reduction in thrombocyte half-life, for autologous platelet survival was diminished in four of five men. However, the fall in platelet count was also considered to be brought about to some extent by their sequestration in the lung. Platelets labelled with ^{51}Cr sequester in the pulmonary vascular bed of rabbits that are decompressed in normoxic and hypoxic conditions (Gray *et al.* 1975).

BLOOD PLATELET STRUCTURE AND FUNCTION

According to Chohan (1984) electron microscopic studies of platelets in patients with high-altitude pulmonary oedema show that the integrity of plasma membrane, capacity for pseudopodia formation, and the ability to degranulate are intact. This suggested to Chohan that blood platelets are structurally sound and active functionally. In these patients there is a rise in immunoglobulins IgG, IgM, and IgA, the first two being adsorbed on the surface of the platelets. This alters their mobility, increases their aggregation, and enhances the release of ADP which in turn promotes the availability of platelet factor 3 (Chohan 1984). In high-altitude pulmonary oedema the electrophoretic mobility of platelets is reduced. Platelet adhesiveness is increased and light microscopy of peripheral blood smears may show larger and young adhesive platelets in aggregates in greater numbers. There is evidence of sequestration of ADP and platelets in the pulmonary vascular bed., Platelet factor 3 provides an active catalytic surface for the interaction of plasma coagulation factors, leading to thrombin generation. The resulting consolidation of platelets leads to their degranulation, with the release of more factor 3 and ADP and more fibrin production.

COAGULATION AND FIBRINOLYSIS IN HIGH-ALTITUDE PULMONARY OEDEMA

In Chapters 13 and 14 we describe how thrombosis in the pulmonary arteries and dural venous sinuses is characteristic of necropsy findings in cases of high-altitude pulmonary oedema and cerebral oedema (Dickinson *et al.* 1983). Studies by Indian workers have suggested that in high-altitude pulmonary oedema there is a breakdown of the fibrinolytic system, resulting in increase in plasma fibrinogen levels and in the time required for lysis of clot in venous blood (Singh *et al.* 1969; Singh and Chohan 1972a, 1973). Both fibrinogen levels and venous clot lysis time were significantly higher during the acute phase of oedema than during convalescence and were regarded by Singh *et al.* (1969) as characteristic of the disease.

It was thought that a combination of altered activity of blood platelets, disturbances of blood coagulation factors as described by Chohan (1984) and described above, and failure of fibrinolysis was responsible for intravascular sludging of erythrocytes and for the formation of fibrin thrombi in the pulmonary capillaries, venules, and arterioles. Nayak *et al.* (1964) studied necropsy specimens of lung from 13 cases of high-altitude pulmonary oedema and found hyaline fibrin thrombi in no fewer than six of them. Usually they appeared as clear homogeneous masses, but sometimes they had an indistinct-laminated appearance with a strongly positive staining reaction with phosphotungstic acid haematoxylin. In one case, multiple fibrin thrombi were not confined to the pulmonary capillary bed but also occurred in the kidney, where they plugged the glomerular and peritubular capillaries. Similar thrombi and small plugs of fibrin strands were found in the hepatic sinusoids. Such minute fibrin thrombi have been considered by Singh *et al.* (1965a) to be involved in the pathogenesis of high-altitude pulmonary oedema.

Twenty years after the original study of Singh *et al.* (1969) the problem of intravascular coagulation and a possible breakdown in the fibrinolytic system was reinvestigated by Bärtsch *et al.* (1989). Their previous study referred to above (Bärtsch *et al.* 1987) revealed elevated fibrinopeptide A with normal levels of fragment E and this led them to investigate if these changes in haemostasis preceded or followed high-altitude pulmonary oedema. They investigated these and a wide range of factors in 25 male mountaineers, of median age 40 years, at low altitude (550 m) and after 6, 18, and 42 hours at an altitude of 4550 m that was climbed in a day. Nine of the subjects studied had a history of a previous attack of high-altitude pulmonary oedema. In 14 subjects symptoms of acute mountain sickness were mild or absent. Eleven subjects had acute mountain sickness and six of them developed radiographically documented high-altitude pulmonary oedema after 18 or 42 hours.

In general terms their study showed that blood coagulation and fibrinolysis are unaltered in healthy mountaineers at rest after rapid ascent to 4550 m. In the subjects free of acute mountain sickness the only abnormalities revealed was a slight decrease in bleeding time. The platelet count did not change and the *in vivo* activation of platelets (β thromboglobulin and platelet factor 4) did not change from baseline values. The observed shortening of the bleeding time could be due to vascular factors such as increased vasoconstriction in the presence of documented elevated levels of noradrenaline at high altitude.

In the subjects with acute mountain sickness the activated partial thromboplastin time fell continuously at high altitude. There were increased factor VIII procoagulant activity and expression of von Willebrand factor antigen to the extent of $57 \pm 12\%$ and $70 \pm 13\%$, respectively. The disproportionately greater increase of the von Willebrand factor suggests an increase of this factor from endothelial cells. Activation of coagulation in acute mountain sickness did not involve platelets as demonstrated by unchanged plasma levels of platelet activators, β thromboglobulin and platelet factor 4. Unchanged plasma levels and normal urinary excretion of fibrinopeptide A demonstrated that the activation of blood coagulation in acute mountain sickness did not lead to fibrin formation.

The early development of high-altitude pulmonary oedema did not bring about changes in blood coagulation significantly different from the partial activation of coagulation associated with acute mountain sickness in the absence of lung oedema noted above. Fibrinopeptide A levels were normal in blood and urine, thus indicating the absence of *in vivo* formation of fibrin in high-altitude pulmonary oedema. Bärtsch *et al.* (1989) believe that activation of blood coagulation leading to *in vivo* fibrin formation most probably occurs only as a consequence of severe high-altitude pulmonary oedema. The levels of β thromboglobulin were normal before and after the onset of lung oedema.

There is some difficulty in comparing baseline levels of fibrinolysis with measurements at high altitude because of diurnal variation showing accelerated euglobulin lysis time in the evening (Bärtsch *et al.* 1989). With the onset of oedema, euglobulin clot lysis time without venous occlusion declined at high altitude compared with low from 289 ± 48 to 201 ± 42 minutes. Bärtsch *et al.* (1989) believe that the prolonged euglobulin clot lysis time could be explained by elevated levels of plasminogen activator inhibitor-1. *In vivo* fibrin formation does not precede high-altitude pulmonary oedema and occurs with severe alveolar oedema only. A normal fibrinolytic response to venous occlusion before the development of lung oedema at low and high altitude indicates a normal release of tissue plasminogen activator in these subjects. Thus, activated coagulation resulting in fibrin formation and decreased fibrinolytic activity are consequences of high-altitude pulmonary oedema and not involved in the pathophysiology initiating the oedema.

THROMBOSIS IN MONGE'S DISEASE

After the hypercoagulability which the Indian studies suggest characterizes the first 2 or 3 weeks at high altitude, the disturbed coagulation factors return to normal. Hence both native highlander and lowlanders acclimatized to mountain conditions show no increased tendency to hypercoagulation and thrombosis. However, highlanders who develop chronic mountain sickness (Chapter 15) after several years' residence at high altitude once again develop abnormalities of coagulation. Chohan (1984) reports in this disease increased plasma fibrinogen, a significant decrease in activated partial thromboplastin time, a fall in platelet count, and significant increases in haemoglobin concentration and haematocrit, all of which indicate a hypercoagulable state. He believes that the peripheral blood smear is characteristic in chronic mountain sickness. The hyperchromatic and large erythrocytes form a mosaic pattern with little plasmatic matrix. Large young platelets seem to be strangulated in the mosaic. Rouleaux formation by erythrocytes is common. These abnormalities in coagulation factors in Monge's disease lead to an increased tendency to thrombosis. This results in a significant difference in the histology of the pulmonary vasculature in chronic mountain sickness compared with that of the healthy native highlander. Widespread thrombosis is superimposed on the muscularization of the terminal portions of the pulmonary arterial tree (Chapter 15).

CAPILLARY FRAGILITY

Increased capillary fragility is found at high altitude. It occurs in high-altitude pulmonary oedema and in cerebral mountain sickness (Chapters 13 and 14). This tendency to bleed also leads to subungual splinter haemorrhages, which are common in healthy native highlanders (see Fig. 25.10(a) and in patients with Monge's disease (see Fig. 25.10(b)). Retinal haemorrhage at high altitude is described in Chapter 27. As early as 1913, Ravenhill reported that epistaxis occurred in some cases of acute mountain sickness. He described having met an elderly man who at high altitude bled 'not only from the nose, but from every mucous membrane of which he was possessed' (Ravenhill 1913). Haemorrhage also occurs readily in the gastric mucosa at high altitude (Chapter 21).

On a visit to the Andes one of us (D.R.W.) developed crops of small haemorrhages up to 2 mm in diameter in the buccal mucosa (Fig. 9.3). Subsequently this observation was confirmed by Hunter *et al.* (1986), who measured the capillary fragility in the mucous membrane on the inner aspect of the lower lip in three healthy White men during an ascent of the Himalayan peak Jogin I (6465 m). The technique employed was that of Stirrups *et al.* (1977) and entailed placing a plastic bell 1 cm in diameter on the mucosa and applying a

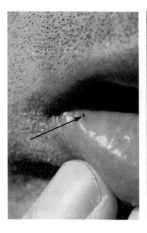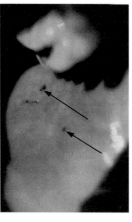

(a)   *(b)*

9.3 *Small haemorrhages (arrows) occurring in one of the authors (D.R.W.) while at Cerro de Pasco in the Andes (4330 m): (a) on the inner aspect of the everted lower lip; (b) on the buccal mucosa.*

negative pressure of 200 mmHg for 1 min, sucking the lip up into the bell. Petechiae proved to be more numerous at high altitude. It is of interest that one of the men during the climb developed two retinal haemorrhages in his right eye and three in his left.

References

Andrew, M., O'Brodovich, H., and Sutton, J. (1987). Operation Everest II: Coagulation system during prolonged decompression to 282 Torr. *Journal of Applied Physiology*, **63**, 1262

Asaji, T., Sakurai, E., Tanizaki, Y., Matsutani, M., Fuzimaku, T., Song, S.Y., and Okeda, R. (1984). Report on medical aspects of Mount Lhotse and Everest expedition in 1983: with special reference to a case of cerebral venous thrombosis in the altitude. *Japanese Journal of Mountain Medicine*, **4**, 98

Bärtsch, P., Schmidt, E.K., and Straub, P.W. (1982). Fibrinopeptide A after strenous physical exercise at high altitude. *Journal of Applied Physiology*, **53**, 40

Bärtsch, P., Waber, U.R.S., Haeberli, A., Maggiorini, M., Kriemler, S., Oelz, O., and Straub, W.P. (1987). Enhanced fibrin formation in high-altitude pulmonary oedema. *Journal of Applied Physiology*, **63**, 752

Bärtsch, P., Haeberli, A., Franciolli, M., Kruithof, E.K.O., and Straub, P.W. (1989). Coagulation and fibrinolysis in acute mountain sickness and beginning pulmonary oedema. *Journal of Applied Physiology*, **66**, 2136

Birks, J.W., Klassen, L.W., and Gurney, C.W. (1975). Hypoxia-induced thrombocytopenia in mice. *Journal of Laboratory and Clinical Medicine*, **86**, 230

Chohan, I.S. (1984). Blood coagulation changes at high altitude. *Defence Science Journal*, **34**, 361

Clarke, C.R.A. (1983). Cerebral infarction at extreme altitude. In *Hypoxia, Exercise and Altitude* (J.R. Sutton, C.S. Houston, and N.L. Jones Eds). New York: A.R. Liss Inc, pp. 453–4

De Gabriele, G. and Penington, D.G. (1967). Physiology of the regulation of platelet production. *British Journal of Haematology*, **13**, 302

Dickinson, J.; Heath, D., Gosney, J., and Williams, D. (1983). Altitude-related deaths in seven trekkers in the Himalayas. *Thorax*, **38**, 646

Evans, R.C. (1956). *Kanchenjunga. The Untrodden Peak*. London; Hodder and Stoughton, p. 169

Fujimaki, T., Matsutani, M., Asai, A., Kohno, T., and Koike, M. (1986). Cerebral venous thrombosis due to high altitude polycythemia. Case report. *Journal of Neurosurgery*, **64**, 148

Genton, E., Ross, A.M., Takeda, Y.A., and Vogel, J.H.K. (1970). Alterations in blood coagulation at high altitude. In *Hypoxia, High Altitude and the Heart* (J.H.K. Vogel, Ed.), Vol. 5, Advances in Cardiology. Basel; Karger, p. 32

Gray, G.W., Bryan, A.C., Freedman, M.H., Houston, C.S., Lewis, W.F., McFadden, D.M., and Newell, G. (1975). Effect of altitude exposure on platelets. *Journal of Applied Physiology*, **39**, 648

Hunter, D.J., Smart, J.R., and Whitton, L. (1986). Increased capillary fragility at high altitude. *British Medical Journal*, **292**, 98

Hyers, T.M., Scoggin, C.H., Will, D.H., Grover, R.F., and Reeves, J.T. (1979). Accentuated hypoxemia at high altitude in subjects susceptible to high-altitude pulmonary edema. *Journal of Applied Physiology*, **46**, 41

Maher, J.T., Levine, P.H, and Cymerman, A. (1976). Human coagulation abnormalities during acute exposure to hypobaric hypoxia. *Journal of Applied Physiology*, **41**, 702

Nayak, N.C., Roy, S., and Narayanan, T.K. (1964). Pathologic features of altitude sickness. *American Journal of Pathology*, **45**, 381

Norton, E.F. (1925). *The Fight for Everest;* London, Arnold, p. 68

Presti, B., Berthrong, M., and Sherwin, R.M. (1990). Chronic thrombosis of major pulmonary arteries. *Human Pathology*, **21**, 601

Pugh, L.G.C.E. (1962). Physiological and medical aspects of the Himalayan scientific and mountaineering expedition 1960–61. *British Medical Journal*, **ii**, 621

Ravenhill, T.H. (1913). Some experiences of mountain sickness in the Andes. *Journal of Tropical Medicine and Hygiene*, **16**, 313

Roborovsky, (1896). The Central Asian Expedition of Capt. Roborovsky and Lt. Kozloff. *Geographical Journal*, **8**, 161

Rowan, R.M. (1985). The blood and bone marrow. In *Muir's Textbook of Pathology*, 12th edn (J.R. Anderson, Ed.). Edward Arnold; London, p. 17.62

Sharma, S.C. (1986). Platelet count on slow induction to high altitude. *International Journal of Biometeorology*, **30**, 27

Shipton, E. (1943). *Upon that Mountain.* London; Hodder and Stoughton, pp. 129–30

Singh, I. (1973). Pulmonary hypertension in new arrivals at high altitude. World Health Organization meeting on Primary Pulmonary Hypertension, Geneva, October

Singh, I and Chohan, I.S. (1972a). Abnormalities of blood coagulation at high altitude. *International Journal of Biometeorology*, **16**, 283

Singh, I. and Chohan, I.S. (1972b). Blood coagulation changes at high altitude predisposing to pulmonary hypertension. *British Heart Journal*, **34**, 611

Singh, I. and Chohan, I.S. (1973). Reversal of abnormal fibrinolytic activity, blood coagulation factors and platelet function in high altitude pulmonary oedema with frusemide. *International Journal of Biometeorology*, **17**, 73

Singh, I., Kapila, C.C., Khanna, P.K., Nanda, R.B., and Rao, B.D.P. (1965a). High altitude pulmonary oedema. *Lancet*, **i**, 229

Singh, I., Khanna, P.K., Lal, M., Hoon, R.S.; and Rao, B.D.P., (1965b). High altitude pulmonary hypertension. *Lancet*, **ii**, 146

Singh, I., Chohan, I.S., and Mathew, N.T. (1969). Fibrinolytic activity in high altitude pulmonary oedema. *Indian Journal of Medical Research*, **57**, 210

Stirrups, D.R., Orth, D.D., and Dinsdale, R.C. (1977). Mucosal petechiometry; a reliable method for the measurement of capillary resistance. *British Journal of Oral Surgery*, **14**, 230

Tilman, H.W. (1948). *Mount Everest 1938.* Cambridge; Cambridge University Press; pp. 93–4

Ward, M. (1975). *Mountain Medicine. A Clinical Study of Cold and High Altitude.* London; Crosby Lockwood Staples

Ward, M.P. (1968). Diseases occurring at altitudes exceeding 17,500 ft. Unpublished MD thesis. University of Cambridge, pp. 66–9

Ward, M.P., Milledge, J.S., and West, J.B. (1989). Vascular disorders. In *High Altitude Medicine and Physiology*. London; Chapman and Hall Medical p. 413

Wohns, R.N.W. (1978). Transient ischaemic attacks at high altitude. In *Hypoxia and Cold* (J.R. Sutton, C.S. Houston, and G. Coates, Eds). New York Praeger, p. 536

10

Pulmonary hypertension

Healthy Quechua and Aymara highlanders, born and living at high altitude in the Andes, have a mild degree of pulmonary arterial hypertension with characteristic remodelling of the pulmonary vasculature. It should be noted that as yet there has been no confirmation that similar haemodynamic and microanatomical changes are to be found in the Tibetan and Sherpa peoples of the Himalaya and Karakorams. The characteristics that we describe in this chapter may not be features of all highlanders. There may be differences related to the ethnic background of the subjects. More probably, the differences are related to the degree of altitude at which the various groups are domiciled.

PULMONARY HYPERTENSION IN QUECHUAS

The pulmonary haemodynamics of 38 healthy adults and 32 healthy children at Morococha (4540 m) and Cerro de Pasco (4330 m) in the Peruvian Andes were studied by Peñaloza et al. (1962, 1963) and by Sime et al. (1963). In the former town the mean barometric pressure is 446 mmHg and the atmospheric partial pressure of oxygen is 80 mmHg, whereas in the latter settlement these values are respectively 455 and 90 mmHg. Compared with an average level of 22/6 mmHg (mean 12 mmHg) for sea-level residents, the adult at high altitude has a mild pulmonary arterial hypertension of 41/15 mmHg (mean 28 mmHg) (Fig. 10.1). The pulmonary wedge pressure is not elevated. The average total pulmonary vascular resistance in the subjects studied by Peñaloza et al. (1962) was found to be increased from a value of 159 dyn/s per cm^{-5} in residents at sea level to 401 dyn/s per cm^{-5} in adult subjects at high altitude.

In young children between the ages of 1 and 5 years, the level of pulmonary arterial pressure is considerably greater. Thus, Sime et al. (1963) found the average pulmonary arterial mean pressure in seven young children to be no less than 45 mmHg, with a systolic pressure as high as 58 mmHg (Fig. 10.1).

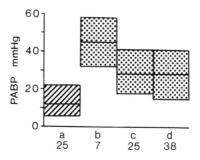

10.1 *Pulmonary arterial blood pressure in adult lowlanders at sea level and in Quechua children and adults at high altitude (4540 m). For each block the top line is the systolic blood pressure, the middle line the mean pressure, and the bottom line the diastolic pressure. Hatched columns are subjects at sea level and stippled columns are acclimatized Quechuas at high altitude. a: 25 adult lowlanders at sea level; b: 7 children, 1–5 years of age, at 4540 m; c: 25 children, 6–14 years of age, at 4540 m; d: 38 adult highlanders at 4540 m (Compiled from data of Peñaloza* et al. *(1962) and Sime* et al. *(1963).)*

However, after the age of 5 years the pulmonary arterial pressure falls to adult levels (Fig. 10.1). The same degree of pulmonary hypertension that persists in Quechua children to the age of 5 years is to be found in infants at sea level only for the first week of life (James and Rowe 1957; Rudolph and Cayler 1958; Rudolph et al. 1961). After only a fortnight of postnatal life at sea level the pulmonary arterial pressure has fallen to adult levels (Keith et al. 1958).

The effects of high altitude on pulmonary haemodynamics are shown in a more pronounced manner on exercise. Peñaloza et al. (1962) found that the average pulmonary arterial mean pressure rose as high as 60 mmHg on exercise in subjects at high altitude, the systolic level being 77 mmHg (Fig. 10.2).

The pulmonary hypertension of high altitude can be partially reversed immediately by the

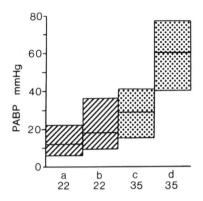

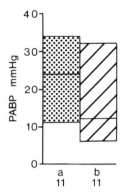

10.2 *Pulmonary arterial blood pressure at rest and on exercise in residents at sea level and in Quechuas at high altitude. For each block the top line is the systolic blood pressure, the middle line the mean pressure, and the bottom line the diastolic pressure. Shading of columns as in Fig. 10.1 a: 22 sea-level residents at rest; b: 22 sea-level residents during exercise; c: 35 high-altitude residents at rest; d: 35 high-altitude residents during exercise. (Compiled from data of Peñaloza et al. (1962).)*

10.3 *Pulmonary arterial blood pressure in Quechuas in their native Andean habitat and after 2 years' residence at sea level. For both blocks the top line is the systolic blood pressure, the middle line the mean pressure, and the bottom line the diastolic pressure. The stippled column represents acclimatized Quechuas at high altitude. The lightly hatched column represents highlanders resident at sea level. a: 11 subjects at 4330 m; b: same 11 subjects after 2 years' residence at sea level. (Compiled from data of Peñaloza et al. (1962).)*

administration of oxygen, but total reversal by removal of the subject to sea level takes a much longer time. Thus the inhalation of oxygen to produce an oxygen tension similar to that found at sea level lowered the pulmonary arterial pressure of highlanders by only 15–20 mm Hg, but this partial reduction took place immediately (Peñaloza *et al.* 1962) In contrast, a halving of the average pulmonary arterial mean pressure from 24 to 12 mmHg in 11 native highlanders from Cerro de Pasco (4330 m) was achieved by taking them to sea level, but it took 2 years to accomplish (Peñaloza *et al.* 1962; see Fig. 10.3)

PERIPHERAL MUSCULARIZATION OF THE PULMONARY ARTERIAL TREE

The mild elevation at rest in adult Quechua Indians in Morococha (4540 m) and Cerro de Pasco (4330 m) is associated with muscularization of the terminal portions of the pulmonary arterial tree (Arias-Stella and Saldaña 1963). The normal pulmonary arteriole of the lowlander has a wall consisting of a single elastic lamina, except at its origin from its parent muscular pulmonary artery where there is commonly a cuff of circularly orientated smooth muscle. In the Andean Indian the pulmonary arterioles have a distinct media of circular muscle sandwiched by inner and outer elastic laminae, so that they come to resemble small pul-

monary arteries or systemic arterioles (Fig. 10.4). This muscularization is associated with the increased pulmonary vascular resistance in the Quechuas and Aymaras. It is easy to mimic this pulmonary vascular remodelling in experimental animals kept in a hypobaric chamber. Thus, Smith *et al.* (1974) subjected Wistar albino rats to a simulated altitude of 5500 m and found that their pulmonary arterioles developed muscular coats. Transverse sections of these vessels revealed that the outer elastic laminae were prominent and clearly represented the original thick elastic lamina of the arteriole. In contrast, the inner elastic laminae were delicate and seemed to be newly formed, internal to the muscle coat (Fig. 10.5). Such histological appearances are more consistent with a hyperplasia of smooth muscle into the pulmonary arterioles than a constriction of pulmonary arteries.

Arias-Stella (Fig. 10.6) has made extensive studies of the histological features of the pulmonary arterial tree of the Quechua Indian. In one investigation he and Saldaña studied what they termed idiosyncratically 'proximal and distal pulmonary arteries', which correspond to what most pathologists, including the authors, would call 'muscular pulmonary arteries and pulmonary arterioles' (Arias-Stella and Saldaña 1963). Arias-Stella and Saldaña found an increase in the number of muscularized pulmonary arterioles

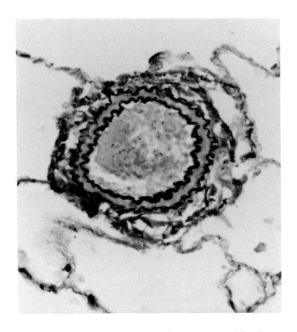

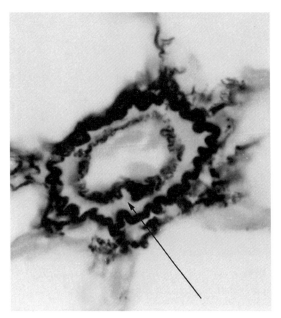

10.4 *Transverse section of a pulmonary arteriole of mean diameter 95 μm, from a male Quechua Indian who lived at Cerro de Pasco (4330 m) in the Peruvian Andes. There is a distinct muscular media sandwiched between internal and external elastic laminae. This muscularization of the terminal portion of the pulmonary arterial tree is in striking contrast to the normal pulmonary arteriole in lowlanders that has a wall consisting of a single elastic lamina. EVG, × 375.*

10.5 *Transverse section of a pulmonary arteriole from a rat exposed for 5 weeks to a simulated altitude of 5500 m. The normal pulmonary arteriole in the rat, as in man, has a wall consisting of a single elastic lamina. The vessel shown here is abnormal, a distinct media of circularly orientated smooth muscle (arrow) having formed internal to the original thick elastic lamina. On the inner aspect of the muscle layer a new thin internal elastic lamina has been laid down. The vessel now resembles a systemic arteriole and is capable of elevating pulmonary vascular resistance to give rise to pulmonary arterial hypertension and right ventricular hypertrophy. EVG, × 1125.*

related to the number of parent muscular pulmonary arteries, and an absolute increase in the amount of arterial muscle in the terminal portions of the pulmonary arterial tree. In their older group of high-altitude subjects there was hypertrophy of the media of the muscular pulmonary arteries. Occasional fasciculi of longitudinally orientated smooth muscle fibres were found in the intima of the pulmonary arteries and arterioles of Quechuas.

This classic study by Arias-Stella and Saldaña (1963) was a major advance in high-altitude pathology but more recent work suggests that it is incomplete. Our own studies of mestizo and Aymara citizens of La Paz (3600 m), Bolivia, a decade apart (Heath *et al*. 1981, 1990 Heath and Williams 1991), have confirmed that muscularization of pulmonary arterioles as small as 30 μm in diameter is very common (Figs 10.7 and 10.8). However, in addition, there is not infrequently the development of a layer of longitudinally orientated smooth muscle in

the intima (Fig. 10.9). This is similar to what occurs in cases of pulmonary emphysema (Hicken *et al.* 1965 Wilkinson *et al.* 1988) where sustained alveolar hypoxia is associated with hypercarbia in contrast to the hypobaric hypoxia of the native highlander. There is limited migration of mature-looking smooth muscle cells from the media into the intima through deficiencies in the inner elastic lamina. Electron-microscopic studies in cases of pulmonary emphysema have revealed the ultrastructure of this limited migration (Smith *et al.* 1992). This is in contrast to events in plexogenic pulmonary arteriopathy, as seen in primary pulmonary hypertension and congenital cardiac shunts, where the migrating vascular smooth muscle cells are electron-dense, dark, and elongated and show a smooth surface with loss of micropinocy-

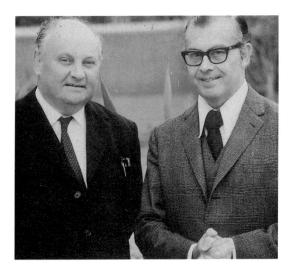

10.6 *Professor J. Arias-Stella (right) with one of the authors (D.H.) in Lima in July 1979.*

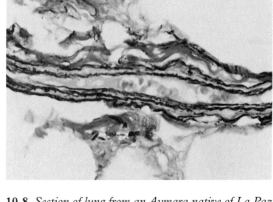

10.8 *Section of lung from an Aymara native of La Paz (3600 m) aged 35 years, showing muscularization of the terminal portions of the pulmonary arterial tree. A minute muscular vessel, only some 25 μm in diameter, has been cut in longitudinal section and shows a distinct media. EVG, × 397.*

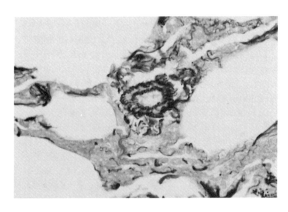

10.7 *Transverse section of a muscularized pulmonary arteriole from a male Aymara resident of La Paz (3600 m) aged 35 years. Although less than 30 μm in diameter, this vessel has a thick muscular coat, an appearance consistent with an elevated pulmonary vascular resistance during life. EVG, × 375.*

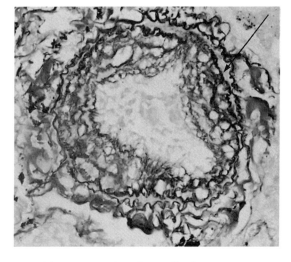

10.9 *Transverse section of a small pulmonary artery from a male mestizo resident, aged 66 years, of La Paz (3600 m) who died of a carcinoma of the stomach. It shows pronounced intimal proliferation of longitudinal smooth muscle with associated elastosis. The original media of circular muscle (arrow) is thin and atrophic. EVG, × 450.*

totic activity (Heath *et al.* 1988). Such dark cells predominate in the inner media and reach the intima by passing by the same route through gaps in the inner elastic lamina as in states of hypoxia. Here they are transformed into myofibroblasts, which migrate freely and extensively into the vascular lumen. It was hitherto thought that the development of intimal longitudinal muscle in the pulmonary arteries in emphysema is the result of physical forces acting on the vessels as they are distended around abnormal air spaces in the lung. Its occurrence in native highlanders as well as in patients with chronic obstructive lung disease suggests rather that it is more likely to be related to chronic alveolar hypoxia. The presence of intimal longitudinal muscle in the

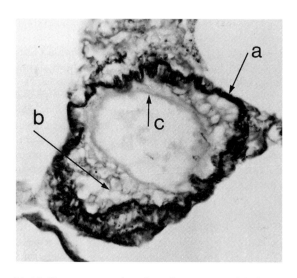

10.10 *Transverse section of a pulmonary arteriole from a male Aymara Indian of 28 years who died from a cerebellar tumour in La Paz (3600 m). From outwards to the lumen its layers consist of a thick elastic lamina (arrow a), a layer of longitudinal muscle (arrow b), and an inner muscular tube (arrow c). EVG, × 745.*

pulmonary arteries in native highlanders never becomes as pronounced as in patients with emphysema.

Another feature of the remodelling of the pulmonary arterial tree in native highlanders is the development of inner muscular tubes (Fig. 10.10). These are far less common than muscularization of pulmonary arterioles or the development of intimal longitudinal muscle. Such inner muscular tubes are also found in chronic obstructive lung disease where, like intimal longitudinal muscle, they occur far more commonly than in native highlanders. Immediately beneath the endothelium of normal pulmonary arteries is a thin layer of circular muscle. With the development of intimal longitudinally orientated muscle, this layer of circular muscle develops around itself inner and outer elastic laminae and forms a circular tube (Smith *et al.*, 1992). In the investigation of 1990 in La Paz we studied 13 Aymara Indians who were born in the city and spent all their lives there. Three of them showed muscularization of pulmonary arterioles, four the development of intimal longitudinal muscle (Fig. 10.9), and only one the formation of inner muscular tubes (Fig. 10.10). In 12 mestizos, two showed arteriolar muscularization, five the development of intimal longitudinal muscle, but none the formation of inner muscular tubes. It is

apparent that a characteristic triad of histological changes may contribute to the remodelling of the human pulmonary arterial tree of the native Quechua and Aymara Indians of the Andes but it is rarely complete.

Thus, remodelling of the pulmonary vasculature in native highlanders of the Andes is far more complex than that envisaged as a simple muscularization of the peripheral portions of the pulmonary arterial tree by Arias-Stella and Saldaña (1963). The components of this remodelling are summarized digrammatically in Fig. 10.11. The venous element of the remodelling is described later in the chapter.

PULMONARY VASCULAR REMODELLING IN DIFFERENT NATIVE HIGHLANDERS

Arias-Stella and Saldaña (1963) entitled their paper 'The terminal portion of the pulmonary arterial tree

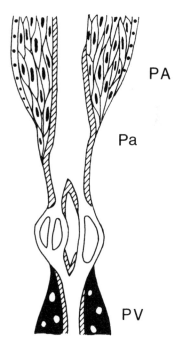

10.11 *Diagram summarizing the remodelling of the pulmonary vasculature in the high-altitude Aymara Indian. In the pulmonary arteries (PA) and arterioles (Pa) longitudinal muscle forms in the intima internal to the media of circular muscle. Inner muscular tubes (indicated by the cross-hatching) line the layer of longitudinal muscle that passes to line intimal proliferation in pulmonary veins. In the pulmonary veins (PV) the pronounced intimal proliferation is composed of smooth muscle cells embedded in a background matrix of collagen.*

in people native to high altitudes', implying that the peripheral muscularization that they reported in the lung was to be anticipated in all subjects born and living at great elevations. This is not so. In our initial study in La Paz (Heath *et al.* 1981) we studied necropsy material from its citizens who comprise Caucasians and mestizos as well as Aymara Indians. In subjects beyond infancy we found muscularization of pulmonary arterioles in five of seven Aymaras, in one of four mestizos, and in one of five Caucasians. This led us to the conclusion that the ethnic background of subjects at high altitude may influence the reaction of their pulmonary circulation to the hypobaric hypoxia.

The pulmonary vasculature of native highlanders from the Himalaya and Karakorams has been far less studied and in fact we are aware of only one published study on the subject (Gupta *et al.* 1992). The authors studied seven subjects coming to necropsy who had lived all their lives at Leh in Ladakh at an altitude of 3600 m. These highlanders had a ratio of right-to-left ventricular weight similar to that found at sea level and showed no muscularization of pulmonary arterioles or proliferation of intimal longitudinal muscle in pulmonary arteries. It was concluded that this was evidence of genetic adaptation to high altitude in a race that has lived in the Himalaya for many thousands of years. They compared their findings with the lack of pulmonary vascular remodelling in indigenous mountain mammals (Chapter 35). We doubt the validity of their conclusions, for the altitude at which their subjects were living was not great and we ourselves have found that rabbits exposed to an altitude of 3370 m for several months in the Rifugio Torino on Monte Bianco in the Italian Alps did not develop pulmonary vascular remodelling (Smith *et al.* 1993). We think it more than likely that the hypoxic stimulus in the Ladakhi highlanders was not strong enough to induce pulmonary vascular remodelling.

Our study of the pulmonary blood vessels of the citizens of La Paz (Heath *et al.* 1981) revealed that age-change intimal proliferation occurs in the muscular pulmonary arteries and pulmonary arterioles of native highlanders, just as it does in lowlanders. Almost certainly the cell responsible for this age change is the myofibroblast. At high altitude the mild pulmonary hypertension of the native highlander remains reversible. There is no tendency for pathological intimal proliferation in the pulmonary arterial tree leading to increasingly irreversible pulmonary hypertension. Indeed this could not be so,

for otherwise man could not survive permanently in a mountain environment.

It seems best to regard the muscularization of the pulmonary arterioles and the development of intimal longitudinal muscle and inner muscular tubes as a physiological remodelling of the pulmonary arterial tree in response to the alveolar hypoxia rather than as a form of pulmonary vascular disease. These changes appear little more than a marker of chronic alveolar hypoxia associated with a mild elevation of pulmonary arterial pressure, which is wholly benign and which does not shorten life or cause morbidity in any way. The development of right ventricular hypertrophy in the absence of a congenital cardiac anomaly or disease of the mitral valve but in the presence of remodelling of the pulmonary arterial tree should not be considered as compatible with a definition of 'cor pulmonale'. It would be absurd to regard the ubiquitous football matches throughout the Andes involving teams of healthy, athletic young Quechuas as being played by 22 cases of cor pulmonale.

PATHOGENESIS OF THE MUSCULARIZATION

It would appear that the muscularization of the periphery of the pulmonary arterial tree is due to a retention of the muscular state of the fetal pulmonary vasculature consequent upon the abnormally low levels of partial pressure of oxygen in the alveolar spaces in infancy and childhood in the mountain environment. As noted in Chapter 23, the intra uterine umbilical arterial oxygen tension is about 20 mmHg, which corresponds to an atmospheric oxygen tension of 61 mmHg, which would be found at an elevation of 7500 m (Mithoefer 1966). In the fetus the lung is solid and there is physiological pulmonary hypertension associated with thick-walled, muscular interlobular and intralobular pulmonary arteries (Civin and Edwards 1951). At birth the lungs suddenly expand and begin to move rhythmically in respiration and, as a consequence, the pulmonary arteries dilate. There is at the same time a sudden relief from the severe degree of hypoxaemia to which the fetal lung is subjected.

At sea level the partial pressure of oxygen in the ambient air and thus in the alveolar spaces is high, and this keeps low the muscular tone of the pulmonary arteries freshly mechanically pulled into dilatation by the expansion of the lung at birth. This thin-walled pulmonary arterial tree is maintained throughout life by the lowlander and with it a low pulmonary arterial pressure and resistance. In sharp contrast, at high altitude the barometric pressure is diminished and with it the partial pressure of oxygen in the ambient air and in the alveolar spaces. As a result, although the pulmonary arteries are mechanically expanded by the inflation of the lung at birth, the terminal portions of the muscular fetal pulmonary vasculature remain in a hypoxic environment. As a result they are not subjected to the stimulus for vasodilatation by oxygen and they remain thick-walled and muscular, retaining a high vascular tone. Even so it has to be realized that, even in a Quechua baby born at 4000 m in the Andes, at the moment of birth it is suddenly brought down in effect from the simulated altitude of 7500 m maintained by the hypoxaemic intra-uterine conditions.

As the infant survives at high altitude and progresses into childhood and adult life, the alveolar hypoxia persists and maintains the muscularization of the pulmonary arterioles. Since the early studies of von Euler and Liljestrand (1946) on the pulmonary circulation of the cat, it has become clear that hypoxia is one of the most powerful constrictors of pulmonary arteries. The mechanism by which hypoxia brings about pulmonary vasoconstriction has always been controversial and it remains so today. Ultrastructural studies of the pulmonary arterioles of rats subjected to simulated high altitude in a decompression chamber confirm and show the fine details of the muscularization (Smith and Heath 1977; see Fig. 10.12). Smooth muscle cells are seen situated between inner and outer elastic laminae. In rats a period of hypoxia as short as 2 weeks will induce the hyperplasia of smooth muscle, which becomes pronounced after 3 weeks (Smith and Heath 1977 see Fig. 10.12). It is not possible to determine whether these new muscle cells arise from division of pre-existing muscle cells, or whether they are the result of an infiltration of primitive mesenchymal cells. It is likely that they are also responsible for secreting the new internal elastic lamina in the same way that smooth muscle cells produce the elastic laminae in the developing aorta (Kadar *et al.* 1971).

MAST CELLS

The part played by mast cells in the lung in the reaction of the pulmonary circulation to hypoxia is controversial. Over a course of several years the debate has resulted in a reversal of the original idea that mast cells are instrumental in bringing about pulmonary vasoconstriction into the concept that in some way they are involved in compensatory pulmonary vascular dilatation. At first it was conceived that alveolar hypoxia brought about pulmonary vasoconstriction through the mediation of some agent lying between alveolar space and pulmonary arteriole that itself received the hypoxic stimulus and converted this into a chemical messenger acting on the vascular smooth muscle. It was postulated that this mediating vasoconstrictor was histamine (Hauge 1968; Hauge and Melman 1968). The choice of histamine as a putative pulmonary vasoconstrictor in the human lung was somewhat surprising, since surveillance of the literature on the pharmacology of the human pulmonary circulation indicates that histamine has always brought about dilatation rather than constriction of pulmonary arteries (Harris and Heath 1986). Nevertheless, since most histamine in the lung is stored in mast cells, they came to be championed as the sought-for tissue mediator. Studies revealed that hypoxia releases histamine from mast cells isolated from the peritoneal cavity without injuring them (Haas and Bergofsky 1972)

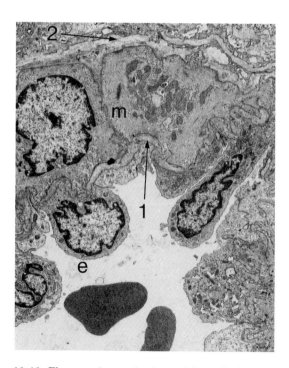

10.12 *Electron micrograph of part of the wall of muscularized pulmonary arteriole from a rat exposed to a simulated altitude of 5500 m for 2 weeks. There is a distinct media of smooth muscle cells (m) bounded by inner (arrow 1) and outer (arrow 2) elastic laminae. Endothelial cells (e) project into the lumen, which contains red cells. × 3750.*

and that perivascular mast cells are degranulated *in vivo* during acute alveolar hypoxia (Haas and Bergofsky 1972). Kay *et al.* (1974) found that the lung mast-cell density doubled in eight rats exposed for 20 days to a diminished barometric pressure of 380 mmHg, simulating an altitude of 5500 m. Our own studies (Williams *et al.* 1977) revealed that the appearance of mast cells in the lungs under these conditions was fleeting, so that the mast cells disappear as soon as the hypoxia is relieved.

Although it is easy to demonstrate a temporary accumulation of mast cells in the lungs under conditions of simulated high altitude, it is far more difficult to come to any conclusion as to what function they are fulfilling. The studies of Mungall (1976) showed that, when rats were exposed to hypoxia, mast cells did not proliferate until after 21 days of exposure, but right ventricular hypertrophy was apparent after only 14 days, a rather unlikely event if the mast cells were instrumental in raising pulmonary vascular resistance leading to right ventricular hypertrophy. Tucker *et al.* (1977) studied the changes in the density and distribution of lung mast cells in six mammalian species (cattle, pigs, rats, sheep, guinea-pigs, and dogs) exposed to an altitude of 4500 m for 19–48 days. Controls were studied at 1600 m. They found considerable accumulations of mast cells, especially around the very muscular pulmonary arteries of cattle and pigs. This led them to postulate that, at high altitude and in other states of hypoxia, the proliferation of mast cells around pulmonary arteries may be more closely related to the muscular changes in those blood vessels than to the existing hypoxia. This in turn suggested to them that mast cells increase in number in response to the pulmonary hypertension rather than induce it. The histamine or other agents liberated by such mast cells may in fact dilate the pulmonary arteries in an attempt to restrain the hypoxic pressor response of high altitude rather than constrict them.

We studied the density of mast cells in various anatomical locations with lungs from a llama and a cow from Cerro de Pasco (4300 m) in the Andes and from a cow from sea level (Williams *et al.* 1981). The total mast-cell density did not differ significantly between the three animals and, in fact, there were more periarteriolar and perivenular mast cells in the llama than in either of the two cows. These data do not support the hypothesis that the perivascular mast cell in the lung is responsible for initiating the vasopressor response to hypoxia. In fact it can be argued that they actually inhibit this response, since a high mast-cell density was found in the llama, an animal that does not develop pulmonary hypertension at high altitude. These data also do not support the findings of Tucker *et al.* (1977), for they show that there may be as many

Table 10.1 Mast-cell density in the lungs of native highlanders of La Paz (3600 m) and in one case of high-altitude pulmonary oedema

Race	Age	Sex	Cause of death, or diagnosis	PVR*	Mast cells/mm²
Caucasian	21	M	Road accident	0	3.8
Caucasian	23	M	"	0	8.8
Caucasian	24	M	"	0	0.6
Caucasian	29	F	Friedreich's ataxia	0	8.8
Mestizo	32	M	Pyelonephritis	0	8.4
Mestizo	27	F	Pyelonephritis	0	3.6
Aymara	42	M	Gastric lymphoma	m	26.0
Aymara	37	M	Ruptured appendix	m	25.6
Aymara	28	M	Cerebellar tumour	mli	25.6
Caucasian	54	M	High-altitude pulmonary and cerebral oedema, Bronchopneumonia	pt	70.1

*PVR, Pulmonary vascular remodelling; m, muscularization of pulmonary arterioles; l, intimal longitudinal muscle; i, inner muscular tubes; pt, pulmonary thrombosis.

mast cells around thin-walled pulmonary arteries as around thick-walled muscular ones.

We have studied the mast-cell density in the lungs of Aymara and mestizo citizens of La Paz (3600 m) and related this to the extent of pulmonary vascular remodelling present (Heath 1992*a*). The data arising from this investigation are shown in Table 10.1. In the native highlanders showing no pulmonary vascular remodelling there was no increase in mast-cell density above levels seen in sea-level controls in Caucasians (Heath 1992*a*).This indicates that the hypobaric hypoxia of high altitude *per se* does not lead to an increased number of mast cells in the lungs. In contrast, in Aymaras and mestizos showing such remodelling there was an increase in the number of mast cells in the lung (Table 10.1). Such data are consistent with the view expressed above that the role of perivascular mast cells in the lung is to relax small pulmonary arteries showing increased muscularity. The increase in number of mast cells is small and is in no way comparable to their vast increase in high-altitude pulmonary oedema (Table 10.1).

EFFECTS OF PULMONARY ARTERIOLAR MUSCULARIZATION

Muscularization of the terminal portions of the pulmonary arterial tree is associated with increased pulmonary vascular resistance and mild pulmonary hypertension. In Quechua children this elevation of pulmonary arterial pressure prevents the loss of neonatal dominance of the right ventricle that occurs in infancy at sea level. Arias-Stella and Recavarren (1962) demonstrated this by comparing the weights of the left and right ventricles of the heart at necropsy in 59 children who lived between 3700 and 4260 m and in 70 children who lived at sea level. The results of their studies are summarized diagrammatically in Fig. 10.13. At sea level the right ventricle weighs as much as the left at birth, but by the age of 4 months the predominance of the left ventricle seen in the adult is already established. In contrast, at high altitude right ventricular hypertrophy persists. This may be associated with some degree of enlargement of the main pulmonary arteries, but it may not be possible to detect this on radiological examination (Fig. 10.14).

With the advent of echocardiography it has become feasible to make more direct measurements of the dimensions of the ventricles and their walls during life. Aparicio-Otero *et al.* (1991) applied M-mode and two-dimensional echocardiography to 50 infants living at high altitude (3800 m) in La Paz

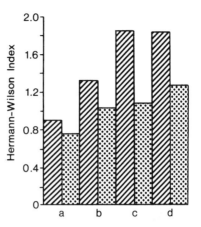

10.13 *Ratio of left to right ventricular weights in newborns and children at sea level and at high altitude. Stippled columns, 59 subjects at high altitude (3700–4260 m). Hatched columns, 70 subjects at sea level. (a) Newborns; (b) 1 day to 3 months; (c) 4–23 months; (d) 2–10 years). (Compiled from data in Arias-Stella and Recavarren (1962).)*

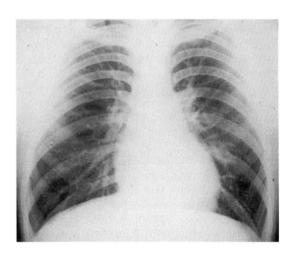

10.14 *Anteroposterior radiograph of the chest from a Quechua Indian aged 42 years living at 4330 m.*

and to 56 infants living at low altitude (400 m) in Santa Cruz, Bolivia. It was found that, at low altitude, the thickness of the anterior wall of the right ventricle decreases during the first month of extrauterine life to a dimension that remains constant for the rest of infancy. Aparicio-Otero *et al.* (1991) found that this thickness at Santa Cruz averaged 0.43 cm in four newly born infants but fell rapidly in the succeeding weeks so that by the end of the first month it had reached an average level of 0.38 cm, which was approximately maintained until the end of the period of observation. At high altitude in La Paz the thickness, 0.45 cm at birth, was similar to that found at low altitude but did not decrease, the average thickness at the end of 1 month being 0.50 cm, which did not diminish during the succeeding 12 months. The ratio of the diameter of the aorta to that of the pulmonary artery was greater at low altitude in all age groups. Their echocardiographic observations are consistent with the persistence of a high pulmonary arterial pressure during infancy at high altitude.

During this investigation the opportunity was taken to note the racial origins of all the infants and it was possible to compare the thickness of the anterior wall of the right ventricle at high altitude in Aymaras and mestizos of mixed Caucasian and Indian blood. There was no statistically significant difference between the two racial groups.

NATIVE LOWLANDERS LIVING PERMANENTLY AT HIGH ALTITUDE

The benign remodelling of the pulmonary arterial tree of native Quechua and Aymara Indians living at high altitude in the Andes is almost certainly a reflection of the fact that over the course of 35 000 years in their mountain environment they have lost their susceptibility to hypobaric hypoxia through genetic selection. This comfortable adjustment to high altitude has to be contrasted sharply with consequences that may follow in the native lowlander who takes up a prolonged sojourn in the mountains. There are mountain communities like Leadville, Colorado (3100 m) that were settled barely a century ago. In them there are probably still individuals who are prone to develop pulmonary hypertension. Vogel *et al.* (1962) identified one family in which five children had pulmonary arterial pressures well above the mean values for that population. Such families in the community account for the disproportionately high mean pulmonary arterial pressure at only 3100 m when compared with the highlanders in the Andes. It has even been reported that, in such communities as Leadville and Climax, Colorado, a few children develop primary pulmonary hypertension. Khoury and Hawes (1963) described two such cases and considered the clinical and haemodynamic data from 11 others. The affected children were usually between 6 weeks and 6 years of age and became cyanosed and breathless. They developed clinical and electrocardiographic ev-

idence of right ventricular hypertrophy and severe pulmonary hypertension. These authors described the pulmonary vascular pathology in two cases. In a female infant of 18 months the muscular pulmonary arteries showed medial hypertrophy with a cellular intimal proliferation, an illustrated example of which is reminiscent of concentric-laminar ('onion-skin') proliferation, which is certainly consistent with a diagnosis of plexogenic pulmonary arteriopathy forming the pathological basis of primary pulmonary hypertension. In a second male infant of 6 months they report severe intimal thickening in a pulmonary arteriole. The medium and small pulmonary arteries and arterioles were also reported to show various degrees of medial necrosis (Khoury and Hawes 1963). Certainly such histological changes are more in keeping with primary pulmonary hypertension than with the purely muscular changes in the terminal portions of the pulmonary arterial tree that were described earlier in the chapter as being characteristic of the native highlanders of the Andes.

An anomalous feature of some of the cases reported by Khoury and Hawes (1963) is that some of the infants from Leadville with moderate to severe pulmonary hypertension improved on descent to lower elevations. This behaviour is different from that expected in a case of primary pulmonary hypertension. It raises the possibility that those sick infants from the Colorado Rockies taken recently up to high altitude by their parents from the plains may be more similar to infants from Tibet who fail to acclimatize to high altitude. This condition is described in Chapter 17. Infants ascending to spend some months in Lhasa (3600 m) may fail to acclimatize to the hypobaric hypoxia and develop muscularization of the pulmonary arteries and arterioles (see Figs 17.4 and 17.5), which elevates pulmonary vascular resistance and leads to right ventricular hypertrophy and dilatation of the pulmonary trunk (see Fig. 17.1). In Chapter 17 we regard the Tibetan condition as the human counterpart of brisket disease in cattle. While this comparison may hold for infants recently taken up to Leadville by their parents from lowland areas it would not be valid for the infants and children of families domiciled at high altitude for one or more generations.

A FATAL LEGACY FOR INFANTS OF LOWLANDERS BORN AND SPENDING THE NEONATAL PERIOD AT HIGH ALTITUDE

We have had experience of two cases that suggest that infants of Caucasian parents born and spending the neonatal period at high altitude may acquire a fatal legacy for the subsequent development of primary plexogenic pulmonary arteriopathy. We studied lung tissues from the case of a female infant of Caucasian parents who was born and spent a stormy infancy with respiratory difficulty in the Andes before coming to sea level in Europe. At the age of 18 years she developed primary pulmonary hypertension, based on plexogenic pulmonary arteriopathy proven on histological examination, from which she died (O'Neill *et al.* 1981). It is conceivable that the early exposure in life to hypobaric hypoxia and its effect on the pulmonary vasculature left a fateful legacy for subsequent years. In a second case a male child was born and spent a difficult infancy at high altitude in the Kenya highlands. As a young child he was returned to low altitude, recovered, and then as a young man entered the Royal Air Force to train as a fighter pilot. This involved further exposure during training to hypobaric hypoxia in a decompression chamber. At the age of 36 years he developed primary plexogenic pulmonary arteriopathy for which he was treated by combined heart–lung transplantation. It has been demonstrated experimentally that Wistar albino rats born and reared in the neonatal period in simulated high altitude in a decompression chamber have pulmonary arteries and arterioles that are unusually sensitive to agents like pyrrolizidine alkaloids that induce vasoconstrictive pulmonary vascular disease (Caslin *et al.* 1991). These clinical pointers and experimental studies suggest that infants of lowlanders born and spending the neonatal period at high altitude may acquire a fatal legacy encouraging the subsequent development of vasoconstrictive and plexogenic pulmonary arteriopathy.

PULMONARY VEINS AND VENULES

It seems that the sustained hypobaric hypoxia of high altitude induces a proliferation of vascular smooth muscle in blood vessels in the entire area adjacent to alveolar spaces. Thus, the process affects pulmonary veins (Fig. 10.15) and venules as well as pulmonary arteries and arterioles. The proliferation of muscle in the intima of small pulmonary veins has a different histological appearance from that in the intima of pulmonary arteries and arterioles (Heath and Williams 1991). In the veins the smooth muscle cells are found largely individually with considerable amounts of collagen separating them, a difference that is probably related to the haemodynamic influences on the two classes of vessel. While alveolar hypoxia appears to be the prime stimulus in in-

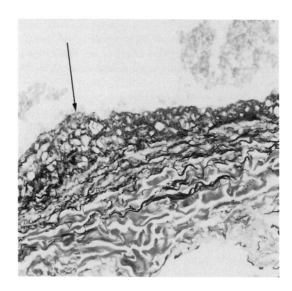

10.15 *Part of an oblique section of a large pulmonary vein from a 28-year-old Aymara resident of La Paz (3600 m) who died from a cerebellar tumour. It shows a striking intimal proliferation, indicated by the arrow, composed of groups of smooth muscle cells appearing as clear areas on a darker background of collagen. EVG, × 322.*

ducing proliferation of vascular smooth muscle cells, the arterial pulsation appears to ensure that initially they retain a compact, overtly muscular nature. In contrast, in the veins where they are not subjected to a comparable pulsatile stimulus, they are widely spaced and separated by much sclerotic tissue.

An increase in the medial thickness of pulmonary veins of 14 residents at high altitude was reported by Wagenvoort and Wagenvoort (1976). It was said to be prominent in five of them. In a subsequent study (1982) these authors stated that they believed such venous muscularization was to be expected in persons living at elevations exceeding 3000 m. In their experience, medial thickening of pulmonary arteries and veins in any one person was proportional, the inference being that the vascular smooth muscle in an individual reacted to the same extent to hypobaric hypoxia. The demonstration of medial hypertrophy of pulmonary veins in highlanders demands the most vigorous application of tissue morphometry (Wagenvoort 1986). Even so, from our own experience, the slight increases in medial thickness in small pulmonary veins that have been reported as occurring in hypobaric hypoxia are commonly so slight and open to technical errors in measurement as not to instil the greatest confidence in the findings. Just as there are difficulties in demonstrating unequivocally the histological effects of hypobaric hypoxia on human pulmonary veins so there are with the lungs of several animal species. Thus, Naeye (1965) reported that in calves and steers exposed to high altitude there was medial hypertrophy of pulmonary veins and he thought this attributable to hypoxic pulmonary vasoconstriction. The difficulty of such observations is that cattle normally have pads of smooth muscle in the walls of pulmonary veins and this muscle winds around the vessel in a spiral fashion (Harris and Heath 1986). As a consequence of this, adjacent sections of the same vein may be free of intimal muscle or show such prominent muscular pads as to compromise the patency of the lumen. Such histological appearances, which are common to all ungulates, render assessment of medial hypertrophy in pulmonary veins all but impossible. Naeye (1965) used only cross-sections with a uniform complete muscular coat for his measurements, but the spiral nature of the muscle must weaken the credibility of his observations. Atwal and Persofsky (1984) induced pulmonary hypertension in cattle by the administration of 3-methylindole. This produced pulmonary oedema and supposedly subsequent alveolar hypoxia. They measured the thickness of the muscular pads projecting into the lumen of pulmonary veins and reported that this was increased.

Rodents present interesting problems in assessing physiological and histological changes in their pulmonary veins. In them, cardiac muscle extends from the wall of the left atrium around pulmonary veins deep into the substance of the lung (Harris and Heath 1986). Thus cardiac and smooth muscle is simultaneously exposed to the stimulus of chronic alveolar hypoxia in rodents living at high altitude. It has been reported that in young mice there is a rapid increase in these perivenous myocardial fibres in a peripheral direction following intermittent exposure to hypoxia (Jarkovská and Ostádal 1983).

ARACHNOID BODIES

We have seen arachnoid bodies closely associated with the pulmonary venules in Aymara and mestizo citizens of La Paz (3600 m) (Heath and Williams 1992; see Figs 10.16 and 10.17). Originally described as multiple minute pulmonary tumours resembling chemodectomas (Korn *et al.* 1960) the constituent round or ovoid cells were later recognized as having ultrastructural features more akin to those of arachnoid cells without dense-core vesicles

but with tangled cytoplasmic fibrils 6–10 nm in width with complex interdigitation between adjoining cells (Kuhn and Askin 1975; Churg and Warnock 1976). The small cellular nodules apparently arise from the interstitial tissues of alveolar walls and pulmonary venules and are found closely adjacent to them (Fig. 10.16). The constituent cells have large round or oval nuclei showing punctate heterochromatin. Their cytoplasm is plentiful and palely eosinophilic and is frequently distended to form large vacuoles that are clustered around the nuclei. In the centres of the nodules are small pulmonary venules. They are lined by flattened endothelial cells with elongated nuclei and occasionally minute channels can be seen lined by such cells linking venule and cellular nodule (Fig. 10.17). Sometimes the nodules are reminiscent of those described by Churg and Warnock (1976) in possessing a central nodule of arachnoid cells with strands extending into the surrounding alveolar walls like a

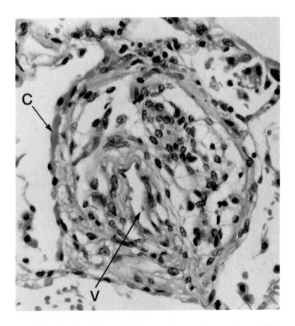

10.16 *Arachnoid nodule from a lung of a mestizo of 32 years who died from pyelonephritis, having spent all his life in Pa Paz. The general configuration of the nodule is shown. It arises from the interstitial tissues of alveolar walls and is covered by pulmonary capillaries (arrow c). In the centre of the body is a venule (arrow v). The substance of the body is formed of arachnoid cells. HE, × 405.*

scirrhus. Adjacent alveolar spaces appear to be increased in size.

Arachnoid bodies occur in the normal lung in about 4% of cases when a special careful search is made for them. Their prevalence in normal lungs suggests that they have a physiological function. In this respect it is of interest to consider in which diseases these nodules become hyperplastic and more noticeable. They are commonly found in various forms of pulmonary vascular disease with pulmonary hypertension and incipient pulmonary oedema such as mitral stenosis and recurrent pulmonary thromboembolism. We have seen them in a case of plexogenic pulmonary arteriopathy (Heath and Smith 1992). It is not surprising, therefore, that they are to be found in native highlanders who show muscular remodelling of their pulmonary vasculature, pulmonary hypertension, and a tendency to develop pulmonary oedema.

We think it possible that the arachnoid-like cells forming the nodules adjacent to the pulmonary venules have a similar function to the arachnoid villi and granulations in the meninges that absorb cerebrospinal fluid and return it to the dural sinuses. It seems likely that oedema fluid of the interstitial tissues of the alveolar walls is absorbed by arachnoid cells that show oedema-vesicles of their cytoplasm. They pass the fluid on through channels found between the arachnoid cells down the streamers of the thickened alveolar walls to the central arachnoid nodule (Fig. 10.18). From here the oedema fluid appears to be passed through conduits lined by elongated, dark cells into the blood in the pulmonary venules. This appears to explain why arachnoid nodules may occur around the pulmonary venules in native highlanders. In the lung at high altitude there is always the risk of incipient oedema, which may become manifested suddenly as high-altitude pulmonary oedema that may become fatal (Chapter 13). It is conceivable that in persons resident in high mountainous areas these arachnoid nodules become

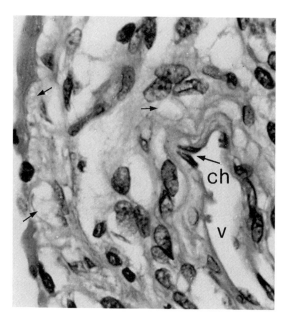

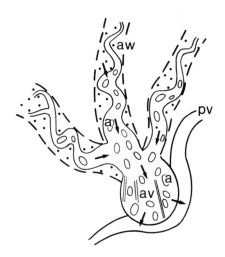

10.17 *Part of the arachnoid body shown in the preceding figure at higher magnification to show cytological detail. Opening into the central venule, v, is a narrow canal (arrow ch) lined by cells with elongated nuclei. Immediately adjacent to these nuclei the underlying cytoplasm contains small vacuoles. The cells around the venule are arachnoid with large round or oval nuclei showing punctate heterochromatin and surrounding vacuolated cytoplasm (small arrows). HE, × 1000.*

10.18 *Schema to illustrate proposed function of arachnoid bodies in the lung. Excess hydration of the interstitial tissue (dotted) of the thickened alveolar walls (aw) passes into the extensions of the arachnoid bodies (wavy lines). In these extensions are arachnoid cells (a) indicated by oval outlines. The flow of fluid is centripetal into the arachnoid-like villus (av) that projects into a pulmonary venule (pv). The direction of flow is shown by black arrows. Drainage channels are indicated by parallel lines.*

active in keeping the hydration of the interstitial tissues of the alveolar walls in safe limits.

PATENT DUCTUS ARTERIOSUS

An interesting complication of the effects of chronic hypoxia and pulmonary hypertension on infants born at high altitude is the higher prevalence in them of patent ductus arteriosus. It is the most frequent form of congenital cardiac anomaly in Mexico City, which is at an altitude of 2380 m (Chavez *et al.* 1953). Natives of the Peruvian Andes show a greater incidence of patent ductus (Alzamora *et al.* 1953: Alzamora-Castro *et al.* 1960). This was confirmed by a screening cardiovascular examination for this condition of 5000 schoolchildren of both sexes, born and living in towns between 3500 and 5000 m above sea level (Marticorena *et al.* 1962). The prevalence of patent ductus arteriosus at these altitudes is 18 times that reported at sea level by different authors (Gardiner and Keith 1951; Richards *et al.* 1955). Between 3500 and 5000 m the prevalence is 30 times greater than at sea level (Peñaloza *et al.* 1964).

One can appreciate the reasons for the greater prevalence of patent ductus at high altitude by considering the normal mechanism of closure of this channel. In the fetus, when the lungs are not yet expanded, the blood pressure in the pulmonary arteries exceeds that in the aorta, so blood flows from right to left through the ductus. Once the umbilical cord has been cut and the lungs expand, the blood pressure falls sharply in the pulmonary arteries and rises in the systemic circulation. As a result richly oxygenated blood now flows from left to right through the ductus, constricting it and leading to its functional closure. Functional closure of the ductus is hindered by hypoxia. Furthermore, if the ductus has already closed functionally, the breathing of hypoxic air or gas mixture leads to pulmonary hypertension and causes the ductus to reopen (Eldridge and Hultgren 1955; James and Rowe 1957; Rowe and James 1957). On the basis of such experimental studies it is readily understood how the breathing of hypoxic ambient air at high altitude will hinder closure of the ductus and lead to the complication of this congenital cardiac anomaly by pulmonary hypertension. Peñaloza *et al.* (1964) note that the clinical picture of patent ductus arteriosus at high altitude is frequently atypical, with the complication of pulmonary hypertension.

Through the kindness of clinicians and pathologists at La Paz (3600 m) we have had the opportunity to study the histology of the pulmonary blood

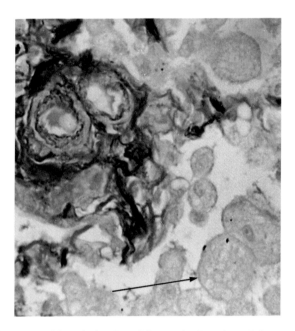

10.19 *Muscularization of the terminal portions of the pulmonary arterial tree in a case of patent ductus arteriosus in a woman of 20 years who was born and lived all her life in Potosi (4000 m). The muscularization extends distally to a remarkable extent to involve minute vessels whose diameter hardly exceeds that of macrophages (arrow) in the surrounding alveolar spaces. EVG, × 600.*

vessels in lung biopsy specimens from cases of patent ductus arteriosus at high altitude. We find evidence of hypertensive pulmonary vascular disease of severity corresponding to grades 1–3 (Fig. 10.19) on the criteria we suggested some years ago (Heath and Edwards 1958).

MUSCULAR EVAGINATIONS IN THE RAT

Throughout this chapter we have seen that the pulmonary vascular remodelling that occurs in the native highlander is a benign process involving a limited migration of smooth muscle cells into the intima of small pulmonary arteries that leads to only slight pulmonary hypertension that does not lead to morbidity or decrease longevity. This is in striking contrast to the response of the pulmonary circulation of the rat to hypobaric hypoxia in decompression chambers. Such exposure leads to intense pulmonary vasoconstriction, which may prove to be rapidly fatal. In the rat there is no evidence of migration of muscle cells into the pulmonary arterioles and arterial intima. Hence the nature and prognosis of the remodelling of the human pulmonary circulation at high altitude are quite distinct from the vasoconstrictive pulmonary vascular disease induced in rats placed in hypobaric chambers (Heath 1992*b*).

The hallmark of this hypoxic vasoconstrictive disease in the rat is the muscular evagination. It is seen at ultrastructural level. Scanning electron microscopy has revealed that when smooth muscle cells constrict they do not simply become shorter and thicker but become covered in bulbous extrusions. This was demonstrated elegantly by the studies of Fay and Delise (1973) on the smooth muscle cells of the stomach wall of *Bufo marinus*. Such prominences are due to evaginations of the cytoplasm of the smooth muscle cells between attachment points in the plasmalemma acting as points of anchorage for the intracellular fibrils of actin and myosin (Heath and Smith 1983; see Fig. 10.20). The clear cytoplasm of the evaginations is devoid of myofilaments and organelles. When vascular smooth muscle cells constrict, the evaginations squeeze through deficiencies in the adjacent inner or outer elastic lamina of the wall of the blood vessel to extend into the intima or adventitia respectively. Since deficiencies in the pulmonary arteries occur naturally in the outer lamina, muscular evaginations in these vessels tend to be into the adventitia. In contrast, in pulmonary veins deficiencies occur mainly in the inner elastic lamina, so that in these vessels the evaginations are found in the intima (Fig. 10.21). In this situation the surface of the muscular evagination presses on the undersurface of the endothelial cells. Since the cyto-

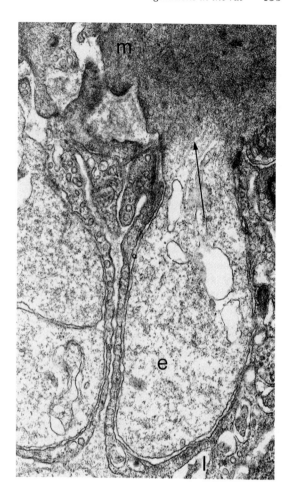

10.21 *Electron micrograph of part of the wall of a pulmonary vein from a rat exposed to severe, acute hypoxia in a hypobaric chamber mimicking conditions at the summit of Mt Everest (8850 m). Vasoconstriction has occurred in response to the hypoxic stimulus with the formation of muscular evaginations (e), the cytoplasm of which is clear being devoid of myofilaments and organelles. The sites of junction of the evaginations with the cytoplasm of the parent smooth muscle cells (m) are indicated by arrows. The edge of the lumen (l) of the vein is seen. × 17 500.*

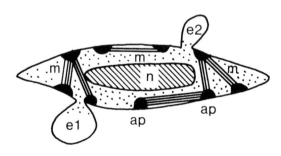

10.20 *Mode of formation of muscular evaginations. On contraction of the myofilaments (m) that connect to 'attachment points' (ap), muscle cell cytoplasm forms evaginations, shown here as e1 and e2. The cytoplasm of these evaginations is clear, being devoid of myofilaments and organelles. The nucleus (n) holds a central position in the cell.*

plasm of muscle and endothelial cell come into such intimate contact, it is possible that substances may pass between these cells and this raises the very interesting possibility that physiological 'conversations' may take place between muscle and endothelium. Muscular evaginations may be readily produced in the lungs of rats by exposing them to simulated high altitude (Dingemans and Wagenvoort 1978), but they must be interpreted with care, and only lungs fixed in distension are satisfactory for examination since muscular evaginations are also readily produced by collapse (Heath and Smith 1983). Muscular evaginations have not been reported in man and hence their possible role in pulmonary vascular remodelling and the adjustment of the human pulmonary circulation to the hypobaric hypoxia of high altitude is not known.

RENIN–ANGIOTENSIN SYSTEM

Over a decade ago it was suggested that the renin–angiotensin system is involved in the development of muscularization of the peripheral segments of the pulmonary arterial tree in chronic hypoxia (Berkov 1974). Renin is formed in the kidney and perhaps even in the same cell that synthesizes erythropoietin where the stimulus is known to be hypoxia (Eepson and McCarry 1968; Gould *et al.* 1968). After release from the kidney, renin acts on an α-globulin in the plasma to split off a decapeptide, angiotensin I. The decapeptide has little effect on smooth muscle, but it can be converted to a highly vasoconstrictor octapeptide, angiotensin II, by the hydrolytic removal of the COOH-terminal dipeptide, as we illustrate elsewhere (Harris and Heath 1986). This conversion is achieved by 'converting enzyme' whose main site of activity is the surface of the pulmonary endothelial cells (Ryan *et al.* 1976). Mice deprived of oxygen developed increased granulation of the juxtaglomerular apparatus and elevated levels of converting enzyme in lungs and serum during the second week of exposure to hypoxia (Molteni *et al.* 1974). After 2–3 days of hypoxia in both man and rats there is a fall in plasma concentration of renin (Gould and Goodman 1970). The infusion of angiotensin I or II into the pulmonary circulation of the dog caused a threefold increase in the vasoconstrictive response to hypoxia (Alexander *et al.* 1976). Zakheim *et al.* (1975) found that blockade of angiotensin I conversion by SQ 20 881, a synthetic nonapeptide, significantly reduced in Sprague–Dawley rats the right ventricular changes of chronic alveolar hypoxia described earlier in this chapter. Since this nonapeptide is a specific competitive inhibitor of converting enzyme, these experimental findings suggest that chronic hypoxia may in part exert its effects through the agency of the renin–angiotensin system. The role of the renin–angiotensin–aldosterone axis in benign acute mountain sickness is considered in Chapter 12.

References

Alexander, J.M., Nyby, M.D., and Jasberg, K.A. (1976). Effect of angiotensin on hypoxic pulmonary vasoconstriction in isolated dog lung. *Journal of Applied Physiology*, **41**, 84

Alzamora, V., Rotta, A., Battilana, G., Abugattas, R., Rubio, C., Bouroncle, J., Zapata, C., Santa-Maria, E., Binder, T., Sabira, R., Paredes, D., Pando, B., and Graham, G.G. (1953). On the possible influence of great altitudes on the determination of certain cardiovascular anomalies. *Pediatrics*, **12**, 259

Alzamora-Castro, V., Battilana, G., Abugattas, R., and Sialer, S., (1960). Patent ductus arteriosus and high altitude. *American Journal of Cardiology*, **5**, 761

Aparicio-Otero, O., Romero-Gutierrez, F., Harris, P., and Anand, I. (1991). Echocardiography shows persistent thickness of the wall of the right ventricle in infants at high altitude. *Cardioscience*, **2**, 63

Arias-Stella, J. and Recavarren, S. (1962). Right ventricular hypertrophy in native children living at high altitude. *American Journal of Pathology*, **41**, 55

Arias-Stella, J. and Saldaña, M. (1963). The terminal portion of the pulmonary arterial tree in people native to high altitudes. *Circulation*, **28**, 915

Atwal, O.S. and Persofsky, M.S. (1984). Ultrastructural changes in intraacinar pulmonary veins. Relationship of 3-methylindole-induced acute pulmonary edema and pulmonary arterial changes in cattle. *American Journal of Pathology*, **114**, 472

Berkov, S. (1974). Hypoxic pulmonary vasoconstriction in the rat. The necessary role of angiotensin II. *Circulation Research*, **35**, 256

Caslin, A., Heath, D., and Smith, P. (1991). Influence of hypobaric hypoxia in infancy on the subsequent development of vasoconstrictive pulmonary vascular disease in the Wistar albino rat. *Journal of Pathology*, **163**, 133

Chavez, I., Espino-Vela, J., Limon, R., and Dorbecker, N. (1953). La persistencia del conducto arterial. Estudio de 200 casos. *Archivos de Instituto de Cardiologia de México*, **23**, 687

Churg, A.M. and Warnock, M.L. (1976). So-called 'minute pulmonary chemodectoma'. A tumor not related to paragangliomas. *Cancer*, **37**, 1759

Civin, W.H. and Edwards, J.E. (1951). The postnatal structural changes in the intrapulmonary arteries and arterioles. *Archives of Pathology*, **51**, 192

Dingemans, K.P. and Wagenvoort, C.A. (1978). Pulmonary arteries and veins in experimental hypoxia. An ultrastructural study. *American Journal of Pathology*, **93**, 353

Eepson, J.H. and McCarry, E.E. (1968). Polycythemia and increased erythropoietin production in a patient with hypertrophy of the juxtaglomerular apparatus. *Blood*, **32**, 370

Eldridge, D.L. and Hultgren, H.N. (1955). The physiologic closure of the ductus arteriosus in the newborn infant. *Journal of Clinical Investigation*, **34**, 987

Fay, F.S. and Delise, C.M. (1973). Contraction of isolated smooth muscle cells: structural changes. *Proceedings of the National Academy of Sciences of the United States of America*, **70**, 641

Gardiner, J.H. and Keith, J.D. (1951). Prevalence of heart disease in Toronto children, 1948–1949. Cardiac registry. *Pediatrics*, **7**, 713

Gould, A.B. and Goodman, S.A. (1970). The effect of hypoxia on the renin:angiotensin system. *Laboratory Investigation*, **22**, 443

Gould, A.B., Keighley, G., and Lowy, P.H. (1968). On the presence of a renin-like activity in erythropoietin preparation. *Laboratory Investigation*, **18**, 2

Gupta, M.L., Rao, K.S., Anand, I.S., Banerjee, A.K., and Bopari, M.S. (1992). Lack of smooth muscle in the small pulmonary arteries of the native Ladakhi. Is the Himalayan highlander adapted? *American Review of Respiratory Disease*, **145**, 1201

Haas, F. and Bergofsky, E.H. (1972). Role of the mast cell in the pulmonary pressor response to hypoxia. *Journal of Clinical Investigation*, **51**, 3154

Harris, P. and Heath, D. (1986). *The Human Pulmonary Circulation*, 3rd edn. Edinburgh; Churchill Livingstone

Hauge, A. (1968). Role of histamine in hypoxic pulmonary hypertension in the rat. I. Blockade or potentiation of endogenous amines, kinins and ATP. *Circulation Research*, **22**, 371

Hauge, A. and Melman, K.L. (1968). Role of histamine in hypoxic pulmonary hypertension in the rat. II. Depletion of histamine, serotonin and catecholamines. *Circulation Research*, **22**, 385

Heath, D. (1992*a*). Mast cells in the human lung at high altitude. *International Journal of Biometeorology*, **36**, 210

Heath, D. (1992*b*). The rat is a poor animal model for the study of human pulmonary hypertension. *Cardioscience*, **3**, 1

Heath, D. and Edwards, J.E. (1958). The pathology of hypertensive pulmonary vascular disease: a description of six grades of structural changes in the pulmonary arteries with special reference to congenital cardiac septal defects. *Circulation*, **18**, 533

Heath, D. and Smith, P. (1983). Electron microscopy of hypertensive pulmonary vascular disease. *British Journal of Diseases of the Chest*, **77**, 1

Heath, D. and Smith, P. (1992). Nodules resembling arachnoid villi in pulmonary venules in plexogenic pulmonary arteriopathy. *Cardioscience*, **3**, 161

Heath, D. and Williams, D. (1991). Pulmonary vascular remodelling in a high-altitude Aymara Indian. *International Journal of Biometeorology*, **35**, 203

Heath, D. and Williams, D. (1992). Arachnoid nodules in the lungs of high altitude Indians. *Thorax*, **48**, 743

Heath, D., Smith, P., Rios-Dalenz, J., Williams, D., and Harris, P. (1981). Small pulmonary arteries in some natives of La Paz, Bolivia. *Thorax*, **36**, 599

Heath, D., Smith, P., and Gosney, J. (1988). Ultrastructure of early plexogenic pulmonary arteriopathy. *Histopathology*, **12**, 41

Heath, D., Williams, D., Rios-Dalenz J., Calderon, M., and Gosney, J. (1990). Small pulmonary arterial vessels of Aymara Indians from the Bolivian Andes. *Histopathology*, **16**, 565

Hicken, P., Heath, D., Brewer, D.B., and Whitaker, W. (1965). The small pulmonary arteries in emphysema. *Journal of Pathology and Bacteriology*, **90**, 107

James, L.S. and Rowe, R.D. (1957). The pattern of response of pulmonary and systemic arterial pressures in newborn and older infants to short periods of hypoxia. *Journal of Pediatrics*, **51**, 5

Jarkovská, D. and Ostádal, B. (1983). Intermittent high altitude hypoxia-induced structural changes in the pulmonary myocardium in young mice. *Virchows Archiv (Cell Pathology)*, **B43**, 327

Kadar, A., Gardner, D.I., and Bush, V. (1971). The relation between the fine structure of the smooth muscle cells and elastogenesis in the chick-embryo aorta. *Journal of Pathology*, **104**, 253

Kay, J.M., Waymire, J.C., and Grover, R.F. (1974). Lung mast cell hyperplasia and pulmonary histamine-forming capacity in hypoxic rats. *American Journal of Physiology*, **226**, 178

Keith, J.D., Rowe, R.D., and Vlad, P. (1958). *Heart Diseases in Infancy and Childhood*. New York; Macmillan

Khoury, G.H. and Hawes, C.R. (1963). Primary pulmonary hypertension in children living at high altitude. *Journal of Pediatrics*, **62**, 177

Korn, D., Bensch, K., Liebow, A.A., and Castleman, B. (1960). Multiple minute pulmonary tumors resembling chemodectomas. *American Journal of Pathology*, **37**, 641

Kuhn, C. and Askin, F.B. (1975). The fine structure of so-called minute pulmonary chemodectomas. *Human Pathology*, **6**, 681

Marticorena, E., Peñaloza, D., Severino, J., and Hellriegel, K. (1962). Incidencia de la persistencia del conducto arterioso en las grandes alturas. *Memorias del IV Congreso Mundial de Cardiologia, México*, **1A**, 155

Mithoefer, J.C. (1966). The respiration of Andean natives. In *Life at High Altitudes*, Scientific Publication No. 140. Washington; Pan American Health Organization, p. 21

Molteni, A., Zakheim, R.M., Mullis, K., and Mattioli, L. (1974). Effects of chronic hypoxia on lung and serum angiotensin-I-converting enzyme activity. *Proceedings of the Society for Experimental Biology and Medicine*, **147**, 263

Mungall, I.P.F. (1976). Hypoxia and lung mast cells: influence of disodium cromoglycate. *Thorax*, **31**, 94

Naeye, R.L. (1965). Pulmonary vascular changes with chronic unilateral pulmonary hypoxia. *Circulation Research*, **17**, 160

O'Neill, D., Morton, R., and Kennedy, J.A. (1981). Progressive primary pulmonary hypertension in a patient born at high altitude. *British Heart Journal*, **45**, 725

Peñaloza, D., Sime, F., Banchero, N., and Gamboa, R. (1962). Pulmonary hypertension in healthy man born and living at high altitudes. *Medicina Thoracalis*, **19**, 449

Peñaloza, D., Sime, F., Banchero, N. Gamboa, R., Cruz, J., and Marticorena, E. (1963). Pulmonary hypertension in healthy men born and living at high altitudes. *American Journal of Cardiology*, **11**, 150

Peñaloza, D., Arias-Stella, J., Sime, F. Recavarren, S., and Marticorena, E. (1964). The heart and pulmonary circulation in children at high altitudes. Physiological, anatomical and clinical observations. *Pediatrics*, **34**, 568

Richards, M.R., Merritt, K.K., Samuels, M.H., and Longmann, A.G. (1955). Congenital malformations of the cardiovascular system in a series of 6053 infants. *Pediatrics*, **15**, 12

Rowe, R.D. and James, L.S. (1957). The normal pulmonary arterial pressures during the first year of life. *Journal of Pediatrics*, **51**, 1

Rudolph, A.M. and Cayler, G.G. (1958). Cardiac catheterization in infants and children. *Pediatric Clinics of North America*, **5**, 907

Rudolph, A.M., Drorbaugh, J.E., Auld, P.A.M., Rudolph, A.J., Nadas, A.S., Smith, C.A., and Hubbell, J.P. (1961). Studies on the circulation in the neonatal period. The circulation in the respiratory distress syndrome. *Pediatrics*, **27**, 551

Ryan, U.S., Ryan, J.W., Whitaker, C., and Chiu, A. (1976). Localization of angiotensin converting enzyme (Kininase II). II Immunocytochemistry and immunofluorescence. *Tissue and Cell*, **8**, 125

Sime, F., Banchero, N., Peñaloza, D., Gamboa, R., Cruz, J., and Marticorena, E. (1963). Pulmonary hypertension in children born and living at high altitudes. *American Journal of Cardiology*, **11**, 143

Smith, P. and Heath, D. (1977). Ultrastructure of hypoxic hypertensive pulmonary vascular disease. *Journal of Pathology*, **121**, 93

Smith, P., Moosavi, H., Winson, M., and Heath, D. (1974). The influence of age and sex on the response of the right ventricle, pulmonary vasculature, and carotid bodies to hypoxia in rats. *Journal of Pathology*, **112**, 11

Smith, P., Rodgers, B., Heath, D., and Yacoub, M. (1992). The ultrastructure of pulmonary arteries and arterioles in emphysema. *Journal of Pathology*, **167**, 69

Smith, P., Heath, D., Williams, D., Bencini, C., Pulera, N., and Giuntini, C. (1993). The earliest histopathological response to hypobaric hypoxia in rabbits in the Rifugio Torino (3370 m) on Monte Bianco. *Journal of Pathology*, **170**, 485

Tucker, A., McMurtry, I.F., Alexander, A.F., Reeves, J.T., and Grover, R.F. (1977). Lung mast cell density and distribution in chronically hypoxic animals. *Journal of Applied Physiology*, **42**, 174

Vogel, J.H.K., Weaver, W.F., Rose, R.L., Blount, S.G., and Grover, R.F. (1962). Pulmonary hypertension and exertion in normal man living at 10,150 feet. In *Normal and Abnormal Pulmonary Circulation* (R.F. Grover, Ed.). Basle; Karger, p. 239

von Euler, U.S. and Liljestrand, G. (1946). Observations on the pulmonary arterial blood pressure in the cat. *Acta Physiologica Scandinavica*, **12**, 301

Wagenvoort, C.A. (1986). The pulmonary veins in hypoxia. In *Aspects of Hypoxia* (D. Heath, Ed.). Liverpool; Liverpool University Press, pp. 20–21

Wagenvoort, C.A. and Wagenvoort, N. (1976). Pulmonary venous changes in chronic hypoxia. *Virchows Archiv*, **A372**, 51

Wagenvoort, C.A. and Wagenvoort, N. (1982). Pulmonary veins in high altitude residents. A morphometric study. *Thorax*, **37**, 931

Wilkinson, M., Langhorne, C.A., Heath, D., Barer, G.R., and Howard, P. (1988). A pathophysiological study of ten cases of hypoxic cor pulmonale. *Quarterly Journal of Medicine, N.S.* **66**, **249**, 65

Williams, A., Heath, D., Kay, J.M., and Smith, P. (1977). Lung mast cells in rats exposed to acute hypoxia and chronic hypoxia and recovery. *Thorax*, **32**, 287

Williams, A., Heath, D., Harris, P., Williams, D., and Smith, P. (1981). Pulmonary mast cells in cattle and llamas at high altitude. *Journal of Pathology*, **134**, 1

Zakheim, R.M., Mattioli, I., Molteni, A., Mullis, K.B., and Bartley, J. (1975). Prevention of pulmonary vascular changes of chronic alveolar hypoxia by inhibition of angiotensin I-converting enzyme in the rat. *Laboratory Investigation*, **33**, 57

11

The pulmonary trunk

The pulmonary trunk and its branches conduct the flow of blood from the right ventricle into the lungs. These large arteries are capacitance vessels able to distend with the influx of an extra volume of blood with each systole. To fulfil this function their medial coat contains a great deal of elastic tissue as well as smooth muscle, and on this account they are commonly referred to as the elastic pulmonary arteries. The structure of this medial coat is modified by the intravascular pressure. Its thickness is increased in the presence of pulmonary hypertension and the pattern of its elastic tissue depends on the time of onset of the raised pulmonary arterial pressure. It was seen in the preceding chapter that native highlanders in the Andes have a mild degree of pulmonary hypertension that is present from birth and exaggerated during infancy and childhood. Thus it comes about that the structure of the pulmonary trunk of the highlander differs from that seen in the resident at sea level.

MEDIAL THICKNESS

Even at sea level, the rapid fall in pulmonary vascular resistance at birth that has been reported in lambs by Dawes *et al.* (1953) does not seem to occur in human newborns. Saling (1960) studied a number of normal infants within 1 hour of birth and found that, as often as not, the mean pulmonary arterial pressure was as high or higher than that in the aorta, the range in the mean pressure in these vessels being 40–80 mmHg. These observations were extended by Emmanouilides *et al.* (1964) who studied normal infants during the first 3 days of life. When the results of these two investigations are put together it becomes clear that the major decrease in the pulmonary arterial mean pressure to a range of 20–50 mmHg has usually occurred during the first 24 hours (Harris and Heath 1986). Rowe and James (1957) published values for the pulmonary arterial pressure in infants with Down's syndrome up to the age of 9 months, from which it seems that, by the end of the first month, it has reached a level that is normal for the rest of

life at sea level. The systemic arterial pressure does not change greatly during the first 9 months of life, so that the pressure in the pulmonary artery becomes considerably less than that in the aorta by the end of the first month.

The physiological pulmonary hypertension in the fetus and in the first month of extrauterine life is associated with a thick-walled pulmonary trunk, the thickness of its media equalling that of the aorta. In the ensuing months of extrauterine life the lowered intravascular pressure in the pulmonary trunk is associated with thinning of its media. As a result, in infants aged between 6 and 24 months the ratio of the thickness of the media of the pulmonary trunk to that of the aorta (PT/A ratio) falls to a range of 0.4–0.8 from the ratio of 1.0 characteristic of fetal life. At sea level the pulmonary arterial pressure achieves by the end of the first month of extrauterine life its low level, which is maintained for the rest of adult life. Associated with this is a PT/A ratio that falls in the range of 0.4–0.7.

In natives at high altitude, pulmonary hypertension persists from birth (Chapter 10); this is moderate in degree during infancy and childhood, but mild for the rest of adult life. Hence the stimulus for the relative thinning of the media of the pulmonary trunk never occurs. Saldaña and Arias-Stella (1963c) studied necropsy specimens of pulmonary trunk in 100 persons who were born and lived permanently at altitudes between 3440 and 4540 m. The subjects studied ranged in age from infancy to 78 years. One hundred control cases from sea level were also studied. The absolute medial thickness of the pulmonary trunk proved to be greater at high altitude than at sea level throughout life. The PT/A ratio was also elevated in native highlanders, but it has to be kept in mind that this was brought about not only by absolute increase in the medial thickness of the pulmonary trunk, but also perhaps by an associated absolute decrease in the thickness of the aortic media associated with the lower systemic blood pressure reported in native highlanders in the Andes (Chapter 18).

In rats exposed to simulated high altitude for a few weeks the media of the pulmonary trunk undergoes rapid hypertrophy in response to the hypobaric hypoxia. In one experiment, within 5 weeks of exposure the PT/A ratio rose from the control value of 0.45 to 0.95 (Heath *et al.* 1973). This rapid hypertrophy regressed almost to normal (PT/A ratio of 0.51) in another group of rats, exposed to hypoxia of the same length and severity, that was then allowed to recover in room air for the same short period of 5 weeks. By analogy with what occurs in rats subjected to simulated high altitude in a decompression chamber (Smith *et al.* 1978) it is possible that an early response of the human pulmonary trunk to natural hypobaric hypoxia is the formation of muscular evaginations (Chapter 10).

ELASTIC TISSUE PATTERN

In the fetus at sea level the pulmonary trunk is subjected to a pressure similar to that found in the aorta, as noted above. As a result, not only is it as thick as the aorta but the pattern of elastic tissue in its media is also aortic in type. The configuration of the elastic fibrils in the fetal pulmonary trunk is so similar to that in the aorta that, at a glance, the two may be confused, but differences do exist that make identification of elastic tissue from the fetal pulmonary trunk clear after careful examination. The fibrils of the pulmonary trunk are fewer and, although mostly parallel to each other, are less regular. They are somewhat coarser and they branch in places; they are shorter than the aortic fibrils, and even very short ones may be found. The thickness of the fibrils is less uniform along their length, the ends of some showing small club-like expansions. These differences are not superficially evident, however, and the configuration of fibrils in the fetal pulmonary trunk appears generally parallel and compact like that in the aorta. Since the similarities of the media of the fetal pulmonary trunk to that of the fetal aorta outweigh the differences, the fetal pulmonary trunk may be said to have an aortic configuration (Heath *et al.* 1959).

This pattern of elastic tissue is seen in the major pulmonary arteries at birth and until the age of about 6 months when changes, which no doubt started at birth, become evident. The elastic fibrils still tend to be parallel, but divide transversely into much more numerous, short, stick-like structures (transitional A pattern in Fig. 11.1), some of which show an accentuation of the clubbed terminations referred to above. As a result of this fragmentation, compactness is lost and the elastic tissue pattern

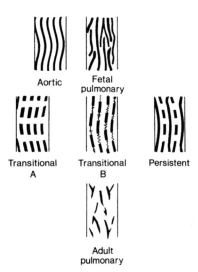

11.1 *Elastic tissue patterns of the pulmonary trunk at high altitude. The elastic tissue of the aortic media is in the form of long elastic fibrils that are parallel to one another and packed together compactly. The elastic tissue of the media of the fetal pulmonary trunk is also packed tightly, but the fibrils are shorter and branched. On the middle line are the transitional forms that are found in the evolution to the adult pulmonary configuration in which the elastic fibrils form an open network of branched, irregularly shaped fibrils. At sea level, transitional forms A and B are found. In form A, the long elastic fibrils fragment into rods; in form B, the rods are still connected by very thin elastic fibrils. At high altitude the 'persistent' configuration is found. In this, long continuous elastic fibrils are found in association with short stick-like rods. These different elastic tissue patterns in the pulmonary trunk are referred to in the text. (Based on data from Saldaña and Arias-Stella (1963a,b).)*

becomes more open and loose. Hence at sea level a glance at a section of the pulmonary trunk in infancy is already sufficient for recognizing it as pulmonary; at the same time the tendency for the fragments of elastic fibrils to be parallel to one another and to retain a fair uniformity of width demonstrates their derivation from an aortic type of elastica. When we originally described this elastic tissue pattern we designated it the *transitional* pattern. Subsequently, Saldaña and Arias-Stella (1963*a*) termed it the 'transitional A' pattern (Fig. 11.1). They described in addition a 'transitional B' pattern in which the zones of apparent fragmentation really correspond to segments of variable length, where the compact elastic fibrils have been replaced by numerous delicate elastic fibrils that maintain the continuity of the long fibres (Fig. 11.1). The physiological basis for the development of the transitional A pattern of elastic fibrils is the normal pronounced postnatal fall of pulmonary arterial pressure to low adult levels at sea level. On the other hand, it seems reasonable to assume that the transitional B pattern is associated with a slower postnatal fall of pulmonary arterial pressure.

By the end of the second year of life at sea level the adult pulmonary type of elastic tissue pattern of the media has become established. In this the elastic tissue is irregular and more sparse than in the aorta. Widely spread, the branched fibrils commonly show expanded terminations (Fig. 11.1). Individual laminae are short and run in all directions and can thus be traced for only short distances, while numerous slender fibrils intervene. This pattern is quite distinct from that of the aorta in that the elastic laminae are not long, parallel, or uniform. Fenestrations are numerous and occasionally clumps of amorphous elastic tissue are found.

At high altitude yet another type of elastic tissue configuration is to be found in the media of the pulmonary trunk. This is the so-called 'persistent' pattern of elastic fibrils. In this, the media of the pulmonary artery shows such a high content of elastic fibres that at first sight it resembles the aorta. However, there is a greater degree of fragmentation. There is a combination of long thick fibres with others that are markedly fragmented, the long ones being more numerous (Fig. 11.1; Saldaña and Arias-Stella 1963*a*). This pattern is seen occasionally at sea level where for some reason or other the postnatal fall in pulmonary arterial pressure has been unusually slow. However, it is characteristic of the pulmonary trunk of native highlanders and in them is almost certainly associated with the pulmonary hypertension that is found to a moderate degree in infants and children and to a slight degree in adults.

In native Quechua highlanders of the Andes it has been demonstrated that the evolution of the elastic configuration of the pulmonary trunk differs notably from that observed at sea level (Saldaña and Arias-Stella 1963*b*). There is an abnormal maintenance of the 'aortic' type of elastic pattern in the pulmonary trunk and a high prevalence of the persistent configuration even into adult life. Saldaña and Arias-Stella (1963*b*) studied the pulmonary trunk of 267 subjects native to the central Andean region of Peru. They found that in communities living between 4040 and 4540 m there is a retention of the aortic

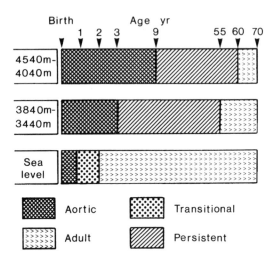

11.2 *Elastic tissue patterns in the media of the pulmonary trunk throughout life at sea level and at high altitude. The two ranges of elevation studied were 4540–4040 and 3840–3440 m. Note that at high altitude the 'persistent' configuration of elastic tissue pattern extends into middle age. (Based on data from Saldaña and Arias-Stella (1963b).)*

type of elastic pattern up to the age of 9 years (Fig. 11.2). This evolves exclusively into the persistent configuration that is commonly observed for the rest of life (Fig. 11.2). These authors report that there may be a conversion of persistent type into the adult type late in middle life, especially after 60 years of age (Fig. 11.2), but the physiological basis for this is not clear to us.

In communities located between 3440 and 3840 m the aortic type of pulmonary trunk is retained up to 3 years (Fig. 11.2) before evolving into the persistent type. This pattern extends through childhood and adolescence into adult life. Once again, Saldaña and Arias-Stella (1963*b*) refer to a late conversion of the persistent configuration into an adult pattern, but the explanation for this is obscure at present.

CHEMICAL COMPOSITION

The different histological appearance of the pulmonary trunk of the highlander is reflected in its chemical composition (Heath 1966; Castillo *et al.* 1967). There is a higher proportion of elastin in the pulmonary trunk with a persistent configuration of elastic tissue. Thus, in 41 specimens showing a normal adult pulmonary configuration of elastic tissue in subjects from Lima at sea level (Fig. 11.3),

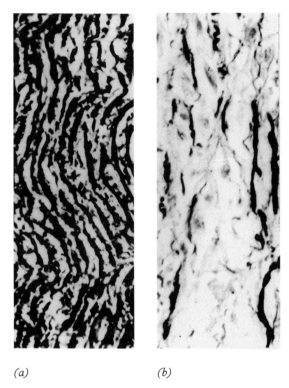

(a)   *(b)*

11.3 *Parts of transverse sections of pulmonary trunks from (a) a native highlander born and bred at an altitude of 4330 m in the Peruvian Andes and (b) a sea-level mestizo. The coastal dweller shows the open network of branched, irregularly shaped fibrils typical of the adult pulmonary trunk. The highlander shows the more compact, 'persistent' configuration of elastic tissue described in the text. EVG, × 150.*

the average elastin content was 27.2% with a tendency for the content to increase with age. In contrast, the elastin contents of the pulmonary trunks showing a persistent configuration of elastic tissue in four highlanders native to 4330 m (Fig. 11.3(a)) were 31.0, 31.4, 37.9, and 40.0%. Moreover, it should be noted that the average age of these four highland subjects was only 22.5 years, compared with an average age of 44.5 years for the low-altitude group (Heath 1966; Castillo *et al.* 1967), so that on the basis of age alone one would have anticipated finding a higher percentage of elastin in the lowlanders.

In contrast, the collagen content of the pulmonary trunk in three native highlanders from 4330 m did not differ appreciably from that in 28 sea-level subjects. The average collagen content in the lowlanders

was 31.0%, whereas that in the three highlanders was , respectively, 28.3, 31.7, and 37.9% (Heath 1966; Castillo *et al.* 1967). When collagen and elastin were both estimated in 27 specimens with an adult pulmonary pattern of elastic tissue, there proved to be a positive relation between the ratio of elastin to collagen and the age of the subject. When this ratio was calculated in specimens from three highlanders native to 4330 m, it was found to be inappropriately high for the age (Heath 1966; Castillo *et al.* 1967).

EXTENSIBILITY

The relation between length and tension in any artery is a curved one, so that the greater the tension applied the less extensible is the vessel (Harris and Heath 1986; see Fig. 11.4). This state of affairs is precisely the reverse of that which occurs in an inorganic material such as a wire. The basis for this was explained by the studies of Roach and Burton (1957), who demonstrated that the initial more horizontal part of the arterial extensibility curve registers the extension of elastic fibrils, whose relaxed length is shorter relative to that of collagen, whereas the later more vertical portion registers the extension of collagen fibres. Hence the arterial extensibility curve is in reality two curves, one for the elastic fibrils and one for collagen fibres (Fig. 11.4). We have previously found that the extensibility of the pulmonary trunk in lowlanders conforms to that of the idealized

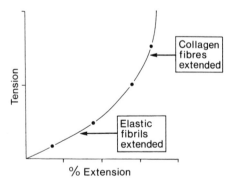

11.4 *Idealized extensibility curve of an artery. The more the artery is stretched, the less extensible it becomes. This is because, when low tension is applied to it, the highly extensible elastic fibrils are stretched. On the other hand, when greater tension is applied, the much less extensible collagen fibres are stretched. Thus it will be seen that the characteristic extensibility curve of an artery is produced by the extension of two sets of fibres.*

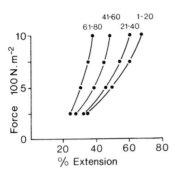

11.5 *Extensibility curves of the pulmonary trunk for different age groups indicated over the curves. It is apparent that this vessel becomes progressively less extensible with increasing age.*

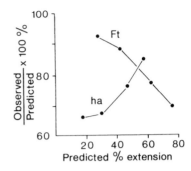

11.6 *Relation between the degree of extension of the pulmonary trunk and the degree of extension expressed as a percentage of that predicted. In high-altitude subjects (ha) the extensibility of this vessel on slight extension is less than would be anticipated and this is because the pulmonary trunk contains excessive amounts of elastic tissue, giving rise to the 'persistent' pattern of elastica in the media. In contrast, in patients with Fallot's tetrad (Ft) the extensibility of this vessel is normal on slight extension, but it is less than would be expected on further extension because the media is composed of excessive amounts of collagen with a sparsity of elastic tissue. The greater the tension applied to the pulmonary trunk of the highlander, the more normal becomes the extensibility of the vessel and this is because it contains normal amounts of collagen.*

arterial extensibility curve, the degree of extension falling with age (Harris *et al.* 1965; see Fig. 11.5). This finding is consistent with the increasing proportion of elastin with age.

In summary, the pulmonary trunk of the native highlander is abnormal in that it contains an excess of elastic tissue, as demonstrated visibly by an 'aortic' or 'persistent' configuration of elastic tissue and chemically by an increased content of elastin. At the same time, the collagen content of the pulmonary trunk of the highlander is no different from that of the sea-level dweller. This being the case, one would anticipate that the extensibility of the pulmonary trunk of the highlander would be abnormally low at a *low* extensile force. This is precisely what one finds. Subjects indigenous to high altitude show an abnormally low extensibility of their pulmonary trunk at a low extensible force of 2.5 N/m^2 (Heath 1966). In one of our investigations (Castillo *et al.* 1967) we found that in Quechuas in the Andes there was an abnormally high ratio of extension at 10 N/m^2 to that at 5 N/m^2 and it seems likely that this is due to the normal proportion of collagen in the pulmonary trunk of the highlander referred to above, coupled with the excess elastic tissue, so that the ratio of elastin to collagen was abnormally high.

When the degree of extension is expressed as a percentage of that predicted, it is found that the pulmonary trunk of the native highlander with an aortic or persistent configuration of elastic tissue shows a maximal decrease in extensibility at a low degree of extension (Fig. 11.6). The extensibility of the pulmonary trunk of the native highlander makes an interesting contrast with that of the patient with

Fallot's tetralogy. In the former, as we have seen, there is an excess of elastic fibrils and no increase in collagen, so that the observed extensibility is lower than anticipated with low levels of tension but rises with increasing tension (curve ha in Fig. 11.6). In Fallot's tetralogy, however, there is a paucity of elastic tissue and increased amounts of collagen, so that the observed extensibility falls with increasing tension (curve Ft in Fig. 11.6).

References

Castillo, Y., Krüger, H., Arias-Stella, J., Hurtado, A., Harris, P., and Heath, D. (1967). Histology, extensibility and chemical composition of pulmonary trunk in persons living at sea level and high altitude in Peru. *British Heart Journal*, **29**, 120

Dawes, G.S., Mott, J.C., Widdicombe, J.G., and Wyatt, D.G. (1953). Changes in the lungs of the newborn lamb. *Journal of Physiology (London)*, **121**, 141

Emmanouilides, G.C., Moss, A.J., Duffie, E.R. Jr., and Adams, F.H. (1964). Pulmonary arterial pressure changes in human newborn infants from birth to 3 days of age. *Journal of Pediatrics*, **65**, 327

Harris, P. and Heath, D. (1986). Form and function in the fetal pulmonary circulation. In *The Human Pulmonary Circulation*, 3rd edn. Edinburgh; Churchill Livingstone, p. 220

Harris, P., Heath, D., and Apostolopoulos, A. (1965). The extensibility of the human pulmonary trunk. *British Heart Journal*, **27**, 651

Heath, D.A. (1966). Morphological patterns: the structure, composition and extensibility of the pulmonary trunk at sea level and high altitude in Peru. In *Life at High Altitudes*, Scientific Publication No. 140. Washington; Pan American Health Organization, p. 13

Heath, D., Wood, E.H., Du Shane, J.W., and Edwards, J.E. (1959). The structure of the pulmonary trunk at different ages and in cases of pulmonary hypertension and pulmonary stenosis. *Journal of Pathology and Bacteriology*, **77**, 443

Heath, D., Edwards, C., Winson, M., and Smith, P. (1973). Effects on the right ventricle, pulmonary vasculature, and carotid bodies of the rat on exposure to, and recovery from, simulated high altitude. *Thorax*, **28**, 24

Roach, M.R. and Burton, A.C. (1957). The reason for the shape of the distensibility curve of arteries.

Canadian Journal of Biochemistry and Physiology, **35**, 681

Rowe, R.D. and James, L.S. (1957). The normal pulmonary arterial pressure during the first year of life. *Journal of Pediatrics*, **51**, 1

Saldaña, M. and Arias-Stella, J. (1963*a*). Studies on the structure of the pulmonary trunk. I. Normal changes in the elastic configuration of the human pulmonary trunk at different ages. *Circulation*, 27, 1086

Saldaña, M. and Arias-Stella, J. (1963*b*). Studies on the structure of the pulmonary trunk. II. The evolution of the elastic configuration of the pulmonary trunk in people native to high altitudes. *Circulation*, 27, 1094

Saldaña, M. and Arias-Stella, J. (1963*c*). Studies on the structure of the pulmonary trunk. III. The thickness of the media of the pulmonary trunk and ascending aorta in high altitude natives. *Circulation*, 27, 1101

Saling, E. (1960). New research results on the blood circulation of the newborn infant immediately after birth. *Archiv für Gynaekologie*, **194**, 287

Smith, P., Heath, D., and Padula, F. (1978). Evaginations of smooth muscle cells in the hypoxic pulmonary trunk. *Thorax*, **33**, 31

12

Benign acute mountain sickness

Some symptoms develop in man immediately on his ascent into the mountains. They are the direct consequences of hypobaric hypoxia and may be regarded as the physiological components of early acclimatization. These adjustments are normal and harmless, but they give rise to unusual bodily sensations that may disturb the timid. There is commonly a feeling of breathlessness on exercise on ascending quickly to mountainous areas, but in our experience the respiratory rate at rest increases only slightly at altitude. In one of us (D.R.W.) during an expedition to the Andes, the rate at rest was 12 breaths/min at 150 m, 12 breaths/min at 3000 m, and 12–16 breaths/min at 4330 m. Forster (1984, 1986) found that astronomers from sea level, ascending to work at 4200 m on the summit of the volcano Mauna Kea in Hawaii, increased their resting respiratory rate from 16.5 to only 18.7 breaths/min (Chapter 30). There has been one report that the hyperventilation on exposure to high altitude involves increase in respiratory rate as well as tidal volume (Chapter 4) but we think that the onset of tachypnoea should be regarded as suspicious of the early onset of high-altitude pulmonary oedema (Chapter 13).

On arrival in the mountains the lowlander may become unduly conscious of his heart's action, a sensation bolstered by awareness of the infrequent ectopic beats that may make their appearance. The heart rate at rest is also surprisingly normal on acute exposure to high altitude, being elevated by only about 10 beats/min above sea-level values. In one of us (D.R.W.) in the Andes, the resting pulse rate was 72 beats/min at Lima (150 m) , between 72 and 80 beats/min at Tarma (3000 m), and 68–84 beats/min at Cerro de Pasco (4330 m). In sea-level astronomers working at 4200 m in Hawaii, the resting pulse rates rose after about 5 hours at the summit to reach a peak on the first day on the mountain, with an average increase of 10 beats/min greater than the count at sea level (Forster 1986; Chapter 30, this volume). The symptoms arising from immediate responses of the body to exposure to high altitude have been succintly termed 'accommodation', in

contrast to the symptom-complex of acute mountain sickness described below.

On arrival in the mountains other signs and symptoms that are not an expression of physiological acclimatization to hypobaric hypoxia may make their appearance. Many who ascend to high altitude develop a persistent non-productive cough, which is due to mouth-breathing and the inhalation of cold, dry mountain air. This becomes increasingly troublesome the higher the altitude. Clarke and Duff (1976) report that high-altitude climbers who use oxygen are particularly affected, especially if no humidifier is included with the oxygen cylinder. Retinal haemorrhages also occur commonly on ascent above about 5000 m (Chapter 27).

ACUTE MOUNTAIN SICKNESS

The sensations directly and immediately related to exposure to hypobaric hypoxia referred to above have to be distinguished sharply from the symptom-complex that develops in susceptible subjects after a time lag of 6 to 96 hours and usually within 12 hours. This constitutes 'acute mountain sickness' which seems to be brought about by retention and redistribution of body water, particularly into the lungs and the brain, rather than by hypoxia *per se*.

Classification and nomenclature

The classification of the different clinical manifestations of acute mountain sickness is controversial. We favour the views of Dickinson (1981) who has had extensive clinical experience of the condition in Nepal. He believes that any classification must indicate the continuity of mild and serious acute mountain sickness, for it is likely that the pathogenesis and pathophysiology of both degrees of severity are the same and the mild may progress into the severe. Dickinson (1981) believes that acute mountain sickness should be considered as benign or malignant, with the latter comprising pulmonary, cerebral, and mixed forms (Table 12.1).

Mild (or 'benign') acute mountain sickness is common in lowlanders going to high altitude and

Table 12.1 Classification of acute mountain sickness (after Dickinson 1981)

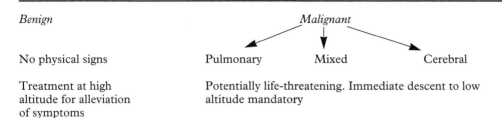

Benign	*Malignant*		
No physical signs	Pulmonary	Mixed	Cerebral
Treatment at high altitude for alleviation of symptoms	Potentially life-threatening. Immediate descent to low altitude mandatory		

presents no physical signs, although those afflicted show a characteristic facies manifesting their malaise (Fig. 12.1). It requires little or no treatment and such as is needed for the alleviation of symptoms can safely be given to the patient on the mountain. In contrast, the serious (or 'malignant') form is potentially life-threatening and immediate descent to low altitude is mandatory. It occurs in two major types, one involving the lungs and the other afflicting the brain, although mixed presentations involving both organs are common. Unfortunately, these forms of malignant acute mountain sickness have been designated 'high-altitude pulmonary oedema' and 'high-altitude cerebral oedema'. These terms carry the erroneous implication that the underlying pathology is solely one of oedema. Although this is an important feature of the patho-

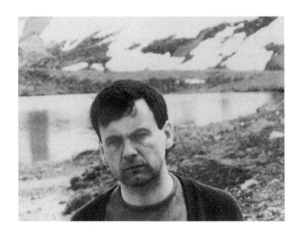

12.1 *One of the authors (D.R.W.) photographed while suffering from benign acute mountain sickness. He had just been driven by car from the coast to the Ticlio pass (4800 m) in the Andes of Central Peru. Although this condition has no clinical signs, it produces a characteristic facies.*

physiology, it ignores the thrombosis that occurs in the pulmonary and cerebral circulations (Chapters 13 and 14). Failure to appreciate that the pathology extends beyond oedema may mislead the clinician into thinking that the ultimate prognosis is always good in these conditions if the oedema is reversed. For this reason we prefer the non-specific designations of 'pulmonary' and 'cerebral mountain sickness'. We use the latter term in this book, but the term 'high-altitude pulmonary oedema' is so entrenched in medical parlance throughout the world that we have retained its use here, while still retaining reservations as to its validity.

Dickinson (1981) makes the excellent point that it is strongly advisable to employ non-technical terms like 'benign' and 'malignant' to provide a rational basis for management of patients in the field by non-medical people. We warmly endorse this viewpoint. The clinical features, prophylaxis, and treatment of benign acute mountain sickness are described in the present chapter. Those for the pulmonary and cerebral forms of malignant acute mountain sickness are described in Chapters 13 and 14, respectively.

CLINICAL FEATURES

Much of our knowledge of the symptomatology of benign acute mountain sickness comes from a study of 840 Indian troops by Singh *et al.* (1969) and of 146 trekkers with the condition in the Himalaya (Hackett *et al.* 1976). The commonest symptoms revealed by the latter study are shown in Table 12.2. Frontal headache is very frequently experienced by the newcomer to high altitude. Few can ascend high mountains without suffering a mild headache and a fuzziness in the head. However, bouts of intense, incapacitating headache may occur. These are commonly frontal and they are often associated with giddiness. When such severe headache is present, there is not infrequently photophobia with some

Table 12.2 Percentage incidence of symptoms in 146 trekkers with benign acute mountain sickness in the Himalaya (after Hackett *et al.* 1976)

Symptom	%
Headache	96
Insomnia	70
Anorexia	38
Nausea	35
Dizziness	27
Headache unrelieved by analgesics	26
Excessive dyspnoea on exercise at rest	25
Reduced urine	19
Vomiting	14
Lassitude	13
Incoordination	11

disturbance of vision, but ophthalmoscopic examination during attacks does not reveal any abnormality.

The cause of the headache is unknown. On ascent to high altitude there is cerebral vasodilatation and an increase in cerebral blood flow (Kety and Schmidt 1948; Severinghaus *et al.* 1966). This vasodilatation overrides the vasoconstriction resulting from hypocarbic alkalosis. Cerebral blood flow is notoriously difficult to measure and hence Hackett (1988) and his group used transcranial Doppler technology to measure the velocity of cerebral blood flow through the middle cerebral artery. In climbers with severe acute mountain sickness the velocity of the blood was increased indicating a higher cerebral flow. Hackett (1988) reports that when oxygen is given during acute mountain sickness cerebral blood flow falls and headache improves. Breathing 3% carbon dioxide stimulates ventilation, improves arterial oxygen saturation, diminishes cerebral blood flow, and improves headache. The inhalation of 7% carbon dioxide stimulates ventilation and increases systemic arterial oxygenation even more but this increases cerebral blood flow and leads to a worsening of headache. The balance is fine and overall it seems likely that any manipulation that increases the product of cerebral blood flow and systemic arterial oxygenation is probably helpful in alleviating the symptomatology of acute mountain sickness but an excessive increase in cerebral blood flow is likely to exaggerate the severity of headache. Reeves *et al.* (1985) took the opposite view that headache at high altitude is not related to internal carotid arterial blood velocity. During attacks of headache there is no elevation of systemic blood pressure. The Birmingham Medical Research Expeditionary Society (BMRES) Mountain Sickness Study Group (1981) reported that during their ascent of Chimborazo (6310 m) in Ecuador all the men who had headache and nausea found that their symptoms were considerably relieved by forced ventilation. This procedure would increase the partial pressure of oxygen in the blood.

Individuals react in an idiosyncratic manner to the hypobaric hypoxia of high altitude, but they react consistently. The existence of good and bad 'acclimatizers' was confirmed objectively in the astronomers manning the British infrared telescope on the summit of Mauna Kea in Hawaii (Chapter 30). Bärtsch *et al.* (1988) confirmed the importance of individual disposition to acute mountain sickness in two studies in which climbers with a history of high-altitude pulmonary oedema occurring in the Alps ascended to the Margherita hut (4560 m) from sea level within 24 hours. Upon ascent to that altitude and a subsequent stay there, 72 and 80%, respectively, of climbers in the two groups developed oedema of the lung again. On the other hand subjects with excellent high-altitude tolerance, proved by prior exposure to elevations above 6000 m, rarely developed high-altitude pulmonary oedema.

Assessment of the severity of acute mountain sickness

There are no reliable clinical signs of benign acute mountain sickness and hence its severity in any individual case has to be assessed on the basis of the evaluation of symptoms as vague as headache and lethargy. This has been a considerable drawback for research into the subject, for careful estimations of such entities as arterial oxygen tension have, in the final analysis, to be related to the presence or absence of a list of symptoms that are commonly assessed by awarding them so many points from a scale according to their severity. Both clinical interviews and peer review have been used, but even in the hands of experienced workers at high altitude, including professionally trained clinical psychologists, this ranking of symptoms leaves much to be desired.

The psychological aspects of acute mountain sickness were studied by Olive and Waterhouse (1979). In order to assess the importance of personality and expectations in the development of acute mountain sickness, three standard personality questionnaires and a mountain sickness-anticipation questionnaire were completed by all 17 members of an expedition before their departure for the Himalaya. Benign acute mountain sickness could not be predicted with these tests and its occurrence, when assessed either by clinical review or peer review, bore no significant relationship to personality. For comparison, daily self-assessment of the symptoms of acute mountain sickness was also conducted throughout the expedition, using graduated and graphic rating scales. The results were found to be unreliable and dependent upon personality factors. Such findings have obvious implications for those assessing others at high altitude.

Duration
Incapacitating illness is likely to be short. In observations on 1925 soldiers between 18 and 53 years of age stationed at altitudes of 3350–5500 m in the Himalaya of Ladakh, Singh *et al.* (1969) found the early phase of severe symptoms to last from only 2–5 days, but complete recovery sometimes took several weeks (Fig. 12.2).

ALTITUDE OF ONSET
The altitude of onset of 57 cases of malignant acute mountain sickness has been provided by Dickinson (1981; see Table 12.3). He reports an exceptional case in which the altitude of onset was as low as 2100 m. At this elevation a young British man of 27 years developed severe headache, lassitude, and unsteadiness. After evacuation he was found to have moderate ataxia and an extensor right plantar reflex. In a second case, developing at moderate altitude below 2500 m, there was pneumonia and emphysema, which must have exaggerated the degree of

Table 12.3 Altitude of onset of 57 cases of malignant acute mountain sickness, seven proving fatal (after Dickinson 1981)

Altitude (km)	Per cent of 57 cases
<3.0	3.5
3.0–3.5	9
3.5–4.0	14
4.0–4.5	33
4.5–5.0	11
5.0–5.5	17.5
5.5–6.0	7
>6.0	5

hypoxaemia. By using a questionnaire on symptoms, Montgomery *et al.* (1989) convinced themselves that 25% of subjects attending a conference held at 2000 m were developing the syndrome. The highest altitude of onset reported by Dickinson (1982) occurred in a 34-year-old Sherpa guide who developed cerebral mountain sickness at 7000 m. Dickinson points out that in two of the fatal cases in his series the victims had reached their highest point and were descending when they became ill.

INCIDENCE
Probably the best indication we have of the incidence of benign acute mountain sickness in lowlanders becoming acutely exposed to high altitude comes from the investigation of Hackett *et al.* (1976). Their data were obtained from 278 questionnaires completed by unacclimatized hikers at Pheriche (4240 m) in the Himalaya of Nepal. The climbers were ascending on the main trekking trail to visit the Mt Everest Base Camp at 5500 m. The overall incidence of acute mountain sickness in these people was 53%, occurring in 53% of men and 51% of women. Of the thousands of climbers making the rapid ascent to the summit of Mt Rainier (4392 m) every year, one-half to three-quarters suffer from acute mountain sickness (Roach *et al.* 1983). The incidence of malignant forms of acute mountain sickness, as described in Chapters 13 and 14, is much lower. It was 4.3% in the series of Hackett *et al.* (1976) and 8.3% in the large series of Indian soldiers reported by Singh *et al.* (1969).

All ages are susceptible to the condition, but younger trekkers are more at risk than older people even if adjustment is made for a slower rate of ascent (Hackett *et al.* 1976). Physical fitness offers no protection against the development of acute mountain

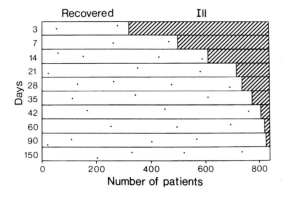

12.2 *Duration of acute mountain sickness in 840 untreated cases studied by Singh* et al. *(1969).*

sickness. As noted by Forster (1984), the computer operator on Mauna Kea (4200 m) in Hawaii who suffered prostrating episodes of benign acute mountain sickness was a non-smoker, a teetotaller, and an active sportsman.

PATHOPHYSIOLOGY

The mechanisms that give rise to the symptoms of acute mountain sickness are not at all clear. It is apparent that the syndrome is not directly and immediately related to the hypobaric hypoxia of high altitude. On exposure to high altitude acute mountain sickness is not of immediate onset. It takes several hours to develop. This lesson has been impressed on us most forcibly during our visits to Peru and the high-altitude volcanoes of the Pacific. When one ascends to Cerro de Pasco at an altitude of 4330 m in the Andes and stops there for a period of days, the onset of acute mountain sickness may be anticipated with some confidence. In contrast, when one ascends to the summit of the volcano Mauna Kea at a very similar altitude of 4200 m in Hawaii and stops there for 4 or 5 hours before return to Hilo on the coast, symptoms related to the altitude may be totally absent. It is clear that there is a lag-period during which the mechanisms leading to acute mountain sickness become operative.

The nature of these mechanisms remains obscure. In some way the course of events seems to be concerned with a retention of body water or a shift of it from intracellular to extracellular compartments. The dependent or periorbital oedema which is sometimes found in sufferers from acute mountain sickness are consistent with this. However, the relation between diuresis and sodium retention and antidiuretic hormone, and the renin–angiotensin–aldosterone system is complex. We consider it in detail in Chapter 20. There is, for example, no straightforward and obvious relation between a rising level of antidiuretic hormone and the onset of acute mountain sickness.

The mechanisms leading to acute mountain sickness are provoked by too rapid an ascent to high altitude. They are also likely to occur more in some individuals than in others. This idiosyncratic response remains on subsequent exposure to the mountain environment. In this respect Milledge (1983) speculates that, in subjects prone to acute mountain sickness, converting enzyme activity does not fall in response to hypobaric hypoxia so that they have raised levels of angiotensin II and aldosterone. This would result in considerable sodium retention and an increase in extracellular fluid volume, together with an increased pressor response in both pulmonary and systemic circulations.

ATRIAL NATRIURETIC PEPTIDE (ANP)

This peptide may be of importance in the genesis of acute mountain sickness. Before considering this suggested relationship we shall consider its nature, origins, and known physiological actions. Granules containing this peptide were found in the atrial myocytes of guinea-pigs in 1956 by Kisch. Jamieson and Palade (1964) found these granules, of 0.3 to 0.4 μm in diameter, to be concentrated in the sarcoplasmic core of the atrial myocytes in intimate association with a central voluminous Golgi complex. De Bold (1979) suggested that atrial specific granules are related to water–electrolyte balance in the body. He demonstrated that, when extracted rat atrial tissue was given intravenously to rats, a very large sodium diuresis promptly occurred (De Bold et al. 1981). The substance in the specific granules was a 24-amino-acid residue rich in glycine, serine, and arginine (Atlas et al. 1984). Hisayuki and Kangawa (1984) isolated from human (h) and rat (r) atrial tissue three bioactive components, a b, and g, ranging in size from 3000 to 13 000 daltons. They identified the major bioactive peptide of the 3000-dalton a-component of human extracts as a 28-amino-acid peptide (hANP). Rat atrial natriuretic peptides (rANPs) terminate in the same C terminal sequence identical with that of a–hANP. These sequences were found to correspond to the C-terminal sequence of the producers of the bioactive a-ANP, namely b-hANP, a 48-residue peptide, and g-hANP consisting of a 126-amino-acid residue. Clearly b- and g-ANPS are precursors of the bioactive a-ANP. Gutkowska et al. (1985) found that, in 59 clinically normal, normotensive subjects, values for plasma ANP were in the range 50–70 pg/ml.

The main physiological actions of atrial natriuretic peptide are to induce diuresis, natriuresis, and vasorelaxation and to inhibit aldosterone production. Both low- and high-molecular-weight forms of ANP are able to induce a powerful diuresis and natriuresis due to an increase in glomerular filtration rate secondary to vasodilatation and a reduction in sodium reabsorption. Thus there is an interplay between renal haemodynamics and the direct tubular action of ANP. This peptide is involved in the control of blood volume. On stretching the walls of the atria of rats the specific granules move from the region of the sarcoplasmic core to the subsarcolemmal region from which secretion of the peptide occurs (Agnoletti et al. 1989). Isoproterenol will also induce release of ANP from rat atrium *in vitro* by stimulation of β adrenoreceptors (Agnoletti *et al.* 1992).

In isolated rat atria a 10°C increase in temperature doubles the output of ANP during stretch, implying the involvement of an enzymatic mechanism (Agnoletti *et al.* 1990).

The peptide binds predominantly to a protein with a molecular mass of 66 000 daltons on the cell surface of cultured bovine aortic smooth muscle cells. Binding sites are found in the zona glomerulosa of the adrenal, on adrenergic and noradrenergic cells of the medulla, and in many other tissues of the body. Sakamoto *et al.* (1986) found ANP in the lung, suggesting it might be a target organ for the peptide. ANP is also to be found in the main branches of the pulmonary veins suggesting that they may be involved in the regulation of plasma volume through the release of the peptide (Matsukura *et al.* 1987). This widespread peptide is also found in the rat in the thyroid, submaxillary gland, brain, and hypothalamus, the latter site suggesting that it may be concerned with the neural regulation of cardiovascular function.

ANP and acute mountain sickness

As noted earlier in this chapter, hypobaric hypoxia greatly influences the fluid balance of the body. The physiological response to acute hypoxia is increased diuresis but in subjects developing acute mountain sickness there is antidiuresis with accumulations of body water and sodium. As we have seen, the release of antidiuretic hormone does not seem to be influenced by the hypobaric hypoxia of high altitude. Recent work, however, suggests that this is not the case with atrial natriuretic peptide. Milledge *et al.* (1989) investigated the mechanisms of acute mountain sickness in 22 subjects at 4300 m on Mount Kenya. They studied a variety of factors including body weight, urine volume over 24 hours, sodium and potassium excretion, and the symptom score for acute mountain sickness. In 15 subjects blood samples were taken for assay of plasma aldosterone and ANP. The combination of ascent to high altitude and exercise resulted in a marked decrease in 24-hour urine volume and sodium excretion. ANP levels were higher on both days at high altitude compared with those of controls. ANP levels at low altitude showed a significant inverse correlation with acute mountain sickness symptom scores on ascent. Winter *et al.* (1987) had previously shown a rise in ANP plasma concentration in rats made chronically hypoxic in a chamber. The elevation of ANP in man at high altitude by Milledge *et al.* (1989) was the first such demonstration and was thought to be due directly to hypoxia or to an increase in right atrial pressure secondary to hypoxic vasoconstriction of the pulmonary arteries. They found a significant inverse correlation between 24-hour sodium excretion and ANP concentration of the day of ascent, and the acute mountain sickness scores. There was also a negative correlation between the ANP levels before ascent to high altitude and subsequent AMS scores. If this finding is confirmed, it would suggest that susceptibility to acute mountain sickness depends upon a subject's normal control value of ANP. The higher of it is, the less chance of developing acute mountain sickness. Resistance to acute mountain sickness may occur as a result of the following events according to Milledge *et al.* (1989). On ascending to high altitude ANP levels rise due to hypoxia and exercise, and there is inhibition of aldosterone excretion and of sodium reabsorption by the kidneys. This results in a sodium-led diuresis or less sodium retention if exercise is taken. This loss of sodium reduces any tendency to oedema formation in the brain or lungs consequent upon other mechanisms initiated by hypoxia.

It is widely believed that the susceptibility to acute mountain sickness is related to a lower initial response to acute hypoxia with a subsequent greater blunting of ventilation. Moore *et al.* (1986) found that of 12 subjects exposed to a simulated altitude of 4800 m, eight developed symptoms of acute mountain sickness and four did not. On previous exposure to natural high altitude, the eight had developed acute mountain sickness whereas the remainder had not. The susceptible subjects had lower minute ventilations and higher end-tidal values of carbon dioxide tension. Hackett *et al.* (1987a) found that climbers whose arterial oxygen saturation was more than one standard deviation below the mean value of the group studied (that is, 77% or less) were more likely to become ill as they ascended further. No fewer than 74% of them developed acute mountain sickness as contrasted to only 34% of those climbers who had a higher systemic arterial saturation. This study led Hackett and his colleagues to use a simple, non-invasive measurement of arterial oxygen saturation, taking some 30 seconds, as a screening test on the mountain to detect those likely to develop acute mountain sickness. They advised susceptible climbers to await normalization of arterial oxygen saturation before ascending further.

While it has been known for some years that subjects with acute mountain sickness have relative hypoventilation (Hackett *et al.* 1982) it has proven to be impossible to detect such diminished levels of ventilation prior to the onset of symptoms. Studies of gas exchange have, however, been more promising. It transpired (Hackett 1988) that in one group of asymptomatic climbers the A–a difference (Chapter 4) was 7.0 (± 1.2) mmHg but 16.0 (± 1.1) mmHg in those with acute mountain sickness (Hackett *et al.* 1987*b*). The assumption is that the increased A–a difference is due to mild interstitial oedema of the lung. A–a difference may be a more sensitive indicator of incipient acute mountain sickness than arterial oxygen saturation itself because some subjects with a big A–a difference may maintain oxygen saturation by hyperventilating. Other groups reporting impaired gas exchange prior to the development of symptoms of acute mountain sickness are Kronenberg *et al.* (1971) and Wagner *et al.* (1987).

Ascent to high altitude involves exposure to hypocarbia as well as to hypoxia and the role of the diminished alveolar partial pressure of carbon dioxide in the mechanisms producing acute mountain sickness has been considered. Maher *et al.* (1975) exposed two groups of subjects to simulated altitude in a hypobaric chamber. One had carbon dioxide added to the atmosphere to raise the partial pressure of the gas at control levels. The other breathed air and became hypocarbic. Hypoxia was similar in the two groups, although to achieve this the group with added carbon dioxide were taken to a lower barometric pressure. The added carbon dioxide made the symptoms of acute mountain sickness worse. It was thought that the worsening of the headache and related symptoms of acute mountain sickness brought about by hypoxia and hypercarbia is due to an increase in the level of cerebral blood flow. In those with a brisk ventilatory response, resulting in increased partial pressure of oxygen in the alveolar spaces but diminished pressure of carbon dioxide, the opposing effects on the cerebral circulation are counterbalanced. Among the test subjects of Maher *et al.* (1975), in the group with little increase of ventilation and added carbon dioxide to bring levels close to sea-level values, there will be dilatation of the cerebral arteries. This may contribute to mild cerebral oedema, a slight rise in intracranial pressure, and the onset of headache and other symptoms of acute mountain sickness.

However, these findings have recently been described as 'controversial assertions' by Pandit (1992) in the correspondence columns of the *British Medical Journal*. He points out that recent studies have not supported the concept of a correlation between a poor ventilatory response and the development of acute mountain sickness (Milledge *et al.* 1988, 1991). Furthermore, neurological symptoms are often worse in subjects who have a higher hypoxic ventilatory response and such symptoms last longer in this group on return to lower altitudes (Hornbein *et al.* 1989). Pandit (1992) thinks it possible that this may be because subjects with a high ventilatory response to hypobaric hypoxia may in fact suffer longer periods of desaturation when they are asleep due to periodic breathing (Chapter 28). He also thinks that a high hypoxic ventilatory response results in a low arterial carbon dioxide pressure, which causes cerebral vasoconstriction and so reduces cerebral blood flow reducing oxygen delivery to the central nervous system. Pandit (1992) also suggests that breathing gas with a high concentration of carbon dioxide (2–5%) can actually improve symptoms of acute mountain sickness. Pollard (1992), however, finds Pandit's view 'a cause for concern'. He states: 'inhaled carbon dioxide should not be recommended in treating altitude illness while there is such strong evidence that it may cause a deterioration in the person's condition. If in doubt go down.'

MANAGEMENT OF BENIGN ACUTE MOUNTAIN SICKNESS

The management of benign acute mountain sickness encompasses three distinct and important aspects. These are prophylaxis against the development of the condition, treatment of established cases on the mountain, and surveillance to ensure that the affected subject is not developing one of the malignant forms of the syndrome.

PROPHYLAXIS

Rate of ascent

There can be few medical conditions where a little forethought and action can avoid so much illness and the occasional deterioration into a life-threatening disease. Mechanical transport by car, train, or aircraft is the worst means of reaching high altitude, for the simple reason that the subject cannot control his rate of ascent. Nevertheless, in the Andes large numbers of tourists travel to high altitude by this means (Fig. 12.3). The cardinal principle is to take one's time and ascend slowly. Houston and Dickinson (1975) refer to the fact that it was previously thought safe to ascend by

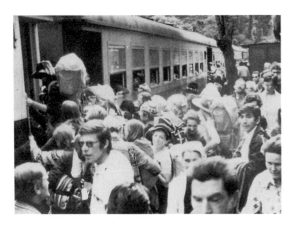

12.3 *A crowd of tourists at Majchu Picchu (2440 m) boarding the train that will transport them rapidly to Cuzco (3400 m). Such mechanical transport is the worst way of reaching high altitude because the individual cannot control the rate of ascent to suit his own needs.*

300 m/day from a starting altitude of 3000 up to 4200 m, but thereafter to ascend by 300 m over 2 days. They have found that the malignant pulmonary and cerebral forms can still occur with this rate of ascent and advocate an even more conservative rate of ascent of 150 m/day from a starting altitude of 2750 m, with days of partial rest at about 4250 and 5500 m. Milledge (1983) offers similar advice. He advocates that care needs to be taken at altitudes exceeding 3000 m, with an ascent of 300 m/day for 2 days followed by an ascent of 300 m over 2 days.

Fig. 12.4 shows the first page of the leaflet issued by the Himalayan Rescue Association to trekkers climbing above an altitude of 3660 m (12 000 feet). Its golden rule is: 'Don't go "too fast too high".' One leaflet says: 'Beware of the "do or die" attitude in the Himalayas. All too often it has meant more "die" than "do".'

Hackett *et al.* (1976) found that acute mountain sickness among 278 trekkers in the Himalaya was commoner in those who did not allow time for acclimatization. Thus it occurred in 60% of those who flew from sea level to 2800 m before climbing higher, but in only 42% of those who walked up from Kathmandu (1200 m). Symptoms were commoner in those who climbed fast or who spent fewer nights acclimatizing on the route. It is wise not to indulge in too much physical activity during the first few days at high altitude and this may be related to endocrinological abnormalities such as the height-

HIMALAYAN RESCUE ASSOCIATION

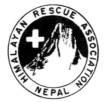

ENJOY YOUR TREK !

ADVICE ON HIGH ALTITUDE SICKNESS
FOR TREKKERS PROCEEDING
ABOVE 12,000 FEET.

THE GOLDEN RULE:

DO'NT GO "TOO FAST TOO HIGH"

Published and distributed by the HIMALAYAN RESCUE ASSOCIATION
Seto Durbar – Durbar Marg KATHMANDU – P. O. B. 283
Telephone : 13854

12.4 *First page of the leaflet issued by the Himalayan Rescue Association to trekkers climbing above an altitude of 3660 m.*

ened renin levels on exposure to high altitude and exercise referred to earlier in the chapter.

Acetazolamide

The measured, conservative ascent into the mountains is too slow for many people today, especially the younger generation. Also the logistics of many trekking parties demand a quicker, more dynamic schedule. Many travellers to high altitude now want acclimatization speeded up and enhanced by chemical means. The drugs that offer this are the diuretics and in particular acetazolamide (Diamox®). This is one of the aromatic and heterocyclic sulfonamides (Fig. 12.5), which are potent inhibitors of carbonic anhydrase. Carbonic anhydrase is concerned with the process of cation exchange in the distal renal tubule, by which there is reabsorption of sodium with simultaneous excretion of an equivalent amount of hydrions and potassium. The hydrions required for exchange with sodium are generated in renal tubular cells by the hydration of carbon

Table 12.4 Effect of acetazolamide on blood gases and arterial and urinary pH at high altitude (after Forster *et al.* 1986)

Altitude (m)	Mean (SD) Pa_{O_2} (mmHg)	Pa_{CO_2} (mmHg)	Arterial pH	Urinary pH
No diuretic				
3000	53.2 (3.4)	26 (2.5)	7.48 (0.02)	6.1 (0.1)
4800	41.9 (3.7)	21.3 (1.4)	7.49 (0.01)	6.2 (0.4)
Acetazolamide				
3000	61.6 (4.6)	21.8 (1.1)	7.39 (0.1)	6.5 (0.4)
4800	47 (2.8)	21.3 (1.8)	7.42 (0.02)	6.6 (0.2)

dioxide to carbonic acid followed by ionization with hydrions and bicarbonate. This process is catalysed by carbonic anhydrase. Acetazolamide inhibits this enzyme and reduces the supply of hydrions. As a result, potassium exchange is enhanced and there is increased renal excretion of bicarbonate. Hence the prophylactic administration of acetazolamide leads to a brisk diuresis, in which the urine is alkaline and rich in bicarbonate, while the body retains the hydrogen ions with a resulting metabolic acidosis (Table 12.4). This induced metabolic acidosis modifies the process of acclimatization that is described in the earlier chapters. The hypoxaemia of high altitude stimulates the carotid bodies to induce hyperventilation, which loses carbon dioxide from the alveolar spaces so that respiratory alkalosis develops. The decrease in the level of bicarbonate in the cerebrospinal fluid re-establishes the central drive to breathing in the face of a lower partial pressure of carbon dioxide in the blood. However, arterial pH is still raised and this limits any increase in ventilatory drive from the carotid bodies which are sensitive to hydrions as well as to hypoxaemia. It is at this point that acetazolamide probably acts by inducing metabolic acidosis, lowering arterial pH.

Acetazolamide

12.5 *Structural formula of acetazolamide.*

This stimulates further the carotid bodies increasing ventilation and with it the partial pressure of oxygen in the alveolar spaces and the blood (Table 12.4).

An early controlled study of the use of acetazolamide as a prophylactic against acute mountain sickness was carried out by Hackett *et al.* (1976). They used the drug in a double-blind study in a dosage of 250 mg twice daily for 4 days. Therapy was started when the climbers were at an altitude of 3440 m, and the authors stressed that acetazolamide must be given at the start of exposure to high altitude if it is to be successful. They concluded from their study that the drug was of benefit, but statistical analysis demonstrated no difference between its ingestion and that of a placebo and the conclusions of the study were criticized (Ramsay 1977). Much earlier, Forwand *et al.* (1968), in a double-blind controlled study of acetazolamide in a dose of 750 mg/day versus placebo, had demonstrated a reduction in the incidence of mild acute mountain sickness, but their study was carried out at an altitude (3900 m) of insufficient magnitude to have anticipated severe affliction by the condition. None of the other studies was properly controlled up to 1981 and hence up to that time there was no convincing evidence of the value of acetazolamide as a prophylactic.

During an expedition to Chimborazo (6310 m) in the Andes of Ecuador, the Birmingham Medical Research Expeditionary Society Mountain Sickness Study Group (1981) carried out a double-blind trial of slow-release acetazolamide by the administration of a daily dosage of 500 mg of the drug versus placebo to men ascending to 5000 m. In the 18 who reached this altitude, those on acetazolamide had fewer symptoms of acute mountain sickness. Ten of the men had been to 5400 m on a previous expedition and on the second study five of them took acetazolamide and five the placebo. Those on the drug performed better than those on placebo and their performance on the second expedition was better. In the group as a whole the symptoms of acute mountain sickness were negatively correlated with arterial oxygen tensions, which were higher in the drug group. Greene *et al.* (1981) carried out a similar double-blind controlled cross-over trial of acetazolamide (500 mg daily) versus placebo during the ascent of Kilimanjaro (5895 m) and Mt Kenya (5186 m). They too recommend the drug as an acceptable and effective prophylactic for acute mountain sickness. Ward *et al.* (1989) make the point that the safety of acetazolamide is confirmed by its widespread use in glaucoma where it is used for years at doses similar to or in excess of that recommended for prophylaxis against acute mountain sickness.

The subsequent investigations of one of the Birmingham group on the astronomers of Mauna Kea (4200 m) (Chapter 30) led him to doubt the earlier conclusion of the group referred to above, that arterial oxygen tension is inversely related to the symptoms of acute mountain sickness (Forster 1986). He found that in commuters ascending each day to the telescope site on the top of the volcano (4200 m) there was a fall in arterial oxygen tension within 3 hours of arrival at the summit, but severe symptoms of acute mountain sickness were not observed. Commuters recorded a lower mean arterial oxygen tension than shiftworkers, but reported fewer symptoms.

Another similar diuretic that has been employed is methazolamide. This has a longer half-life and produces fewer side-effects than acetazolamide, which can induce peripheral paraesthesiae in up to 75% of subjects treated. A trial of the effect of methazolamide at high altitude was performed on seven staff manning the infrared telescope on the summit of Mauna Kea (4200 m) (Forster 1983; Chapter 30, this volume). Arterial oxygen tension was higher during the course of methazolamide. On the first day at high altitude it was 44.2 mmHg, as contrasted to a control value of 40.9 mmHg; on the fifth day at high altitude it was 48.3 mmHg, as contrasted to the control value of 44.4 mmHg. Two of the seven subjects experienced peripheral paraesthesiae and two complained of an abnormal flat taste with carbonated drinks while methazolamide was being taken. This is due to the inhibition of carbonic anhydrase

in the tongue so that the conversion of carbon dioxide to carbonic acid fails to take place in the time available as the drink passes over the tongue, and the acid-sensing buds are not stimulated (Ward *et al.* 1989). Methazolamide, like acetazolamide, decreases the loss of hydrogen ions in the urine and restores serum hydrogen ion concentration to normal. It stimulates the respiratory drive, increasing oxygen uptake. It is given in a dose of two 50-mg tablets twice a day. The course of the drug is commenced 24 hours before the ascent to high altitude. Side-effects listed by Forster (1983) include a mild increase in urine output, lasting 24–48 hours, and intermittent tingling ('pins and needles') in the hands and feet. There may be mild nausea and indigestion with loss of appetite. Lethargy is sometimes complained of. Sensitivity reactions such as a skin rash have been reported. There is the very characteristic complaint of the change in taste of carbonated drinks. Chronic use may lead to the formation of renal calculi.

Other more powerful and more rapidly acting diuretics have been advocated, particularly by Singh *et al.* (1969), who dealt with the massive outbreak of acute mountain sickness among Indian troops in Ladakh. An example is frusemide. This was used mainly to combat cerebral mountain sickness (Chapter 14) and we shall consider the drug there. Suffice it to say here that many are highly critical of its use, particularly as it is thought to cause haemoconcentration and hence to induce thrombosis which is a serious part of the pathology of the pulmonary and cerebral forms of malignant acute mountain sickness, as will be seen in Chapters 13 and 14.

Hypobaria *per se* and acute high-altitude illness

A recently introduced alternative to rapid descent in the treatment of acute mountain sickness is the use of hyperbaria by portable compression chambers. Before considering the role for hyperbaric therapy in acute high-altitude illness we should first consider the role of hypobaria *per se* as contrasted to hypobaric hypoxia in the genesis of acute high-altitude sickness.

Roach and Hackett (1992) have recently raised once again the much-discussed problem as to why syndromes like those of acute mountain sickness are not recognized at low altitude in patients who become hypoxic for hours or days due to illness or injury. It is possible that the hypoxia of illness causes symptoms that obscure those similar to features of acute mountain sickness. On the other hand, it is well known that it is virtually impossible to produce animal models of high-altitude disease by the use of normobaric hypoxia alone at low altitude. It has to be kept in mind that hypobaria *per se* may be of importance in the mechanism of high-altitude illness.

Interest in the physiological effects of hypobaria *per se* increased because of American manned space flight (Roach and Hackett 1992). Until the fire in a spacecraft in 1967, the atmosphere in the early space flight missions was hypobaric but not hypoxic. Epstein and Saruta (1972) exposed eight men to a hypobaric chamber pressure of 258 mmHg without hypoxia for 9 days. They found that prolonged exposure to hypobaria without hypoxia led to a progressive decrease of creatinine clearance starting on the second day of exposure to a maximal decrement of 40% on day eight and a return to baseline by the third day of recovery. Compared to control values this resulted in a decrease in the filtered load of sodium and a positive sodium and potassium balance. Aldosterone excretion was found to be higher during hypobaria. None of the men developed symptoms of acute mountain sickness but Epstein and Saruta (1972) wondered if these physiological changes could contribute to the development of acute mountain sickness. A suggestion of decreased creatinine clearance was also found in a previous hypobaric exposure to an oxygen–helium atmosphere (Glatte and Gianetti 1966). Tucker *et al.* (1983) found that hypobaria *per se* did not stimulate the chemosensitivity of the chemoreceptors and, in the absence of hypoxia, the ventilatory response was nearly abolished. When oxygen was removed from the chamber the ventilatory response to hypoxia returned.

Hyperbaric therapy in the treatment of acute high-altitude illness

According to Roach and Hackett (1992) hyperbaric treatment has been used for about 15 years in cases of acute mountain sickness, high-altitude pulmonary oedema, and cerebral mountain sickness in trekkers reporting to the medical clinic of the Himalayan Rescue Association in Pheriche, Nepal (4250 m), where the first portable chamber was used and found to be useful. A large, non-portable chamber was used to study 15 patients with acute mountain sickness including four cases of cerebral oedema and one mixed type of cerebral and pulmonary oedema (Takei *et al.* 1988). These patients were compressed some 200 mmHg above ambient pressure. The inner pressure was compressed to 620 mmHg within 20

minutes initially, maintained at 620 mmHg for 10 minutes, and then decompressed immediately. They were able to confirm that hyperbaria mimics descent and is thus very effective for the treatment of high-altitude diseases. There was a significant improvement of oxygen saturation level from a pre-treatment level of 67.6% to a post-treatment level of 83.9%. Since the late 1980s portable fabric hyperbaric chambers, as described below, have become commercially available for the treatment of acute mountain sickness and its serious pulmonary and cerebral variants. Clinical studies in the field by King and Greenlee (1990) confirmed that hyperbaria, when administered alone or in combination with other treatments, was equally and rapidly effective in combating acute mountain sickness.

Hackett *et al.* (1990) used a randomized crossover design of clinical trial with hyperbaria and oxygen breathing in eight climbers with high-altitude pulmonary oedema on Mt McKinley. The hyperbaria applied was some 200 mmHg above ambient pressure for 2 hours, and oxygen was titrated, to match that provided by the hyperbaria. They found that both treatments were successful in reversing the signs and symptoms of the condition but hyperbaria was no more effective than oxygen in treating the patients with high-altitude pulmonary oedema. They found a decreased haemoglobin concentration with both treatments, consistent with a shift in fluids into the intravascular compartment. The comparison of hyperbaria with oxygen in the treatment of acute mountain sickness was also made by Kasic *et al.* (1991) and hyperbaria was found to come out well in this comparison. Roach and Hackett (1992) refer to an unpublished study by Robertson and Shlim who compared the effectiveness of hyperbaria and acetazolamide in treating acute mountain sickness. They compared 100 mmHg above ambient pressure to one dose of 250 mg acetazolamide in trekkers reporting to a Himalayan Rescue Association Aid Post at Menang, Nepal. They reported that hyperbaria was more effective than the single dose of acetazolamide.

The Gamov bag, developed by Dr Igor Gamov, of Boulder, Colorado, is a portable lightweight (6.6 kg) airtight nylon bag with an airtight zipper. The patient is zipped inside the bag. A foot-pump is then attached to an inlet valve, and air is pumped into the bag to a pressure of 110 mmHg (2 lb per square inch). Air is pumped into the bag continuously to prevent carbon dioxide buildup, and a pop-off valve bleeds air when the pressure exceeds 2 lb per square inch (King *et al.* 1989). During the Wyoming

Centennial Everest expedition to Mt Everest in 1988 the Gamov bag was employed on a 33-year-old mountaineer with high-altitude pulmonary oedema. He was placed in the bag at an altitude of 5200 m and pressure was inflated to 2 lb per square inch to simulate an altitude of 3200 m. Within 3–4 minutes his headache had gone and there was an increase in oxygen saturation. After 2 hours in the bag he was removed and returned to the altitude of 5200 m. He had renewed but less severe symptoms within a half hour (King *et al.* 1989).

It is clear that such treatment could obviate the need for storing large quantities of oxygen at high-altitude work studies such as the United Kingdom Infrared Telescope on the summit of Mauna Kea (Chapter 30; Forster 1994). However, it is not to be recommended as a substitute for descent. Further clinical trials are necessary to determine the length of hyperbaric treatment necessary for complete resolution of acute mountain sickness, and the length of treatment that allows safe re-entry to higher altitudes (Roach and Hackett 1992). Roach and Hackett agree that hyperbaria should be used as a temporizing measure until descent is feasible.

Dexamethasone

This drug is the treatment of choice for cerebral mountain sickness but Ferrazzini *et al.* (1987) and Oelz (1988) believe that it also has a role to play as an emergency treatment for severe acute mountain sickness to facilitate safe descent to a lower altitude. Such a simple drug regimen is desirable when rapid descent is prevented by weather or avalanche conditions. They carried out a double-blind, randomized, placebo-controlled trial of treatment with the drug at an altitude of 4550 m in the Valais Alps. They gave 8 mg dexamethasone initially followed by 4 mg every 6 hours. After 12–16 hours' treatment the mean acute mountain sickness scored decreased significantly. Eight of the 17 patients became totally asymptomatic. Thus one of the features of benign acute mountain sickness is that it can be safely treated on the mountainside. Dexamethasone is more effective in treating the cerebral form of acute mountain sickness (Chapter 14). The pulmonary vasodilator nifedipine, on the other hand, has been employed in cases of acute mountain sickness merging into high-altitude pulmonary oedema. It brings about a decrease in pulmonary arterial pressure and a prompt reduction in the size of the right heart (Chapter 13).

Reassurance

In the experience of the authors, many subjects who visit high altitude for the first time, especially if they are of a timid disposition, find the symptoms of acute mountain sickness disturbing. Many lowlanders expect to become ill, especially if they are familiar with the dreaded reputation of *soroche*, as is the Peruvian coastal dweller. In a delightful aside, Ravenhill (1913) noted that the railway on the Bolivian border of Chile rose to its greatest elevation at Ascotan (3960 m), a fact advertised on a notice board at the side of the railway-line which immediately induced acute mountain sickness in many travellers. The difference in psychological approach to a journey to high attitude may *in part* account for the different susceptibilities of individuals to acute mountain sickness. However, in Chapter 30 evidence is produced to show that individual response to hypobaric hypoxia has a physiological basis.

Singh (1964) expressed the opinion that individuals of nervous temperament and psychological instability are not likely to do well in high mountains. On the other hand, subjects like mining engineers, who wish to get on with their duties as soon as possible, will tend to accept acute mountain sickness as a necessary but transient discomfort. It is not possible to predict the behaviour of a sea-level subject at high altitude and there is no sure method for the selection of individuals suitable for travel or employment at great heights. Most subjects who experience symptoms on travelling to high altitude need little more than the reassurance of their companions and the time to allow themselves to accommodate to the new environment and the novel and unpleasant bodily sensations it induces. After a few days the symptoms will lessen and disappear. On the other hand, in about 5% of cases the symptoms may persist or get worse and under those circumstances consideration has to be given to the possibility that the disease has entered a malignant phase of either pulmonary or cerebral form.

Analgesics and sedatives

Headache is the most troublesome and persistent symptom of benign acute mountain sickness. Voluntary hyperventilation will raise arterial oxygen tension, diminish cerebral vasodilation, and ameliorate headache. Simple analgesics may give some relief. Sedatives are best avoided, for they will depress respiration and make the hypoxia worse, especially during sleep. Problems related to difficulty in sleeping are considered in Chapter 28.

Oxygen

Since there is no direct relation between hypoxia and acute mountain sickness, the role of oxygen in the treatment of the condition is not as straight forward as it might at first seem.Houston and Dickson (1975) found that the benefit of oxygen is less striking than might be anticipated. In our experience, severe bouts of headache may be relieved by its use. Breathing oxygen at night may prove effective in preventing morning headaches. Frequent intermittent use of small amounts of oxygen should be avoided, for this will delay rather than aid acclimatization. In contrast, voluntary hyperventilation often helps and probably does promote acclimatization (Ward *et al.* 1989).

Historical remedies

Whymper, who first climbed the Matterhorn in 1865 and opened the way to the conquest of peaks throughout the world, mentions in his book, *Travels Amongst the Great Andes of the Equator*, that his doctor recommended potassium chloride to him as an antidote to mountain sickness from which he suffered severely (Whymper 1892). It is of interest that many year later Waterlow and Bunjé (1966) came to believe that potassium depletion may be a factor in inducing acute mountain sickness. They considered that potassium supplements should be given. Their view were based on trials carried out during four expeditions to the Sierra Nevada de Santa Maria in Colombia (3660–4270 m), when the efficacy of potassium supplements versus lactose was tested. Ravenhill (1913) recorded that the Quechua and Aymara Indians of Peru and Bolivia had great faith in several herbs for the relief of *soroche* or *puna*. Of these, 'chaca como' and 'flor de puna' were most used in the form of an infusion. Another herb employed was 'huamanripu'.

SURVEILLANCE

The reassurance that may be necessary for the nervous traveller to high altitude was referred to earlier in this chapter. On the other hand, reference was also made to the danger of the 'do or die' attitude, the determination to push ahead with the ascent regardless of the consequence, and the willingness to hide symptoms that might in fact be worsening. The leader or doctor of a group at high altitude must be keenly aware that a small proportion of cases of benign acute mountain sickness, say 5%, may slowly or explosively change into either pulmonary or cerebral types of the malignant form of the disease, which are described in the following two chapters. He must keep the members of the party under close surveillance, unobtrusively to avoid causing any apprehension, so that, should the tell-tale signs and symptoms appear, immediate evacuation of the subject to low altitude can take place to avoid a life-threatening situation.

Reference

Agnoletti, G., Ferrari, R., Slade, A.M., Severs, N.J., and Harris, P. (1989). Stretch-induced centrifugal movement of atrial specific granules — a preparatory step in atrial natriuretic peptide secretion. *Journal of Molecular and Cellular Cardiology*, **21**, 235

Agnoletti, G., Cornacchiari, A., Ferrari, R., and Harris, P. (1990). Effects of temperature and osmolality on the release of atrial natriuretic peptide. *Biochemical and Biophysical Research Communications*, **167**, 1001

Agnoletti, G., Rodella, A., Cornacchiari, A., Panzali, A.F., Harris, P., and Ferrari, R. (1992). Isoproterenol induces release of atrial natriuretic peptide from rat atrium in vitro. *American Journal of Physiology*, **262**, H285

Atlas, S.A., Kleinert, H.D., Camargo, M.J., Januszewics, A., Sealey, J.E., Laragh, J.H., Schilting, J.W., Lewicki, J.A., Johnson, L.K., and Maack, T. (1984). Purification, sequencing and synthesis of natriuretic and vasoactive rat atrial peptide. *Nature*, **309**, 717

Bärtsch, P., Shaw, S., Franciolli, M., Gnädinger, M.P., and Weidmann, P. (1988). Elevated atrial natriuretic peptide in acute mountain sickness. *Journal of Applied Physiology*, **65**, 1929

Birmingham Medical Research Expeditionary Society Mountain Sickness Study Group (1981). Acetazolamide in control of acute mountain sickness. *Lancet*, **i**, 180

Clarke, C. and Duff, J. (1976). Mountain sickness, retinal haemorrhages, and acclimatization on Mount Everest in 1975. *British Medical Journal*, **ii**, 495

De Bold, A.J. (1979). Heart atria granularity. Effects of changes in water–electrolyte balance. *Proceedings of the Society for Experimental Biology and Medicine*, **161**, 508

De Bold, A.J., Borenstein, H.B., Veress, A.T., and Sonrenberg, H. (1981). A rapid and potent natriuretic response to intravenous injection of atrial myocardial extract in rat. *Life Sciences*, **28**, 891

Dickinson, J.G. (1981). Acute mountain sickness. A dissertation based on eleven years' experience in the Nepal Himalaya. Unpublished D.M. thesis, University of Oxford

Dickinson, J.G. (1982). Terminology and classification of acute mountain sickness. *British Medical Journal*, **285**, 720

Epstein, M. and Saruta, T. (1972). Effects of simulated high altitude on renin–aldosterone and Na homeostasis in normal man. *Journal of Applied Physiology*, **33**, 204

Ferrazzini, G., Maggiorini, M., Kriemler, S., Bärtsch, P., and Oelz, O. (1987). Successful treatment of acute mountain sickness with dexamethasone. *British Medical Journal*, **294**, 1380

Forster, P.J.G. (1983). Work at high altitude: a clinical and physiological study at the United Kingdom Infrared Telescope, Mauna Kea, Hawaii. *Occasional Reports of the Royal Observatory*, Edinburgh

Forster, P.J.G. (1984). Health and work at high altitude: a study at the Mauna Kea observatories. *Publications of the Astronomical Society of the Pacific*, **96**, 478

Forster, P. (1986). Telescopes at high altitude. In *Aspects of Hypoxia* (D. Heath, Ed.). Liverpool; Liverpool University Press, p. 227

Forster, P.J.G. (1994). Working at high altitude. In *Hunter's Diseases of Occupations*, 8th edn (P.A.B. Raffle, P.H. Adams, P.J. Baxter, and W.R. Lee, Eds.) London; Edward Arnold, p. 363

Forster, P.J.G., Nuki, G., Rylance, H.J., and Wallace, R.C. (1986). Effect of high altitude and acetazolamide on human serum and urine purines. *Advances in Experimental Medicine and Biology*, **195**, 601

Forwand, S.A., Landowne, M., Follansbee, J.N., and Hansen, J.E. (1968). Effect of acetazolamide on acute mountain sickness. *New England Journal of Medicine*, **279**, 839

Glatte, H.V. and Gianetti, C.L. (1966). Study of man during a 56-day exposure to an oxygen–helium atmosphere at 258 mmHg total pressure: III Renal response. *Aerospace Medicine*, **37**, 559

Greene, M.K., Kerr, A.M., McIntosh, I.B., and Prescott, R.J., (1981). Acetazolamide in prevention of acute mountain sickness: a double-blind controlled cross-over study. *British Medical Journal*, **283**, 811

Gutkowska, J., Bourassa, M., Roy, D., Thibault, G., Garcia, R., Cantin, M., and Genest, J. (1985). Immunoreactive atrial natriuretic factor (ir-ANF) in human plasma. *Biochemical and Biophysical Research Communications*, **128**, 1350

Hackett, P.H. (1988). Medical research on Mount McKinley. *Annals of Sports Medicine*, **4**, 232

Hackett, P.H., Rennie, D., and Levine, H.D. (1976). The incidence, importance and prophylaxis of acute mountain sickness. *Lancet*, **ii**, 1149

Hackett, P.H., Rennie, D., Hofmeister, S.E., Grover, R.F., Grover, E.B., and Reeves, J.T. (1982). Fluid retention and relative hypoventilation in acute mountain sickness. *Respiration*, **43**, 321

Hackett, P.H., Roach, R.C., Hollingshead, K.F. *et al.* (1987*a*). Arterial oxygen saturation reveals impending acute mountain sickness during ascent to high altitude. In *Hypoxia and Cold* (J.R. Sutton, C.S. Houston, and G. Coates, Ed.). New York; Praeger, p. 544

Hackett, P.H., Roach, R.C., Swenson, R.C., *et al.* (1987*b*). Subclinical pulmonary oedema in acute mountain sickness. In *The Tolerable Limits of Hypoxia* (J.R. Sutton and C.S. Houston, Ed.). Indianapolis; Benchmark Press, p. 383

Hackett, P.H. , Roach, R.C., Goldberg, S., Greene, E.R., Selland, M., Wilson, N., and Feil, P. (1990). A portable, fabric hyperbaric chamber for treatment of high altitude pulmonary edema (Abstract). In *Hypoxia: The Adaptations* (J.R. Sutton, G. Coates and J.E. Remmers, Eds), Philadelphia, B.C. Dekker, p. 291

Hisayuki, M. and Kangawa, K. (1984). Human and rat atrial natriuretic polypeptides (h ANP and r ANP). Purification, structure and biological activity. *Clin. Exp. Theor. Pract.* **A6**, 1717

Hornbein, T.F., Townes, B.D., Schoene, R.B., Sutton, J.R., and Houston, C.S. (1989). The cost to the central nervous system of climbing to extremely high altitude. *New England Journal of Medicine*, **321**, 1714

Houston, C.S. and Dickinson, J. (1975). Cerebral form of high altitude illness. *Lancet*, **ii**, 758

Jamieson, J.D. and Palade, G.E. (1964). Specific granules in atrial muscle cells. *Journal of Cell Biology*, **23**, 151

Kasic, J.F., Yaron, M., Nicholas, R.A., Lickteig, J.A., and Roach, R.C. (1991). Treatment of acute mountain sickness: hyperbaric versus oxygen therapy. *Annals of Emergency Medicine*, **20**, 1109

Kety, S.S. and Schmidt, C.F. (1948). The effects of altered arterial tensions of carbon dioxide and oxygen on cerebral blood flow and cerebral oxygen consumption of normal young men. *Journal of Clinical Investigation*, **27**, 484

King, S.J. and Greenlee, R.R. (1990). Successful use of the Gamov Hyperbaric Bag in the treatment of altitude illness at Mount Everest. *Journal of Wilderness Medicine*, **1**, 193

King, S.J., Greenlee, R., and Goldings, H.J. (1989). Acute mountain sickness. *New England Journal of Medicine*, **320**, 1492

Kisch, B. (1956). Electron microscopy of the atrium of the heart: guinea pig. *Experimental Medicine and Surgery*, **14**, 99

Kronenberg, R.S., Safer, P., Lee, J., Wright, F., Noble, W., Wahrenbrock, E., Hickey, R., Nemota, E., and Severinghaus, J.W. (1971). Pulmonary artery pressure and alveolar gas exchange in man during acclimatization to 12,470 ft. *Journal of Clinical Investigation*, **50**, 827

Maher, J.T., Cymerman, A., Reeves, J.T., Cruz, J.C., Denniston, J.C., and Grover, R.F. (1975). Acute mountain sickness: increased severity in eucapnic hypoxia. *Aviation, Space, and Environmental Medicine*, **46**, 826

Matsukura, S., Kangawa, K., and Matsuo, H. (1987). Presence of atrial natriuretic polypeptide in the pulmonary veins and vena cava. *Biochemical Research Communications*, **146**, 1465

Milledge, J.S. (1983). Acute mountain sickness. *Thorax*, **38**, 641

Milledge, J.S., Thomas, P.S., Beeley, J.M., and English J.S.C., (1988). Hypoxic ventilatory response and acute mountain sickness. *European Respiratory Journal*, **1**, 948

Milledge, J.S., Beeley, J.M., McArthur, S., and Morice, A.H. (1989). Atrial natriuretic peptide, altitude and acute mountain sickness. *Clinical Science*, **77**, 509

Milledge, J.S., Beeley, J.M., Broome, J. Luff, N., Pelling, M., and Smith, D. (1991). Acute mountain sickness: susceptibility, fitness and hypoxic ventilatory response. *European Respiratory Journal*, **1**, (4), 1000

Montgomery, A.B., Mills, J., and Luce, J.M. (1989). Incidence of acute mountain sickness at intermediate altitude. *Journal of the American Medical Association*, **261**, 732

Moore, L.G., Harrison, G.L., McCullough, R.E., McCullough, R.G., Micco, A.J., Tucker, A., Weil, J.V., and Reeves, J.T. (1986). Low acute hypoxic ventilatory response and hypoxic depression in acute altitude sickness. *Journal of Applied Physiology*, **60**, 1407

Oelz, O. (1988). Research in acute mountain sickness in the Swiss Alps. *Annals of Sports Medicine*, **4**, 255

Olive, J.E. and Waterhouse, N. (1979). Birmingham Medical Research Expeditionary Society 1977 Expedition: psychological aspects of acute mountain sickness. *Postgraduate Medical Journal*, **55**, 464

Pandit, J.J. (1992). Altitude induced illness. *British Medical Journal*, **304**, 1633

Pollard, A.J. (1992). Response to above letter. *British Medical Journal*, **304**, 1633

Ramsay, L.E. (1977). Prophylaxis of acute mountain sickness. *Lancet*, **i**, 540

Ravenhill, T.H. (1913). Some experience of mountain sickness in the Andes. *Journal of Tropical Medicine and Hygiene*, **16**, 313

Reeves, J.T., Moore, L.G., McCullough, R.E., McCullough, R.G., Harrison, G., Tranmere, B.I., Micco, A.J., Tucker, A., and Weil, J.V. (1985). Headache at high altitude is not related to internal carotid arterial blood velocity. *Journal of Applied Physiology*, **59**, 909

Roach, R., and Hackett, P.H. (1992). Hyperbaria and high altitude illness. In *Hypoxia and Mountain Medicine* (J.R. Sutton, G. Coates, and C.S. Houston, Ed.), Oxford; Pergamon Press, p. 266

Roach, R.C., Larson, E.B., Hornbein, T.F., Houston, C.S., Bartlett, S., Hardestry, J., Johnson, D., and Perkins, M. (1983). Acute mountain sickness, antacids and ventilation during rapid, acute ascent of Mount Rainier. *Aviation, Space and Environmental Medicine*, **54**, 397

Sakamoto, M., Nakao, K., Morii, N., Sugawara, A., Yamada, T., Itah, I., Shiono, S., Saito, Y., and Imura, H. (1986). The lung as a possible target organ for atrial natriuretic polypeptide secreted from the heart. *Biochemical and Biophysical Research Communications*, **135**, 515

Severinghaus, J.W., Chiodi, H., Eger, E.I., Brandstater, B., and Hornbein, T.F. (1966). Cerebral blood flow in man at high altitude. *Circulation Research*, **19**, 274

Singh, I. (1964). Medical problems during acclimatization to high altitude. In *Physiological Effects of High Altitude* (W.H. Weihe, Ed.). Oxford; Pergamon Press, p. 333

Singh, I., Khanna, P.K., Srivastava, M.C., Lal, M., Roy, S.B., and Subramanyam, C.S.V. (1969). Acute mountain sickness. *New England Journal of Medicine*, **280**, 175

Takei, S., Kamio, S., Uehara, A., Naitch, J., and Hayata Y. (1988). Treatment of acute mountain sickness using a compression chamber. In *High Altitude Medical Science* (G. Ueda, S. Kusama, and N. Voelkel, Ed.). Matsumoto, Japan; Shinshu University Press, p. 284

Tucker, A., Reeves, J.T., Robertshaw, D., and Grover, R.F. (1983). Cardiopulmonary response to acute altitude exposure. Water loading and denitrogenation. *Respiration Physiology*, **54**, 363

Wagner, P.D., Sutton, J.R., Reeves, J.T., Cymerman, A., Groves, B.M., and Malconian, M.K. (1987). Operation Everest II: pulmonary gas exchange during a simulated ascent of Mt. Everest. *Journal of Applied Physiology*, **63**, 2348

Ward, M.P., Milledge, J.S., and West, J.B. (1989). Acute mountain sickness (AMS). In *High Altitude Medicine and Physiology*. London; Chapman and Hall Medical, p. 369

Waterlow, J.C. and Bunjé, H.W. (1966). Observations on mountain sickness in the Colombian Andes. *Lancet*, **ii**, 655

Whymper, E. (1892). *Travels Amongst the Great Andes of the Equator*. London; John Murray

Winter, R.J.D., Meleagros, J., Perrez, S., Krausz, T., Polak, J.M., and Bloom, S.R. (1987). Plasma atrial natriuretic factor and ultrastructure of atrial specific granules following chronic hypoxia in rats. *Clinical Science*, **73** (Suppl. 17), 26P

13

High-altitude pulmonary oedema

About half of all lowlanders who ascend rapidly to altitudes above 3000 m develop symptoms and signs of benign acute mountain sickness. In most people this condition is more in the nature of an inconvenience than an illness but in a minority of cases it rapidly escalates into serious, and commonly life-threatening, pulmonary or cerebral oedema. Sometimes these frightening manifestations appear suddenly without an earlier benign phase. This is particularly true of lung oedema and this has prompted some into considering whether benign acute mountain sickness and high-altitude pulmonary oedema are fundamentally distinct conditions. The central feature of this condition is the sudden overwhelming onset of oedema of the lung but there are often other important aspects to the underlying pathology such as pulmonary thrombosis and even infarction. Nevertheless, since the condition is so widely known as 'high-altitude pulmonary oedema', we shall retain this term in this account.

RECOGNITION OF HIGH-ALTITUDE PULMONARY OEDEMA AS A DISTINCT ENTITY

Until about 1950 the acute onset of severe breathlessness far beyond what one would expect to occur in acute mountain sickness was regarded as due to pneumonia. More than a decade earlier, however, Hurtado had suspected that the dyspnoea was due to the sudden onset of lung oedema (Hurtado 1937). Then early reports by Peruvian doctors began to appear with increasing recognition of the of the true nature of the condition (Lundberg 1952; Bardales 1955; Lizarraga 1955). The first clear account of high-altitude pulmonary oedema in the English language was given by Houston (1960) who described its onset in an athletic student of 21 years carrying a heavy pack in deep snow and cold weather at an altitude of 3600 m. He also referred briefly to four other cases, but the brevity of these reports does not detract from the dramatic nature of the condition that he described as a distinct clinical

entity. Thus, he reports the companion of one of his subjects who died from pulmonary oedema as saying: 'He sounded as though he were literally drowning in his own fluid with an almost continuous loud bubbling sound as if breathing through liquid. I noticed that a white froth resembling cotton candy had appeared to well up out of his mouth.' Subsequently, with other colleagues (Hultgren et al. 1961), he presented data from 15 patients with high-altitude pulmonary oedema at La Oroya (3750 m) in Peru and added information on 14 patients collected by Lizarraga (1955) and on 12 cases studied by Bardales (1955). This review and analysis of 41 cases formed the first major account of high-altitude pulmonary oedema in the English language. Thirty-six cases were reported soon after by Marticorena et al. (1964) and since that time an extensive literature on the disease has accumulated.

PREDISPOSING FACTORS

The altitude at which the risk of developing oedema of the lung begins has been reported as about 3350 m in the Himalaya (Singh et al. 1965), 3660 m in the Andes, and somewhat lower (2590 m) in the Rockies. Sophocles (1986) reported the 47 cases of high-altitude pulmonary oedema that occurred in Vail, Colorado (2500 m) during the period 1975–82. The average total ascent was 2330 m in less than 1 day from 170 m. High-altitude pulmonary oedema is a disease affecting young healthy people. Children and teenagers are especially at risk, but this is not to say that the condition does not occur in the middle-aged, especially those who venture too quickly up to the high mountainous regions on 'adventure holidays'. The susceptibility of young people in the second or third decades to the disease has been reported by many investigators (Marticorena et al. 1964; Menon 1965; Scoggin et al. 1977). The age range of patients in the series of 15 cases collected by Hultgren and co-workers was 4–42 years, the mean age being as low as 16.1 years. The larger reviewed series of 41 cases was composed of 35 males and six females. The person most at risk is the young male and many afflicted are of athletic disposition and totally free of heart and lung disease (Houston 1960). There is nothing to suggest that any preceding respiratory infection is involved. This is an important point to bear in mind, for it indicates that the most meticulous clinical examination of persons planning to go to high altitude will not pick out those who will subsequently develop high-altitude pulmonary oedema. A clean bill of health at sea level in no way guarantees exemption from the development of lung oedema.

The condition commonly afflicts the unacclimatized subject exposed to diminished barometric pressure who engages too quickly in strenuous physical exercise on arrival. It is thus a hazard for the mountain climber and skier (Fred *et al.* 1962). However, exercise is not an essential predisposing factor and many cases of high-altitude pulmonary oedema occur in people arriving for the first time in mountainous areas by aircraft. The condition may occur while the subject is at rest (Singh *et al.* 1965) or even asleep (Marticorena *et al.* 1964; Peñaloza and Sime 1969).

There appears to be a distinct individual predisposition to the development of the condition, since some patients have repeated attacks of *soroche* and pulmonary oedema occurring each time they return to the mountains after a sojourn at lower altitudes (Hultgren *et al.* 1961). One of the patients reported by these authors had four attacks of pulmonary oedema in 6 years. There may be inherited familial predisposition as well as individual susceptibility (Hultgren *et al.* 1961; Fred *et al.* 1962). There do not appear to be racial differences in predisposition to lung oedema.

A most important predisposing factor is re-entry to hypoxia, with the lung oedema occurring in the highlander returning to his mountain home after a period spent at a lower altitude. Thus, although two-thirds of the 332 cases reported in India by Singh *et al.* (1965) were in fresh inductees to high altitude, over 80 cases were in hill people who had been at lower altitudes for from 1 day to 6 months. Hultgren *et al.* (1961) found that only one of the 41 cases they reviewed had not recently been to a lower altitude prior to his illness. Furthermore, only nine had developed pulmonary oedema during their first visit to the mountains. Menon (1965) also found that 65 of his 101 cases occurred in people re-entering high altitude. Marticorena *et al.* (1964) elicited a history of a recent visit to low altitude in 33 of their 36 cases of lung oedema. The length of stay at a lower elevation prior to subsequent development of the disease was

5–21 days in one series of cases (Hultgren *et al.* 1961). Previous acclimatization will not necessarily guard against development of the condition (Singh *et al.* 1965) and ascent for as little as an extra 300 m may induce it. In Peru the condition is commonest in January. At first one might be tempted to relate this to the rain and snow in the mountains at that time, but this is also the season when the highlanders tend to take their vacation at the coast. Hence, January is the month when the number of re-entries to the hypoxia of high altitude is greatest.

A study from Colorado underlines the importance of re-entry into high altitude in the development of lung oedema and reveals in a striking manner just how brief needs to be the visit to low altitude to put the highlander at risk on his return to the mountains. Leadville, Colorado (3100 m) is of unusual interest in illustrating the importance of re-entry to the hypoxia of high altitude in the pathogenesis of high-altitude pulmonary oedema. It has a resident population of only 8300, but is visited annually by no fewer than 100 000 tourists. This offers a unique opportunity of contrasting the incidence of lung oedema in newcomers to the area with that in long-term residents re-entering their mountain home after a brief visit to low altitude. During a period of 7 years and 3 months there were 58 suspected cases and, of these, 39 episodes in 32 patients met strict diagnostic criteria for high-altitude pulmonary oedema (Scoggin *et al.* 1977). This group consisted of 18 males and 14 females, ranging in age from 3 to 41 years with an average age of only 12 years. Nineteen patients with shortness of breath were excluded only because of lack of radiographic evidence of oedema. All but two cases occurred in long-term residents at high altitude and represented 0.9% of the population 1–14 years of age. All but one of the 30 cases occurring in residents of Leadville developed after they had returned from a visit to low altitude. These visits needs only to be brief and in three instances lasted for only 1 day (Fig. 13.1). In five patients there was more than one attack of lung oedema. In four instances, the recurrences followed a return from a low-altitude visit and in the fifth it followed still higher ascent from the normal altitude of residence. Some residents at high altitude may make repeated trips to low altitude without developing pulmonary oedema in their re-ascent. However, many of the patients studied volunteered that they often had symptoms of respiratory distress similar to their recognized episodes of high-altitude pulmonary oedema, but that these symptoms resolved spontaneously in a few hours and did not require medical

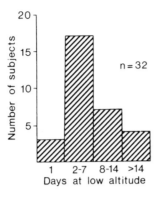

13.1 *Number of days spent at low altitude preceding the development of high-altitude pulmonary oedema at Leadville, Colorado (3100 m) in 32 subjects.*

attention. A possible familial tendency for this condition was suggested by the occurrence of high-altitude pulmonary oedema in a 21-year-old woman from Leadville and, 3 years later, in her 3-year-old daughter.

The conclusions from this clinical study are striking. The disease is not rare. It occurs on re-entry to high altitude of those already living at such elevations, rather than in newcomers to the environment. It affects the young predominantly and is a special risk for children. Even brief exposure to low level

puts the susceptible at risk; it is usually less than 1 week and may only be 1 day. Subjects who fall prey to this dangerous illness are otherwise in excellent health. Scoggin *et al.* (1977) concluded that 'high-altitude pulmonary oedema is a serious health problem for high-altitude dwellers in North America, and re-emphasises the point that acute changes in oxygen tension have profound effects on lung function'.

INCIDENCE

The incidence of high-altitude pulmonary oedema depends on the method used to detect the condition and, most importantly, on the antecedent medical history. Reports from the literature suggest that in a population of trekkers, climbers, soldiers stationed at high altitude, and residents at high altitude returning to their home after a period at low altitude, the incidence of lung oedema *diagnosed clinically* is less than 1.5% (Table 13.1). Some authorities believe the incidence of the condition to be somewhat higher. Thus, Hultgren and Marticorena (1978) investigated 97 residents of La Oroya (3750 m) in central Peru by means of a questionnaire and came to the conclusion that the incidence including mild cases was as high as 6.1%. Hackett (1988) believes that the incidence of high-altitude pulmonary oedema is higher on Mt McKinley where it occurs in one of every 30–50 climbers than in

Table 13.1 Incidence of severe episodes of high-altitude pulmonary oedema (HAPO) in adults in various mountainous regions of the world (after Hultgren and Marticorena 1978)[*]

Area	Altitude (m)	Subjects	Incidence of HAPO (%)[*]	Reference
Himalaya	3050–5490	Indian troops	0.57	Menon (1965)
Mt Kenya	5200	7500 climbers	0.44	Houston (quoted by Hultgren and Marticorena 1978)
Himalaya	2800–5500	522 trekkers	1.50	Hackett and Rennie (1976)
Mt Rainier	4400	141 climbers	0.50	Houston (1976)
Mt McKinley	6195	587 climbers	1.00	Wilson (quoted by Hultgren and Marticorena 1978)
La Oroya, Central Peru	3750	97 residents in mining community	0.60	Hultgren and Marticorena (1978)

[*]It will be seen from the table that the incidence of high-altitude pulmonary oedema diagnosed clinically in a population of trekkers, climbers, soldiers, and residents at high altitude is less than 1.5%. However, this incidence rises to 12.5% when subjects without a history of previous HAPO are examined radiographically within a day of ascent to 4550 m (Vock *et al.* 1989). It increases to a remarkable 66% in subjects who have had a previous attack of the condition and in whom lung oedema is detected radiographically with ascent to 4550 m (Vock *et al.* 1989).

other locations and he relates this to the extreme cold in this particular mountain area. The studies of Scoggin *et al.* (1977) on highland residents of Leadville, Colorado convinced them that the disease is commoner than hitherto thought. In this respect Norboo and Ball (1988) reported that no fewer than 40 cases were seen at the Sonam Memorial Hospital in Leh, Ladakh (3500 m) between June 1981 and August 1986. The affected subjects comprised tourists from Europe, Japan, and lowland India. Eleven of them were residents of Ladakh returning home after visiting lowland India. Most of those afflicted were between 20 and 59 years of age.

When subclinical cases are *diagnosed radiographically* the incidence of high-altitude pulmonary oedema rises sharply. When Vock *et al.* (1989) studied the chest radiographs of subjects without a history of a previous attack of the condition within a day of ascent to an altitude of 4550 m they found the incidence to be 12.5%. When they carried out the same procedure on subjects with a medical history of such an attack, they found that the incidence of high-altitude pulmonary oedema was a remarkable 66%.

CLINICAL FEATURES

Most of the cases that have been reported from the Peruvian Andes have occurred acutely within 3–48 hours of the ascent (Arias-Stella and Krüger 1963; Marticorena *et al.* 1964). However, in the Indian cases reported by Singh *et al.* (1965), whereas two-thirds of the cases admittedly occurred within 3 days of arrival at high altitude, many were delayed for up to 10 days. There are initial symptoms of a dry cough associated with breathlessness, palpitation, and precordial discomfort. Headache, nausea, and vomiting occur commonly. Pronounced weakness and fatigue are common early symptoms. The patient then becomes extremely breathless and begins to cough up foamy pink sputum. Haemoptysis may occur (Hultgren *et al.* 1961). There is pronounced peripheral vasoconstriction, with pallor of the face and coldness and clamminess of the skin. On clinical examination widespread crepitations are heard throughout the lungs. Singh *et al.* (1965) recognize several clinical variants. Thus in some cases the onset is insidious with premonitory malaise, headache, insomnia, and anxiety. Only later are these symptoms followed by dry cough and dyspnoea. In others the conditions start more dramatically with acute respiratory symptoms.

Bonington (1971) gives a graphic account of the onset of what appears to have been a case of high-altitude pulmonary oedema in one of his fellow climbers during the ascent of Annapurna: 'Mike's condition worsened. His breathing seemed to have got out of control, rising to a crescendo of raucous pants. He was convinced he was dying; it was as if his heart and lungs were exploding.' Such patients develop progressive cough, productive of large quantities of frothy pink sputum, with dyspnoea and cyanosis and may become moribund. Haemoptysis, sometimes involving fairly large quantities of blood, is seen in about 20% of severe episodes. Some patients first show signs of the condition by developing oliguria. Some cases are complicated by cerebral oedema (Chapter 14) when they become giddy and increasingly apprehensive of death. They may become incoherent or irrational or experience hallucinations. Coma may follow and death is then likely to occur in very few hours.

On clinical examination patients with high-altitude pulmonary oedema commonly have tachycardia and low-grade fever. Tachypnoea up to 40 breaths/min may develop. Cyanosis of the lips and extremities may be pronounced. The systemic blood pressure may be low. Early harshness of expiration in the interscapular region is soon followed by crepitations and bubbling rales. In severe cases gurgling sounds can be heard without a stethoscope. The second sound in the pulmonary area is often loud and even palpable (Singh *et al.* 1965). There are no murmurs and there is no clinical evidence of cardiac failure. There is commonly an elevated haematocrit and an acid urine with a high specific gravity compatible with haemoconcentration. Signs of infection are absent, with only a minor rise in temperature. There is a normal white cell count and a normal sedimentation rate. Studies at 4200 m on Mt McKinley using contrast echocardiography have revealed that in some cases of high-altitude pulmonary oedema there may be prominent right-to-left shunting across the interatrial septum through a patent foramen ovale (Levine *et al.* 1991). Similar shunting has been demonstrated in patients with acute mountain sickness, and in well-acclimatized climbers (Levine *et al.* 1991).

RADIOLOGICAL FEATURES

Radiological examination demonstrates the pulmonary oedema as a coarse mottling that is commonly confluent and prominent in the parahilar regions (Marticorena *et al.* 1964). Singh *et al.* (1965) and Menon (1965) reported that the shadowing was at first pronounced in the upper and middle lobes, especially on the right side. However, Hultgren *et al.*

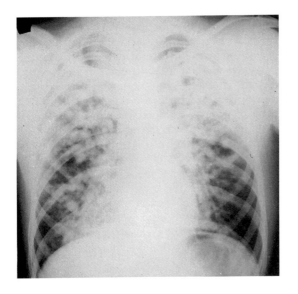

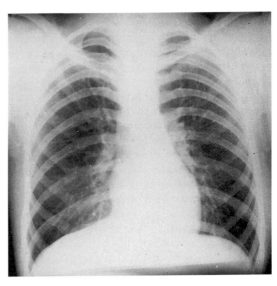

(a)   *(b)*

13.2 *(a) Radiograph of the chest from a Peruvian youth of 17 years returning to an altitude of 4330 m after 1 week's residence at sea level. There is coarse mottling of the lung fields indicative of high-altitude pulmonary oedema. The changes are bilateral and most pronounced at the apices. (From Peñaloza and Sime (1969).) (b) Radiograph of the chest from the same case taken 3 days later. There has been clearing of the pulmonary oedema.*

(1961) found there was no predilection of the process for either lung or any area of the lung. This is certainly our experience. In some cases that we have seen, the oedema presents as a coarse mottling which is bilateral and most pronounced at the apices (Fig. 13.2). In others the oedema is confined to one lung and most pronounced at the base (Fig. 13.3). The typical symmetrical butterfly distribution of pulmonary oedema, as seen frequently in uraemia and left ventricular failure, was not seen in the cases of Lizarraga (1965) and Bardales (1955), and in only two of the cases of Hultgren *et al.* (1961). Basal horizontal lines (Kerley B lines) and pleural effusions are rarely seen.

The pulmonary conus is usually prominent and the hilar and major pulmonary arteries are dilated in most cases, such dilatation being consistent with elevation of pulmonary arterial pressure. With clinical improvement of the oedema, the shadowing in the lung fields disappears within 6–48 hours (Singh *et al.* 1965; see Fig. 13.2). At the same time the fullness of the hilar vessels recedes. After clinical recovery Hultgren and co-workers found no consistent change in heart size, which was often unchanged by the onset of pulmonary oedema. In some cases recovery from the attack was followed by a decrease in

the cardiothoracic ratio; in others it was increased. The right atrial shadow tends to get smaller after clinical recovery from the oedema. Chest radiographs may reveal exudates persisting for days or even a fortnight after clinical recovery. Hence radiological examination is important to ensure a return to normal in patients who are symptom-free.

The development of radiographic features of lung oedema at high altitude was studied by Vock *et al.* (1989) in 25 male volunteers 6, 18, and 42 hours after arrival at 4550 m. Nine had a history of high-altitude pulmonary oedema. Baseline studies were obtained at 550 m. As soon as 6 hours after arrival, and independently of the consecutive presence of lung oedema, the diameters of the central pulmonary arteries increased by 10–30%. After 18 hours and increasingly at 42 hours, radiographic evidence of lung oedema appeared in eight subjects, six of whom had a history of a previous attack of high-altitude pulmonary oedema. The radiographic signs of oedema were most severe peripherally and their characteristics were compatible with permeability/overperfusion oedema. Radiography could detect oedema in subjects with normal findings on lung auscultation. This study demonstrated a significant individual susceptibility of low-

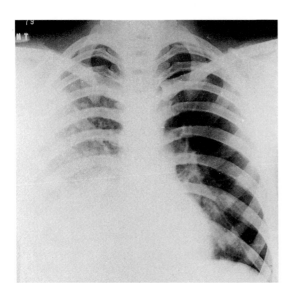

13.3 *Radiograph of the chest from a French student of 24 years who developed high-altitude pulmonary oedema while on a trekking holiday in the Bolivian Andes at an altitude of around 3800 m. In this instance the oedema is unilateral, being confined to the right lung, and most pronounced at the right base.*

landers with a history of high-altitude pulmonary oedema to develop the condition again on re-exposure to hypobaric hypoxia, with a remarkable recurrence rate of 66%. In one patient with high-altitude pulmonary oedema reported by Kobayashi *et al.* (1987) lung scintiscans with technetium-99m-macroaggregated albuminin showed decreased perfusion in the area of radiographic infiltrates.

ELECTROCARDIOGRAPHIC FEATURES

The majority of subjects who develop high-altitude pulmonary oedema have electrocardiographic evidence suggestive or characteristic of right ventricular hypertrophy, since they are mountain dwellers re-entering high altitude. Peñaloza and Sime (1969) recorded in two cases sinus tachycardia, right deviation of Â QRS, and tall peaked T waves over the right precordial leads. Marticorena *et al.* (1964) reported sinus tachycardia, slight peaked P waves, tall R waves in aVR, Rs complexes in V3R, and deep S waves in V6. They also recorded positive displacement of the RS–T segment and tall, peaked T waves. In one severe case reported by Singh *et al.* (1965) there were similar electrocardiographic findings with right-axis deviation, clockwise rotation,

T-wave inversion in leads V1–V5, a prominent R in leads aVR and V1, and peaked P waves. Some patients, however, have a normal electrocardiogram during an attack of high-altitude pulmonary oedema. On recovery there is a decrease in heart rate, a lowering of the P wave, and a decrease in the degree of right ventricular strain (Hultgren *et al.* 1961). After clinical recovery the electrocardiogram may take 3–6 weeks to return to normal (Singh *et al.* 1965).

PATHOLOGY

The pathology of this condition is more complex than merely one of oedema of the lung. There is commonly associated pulmonary thrombosis and infarction of the lung. Sometimes there is bronchopneumonia. Cases of malignant pulmonary acute mountain sickness are often combined with the cerebral form (Houston and Dickinson 1975) described in Chapter 14. For such reasons we believe that the customary term of 'high-altitude pulmonary oedema' is inclined to be misleading both as regards prognosis and treatment. It should not be expected that the rapid collection of fluid in the lung can be dispelled just as easily and it should not be imagined that the outcome of every treated case will be successful.

The early paper of Arias-Stella and Krüger (1963) concentrates on the features of the oedema. They report that in this condition the lungs at necropsy do not collapse and are congested, so that on pressure they yield a foamy pink fluid. Histological examination shows dilatation of pulmonary capillaries leading to thickening of the alveolar septa. Oedema coagulum is found in the alveolar ducts and space (Figs 13.4 and 13.5). There are hyaline membranes in close contact with the alveolar walls, and their histochemistry is identical to that of membranes found in the respiratory distress syndrome of the newborn. There may be haemorrhage into alveolar spaces. There is dilatation of pulmonary lymphatics and interstitial pulmonary oedema.

The state of the muscularization of the pulmonary arterial tree and of the right ventricle will depend on the background of the subject concerned. Thus, in affected highlanders there will be muscularization of the pulmonary arterioles and right ventricular hypertrophy, as described in Chapter 10 (Fig. 13.6). This muscularization is a feature of the native highlander, and, while a sudden exacerbation of pulmonary arterial hypertension is almost certainly involved in the aetiology of high-altitude pulmonary oedema, the muscular pulmonary arterioles are probably more a

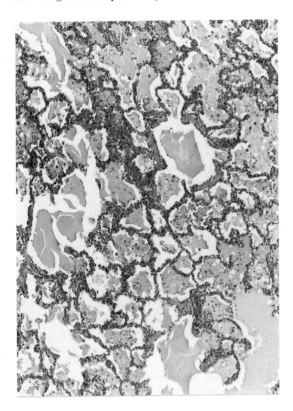

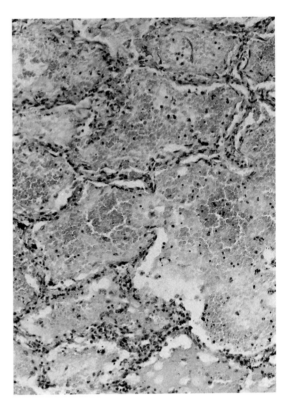

13.4 *Section of lung from a case of high-altitude pulmonary oedema occurring in a mestizo male aged 29 years. A native of Huanuco (3410 m), he lived for 1 month at sea level before returning to an altitude of 4330 m. There is excessive filling of the alveolar spaces by oedema coagulum. HE, × 55.*

13.5 *Section of lung from a case of high-altitude pulmonary oedema occurring in a 62-year-old Austrian doctor trekking to Gorakshep (5200 m) in Nepal. The alveolar spaces are distended with blood-stained oedema fluid. HE, × 150.*

marker of the chronic hypobaric hypoxia inherent in life in the mountains rather than a feature of the onset of pulmonary acute mountain sickness. In contrast, in seven Caucasian trekkers dying from malignant pulmonary acute mountain sickness, the pulmonary arteries were thin-walled, their mean medial thickness being in the range 2.8–6.0% (Dickinson *et al.* 1983). Such data suggest that the muscularity of the pulmonary vasculature may aid the elevation of pulmonary arterial pressure involved in the development of high-altitude pulmonary oedema, but it is not essential for its development.

We had the opportunity to study blocks of tissues taken at necropsy in seven trekkers in the Himalaya who died from malignant acute mountain sickness. The pathological findings in the lungs and brain

from these cases are shown in Table 13.2. Pulmonary arterial thrombosis was present in five and prominent in four of the seven cases (Fig. 13.7) and in one case deep vein thrombosis had occurred in addition. There were red infarcts of the lung in three instances (Fig. 13.7). Pulmonary oedema was present in four cases and was prominent in three. Inspection of Table 13.2 shows how commonly thrombosis, haemorrhage, and oedema in the lungs and brain are associated.

Bronchopneumonia was found in no fewer than six cases and in two it was severe (Fig. 13.8). Most patients with high-altitude pulmonary oedema, if it is not reversed, develop bronchopneumonia. Infection may be secondary to pulmonary thrombosis. Bronchopneumonia may on the other hand be the direct result of exposure to the harsh mountain environment or bathing in glacial rivers.

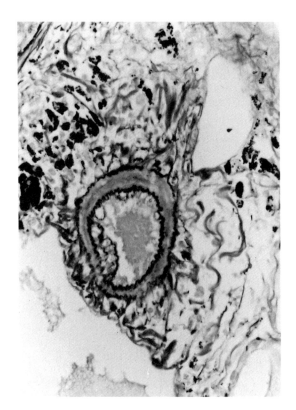

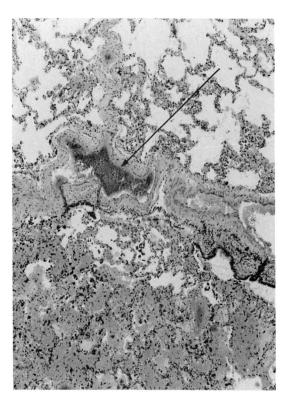

13.6 *Section of lung from the case illustrated in Fig. 13.4. It includes a transverse section of a small muscular pulmonary artery. This shows medial hypertrophy and crenation of elastic laminae consistent with pulmonary vasoconstriction. Such histological appearances are anticipated in native highlanders developing high-altitude pulmonary oedema. The muscularization typical of the native highlander (see Chapter 10) aids the development of significant pulmonary arterial hypertension and the development of lung oedema. EVG, × 335.*

13.7 *Section of lung from a case of malignant pulmonary acute mountain sickness occurring in a man of 38 years trekking to Gorakshep (5200 m) in Nepal. A muscular pulmonary artery contains a recent thrombus (arrow). Beneath the vessel is the edge of a red infarct. HE, × 60.*

HAEMODYNAMICS

Some insight into the mechanism of production of high-altitude pulmonary oedema is obtained from the results of cardiac catheterization carried out during an attack. Fred *et al.* (1962) studied the pulmonary haemodynamics of a 48-year-old doctor who had an attack of pulmonary oedema after 2 days of vigorous skiing at altitudes between 2600 and 3125 m. They found a raised pulmonary arterial mean pressure of 46 mmHg with normal left atrial and pulmonary venous pressures, the latter being obtained by advancing the catheter through a probe-patent foramen ovale into the left atrium and thence

into a pulmonary vein. Peñaloza and Sime (1969) reported findings at cardiac catheterization in two young men, aged 17 and 21 years, who developed high-altitude pulmonary oedema on returning to their homes at 4330 m after a brief visit to sea level. During the attack both were found to have severe hypoxaemia, and pulmonary arterial mean blood pressures of 62 and 63 mmHg, respectively. These findings were associated with low cardiac output and pulmonary wedge pressure. The degree of pulmonary arterial hypertension was significantly reduced after inhalation of 100% oxygen. Following recovery, physiological observations were similar to those seen in healthy residents well acclimatized to high altitude. The data were regarded by Peñaloza and Sime (1969) as indicating pulmonary arteriolar constriction at the precapillary level due to severe hypoxia. As this constriction occurs proximal to the

Table 13.2 Pathological findings in the lungs and brain of seven trekkers in the Himalaya dying from malignant acute mountain sickness, including the pulmonary form

Case no.	Age (years)	Lungs				Brain			Deep vein thrombosis
		Pulmonary thrombosis	Red infarcts	Broncho pneumonia	Oedema	Thrombosis	Haemorrhage	Oedema	
1	54	+	0	++	+	0	0	++	0
2	38	++	++	+	0	Subarachnoid venous with haemorrhage Petechiae	+	0	0
3	27	++	++	+	0	Venous with subarachnoid haemorrhage Posterior dural venous sinuses	+	+	0
4	54	++	+	++	0	0	0	+	+
5	41	0	0	0	++	0	+	++	0
6	46	0	0	+	++	0	0	++	0
7	62	++	0	+	++				0

+ = present; ++ = severe.

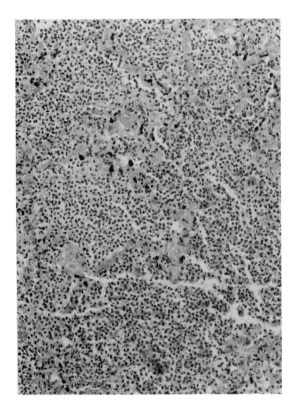

13.8 *Section of lung from a man aged 54 years who ascended to Namche Bazaar (3440 m) in Nepal. There is confluent bronchopneumonia, the alveolar spaces being packed with neutrophil polymorphonuclears. HE, × 60.*

pulmonary capillary bed it would not explain the development of pronounced pulmonary oedema. Fred and co-workers argue that to explain the coexistence of acute pulmonary arterial hypertension and acute pulmonary oedema in the presence of normal left atrial and pulmonary venous pressure, one must postulate some increased vascular resistance situated in either the pulmonary venous capillaries or venules. Roy *et al.* (1969) studied six subjects with high-altitude pulmonary oedema and also found pulmonary arterial hypertension with normal left atrial and pulmonary capillary pressure.

RHEOLOGICAL FACTORS

It would appear that rheological abnormalities can be excluded as an initiating event in the development of acute mountain sickness and high-altitude pulmonary oedema. Reinhart *et al.* (1991) studied 23 volunteers at low altitude (490 m) and at 2 and

18 hours after arrival at 4550 m. Eight remained healthy, seven developed acute mountain sickness, and eight lung oedema after their arrival at high altitude. Haematocrit, whole blood viscosity, plasma viscosity, erythrocyte aggregation, and erythrocyte deformability were measured. Plasma viscosity and erythrocyte deformability remained unaffected. The haematocrit level was lower 2 hours after arrival at high altitude and higher after 18 hours, compared with low altitude. Whole blood viscosity changed according to the haematocrit. There were no significant differences in any rheological parameters between healthy individuals and those with high-altitude pulmonary oedema either before or during the illness.

CHARACTER OF THE OEDEMA FLUID

Schoene *et al.* (1986) carried out bronchopulmonary lavage at 4400 m on Mt McKinley on three climbers suffering from high-altitude pulmonary oedema. The results of the analysis of the fluid were compared with those from lavage fluid obtained from three of the investigators at the same elevation. The fluid from the cases of high-altitude pulmonary oedema showed a pronounced increase in proteins of high molecular weight and contained many red and white cells, the latter consisting predominantly of macrophages (Table 13.3). It also contained traces of leukotriene B_4 and other lipoxygenase products of arachidonic acid metabolism. Complement fragments (C5a), inhibitors of neutrophil chemotaxis, and acid proteases were also present. There was no hydroxyproline. Despite the presence of two potent mediators of inflammation, leukotriene B_4 and C5a, high-altitude pulmonary oedema is not characterized by the intense neutrophil accumulation that is typical of other forms of acute lung injury.

Hackett *et al.* (1986) described the case of a male skier aged 45 years in southern California who developed typical high-altitude pulmonary oedema at an altitude of 3300 m. They performed bronchoscopy when he was brought down to a hospital at 1265 m. They measured the total protein content in the oedema fluid, undiluted by lavage, and found it to be the same as that in the serum. Total protein values were 5.9 g/dl in the serum, 4.8 g/dl in the right middle lobe, and 6.3 g/dl in the left lower lobe. The resultant ratio of the total protein in oedema fluid to that in serum was thus 0.8 for the right middle lobe and 1.1 for the left lower lobe. The ratio for hydrostatic oedema should be <0.5 and for permeability oedema should be >0.7.

Table 13.3 Features of bronchoalveolar lavage fluid in three cases of high-altitude pulmonary oedema at 4400 m contrasted to those of lavage fluid from three controls at the same altitude (from Schoene *et al.* 1986) *Journal of the American Medical Association*, **256**, 63–9. Copyright 1986, American Medical Association.

	Control (*n* = 3)	High-altitude pulmonary oedema (*n* = 3)
Age	25.3 ± 0.9 yr	32.7 ± 6.7 yr
Cells × 10⁴ ml (× 10⁷ litre)		
Red blood cells	1.1 ± 0.5	261.4 ± 243.4
White blood cells	4.3 ± 1.4	36.7 ± 16.5
Alveolar macrophages*	4.0 ± 1.3	28.4 ± 12.7†
	(92.7% ± 3.3%)	(78.7% ± 3.5%)
Neutrophils*	0.1 ± 0.1	2.6 ± 1.1
	(3.0% ± 1.0%)	(8.0% ± 2.7%)
Lymphocytes*	0.3 ± 0.1	5.7 ± 2.9
	(4.3% ± 2.3%)	(13.3% ± 6.1%)
Proteins, mg/dl (g/l)	11.7 ± 2.3	673.0 ± 234.6†
Total protein	(0.12 ± 0.02)	(6.73 ± 2.35)
Albumin	6.4 ± 0.9	390.0 ± 141.8†
	(0.06 ± 0.01)	(3.90 ± 1.42)
IgG	(0.5 ± 0.1)	85.7 ± 33.7†
	(0.01 ± 0.00)	(0.86 ± 0.34)
IgA	0.3 ± 0.1	14.9 ± 5.7†
	(0.003± 0.00)	(0.15 ± 0.06)
IgM	ND‡	5.3 ± 0.9
		(0.05 ± 0.01)
α₁-Antitrypsin	ND‡	32.9 ± 7.3
		(0.33 ± 0.07)

*Values in parentheses indicate percentage of each cell type in the differential cell count.
† *p* <0.05 in comparison to controls.
‡ ND, Not detectable.

PATHOGENESIS

The presence of high concentrations of proteins of high molecular weight in the lavage fluid from cases of high-altitude pulmonary oedema suggests that the integrity of the endothelial–epithelial barrier has been lost and that permeability leak has occurred (Schoene *et al.* 1986). Inflammatory mechanisms do not appear to be involved, since the lavage fluid contains macrophages rather than the neutrophil polymorphs that occur with proteinous lavage fluids in such conditions as the adult respiratory distress syndrome. Clearly, the pathogenesis of high-altitude pulmonary oedema involves a transient 'large pore' leak in the pulmonary circulation without major activation of inflammatory mechanisms (Schoene *et al.* 1986). The findings of Hackett *et al.* (1986) also strongly support the concept that high-altitude pulmonary oedema is a transient permeability oedema. The increased permeability of the vascular endothelium appears to be brought about by shear forces re-sulting from a sudden elevation of pulmonary arterial pressure.

Many subjects who develop high-altitude pulmonary oedema are native highlanders who have mild chronic pulmonary arterial hypertension associated with the expected muscularization of the peripheral portions of the pulmonary vasculature that we have described in Chapter 10, and which are reported in the necropsy findings of Arias-Stella and Krüger (1963; Fig. 13.6). It is clear that the increased amount of muscle in the walls of the pulmonary arterioles and the associated hypertrophy of the right ventricle make a sudden and considerable increase in pulmonary arterial pressure possible. This would explain why the illness is most likely to afflict native highlanders returning to high altitude after a brief sojourn at sea level. Although this theory fits well the case of the Quechua or Aymara developing pulmonary oedema on re-ascent into the mountains, it does not seem to offer an explanation for the lowlanders with very thin-walled pulmonary arteries and a normal right ventricle. Yet such people develop the condition. Menon (1965) refers to its development in travellers arriving for the first time at high altitude by aircraft. Indeed the haemodynamic studies of Fred *et al.* (1962) referred to above confirm that even in lowlanders at the time of an attack the pulmonary arterial blood pressure is raised significantly.

Exercise raises the pulmonary arterial pressure even further and is thus of importance in inducing high-altitude pulmonary oedema. Whayne and Severinghaus (1968) showed that the breathing of 8% oxygen would cause pulmonary oedema in rats after 8 hours at rest, but after only 10 minutes if the animals were forced to exercise. The oedema liquid in these animals appeared to reach the alveolar walls and spaces secondarily from its appearance in the perivascular spaces around arterial vessels. There is, however, no evidence that oedema of these perivascular spaces is a feature of the pathology of high-altitude pulmonary oedema in man (Arias-Stella 1971). Whayne and Severinghaus (1968) thought that the leakage was not a general transarterial migration of matter down a hydrostatic gradient, but rather a focal rupture or separation of elements of the arterial wall that permits the passage of plasma or blood into the extravascular spaces. Severinghaus (1971) refers to this as 'discrete focal damage' in small elastic and muscular pulmonary arteries, but he does not describe the nature of this pulmonary vascular pathology. Like Arias-Stella (1971), we are not familiar with a focal arterial lesion of this type in states of chronic hypoxia, at least at the level of light microscopy.

Staub (1982) proposed that the pulmonary oedema induced by high altitude is similar to that brought about by multiple emboli to the lung. He thought that there was a disseminated obstruction of small pulmonary arteries by uneven vasoconstriction or by occlusion with fibrin, platelets, or white cells. Certainly, platelet and fibrin agglutination and microthrombi have been found in the pulmonary capillaries in individuals dying from high-altitude pulmonary oedema (Hultgren *et al.* 1962; Arias-Stella and Krüger 1963; Nayak *et al.* 1964). The acute pulmonary hypertension induced by hypoxic vasoconstriction would generate high shear stresses, which would lead to an extravasation of oedema fluid from unobstructed and unprotected microvessels. This harks back to the original suggestion of Hultgren (1967) that high-altitude pulmonary oedema is a consequence of hypoxic vasoconstric-

tion in some vessels and overperfusion of the remainder, which are unprotected by arteriolar vasoconstriction. This idea is made more plausible by the finding that persons born with only one pulmonary artery are highly susceptible to high-altitude pulmonary oedema (Hackett *et al.* 1980).

There is controversy as to whether or not susceptibility to high-altitude pulmonary oedema can be reliably detected by testing pulmonary vasoreactivity to hypoxia at sea level. Thus, Naeije *et al.* (1986) reported the case of a mountaineer of 51 years who developed pulmonary oedema in the mountains. When his pulmonary vascular reactivity to hypoxia was tested at sea level 11 months before and 3 weeks after the incident, it was found to be normal. Similarly, a man of 40 years developing high-altitude pulmonary oedema during a climbing expedition to the Ruwenzori mountain range in Uganda was known to have been studied by right heart catheterization 6 years before as a healthy volunteer during hypoxic breathing at sea level. His pulmonary vascular reactivity had been within the normal range for 32 healthy subjects (Naeije and Mélot 1990). On the other hand, Fasules *et al.* (1985) found evidence of such increased pulmonary vasoreactivity in seven children from Leadville, Colorado after recovery from high-altitude pulmonary oedema. All were life-long residents at elevations above 3000 m. Three of the seven had developed pulmonary oedema without antecedent travel to low altitude, but had an upper respiratory infection. Response of pulmonary arterial pressure to 16% inspired oxygen in all seven was compared with that in six well children who resided at similar altitude and had no history of high-altitude pulmonary oedema. With hypoxia, the susceptible patients had a greater mean pulmonary arterial pressure (56.3 ± 23.8 mmHg) than the non-susceptible children (18.8 ± 3.9 mmHg). This suggested to the authors that, in children from high altitudes, increased pulmonary vasoreactivity to hypoxia may play a role in the pathogenesis of high-altitude pulmonary oedema. The finding of right ventricular hypertrophy on an electrocardiogram in children from high altitudes may be predictive of their susceptibility to high-altitude pulmonary oedema.

Earlier suggestions that high-altitude pulmonary oedema was due to left ventricular failure (Menon 1965) were negated by the finding of normal levels of pulmonary venous or left atrial pressure. The normal wedge pressure does not necessarily rule out the suggestion (Fred *et al.* 1962) that the oedema is due to constriction of small pulmonary veins, but it renders this theory unlikely.

Another factor that may lead to an increased pressure in pulmonary capillaries is a redistribution of blood from the systemic to the pulmonary circulation and the changes in total blood volume induced by high altitude. As will be seen in Chapter 18, prolonged exposure to high altitude results in an increase in blood volume of as much as 30%. This level is reached after about 6 weeks' continuous exposure and may increase slowly for up to 1 year. Much of it is due to an increase in the red cell volume. On return to sea level there is a rapid decrease in red cell mass, as described in Chapter 33, and this is accompanied by a compensatory rise in plasma volume. Hultgren *et al.* (1961) believe this may be of importance in the pathogenesis of high-altitude pulmonary oedema in native highlanders. They emphasize that subjects who have lived at a high elevation and then returned to sea level may have, after about 1 week, a higher than normal plasma volume that persists for an unknown period of time. If such a person returns to high altitude during this time, he may well be more susceptible to the development of pulmonary oedema than the total newcomer to the mountains who will have a lower plasma volume. This may be a contributory factor in explaining why many subjects with lung oedema at high altitude develop the condition after spending some time at sea level. Some believe that the condition is a form of neurogenic pulmonary oedema (Theodore and Robin 1975). A massive central sympathetic discharge might shift blood from the high-resistance systemic to the low-resistance pulmonary circulation, with resultant pulmonary hypertension, lung haemorrhage and increased capillary permeability, malperfusion, and maldistribution of ventilation (*Lancet* Annotation 1976). Hackett *et al.* (1988) believe that victims of this disease have a markedly blunted ventilatory response to hypoxia that remains low after recovery from the oedema.

ULTRASTRUCTURE OF PULMONARY CAPILLARIES AND VEINS OF RATS SUBJECTED TO SIMULATED HIGH ALTITUDE

We have studied the ultrastructure of pulmonary capillaries in rats exposed for 12 hours in a hypobaric chamber to a subatmospheric pressure of 265 mmHg that simulates a high altitude roughly corresponding to the summit of Mt Everest (Heath *et al.* 1973). Under these conditions there is a formation of multiple endothelial vesicles that protrude into the pulmonary capillaries (Fig. 13.9). When seen in a longitudinal section these vesicles have an elongated shape that accommodates itself to the confines of the capillary into which it projects. These extrusions are large enough to occlude the pulmonary capillaries into which they project. They arise by pedicles from localized widened areas of the fused basement membranes of the alveolar wall where there seems to be an accumulation of fluid. The oedema vesicles are covered by an exceedingly thin layer of cytoplasma which consists of part of the overlying endothelial cell of the pulmonary capillary stretched by the localized accumulation of fluid. When an oedema vesicle is cut in transverse section without fortuitously including its pedicle, it appears to be a round body covered by a double membrane and gives the spurious appearance of lying free in the pulmonary capillary (Fig. 13.9). In conditions of

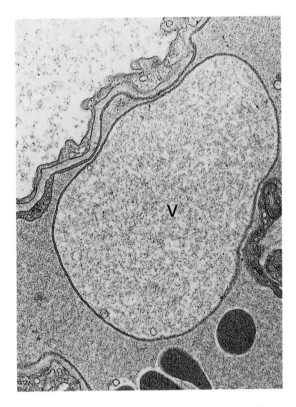

13.9 *Electron micrograph of pulmonary capillary from a Wistar albino rat subjected for 12 hours to a barometric pressure of 265 mmHg, simulating the altitude of the summit of Mt Everest. An endothelial vesicle (v) projects into the capillary from the alveolar-capillary wall. The vesicle is covered by an attenuated cytoplasmic lining derived from the pulmonary endothelial cell. × 12 500.*

simulated high altitude, many capillaries in the lungs contain oedema vesicles that reduce the diameter of the capillaries thus distorting erythrocytes.

These oedema vesicles are in no sense specific. In the thinner portions of the alveolar wall over the convexities of the pulmonary capillaries they have in the past been regarded as characteristic of pulmonary oedema produced by toxic substances. Thus they have been produced by ammonium sulfate (Hayes and Shiga 1970), alpha naphthyl urea (Meyrick *et al.* 1972), and the seeds of *Crotalaria spectabilis* containing monocrotaline (Kay *et al.* 1969). Clearly, one must exercise considerable caution before ascribing functional significance to structural change in the absence of physiological data. However, the lesions described by Heath *et al.* (1973) are composed largely of oedema fluid and could form rapidly and thus account for the very sudden onset of the symptoms of high-altitude pulmonary oedema. Likewise they could shrink equally rapidly on return to low altitude or on the administration of oxygen. These oedema vesicles could produce a haemodynamic effect by protruding into pulmonary venous capillaries. This would meet the requirements laid down by Fred *et al.* (1962) to explain the coexistence of acute pulmonary arterial hypertension and acute pulmonary oedema in the presence of normal left atrial and pulmonary venous pressure. It would be possible to object to the view that these oedema vesicles are of functional significance on the grounds that the pulmonary capillary bed has an enormous reserve capacity, but we are unable to assess the validity of this objection without knowing what percentage of capillaries is involved by these intraluminal projections.

J RECEPTORS AND PULMONARY OEDEMA AT HIGH ALTITUDE

At high altitude, J receptors in the alveolar walls appear to be stimulated by pulmonary oedema. Lying in the interstitial tissue of the alveolar walls are minute sensory nerve fibres with a diameter of the order of 0.1–0.3 μm (Paintal 1970). Due to the position of the pulmonary capillaries lying on a connective tissue scaffolding, they have two distinct microanatomical aspects (see Fig. 4.5). One is bordered by a very thin wall composed of the attenuated cytoplasmic extensions of membranous pneumonocytes, the fused basement membrane of alveolar epithelium and pulmonary capillary, and the ultra-thin cytoplasm of the endothelium of the pulmonary capillary (Fig. 4.5). This part of the alveolar-capillary membrane is concerned with the exchange of respiratory gases. The other aspect of the alveolar-capillary membrane is composed of the pulmonary capillary endothelium, its basement membrane, interstitial tissues of collagen and reticulin, the basement membrane of the alveolar epithelium, and the epithelium itself (Fig. 4.5). This thicker part of the alveolar-capillary wall is concerned with the movement of the interstitial fluid of the lung. The designation 'J receptors' is an abbreviation of 'juxta-pulmonary capillary receptors' which refers to their anatomical position. They are rapidly stimulated by injection of phenyl diguanide into the right atrium or ventricle, or insufflation of volatile anaesthetics into the lungs, consistent with their postulated situation in the alveolar wall.

J receptors lie in the interstitial tissue (Fig. 4.5) and are perhaps connected to collagen fibres. They are stimulated when more fluid enters the interstitial tissue, which acts like a sponge. Even a small increase in pulmonary capillary pressure might be expected to cause a slight increase in interstitial volume, stimulating the endings. Paintal (1970) is of the opinion that the increased pulmonary arterial pressure and plasma volume that occur in subjects at high altitude, especially on exercise, produce congestion and hypertension in the pulmonary capillaries that in a minority of cases progress to pulmonary oedema. He cites the experience of Vogel *et al.* (1963) who found that, during exercise in 28 healthy residents between 13 and 17 years of age at Leadville, Colorado (3100 m), the pulmonary arterial pressure rose from 25 to 54 mmHg. Paintal (1970) believes that exercise at high altitude leads to a rise in pulmonary capillary pressure with an increase in interstitial pulmonary volume. The J receptors in the alveolar walls are stimulated and a feeling of breathlessness ensues.

MANAGEMENT OF HIGH-ALTITUDE PULMONARY OEDEMA

Familiarity with the clinical features of high-altitude pulmonary oedema and with the means of avoiding and treating it is becoming of increasing importance. There have always been small mining communities at high altitude, such as at La Oroya (3750 m) in Peru, where the physicians have had to be aware of the dangers of too rapid an ascent into the mountains or of a return to great heights after a period at lower elevations. La Oroya is situated on the main route from Lima and the coastal strip to the Amazon and this route through the Andes is a major economic lifeline for the nation. The road past the hospital carries a never-ending stream of buses and *collectivos* (a type of communal taxi), so that the physicians gain an extensive experience of the condition. In recent years the growing popularity of adventure and trekking holidays in such areas as the Himalaya has made it very desirable for family doctors to be able to advise their patients about to take such vacations as to how to avoid developing the condition. Occasionally, special circumstances arise where medical advice is sought as to a safe code of practice for groups of sea-level subjects being sent to work at high altitude; an example of this is the manning of the new UK infrared telescope on the summit of Mauna Kea in Hawaii (Chapter 30). For all these differing groups of subjects the clear message should be that avoidance is much better than cure.

PROPHYLAXIS

Most cases of high-altitude pulmonary oedema can be avoided if the subject does not attempt to ascend too rapidly and if he is not tempted to undertake too much exertion soon after arrival at high altitude. We have already considered in the previous chapter what constitutes a safe rate of ascent. Over-exertion should be avoided during the early hours and days of arrival at high altitude. It should be kept in mind that children and adolescents are peculiarly prone to high-altitude pulmonary oedema. Acclimatized subjects returning to the mountains after a few days at sea level are more at risk than newcomers to high altitude. Those who have experienced a previous attack of high-altitude pulmonary oedema should be especially careful.

TREATMENT

Early diagnosis

Prompt recognition of the condition is vital. The onset of repeated coughing and the early symptoms described earlier in this chapter should be viewed seriously. If anyone looks uncharacteristically weak or fatigued he should be brought down the mountain immediately (*Lancet* Annotation 1976). One should not wait for obvious rales or bubbling to indicate the onset of undeniable and severe pulmonary oedema. The subject with early suggestive symptoms should be taken down the mountain quickly and intellectual debate on the validity of the diagnosis can then take place at a lower and safer altitude.

Descent

Delaying descent for anything but the mildest cases is likely to be highly dangerous. The conditions of descent should be made as comfortable as can be managed to avoid all unnecessary exertion. Although prompt evacuation to levels below 2400 m usually brings about rapid recovery, this cannot be relied upon. We have already pointed out that the underlying pathology of the condition may involve pulmonary thrombosis and red infarction of the lung in severe cases, together with associated cerebral venous thrombosis and petechial haemorrhages into the brain in some cases. Dickinson (1979), speaking at a Symposium on Acute Mountain Sickness at the University of Birmingham, reported the case of a middle-aged doctor who was diagnosed immediately on the appearance of pulmonary oedema and urgently taken down the mountain to 'safe' levels, but who died in spite of such prompt recognition and treatment.

Oxygen

Oxygen is a vital component in treatment. Its administration lowers pulmonary arterial pressure dramatically. High flow rates are necessary. Thus, Menon (1965) gave the gas continuously at 6–8 l/min, finding that an intermittent flow below 4 l/min was ineffective. He found that there was a response to oxygen therapy within 30 minutes to 2 hours, with relief of cough, cyanosis; and chest pain, and a diminution of pulse rate. Oxygen treatment was tapered off after 8–12 hours. Some patients may show no improvement even after inhalation of the gas for 12–48 hours and cyanosis may persist. Wilson (1973) recommends that oxygen should be delivered through a tight-fitting mask for at least 24 hours. He also recommends that the rate of flow should be 6–8 l/min, but is of the opinion that, if supplies of oxygen are small, lower flows may still prove beneficial. Hultgren *et al.* (1961) recommend that all parties climbing above about 4570 m should have available emergency oxygen sufficient to provide a minimum of 4 l/min for several days. They should also have appropriate tools and spare parts to utilize additional oxygen if it is dropped by plane. Wilson (1973) points out that efforts to arrange descent should not await oxygen therapy, which can be continued *en route*.

Diuretics

Frusemide

The use of frusemide in the aborting or treatment of a case of high-altitude pulmonary oedema is controversial. It is powerful and rapid in its action and, while this may produce very rapid effects in clearing pulmonary oedema, it has to be kept in mind that on the mountainside the production of torrents of urine can be distressing. Bonington (1971) gives an account of the effects of such prophylaxis by dehydration on one of his companions during the climbing of Annapurna: 'The pills in Dave's box had the effect of dehydrating the patient by making him want to urinate, and hence reducing the likelihood of fluids forming in the lung. Mick decided to try out the treatment and took the prescribed dose. As a result he had to get out of bed every half hour or so through the night, a grim and exhausting experience in sub-zero temperatures.'

Indian physicians have claimed that frusemide in a dosage of 80 mg daily for 2 days or more may prevent high-altitude pulmonary oedema but others have found that such a dose gave rise to headache, vomiting, ataxia, and even coma (Wilson 1973). More warranted is the cautious use of the drug in a dosage of 20 mg every 12–24 hours. It has to be kept in mind that frusemide may lead to haemoconcentration, with the associated risk of initiating thrombosis, which as we have seen may characterize the pathology of severe cases of high-altitude pulmonary oedema. Dickinson (1981) uses at least one dose of intravenous frusemide and is prepared to accept evidence of mild peripheral dehydration in the process of attempting to reduce pulmonary oedema, but the patient must be monitored for signs of hypovolaemia.

Bumetanide

Bumetanide is a derivative of metanilamide which is as effective a diuretic as frusemide at only one-fortieth of the molar dose (Seth *et al.* 1975). When the drug was given intravenously in a dose of 1–3 mg to 35 patients with pulmonary oedema of different aetiology, it had a diuretic action within 20 minutes and continued to do so for about 5 hours. Bumetanide is more effective in acute than chronic pulmonary oedema and hence might be expected to be of value in the treatment of high-altitude pulmonary oedema. Pines (1974) reported the effects of the drug in two cases of acute oedema developing in subjects at high altitude. The cases he treated occurred among 30 climbers scaling peaks up to 7450 m in the Hindu Kush range of Afghanistan. An oral dose of 2 mg of bumetanide caused clearance of the oedema.

Nifedipine

High-altitude pulmonary oedema can be prevented by lowering pulmonary arterial pressure with nifedipine (Oelz *et al.* 1989; Bärtsch *et al.* 1991). The general use of this medication in subjects susceptible to the condition is not advocated because of its potentially harmful side-effects (Bärtsch *et al.* 1991). The best management of a case of high-altitude pulmonary oedema is immediate descent as noted above but occasionally this is not possible because of bad weather or avalanche conditions, or because the patient is too ill to move and beyond the reach of rescue services. In a retrospective analysis of 166 cases the overall mortality rate was 11% but, when descent was impossible, and no supplementary oxygen was available this rose to 44% (Lobenhoffer *et al.* 1982). Under such dire circumstances a simple drug treatment for emergency conditions would be highly desirable. As we note above, the analysis of the oedema fluid in this disease indicates that the egress of fluid has a basis in enhanced permeability of the alveolar-capillary membrane. We have also referred above to the fact that hypoxic pulmonary vasoconstriction seems to be of importance in enhancing the flow of fluid across the damaged endothelial cells. In the rat hypoxic pulmonary hypertension can be reversed by calcium antagonists and Oelz *et al.* (1989) came to the conclusion that by lowering pulmonary arterial pressure a calcium antagonist might slow up further oedema formation. Elsewhere we give an analysis of the powerful vasodilator effects of nifedipine in the lungs of patients with chronic respiratory disease and severe arterial hypoxaemia (Harris and Heath 1986). The drug exerts a powerful vasodilator effect in the lungs.

Oelz *et al.* (1989) originally studied six men between the ages of 27 and 51 years in a laboratory at 4550 m in the Valais Alps. Five of the six had experienced high-altitude pulmonary oedema, documented radiographically in the past 4 years. They ascended to high altitude within 24 hours and within 12–36 hours of arrival all six developed lung oedema. They were given 10 mg of nifedipine sublingually and 20 mg of a slow-release preparation of the drug. Subsequently, they received 20 mg of slow-release nifedipine every 6 hours of their entire time at high altitude. The patients experienced no unpleasant side-effects from the drug. Shortness of breath was relieved within 1 hour of taking the drug and usually within 15 minutes. Systemic arterial oxygen tension and saturation were much more hypoxaemic in the patients than in the controls before treatment, but they improved on treatment with nifedipine, although they remained lower than in the controls. The raised alveolar-arterial oxygen gradient was strikingly raised in the oedematous subjects and declined in all of them during the first 12 hours of treatment. The radiographic manifestations of high-altitude pulmonary oedema regressed during treatment. In the control subjects there was pronounced hypoxic pulmonary hypertension with a mean systolic pulmonary arterial pressure of 63.9 mmHg. In the subjects who developed lung oedema the corresponding pressure rose to 133.7 mmHg. Upon initiation of treatment with nifedipine pulmonary arterial pressure dropped to within the range seen in control subjects and remained there. There was a significant reduction in the size of the right atrium and right ventricle. All in all, nifedipine had clearly reduced pulmonary arterial and right ventricular pressure and led to resorption of oedema fluid. Improvement under the difficult circumstances referred to above should be exploited to allow descent rather than to allow continued activities at high altitude.

In a further investigation the same group (Bärtsch *et al.* 1991) studied 21 mountaineers, 20 men and one woman, ranging in age from 20 to 60 years, with a history of radiographically documented high-altitude pulmonary oedema. Seven of the 11 who received only a placebo developed lung oedema but only one of the 10 who received a slow-release preparation of nifedipine at 4550 m every 8 hours during the ascent and during the following 3 days at this altitude developed lung oedema. Subjects receiving the drug had a significantly lower mean systolic pulmonary arterial pressure (41 ± 8 mmHg) compared to controls receiving only a placebo (52 ± 16 mmHg). The A–a difference was also significantly lower at 6.6 ± 3.8 mmHg compared to controls receiving the placebo (11.8 ± 4.4 mmHg). The observation that high-altitude pulmonary oedema can be prevented by lowering pulmonary arterial pressure with nifedipine adds support to the view that hypoxic pulmonary vasoconstriction is important in the pathophysiology of this disease.

Morphia

Morphia has a traditional use in the treatment of pulmonary oedema with a cardiac basis. However, in high-altitude pulmonary oedema unwanted depression of respiration can occur, particularly if cerebral oedema is present. The use of morphine has met with favour with Indian physicians, but there has been less confidence in it elsewhere. Some authors (Wilson 1973) believe that parenteral morphine, in a dose of 10–15 mg, may be helpful because it calms the victim and dilates peripheral veins, pooling blood there. Others, like Hultgren,

point out that there have been no controlled studies of its use in high-altitude pulmonary oedema and believe that its use should be avoided.

Antibiotics

Necropsy studies of subjects dying from malignant pulmonary acute mountain sickness commonly show evidence of bronchopneumonia (see Table 13.2). Antibiotics may be needed to control superadded respiratory infection in high-altitude pulmonary oedema.

PROGNOSIS

If high-altitude pulmonary oedema is not treated promptly and effectively, it may prove fatal. On the other hand, if it is treated adequately, in the majority of cases the prognosis is excellent, with the oedema of the lung proving totally and rapidly reversible. Clinical improvement should follow within 30 minutes to 2 hours. Singh *et al.* (1965) found that the lungs were free of oedema in 4 days and the chest radiograph was clear in 5 days. However, a few patients will die even though diagnosis is made early and rapid descent is organized to low altitude where prompt and vigorous treatment is given (Dickinson 1979). Such cases will be afflicted by the thrombotic events in the lung described above. It is also wise to warn a patient who has recovered from high-altitude pulmonary oedema that he should be very careful if he returns to the mountains. In his series of 101 cases, Menon (1965) found that two patients developed high-altitude pulmonary oedema for a second time. Naeije and Melót (1990) reported the case of a man of 40 years who developed high-altitude pulmonary oedema in the 'mountains of the moon' in the Ruwenzori mountain range some 30 km north of the equator on the Uganda/Zaire border. This was in spite of the fact that he had taken acetazolamide in a dosage of 500 mg per day and high doses of dexamethasoze in an initial dose of 8 mg then 4 mg every 6 hours.

References

Arias-Stella, J. (1971). Discussion of paper by Severinghaus, J.W. quoted below. In *High Altitude Physiology: Cardiac and Respiratory Aspects*, a Ciba Foundation Symposium (R. Porter and J. Knight, Eds), Edinburgh; Churchill Livingstone, p. 73

Arias-Stella, J. and Krüger, H. (1963). Pathology of high altitude pulmonary oedema. *Archives of Pathology*, **76**, 147

Bardales, A. (1955). Algunos casos de edema pulmonar aguda por soroche grave. *Anales de la Facultad de Medicina, Universidad Nacional Mayor de San Marcos*, **38**, 232

Bärtsch, P., Maggiorini, M., Ritter, M., Noti, C., Vock, P., and Oelz, O. (1991). Prevention of high-altitude pulmonary edema by nifedipine. *New England Journal of Medicine*, **325**, 1284

Bonington, C. (1971). *Annapurna South Face*. London; Cassell, p. 172

Dickinson, J.G. (1979). Severe acute mountain sickness. *Postgraduate Medical Journal*, **55**, 454

Dickinson, J.G. (1981). Acute mountain sickness. A dissertation based on eleven years' experience in the Nepal Himalaya. Unpublished D.M. thesis, University of Oxford.

Dickinson, J., Heath, D., Gosney, J., and Williams, D. (1983). Altitude-related deaths in seven trekkers in the Himalayas. *Thorax*, **38**, 646

Fasules, J.W., Wiggins, J.W., and Wolfe, R.R. (1985). Increased lung vaso-reactivity in children from Leadville, Colorado, after recovery from high-altitude edema. *Circulation*, **72**, 957

Fred, H.L., Schmidt, A.M., Bates, T., and Hecht, H.H. (1962). Acute pulmonary edema of altitude. Clinical and physiologic observations. *Circulation*, **25**, 929

Hackett, P.H. (1988). Medical research on Mount McKinley. *Annals of Sports Medicine*, **4**, 232

Hackett, P. and Rennie, D. (1976). The incidence, importance, and prophylaxis of acute mountain sickness. *Lancet*, **ii**, 1149

Hackett, P.H., Creagh, C.E., Grover, R.F., Honigman, B., Houston, C.S., Reeves, J.T., Sophocles, A.M., and Van Hardenbroek, M. (1980). High altitude pulmonary edema in persons without the right pulmonary artery. *New England Journal of Medicine*, **302**, 1070

Hackett, P.H., Bertman, J., and Rodriguez, G. (1986). Pulmonary edema fluid protein in high altitude pulmonary edema. *Journal of the American Medical Association*, **256**, 36

Hackett, P.H., Roach, R.C., Schoene, R.B., Harrison, G.L., and Mills, W.J. (1988). Abnormal control of ventilation in high altitude pulmonary oedema. *Journal of Applied Physiology*, **64**, 1268

Harris, P. and Heath, D. (1986). Pharmacology of the pulmonary circulation. In *The Human Pulmonary Circulation*, 3rd edn. Edinburgh; Churchill Livingstone.

Hayes, J.A. and Shiga, A. (1970). Ultrastructural changes in pulmonary oedema produced experimentally with ammonium sulphate. *Journal of Pathology*, **100**, 281

Heath, D., Moosavi, H., and Smith, P. (1973). Ultrastructure of high altitude pulmonary oedema. *Thorax*, **28**, 694

Houston, C.S. (1960). Acute pulmonary edema of high altitude. *New England Journal of Medicine*, **263**, 478

Houston, C. (1976). High altitude illness: disease with protean manifestations. *Journal of the American Medical Association*, **236**, 2193

Houston, C.S. and Dickinson, J. (1975). Cerebral forms of high altitude illness, *Lancet*, **ii**, 758

Hultgren, H.N. (1967). High altitude pulmonary edema. In *Biomedical Problems of High Terrestrial Altitudes*. Springfield, Virginia; Federal Scientific and Technical Information, p. 131

Hultgren, H.N. and Marticorena, E. (1978). High altitude pulmonary edema. *Chest*, **74**, 372

Hultgren, H.N., Spickard, W.B., Hellriegel, J., and Houston, C.S. (1961). High altitude pulmonary edema. *Medicine*, **40**, 289

Hultgren, H., Spickard, W., and Lopez, C. (1962). Further studies of high altitude pulmonary oedema. *British Heart Journal*, **24**, 95

Hurtado, A. (1937). *Aspectos Fisologicos y Patologicos de la Vida en la Altura*. Lima; Imp. Edit. Rimac

Kay, J.M., Smith, P, and Heath, D. (1969). Electron microscopy of *Crotalaria* pulmonary hypertension. *Thorax*, **24**, 511

Kobayashi, T., Koyama, S., Kubo, K., Fukushima, M., and Kusama, S. (1987). Clinical features of patients with high-altitude pulmonary edema in Japan. *Chest*, **92**, 815

Lancet Annotation (1976). See Nuptse and die. *Lancet*, **ii**, 1177

Levine, B.D., Grayburn, P.A., Voyles, W.F., Greene, E.R., Roach, R.C., and Hackett, P.H. (1991). Intracardiac shunting across a patent foramen ovale may exacerbate hypoxaemia in high-altitude pulmonary edema. *Annals of Internal Medicine*, **114**, 569

Lizarraga, L. (1955). Soroche agudo: edema agudo del pulmon. *Anales de la Facultad de medicina,*

Universidad Nacional Mayor de San Marcos, **38**, 244

Lobenhoffer, H.P., Zink, R.A., and Brendel, W. (1982). High altitude pulmonary oedema: analysis of 166 cases. In *High Altitude Physiology and Medicine*. (W. Brendel and R.A. Zink, Ed.). New York Springer, p. 219

Lundberg, E. (1952). Edema agudo del pulmón en el soroche. Conferencia sustenada en la Asociación Medica de Yauli, Oroya

Marticorena, E., Tapia, F.A., Dyer, J., Severino, J., Banchero, N., Gamboa, R., Krüger, H., and Peñaloza, D. (1964). Pulmonary edema by ascending to high altitudes. *Diseases of the Chest*, **45**, 273

Menon, N.D. (1965). High-altitude pulmonary edema. *New England Journal of Medicine*, **273**, 66

Meyrick, B., Miller, J., and Reid, L. (1972). Pulmonary oedema induced by ANTU, or by high or low oxygen concentrations in rat — an electron microscopic study. *British Journal of Experimental Pathology*, **53**, 347

Naeije, R. and Mélot, C. (1990). Acute pulmonary oedema on the Ruwenzori mountain range. *British Heart Journal*, **64**, 400

Naeije, R., Mélot, C., and Lejeune, P. (1986). Hypoxic pulmonary vasoconstriction and high altitude pulmonary edema. *American Review of Respiratory Disease*, **134**, 332

Nayak, N.C., Roy, S., and Narayanan, T.K. (1964). Pathologic features of altitude sickness. *American Journal of Pathology*, **45**, 381

Norboo, T. and Ball, K. (1988). High altitude pulmonary oedema in the Himalayas: a preventable condition. *The Practitioner*, **232**, 557

Oelz, O., Maggiorini, M., Ritter, M., Waber, U., Jenni, R., Vock, P., and Bärtsch, P. (1989). Nifedipine for high altitude pulmonary oedema. *Lancet*, **ii**, 1241

Paintal, A.S. (1970). The mechanisms of excitation of type J receptors, and the J reflex. In *Breathing*, Hering-Breuer Centenary Symposium. London; Churchill, p. 59

Peñaloza, D. and Sime, F. (1969) Circulatory dynamics during high altitude pulmonary edema. *American Journal of Cardiology*, **23**, 369

Pines, A. (1974). Oedema of mountains. *British Medical Journal*, **4**, 233

Reinhart, W.H., Kayser, B., Singh, A., Waber, U., Oelz, O., and Bärtsch, P. (1991). Blood rheology in acute mountain sickness and high-altitude pulmonary edema. *Journal of Applied Physiology*, **71**, 934

Roy, S.B., Guleria, J.S., Khanna, P.K., Manchanda, S.C., Pande, J.N., and Subba, P.S. (1969). Haemodynamic studies in high altitude pulmonary oedema. *British Heart Journal*, **31**, 52

Schoene, R.B., Hackett, P.H., Henderson, W.R., Sage, H., Chow, H., Roach, R.C., Mills, W.J., and Martin, T.R. (1986). High-altitude pulmonary edema. Characteristics of lung lavage fluid. *Journal of American Medical Association*, **256**, 63

Scoggin, C.H., Hyers, T.M., Reeves, J.T., and Grover, R.F. (1977). High-altitude pulmonary edema in the children and young adults of Leadville, Colorado. *New England Journal of Medicine*, **297**, 1269

Seth, H.C., Coulshed, N., and Epstein, E.J. (1975). Intravenous bumetanide in the treatment of acute and chronic pulmonary oedema. *British Journal of Clinical Practice*, **29**, 7

Severinghaus, J.W. (1971). Transarterial leakage: a possible mechanism of high altitude pulmonary oedema. In *High Altitude Physiology: Cardiac and Respiratory Aspects*, a Ciba Foundation Symposium (R. Porter and J. Knight, Eds). Edinburgh; Churchill Livingstone, p. 61

Singh, I., Kapila, C.C., Khanna, P.K., Nanda, R.B., and Rao, B.D.P. (1965;). High-altitude pulmonary oedema. *Lancet*, **i**, 229

Sophocles, A.M. (1986). High-altitude pulmonary edema in Vail, Colorado, 1975–1982. *Western Journal of Medicine*, **144**, 569

Staub, N.C. (1982). Mechanisms of pulmonary edema following uneven pulmonary artery obstruction and its relationship to high altitude lung injury. In *High Altitude Physiology and Medicine* (W. Brendel and R.A. Zink, Eds). New York; Springer Verlag, p. 255

Theodore, J. and Robin, E.D. (1975). Pathogenesis of neurogenic pulmonary oedema. *Lancet*, **ii**, 749

Vock, P., Fretz, C., Franciolli, M., and Bärtsch, P. (1989). High-altitude pulmonary edema: findings at high-altitude chest radiography and physical examination. *Radiology*, **170**, 661

Vogel, J.H.K., Weaver, W.F., Rose, R.L., Blount, S.G., and Grover, R.F. (1963). Pulmonary hypertension on exertion in normal man living at 10,150 feet (Leadville, Colorado). In *Progress in*

Research in Emphysema and Chronic Bronchitis, Vol. I (R.F. Grover and H. Herzog. Ed.). New York; Karger, pp. 269, 285

Whayne, T.F. Jr. and Severinghaus, J.W. (1968). Experimental hypoxic pulmonary edema in the rat. *Journal of Applied Physiology*, **25**, 729

Wilson, R. (1973). Acute high-altitude illness in mountaineers and problems of rescue. *Annals of Internal Medicine*, **78**, 421

14

Cerebral mountain sickness

When Ravenhill (1913) went to work in the Andes as medical officer in a mining district, he soon came into contact with acute mountain sickness which the Quechua Indians in Peru called 'soroche' and the Aymara Indians around Lake Titicaca on the border with Bolivia called 'puna'. According to Dickinson (1981) these Indian names mean lead or antimony and reflect their belief that the disease of the mountains was caused by vapours from ore-bearing rocks. Ravenhill (1913) appears to have been a very astute clinician, for he was able to distinguish clearly three forms of the mountain disease. The first he called 'puna of the normal type' and today this is usually referred to as benign acute mountain sickness (Chapter 12). The second he called 'puna of a cardiac type' and this corresponds to high-altitude pulmonary oedema (Chapter 13). The third, which he regarded as a rare variant, he called 'puna of a nervous type' which is the subject of this chapter as 'cerebral mountain sickness'. He refers to affected subjects showing nervous excitation, with twitching of the lips and trembling of the limbs. In one young Chilean male of 19 years the movements of the limbs were violent and spasmodic and it is conceivable that they were hysterical in origin. Ravenhill reported convulsions in a young Englishman and refers to the symptom of vertigo in some of the patients. It is a remarkable fact that the first case of cerebral mountain sickness was not reported in the American literature until half a century later (Fitch 1964).

When thousands of Indian soldiers were speedily air-lifted to the airfield at Leh (3500 m), the capital of Ladakh, to face the acclimatized Chinese troops approaching by the high Tibetan plateau, many were overcome by acute mountain sickness. This military operation produced no fewer than 1925 cases for study (Singh et al. 1969). As already seen in Chapter 12, headache is one of the commonest and most persistent symptoms of acute mountain sickness and so it proved among the Indian troops. As a result it has no diagnostic value in distinguishing a predominantly cerebral form of the disease. However, a small minority of the Indian soldiers had hysterical outbursts and other disorders of behaviour, usually during exertion involving exposure to severe cold and winds at heights above 4500 m. These events were reminiscent of the initial report by Ravenhill half a century earlier. Nevertheless, in this large series some of the victims went beyond nervous excitation and movements of the limbs to unequivocal neurological signs indicative of disease of the nervous system and of such severity in some instances as to lead to paralysis, coma, and death.

INCIDENCE

The data from Singh et al. (1969) probably reflect accurately the incidence of the cerebral form in a large number of cases of acute mountain sickness as seen in the field. Thus they report dimness of vision, blurring of disc margins, and frank papilloedema in just four of the 1925 cases, and the development of papilloedema, stupor, paralysis, and coma in a further 24. These figures suggest that cerebral mountain sickness is indeed a rare variant when seen against the background of a large number of cases of acute mountain sickness ranging from the mild to the fatal. On the other hand, in his dissertation on acute mountain sickness based on 11 years' experience in the Nepal Himalaya, Dickinson (1981) reviews a much smaller series of 57 subjects with very severe symptoms (including cases of high-altitude pulmonary oedema and cerebral mountain sickness) who were evacuated from the high mountain ranges of the Himalaya to Kathmandu (1350 m). Seven of these patients were so ill that they could not be saved. Clearly, this group of subjects was highly selected because of the severity of their illness and urgent need to benefit from the special diagnostic and therapeutic expertise available at the Shanta Bhawan hospital. Since the epidemiological denominator was missing, it is not surprising that cerebral mountain sickness figures prominently in his series (Dickinson 1979). Thus, of the 50 patients in his series who survived, no fewer than 11 had purely cerebral mountain sickness, and 33 had clinical manifestations of both the cerebral form and high-altitude pulmonary oedema; only six had purely pulmonary sickness. It is likely that this undue prominence of cerebral symptomatology is an indication that it represents the hard core of very ill patients with the worst prognosis and the greatest need for skilled and intensive treatment. Wherever incidence of cerebral mountain sickness is referred to in this chapter, the nature of the series from which the data are derived must be kept in mind.

CLINICAL FEATURES

We have already noted that headache is such a common feature of acute mountain sickness of all manner of severity that it is worthless as an indicator of cerebral mountain sickness. In the same way, engorgement of retinal veins is so commonplace in all those who ascend to high altitude (Chapter 27) that it cannot be regarded as a sign of prognostic import. Forster (1986) found that this occurred even in fit young astronomers ascending the volcano Mauna Kea (4200 m) in Hawaii (Chapter 30). Nevertheless, Singh *et al.* (1969) report engorgement of retinal veins specifically in 17 of their 1925 cases. One suspects that this is because in these troops fundoscopic examination was restricted to the minority of subjects with symptoms related to the nervous system. The significance of retinal haemorrhages can be similarly discounted. They are very common in subjects ascending to high altitude, even when they are symptom-free (Chapter 27). Retinal haemorrhages occurred in 57% of Dickinson's series of 50 cases of cerebral mountain sickness but he thought this was of no importance.

In contrast, the development of papilloedema is strong evidence for cerebral mountain sickness and Dickinson (1981) found it in 23 of 44 cases in the highly selected group of very ill patients with pure or mixed acute mountain sickness sent down from high altitude for urgent treatment (Table 14.1). In the massive series of just under 2000 cases of acute mountain sickness in Indian troops in the Himalaya, Singh *et al.* (1969) found that dimness of vision, and blurring of the margins of the optic disc or frank papilloedema were the prominent features in just four cases, and vitreous haemorrhages were present in three of these. Dickinson makes the important clinical observation that 12 of his cases with mild or moderate disturbance of consciousness showed no papilloedema. It is thus clear that the absence of papilloedema does not preclude the diagnosis of cerebral mountain sickness. It suggests too that there is more to the pathology of the condition than oedema alone and we shall return to this point below.

Table 14.1 Percentage incidence of neurological signs in 44 non-fatal cases of cerebral and mixed mountain sickness (after Dickinson 1981)

Sign	%
Disturbed consciousness	70
Ataxia	68
Papilloedema	53
Bladder dysfunction	48
Abnormal plantar reflexes	36
Abnormal limb tone or power	14
VIth nerve palsy	5
Pupil difference	5
Visual field loss	5
Speech difficulty	2
Flapping tremor	2
Hearing loss	2

Retinal haemorrhages were absent in one-third of the 23 patients in Dickinson's series who developed papilloedema.

Ataxia was inferred from the history or observed clinically in two-thirds of Dickinson's patients with pure or mixed cerebral sickness (Table 14.1). Disturbances of consciousness were noted in 31 of these 44 subjects. Recovery from this is commonly rapid on entry to hospital, but this is not always the case. Dickinson (1981) refers to two of his patients, one Japanese and one Korean, who lost consciousness for 3 weeks, and then experienced a further 3 weeks of vagueness and irrationality to be left with mild degrees of residual mental impairment. These clinical features are more suggestive of a disease with pathological components more persistent than an ephemeral oedema of the brain and below we consider the organic lesions concerned.

In 24 of the Indian soldiers caught up in the epidemic of acute mountain sickness in Ladakh, increasing headache was followed by the development of serious neurological manifestations such as stupor and paralysis ending in coma. In Dickinson's cases there were examples of flaccid left hemiparesis and disturbance of limb tone such as generalized rigidity or flaccidity of both legs. Incontinence or retention of urine were commonly associated with disturbances of consciousness. Unilateral or bilateral extensor plantar responses were found in 15 of the patients in his series (Table 14.1). Cranial nerve palsies were reported in both the Indian and European subjects. Paresis of the left sixth cranial nerve was found in two of Dickinson's patients

(Table 14.1), while one of the Indian troops developed palsies of the sixth and seventh cranial nerves. Convulsions were not reported or observed in the European trekkers, but 'seizures' were said to have occurred in the Indian soldiers.

Clarke (1988) notes that acute cerebral mountain sickness may occur with great rapidity at extreme altitudes above 7000 m. During the British expedition to the south-west face of Mt Everest in 1975 a 28-year-old Sherpa suddenly became unwell at 7500 m. He had spent 4 weeks above 5000 m and had not suffered from acute mountain sickness. Suddenly he developed severe headache, neck stiffness, drowsiness, and severe bilateral papilloedema and was unable to stand. The clinical picture resembled that of a subarachnoid haemorrhage. He was evacuated to base camp and treated with dexamethasone. A week after the onset of his illness he was symptom-free. Clarke (1988) reports two other similar case histories. One of the patients reported went into coma and died underlining the fact that the condition can be rapidly fatal.

NEUROLOGICAL INVESTIGATIONS
Lumbar puncture in this disease reveals an elevated cerebrospinal fluid pressure. Singh *et al.* (1969) found it raised by 60–210 mmH$_2$O in the 34 soldiers with cerebral mountain sickness on whom they carried out this procedure. The fluid is clear and colourless, with a normal content of sugar and protein (Singh *et al.* 1969; Dickinson *et al.* 1983). Queckenstedt's test is negative.

Hackett (1988) refers to two cases of acute cerebral mountain sickness in which magnetic resonance imaging (MRI) of the brain revealed diffuse white matter oedema especially of the corpus callosum and the splenium. Control MRI in asymptomatic subjects at high altitude showed no evidence of oedema. Cerebral oedema was demonstrated by computed tomograms of the brain in eight of nine cases of high-altitude pulmonary oedema studied by this technique (Kobayashi *et al.* 1987). They were from a series of 27 patients with lung oedema transported from the Japan Alps (2680–3190 m) to Shinshu University Hospital, Matsumoto, Japan. The computerized tomography showed small cerebral ventricles and cisterns, with disappearance of sulci, and diffuse low density of the cerebrum indicating cerebral oedema. In the following year Koyama *et al.* (1988) reported again identical findings on computed tomography in high-altitude cerebral oedema. These authors believe that the oedema of the brain is partly responsible for increased sympathoadrenal

activity which generates neurogenic pulmonary oedema such as we describe in Chapter 13. On the hypothesis of Theodore and Robin (1975) neurogenic pulmonary oedema results from a massive centrally mediated sympathetic discharge, leading to intense generalized vasoconstriction with a shift of blood from the high-resistance systemic circulation to the low-resistance pulmonary circulation. They found that on admission patients with high-altitude pulmonary oedema showed a four fold elevation of urinary catecholamine secretion reflecting sympathoadrenal activity over a whole day. There was also a two fold increase of plasma noradrenaline.

PATHOLOGICAL FINDINGS
We were privileged to examine the necropsy material from the seven subjects from the Nepal series who died from mountain sickness (Dickinson *et al.* 1983). In two cases there was thrombosis in cerebral venous sinuses with subarachnoid haemorrhage. In one of them, a man of 38 years, there were several haemorrhages into the subarachnoid space, the largest being in the Sylvian and inferior Rolandic fissures and measuring 5 × 3.5 cm. There was a haemorrhage, 17.8 × 8 mm, in the subcortical matter of the right parietal lobe. Foci of degeneration were seen in the adjacent brain substance. Smaller haemorrhages and petechiae were found in the subcortical white matter of the cerebrum, corpus callosum, pons, and cerebellum. Sites of older haemorrhage were indicated by focal collections of compound granular corpuscles and haemosiderin. In the second case, a man of 27 years, the posterior and transverse dural venous sinuses on both sides contained thrombus. Veins in the subarachnoid space overlying the cerebral cortex were distended by thrombus (Fig. 14.1) and there was much haemorrhage into the subarachnoid space. The brain showed swelling and flattening of the gyri with compression of the sulci. There was moderate bulging of the unci, cingulate gyri, and cerebellar tonsils. All parts of the brain were oedematous with a variable degree of spongiosis of the tissues, greatest in the basal ganglia and white matter generally. There were extensive areas of haemorrhagic infarction and associated oedema in the cerebral cortex, subcortical white matter, and brainstem.

In five of the cases the brain was oedematous with swelling and flattening of gyri, and narrowing and compression of sulci. Commonly there was herniation of the cerebellar tonsils, unci, and cingulate gyri. Spongiosis was prominent in the white matter of the brain, including cerebral hemispheres,

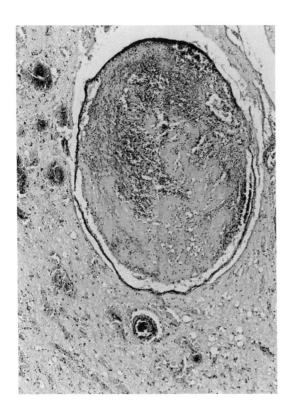

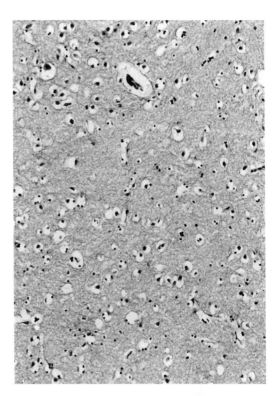

14.1 *A Swiss physician aged 27 years acted as medical officer to a climbing party that ascended to Pumori base camp in the Nepal Himalaya (5180 m). He became unconscious with fixed dilated pupils, papilloedema, and retinal haemorrhages. He died despite treatment with oxygen, mannitol, dexamethasone, and intravenous acetazolamide. The section shows a vein in the subarachnoid space overlying the cerebral cortex. It is distended by thrombus. There was much haemorrhage into the subarachnoid space. The brain is oedematous and shows spongiosis. HE, × 60.*

14.2 *A man of 54 years climbed to Namche Bazaar (3440 m) in the Nepal Himalaya. He developed bronchopneumonia and red infarcts of the lower lobes of the lungs. Clinically he developed tremor and a right extensor plantar response. At necropsy he was found to have cerebral oedema. A section of the brain shows spongiosis. HE, × 150.*

medulla, and various nuclei (Fig.14.2). Numerous petechiae and haemorrhages with focal destruction of brain tissue were commonly associated (Fig.14.3).

The salient fact that arises from this study (Dickinson *et al.* 1983) is that the underlying pathology of cerebral mountain sickness is not merely cerebral oedema but also comprises thrombosis in cerebral venous sinuses, subarachnoid haemorrhage, and petechial haemorrhages with focal areas of degeneration throughout the brain. The implication is that several of these changes are serious and not totally reversible and they may leave residual damage. It must not be assumed that cerebral

mountain sickness will be successfully treated by a reversal of cerebral oedema alone.

PATHOPHYSIOLOGY

The malignant cerebral variant of mountain sickness is commonly associated with high-altitude pulmonary oedema and probably shares with it a common pathophysiology. As with the pulmonary form, the pathology of cerebral mountain sickness is not confined to oedema, but encompasses both haemorrhages into the brain and thrombosis in the cerebral venous sinuses. Nevertheless, cerebral oedema is an important component, as evidenced clinically by papilloedema and pathologically by a swollen brain at necropsy and spongiosis in histological sections of the brain. The symptoms of cerebral

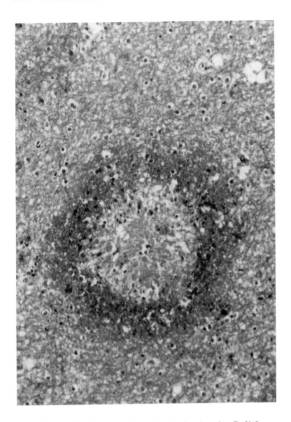

14.3 *Petechial haemorrhage in the brain of a Polish doctor aged 41 years who died from cerebral and pulmonary oedema while climbing in the vicinity of Pangboche in the Everest area. His condition became worse at Pheriche (4260 m) which was the highest point he reached. He was dead by the time he reached Shanta Bhawan hospital in Nepal. HE, × 150.*

mountain sickness are almost certainly due to compression of brain cells brought about by increased hydration of the organ.

The basis for the oedema in the brain is likely to be the same as for that in the lung and the reader is referred to the discussion on the pathophysiology of oedema in benign acute mountain sickness (Chapter 12) and high-altitude pulmonary oedema (Chapter 13). Thus both increased production of antidiuretic hormone and activation of the renin–angiotensin–aldosterone axis may be involved. Local factors are also likely to be involved in the genesis of cerebral mountain sickness. One of these is cerebral blood flow which Singh *et al* (1969) found to undergo a transient increase of 40% within 12–36 hours of exposure to high altitude, thereafter falling back to

normal values by the fifth day in the mountains. Shimojyo *et al.* (1968) thought that cerebral blood flow was significantly increased only at altitudes over 5000 m when arterial oxygen tension fell to 30 mmHg. They felt that only at such altitudes did this hypoxic stimulus override the vasoconstricting effect of hypocarbia. Such a fall in arterial oxygen tension could be produced during sleep or in the presence of high-altitude pulmonary oedema. Although most workers (Fishman 1975; Houston and Dickinson 1975) believe the oedema of the brain to be primarily vasogenic, others (Lassen and Harper 1975; Sutton and Lassen 1979) think it to be histiotoxic in origin.

Acetazolamide reduces the largely cerebral symptoms of benign acute mountain sickness. The drug increases ventilation and also causes a considerable increase in cerebral blood flow a few minutes after intravenous injection of the drug (Friis *et al* 1980; Vorstrup *et al.* 1984). Both factors would be beneficial in tending to augment cerebral oxygen supply. Lassen *et al.* (1987) found that oral administration of 1 g acetazolamide to eight normal subjects studied at sea level and in normoxia caused an acute increase in cerebral blood flow.

CORTICAL BLINDNESS

This condition reported by Hackett *et al.* (1987) and Hackett (1988) has been described as an example of 'focal neurological deficit' that has been found on Mt McKinley. The condition consists of bilateral blindness with intact papillary reflexes. It is intermittent in nature, but sometimes lasts for 2–3 hours. Most climbers misdiagnose the condition as high-altitude cerebral oedema. Descent and the administration of oxygen and carbon dioxide both relieve the symptoms. The mechanism of the condition is unclear but it seems likely that vascular spasm in the occipital cortex is responsible (Hackett 1988). Migraine-type attacks consisting of unilateral hemiparesis, hypoaesthesia, unilateral visual changes, and ophthalmic migraine have been reported at high altitude (Hackett 1988).

MANAGEMENT OF CEREBRAL MOUNTAIN SICKNESS

RAPID DESCENT

The most urgent and effective treatment of cerebral mountain sickness, as with high-altitude pulmonary oedema, is immediate and rapid descent to a lower altitude. In our experience this is an easier practical proposition in the Andes than in the Himalaya, for the road system in the former mountain ranges is better developed. Many areas in such regions as Ladakh and the Karakorams are remote, difficult to get into, and difficult to get out of. Even the established airfield at Leh, the capital of the region, offers an erratic service, with aircraft not landing or leaving for days at a time. A very sick patient is not in a position to wait until the abatement of winds makes it possible for a plane to land in a few days' time. Descent may have to be made immediately by car by dirt-track roads, no matter how hazardous.

For those in remote mountainous areas the case for urgent descent was expressed forcibly by Dickinson (1979) who has an unrivalled clinical experience of treating the disease.

The current recommendation in Nepal, no matter how serious the case, is to start evacuation by foot. If the patient is able to walk, he may do so, otherwise he must be carried on a porter's back or on a yak. This is generally simpler on mountain trails than using a stretcher. If necessary, the descent should not be delayed until morning, but undertaken by moonlight or torchlight. Using these methods it is rarely necessary to go to the expense of helicopter evacuation, which in any case may be much delayed because of slow communications. Even if a helicopter is summoned, arrangements should be made for foot evacuation in the meanwhile and the helicopter service advised of various possible picking-up points.

North (1988) reported a case of cerebral oedema developing in a fit soldier of 32 years who was a member of an Army Mountaineering Association expedition climbing in the Huascarán region of Peru. He was brought down rapidly by mule and survived.

Failure to follow 'the cardinal principle of retreat' (Wilson 1973) is exemplified by his report of the case of a 21-year-old climber on Mt McKinley in 1971 who became ill at 4400 m. He was taken to a nearby but higher shelter at 5200 m, rather than take the longer journey down to base camp. He died. It is important to bear in mind that it may be dangerous to transport volunteers engaged in a rescue attempt abruptly from sea level to any elevation above 2400 m. On a rescue operation on Mt McKinley in 1960, two of the rescuers developed acute high-altitude pulmonary oedema (Wilson 1973). For this reason, groups of rescuers should be at least three in number.

PORTABLE HYPERBARIC CHAMBERS

Treatment of acute mountain sickness by simulated descent can be mimicked by the use of portable compression chambers as we describe in Chapter 12. Treatment of acute mountain sickness in 64 climbers at 4559 m above sea level including the use of hyperbaric portable chambers was carried out by Bärtsch *et al.* (1993). They found this 1 hour of treatment with a pressure of 193 mbar corresponding to a descent of 2250 m leads to greater relief of symptoms of acute mountain sickness after treatment than control treatment at rest in supine position. This short-term beneficial effect may be attributed to improvement of oxygenation. There was, however, no significant beneficial long-term effect that could be attributed to the hyperbaric treatment.

There has been limited experience of the use of use of hyperbaric chambers in the treatment of cerebral mountain sickness (Forster *et al.* 1990). Roach and Hackett (1992) reported the treatment of cases of high-altitude cerebral oedema occuring in trekkers reporting to the medical clinic of the Himalayan Rescue Association in Pheriche, Nepal (4250 m). In their series of cases of 15 patients with acute mountain sickness Takei *et al.* (1988) included four cases of cerebral oedema and one with mixed pulmonary and cerebral oedema. Thus there is limited experience of the use of hyperbaria in the treatment of cerebral mountain sickness and at present it seems to be that hyperbaria should be used only as a temporizing measure until very early descent is feasible.

CORTICOSTEROIDS

Corticosteroids such as betamethasone and dexamethasone are efficacious in reversing cerebral oedema and constitute the treatment of choice for the condition. Clarke (1988) advocates that the latter may be given orally or parenterally in the usual adult dose of 9–16 mg a day. Dickinson (1979) employed a parenteral dosage of 40 mg/day until improvement was obvious. He points out that it is difficult to separate the effects of these agents from the effect of evacuation to a lower altitude. A more direct attack by the rapid injection of hyperosmolar solutions of 50% saline, 50% sucrose or mannitol has been employed (Houston and Dickinson 1975). Glycerol by nasogastric tube has been used to achieve the same result.

Frusemide

The role of powerful diuretics in treating this condition is controversial. The compound that has been used most frequently is frusemide (Lasix[R]). This is a more powerful and rapidly acting diuretic than acetazolamide. Being related to the thiazides it exerts a powerful depressant action on distal tubular reabsorption (Burgen and Mitchell 1972). In addition it contains a sulfonamide group (Fig.14.4) and is thus, like acetazolamide, a carbonic anhydrase inhibitor. When given orally it is rapid in action, with a peak effect leading to copious outpouring of alkaline urine with potassium loss. At first sight this may seem to be an ideal agent for clearing cerebral oedema, but it has to be kept in mind that the resulting haemoconcentration may induce thrombosis. As we have seen, the pathology of cerebral mountain sickness embraces thrombosis as well as oedema, so one may unwittingly make the condition worse. Dickinson (1979) recognizes the problem of bringing about an undesirable contraction of the plasma and extracellular fluid space when dehydration is already one of the drawbacks of sojourn at high altitude. He believes it reasonable to accept some degree of peripheral dehydration for the sake of drawing fluid from the brain and lungs, provided a careful watch is kept for evidence of hypovolaemia.

Singh *et al.* (1969) were enthusiastic in their use of frusemide, which they gave in a heavy dosage of 80 mg every 12 hours for 2 days. They claimed that on this regimen the symptoms of acute mountain sickness were relieved within 6 to 48 hours. When there were associated neurological manifestations, betamethasone was given with the frusemide. Such therapy relieves headache and vomiting within 3 days, although papilloedema took up to 1 month to resolve. They point out that, in the cases of cerebral mountain sickness in Indian troops seen before the combination of frusemide and betamethasone was used, three died after routine treatment and two survived with optic atrophy.

Other clinicians were not nearly so convinced of the efficacy or wisdom of this therapy. It was pointed out that the dosage of frusemide advocated by Singh and co-workers was heavy. Wilson (1973) thought it illogical to provoke diuresis in individuals already dehydrated from the effort of climbing, by the low humidity, and from vomiting. He thought the improvement in the cerebral condition was more likely to have been brought about by the betamethasone than the frusemide. Gray *et al.* (1971) noted that severe ataxia developed in five subjects given frusemide in a study to test the efficacy of the agent for preventing acute mountain sickness. They thought that frusemide may be dangerous and considered that doses over 200 mg should be avoided. Wilson (1973) reported that in one case of *soroche* occurring in a man of 22 years, 80 mg of frusemide produced copious, incontinent urination but did not relieve his headache. Aoki and Robinson (1971) also found frusemide to be ineffective in relieving symptoms on ascent to high altitude.

Oxygen

Administration of oxygen should not be regarded as an effective substitute for evacuation to a lower altitude.

In spite of the serious nature of cerebral mountain sickness, Dickinson (1981) found that improvement was generally rapid once treatment was instituted at a hospital at low altitude. Of his series of 57 patients, 46 were admitted to hospital and the average duration as an in-patient was only 6.7 days. Three patients were obliged to remain for over 2 weeks but, if they are excluded, the average length of stay was only 5.3 days. While such data indicate the rapidity of recovery of most cases of cerebral mountain sickness, it has to be kept in mind that oedema comprises only part of the pathology of the condition, and thrombosis of cerebral venous sinuses and haemorrhages into the brain may play a significant part in individual cases. Descent from high altitude or the other measures referred to above will not resolve these vascular lesions. Dickinson's series comprised 57 subjects, highly selected because they were very ill and sent to Shanta Bhawan hospital for urgent treatment. On receipt of this, 50 enjoyed a rapid reversal of their condition. The remaining seven, however, died.

Sedatives should not be given at high altitude. They block the hypoxic ventilatory response and exaggerate arterial desaturation during sleep. This may predispose to cerebral mountain sickness or high-altitude pulmonary oedema (Sutton *et al.* 1979).

Clarke (1988) notes that acute cerebral mountain sickness may be confused clinically with meningitis

Frusemide

14.4 *Structural formula of frusemide.*

or with subarachnoid haemorrhage. The temptation to carry out a lumbar puncture should be avoided for the procedure is potentially lethal if there is a tonsillar herniation. If bacterial meningitis seems likely in the field, treatment with parenteral antibiotics is suggested without further investigation.

References

Aoki, V.S. and Robinson, S.M. (1971). Body hydration and the incidence and severity of acute mountain sickness. *Journal of Applied Physiology*, **31**, 363

Bärtsch, P., Merki, B., Hofstetter, D., Maggiorini, M., Kayser, B., and Oelz, O. (1993). Treatment of acute mountain sickness by simulated descent: a randomised controlled trial. *British Medical Journal*, **306**, 1098

Burgen, A.S.V. and Mitchell, J.F. (1972). *Gaddum's Pharmacology*, 7th edn. London; Oxford University Press

Clarke, C. (1988). High altitude cerebral oedema. In *High Altitude Medical Science* G. Ueda, S. Kusama, and, N. Voelkel Eds. Matsumoto, Japan; Shinshu University Press, p. 257

Dickinson, J.G. (1979). Severe acute mountain sickness. *Postgraduate Medical Journal*, **55**, 454

Dickinson, J.G. (1981). Acute mountain sickness. A dissertation based on eleven years' experience in the Nepal Himalaya. Unpublished, D.M. thesis, University of Oxford

Dickinson, J., Heath, D., Gosney, J., and Williams, D. (1983). Altitude-related deaths in seven trekkers in the Himalayas. *Thorax*, **38**, 646

Fishman, R.A. (1975). Brain edema. *New England Journal of Medicine*, **293**, 706

Fitch, R.F. (1964). Mountain sickness: a cerebral form. *Annals of Internal Medicine*, **60**, 871

Forster, P. (1986). Telescopes in high places. In *Aspects of Hypoxia* (D. Heath, Ed.). Liverpool; Liverpool University Press, p. 221

Forster, P.J.G., Bradwell, A.R., Winterborn, M.J., Delamere, J.P., Harrison, G., and Birmingham Medical Research Expeditionary Society (1990). Alleviation of hypoxia at high altitude: a comparison between oxygen, oxygen and carbon dioxide inhalation and hyperbaric compression. *Clinical Science*, **79**, 1P

Friis, M.L., Paulson, O.B., and Hertz, M.M. (1980). Carbon dioxide permeability on the blood–brain barrier in man. *Microvascular Research*, **20**, 71

Gray, G.W., Bryan, A.C., Frayser, R., Houston, C.S., and Rennie, I.D.B. (1971). Control of acute mountain sickness. *Aerospace Medicine*, **42**, 81

Hackett, P.H. (1988). Medical research on Mount McKinley. *Annals of Sports Medicine*, **4**, 232

Hackett, P.H., Hollingshead, K.F., Roach, R., Schoene, R.B., and Mills, W.J. (1987). Cortical blindness in high altitude climbers and trekkers — a report of 6 cases. In *Hypoxia and Cold* (J.R. Sutton, C.S. Houston, and G. Coates, Ed.). New York; Praeger, p. 536

Houston, C.S. and Dickinson, J. (1975). Cerebral form of high altitude illness. *Lancet*, **ii**, 758

Kobayashi, T., Koyama, S., Kubo, K., Fukushima, M., and Kusama, S. (1987). Clinical features of patients with high-altitude pulmonary edema in Japan. *Chest*, **92**, 815

Koyama, S., Kobayashi, T., Kubo, K., Fukushima, M., Yoshimura, K., Shibamoto, T., and Kusama, S. (1988). The increased sympathoadrenal activity in patients with high altitude pulmonary edema is centrally mediated. *Japanese Journal of Medicine*, **27**, 10

Lassen, N.A. and Harper, A.M. (1975). High altitude cerebral oedema. *Lancet*, **ii**, 1154

Lassen, N.A., Friberg, L., Kastrup, J., Rizzi, D., and Jensen, J.J. (1987). Effects of acetazolamide on cerebral blood flow and brain tissue oxygenation. *Postgraduate Medical Journal*, **63**, 185

North, J.P. (1988). Cerebral oedema at high altitude. *Journal of the Royal Army Medical Corps*, **134**, 98

Ravenhill, T.H. (1913). Some experience of mountain sickness in the Andes. *Journal of Tropical Medicine and Hygiene*, **16**, 313

Roach, R. and Hackett, P.H. (1992). Hyperbaria and high altitude illness. In *Hypoxia and Mountain Medicine* (J.R. Sutton, G. Coates, and C.S. Houston, Ed.). Oxford; Pergamon Press, p. 266

Shimojyo, S., Scheinberg, P., Kogure, K., and Reimuth, O.M. (1968). The effect of graded hypoxia upon transient cerebral blood flow and oxygen consumption. *Neurology*, **18**, 127

Singh, I., Khanna, P.K., Srivastava, M.C., Lal, M., Roy, S.B., and Subramanyam, C.S.V. (1969). Acute mountain sickness. *New England Journal of Medicine*, **280**, 175

Sutton, J.R. and Lassen, N. (1979). Pathophysiology of acute mountain sickness and high altitude pulmonary oedema: an hypothesis. *Bulletin Européen de Physiopathologie Respiratoire*, **15**, 1045

Sutton, J.R., Powles, A.C.P., Gray, J.W., and Houston, C.S. (1979). Insomnia, sedation and high altitude cerebral oedema. *Lancet*, **i**, 165

Takei, S., Kamio, S., Uehara, A., Naitoh, J., and Hayata, Y. (1988). Treatment of acute mountain sickness using a compression chamber. In *High Altitude Medical Science* (G. Ueda, S. Kusama, and N. Voelkel, Ed.). Matsumoto, Japan; Shinshu University Press, p. 284

Theodore, J. and Robin, E.D. (1975). Pathogenesis of neurogenic pulmonary oedema. *Lancet*, **ii**, 749

Vorstrup, S., Henriksen, L., and Paulson, O.B. (1984). Effect of acetazolamide on cerebral blood flow and cerebral metabolism rate for oxygen. *Journal of Clinical Investigation*, **74**, 1634

Wilson, R. (1973). Acute high altitude illness in mountaineers and problems of rescue. *Annals of Internal Medicine*, **78**, 421

15

Monge's disease

In the preceding chapters we have described the clinical features, pathogenesis, and treatment of the various forms of acute mountain sickness, which usually make their appearance within a few hours of exposure to the hypobaric hypoxia of high altitude in lowlanders or in highlanders re-entering the mountain environment. Here we give an account of the features of 'chronic mountain sickness', which develops in some native highlanders after many years' residence at high altitude. It has been reported most commonly in Quechuas and Aymaras living above 4000 m in the Andes but increasing numbers of cases are now coming to light in Tibet and the western Himalaya. Affected subjects develop a complex clinical picture in which haematological, cardiovascular, and respiratory elements are all represented. In the untreated cases, which were allowed to run their full clinical course before the condition was recognized for what it was, serious psychological disorders were also described. This clinical syndrome was first described in 1928 by Carlos Monge-Medrano as 'la enfermedad de los Andes' and it has since come to be termed 'chronic mountain sickness' or 'Monge's disease' in his honour (Fig. 15.1). In this chapter we shall consider its clinical and pathological features and the concept of the condition as a distinct disease entity. Peñaloza et al. (1971) have made a special study of Monge's disease and in this account we shall draw heavily on their unique experience of the clinical features.

SYMPTOMS

Most patients with the disease are young or middle-aged men, but the mean age approaches 40 years (Sime et al. 1975; see Fig. 15.2(a)). Thus, in the study described by Peñaloza and Sime (1971) and Peñaloza et al. (1971), all 10 subjects were males between 22 and 51 years of age and the mean age was 38 years. The cases of Hurtado (1942) were all men between 24 and 44 years. The disease occurs rarely in women and the exemption may be ascribed to menstrual loss. It is not found in children.

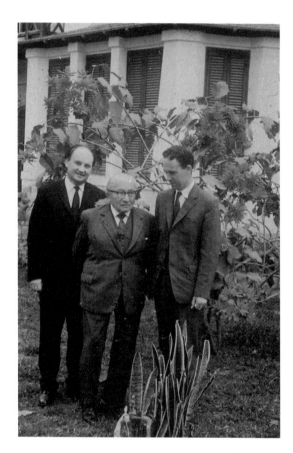

15.1 *Professor Carlos Monge-Medrano (centre) with Professor Peter Harris (right) and one of the authors, D.H. (left), in the garden of his home in Lima in July 1965. The distinguished Peruvian physician was the first person to recognize, in 1928, chronic mountain sickness as a distinct clinical syndrome, which has since come to bear his name.*

Symptoms related to the nervous system are common and frequently take the form of headaches, dizziness, paraesthesiae, and somnolence (Peñaloza and Sime 1971). Winslow and Monge (1987) refer to confusion and a feeling of congestion of the head.

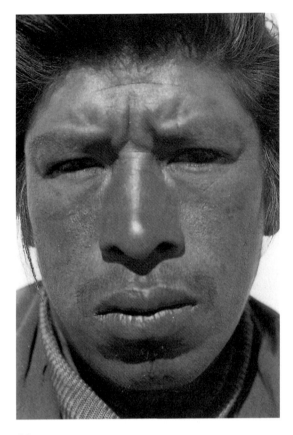

(a)

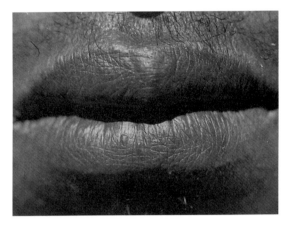

(b)

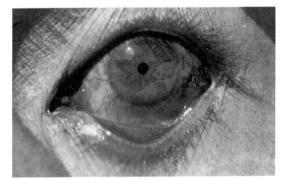

(c)

15.2 *(a) Young male Quechua Indian, aged 35 years, who resided at 4330 m and developed Monge's disease; (b) lips appear almost black due to a combination of greatly elevated haematocrit and diminished arterial oxygen saturation, this giving the designation 'cardiac negro'; (c) conjunctival vessels are suffused and congested and dark wine-red in colour, this being the consequence of the greatly elevated haematocrit and diminished arterial oxygen saturation; (d) fingers are clubbed.*

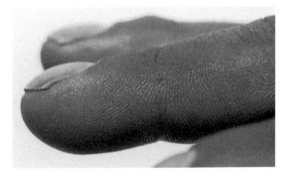

(d)

The earliest reports stressed such symptomatology and Monge and Monge (1966) present an imposing list of neurological and psychological symptoms ranging from depression and irritability to hallucinations. Untreated early cases sometimes presented with cerebral crises, which over a period of hours or even minutes deteriorated through drowsiness to coma, which occasionally proved fatal. In present times, when the effective treatment is known to be removal to sea-level and when transport is readily available, such serious developments are virtually unknown. Patients with Monge's disease tire easily and have a decreased exercise tolerance. Breathlessness is not a common symptom.

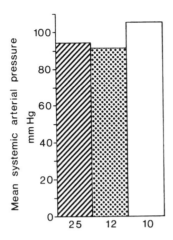

15.3 *Mean systemic arterial pressure (mmHg) in
25 healthy residents at sea level (hatched column), in
12 healthy highlanders (stippled column), and in
10 cases of Monge's disease (open column). The levels
are significantly higher in the cases of chronic mountain
sickness. (The data presented diagrammatically in
Figs 15.3 and 15.5–15.8 are derived from Peñaloza
et al (1971). Their study was carried out at an altitude
of 4375 m, with a mean barometric pressure of
446 mmHg and an atmospheric* PO_2 *of 90 mmHg.*

Haemoptysis is said to occur (Hurtado 1942; Monge
and Monge 1966). Bone pain is said to be characteristic and this may be related to the excessive hyperplasia of the bone marrow (Winslow and Monge
1987).

SIGNS
Physical examination must take into account the altitude at which the patient lives, for the higher the
location the more erythraemic and cyanosed will the
normal healthy residents look. Only when this comparison is made will it be appreciated that in
Monge's disease there is a change from the ruddy
erythraemic colour of the normal healthy residents
to a frankly cyanotic appearance. The combination
of the virtually black lips and wine-red mucosal surfaces against the greenish tinge of the Indian skin
give the patient with Monge's disease a striking
appearance (Fig. 15.2(a)). The greatly elevated
haematocrit and diminished arterial oxygen saturation described below give the lips a deeply cyanosed,
almost black colour (Fig. 15.2(b)). The ear lobes
and facial skin may also appear very dark. The conjunctivae are dark red in colour and look very suffused and congested (Fig. 15.2(c)). The fingers are

commonly clubbed (Fig. 15.2(d). In our experience,
haemorrhages in the finger nails are characteristic of
the condition (Chapter 25).

When cyanosis is severe, there may be signs of
mild congestive cardiac failure. On examination of
the chest there may be increased loudness of the
second sound in the pulmonary area, suggestive of
an exaggeration of the degree of pulmonary hypertension normal for highlanders at the altitude in
question. An associated midsystolic murmur may be
present. There is a slight but significant elevation of
systemic diastolic and mean pressure according to
Peñaloza *et al.* (1971) (Fig. 15.3). Other authors
have commented that the systemic blood pressure is
normal or low (Monge and Monge 1966). The fundi
show tortuosity and dilatation of venous vessels. It is
reported that the barrel-shaped chest of the
Quechua Indian is exaggerated when he develops
symptoms and signs of chronic mountain sickness
(Monge and Monge 1966), but this seems unlikely
to us.

RADIOLOGICAL CHANGES
Radiological examination of the chest in chronic
mountain sickness reveals cardiac enlargement due
to increase in size of the right cardiac chambers (Fig.
15.4). In a minority of cases in which the heart is
greatly enlarged, the left ventricle is also involved
(Fig. 15.4). The mean values per square metre of
body surface of the transverse diameter of the heart,
frontal area, and heart volume in patients with
Monge's disease, compared with healthy highlanders, are shown in Fig. 15.5. Prominence of the
pulmonary artery and accentuation of the pulmonary vascular markings is found in all patients
with Monge's disease, but they are especially pronounced when the cardiac enlargement is great. On
descent to sea level, the cardiac size and the
pulmonary vascular markings decrease with the
passage of time.

ELECTROVECTORCARDIOGRAPHY
Peñaloza and Sime (1971) have described the electrocardiograms and vectorcardiograms in 10 cases of
chronic mountain sickness. Peaked P waves with increased voltage were often observed in leads II, III,
and aVF as well as in the right precordial leads. The
mean voltage of the P wave in lead II was 2.9 mm,
compared with 1.0 mm obtained in a group of 12
healthy residents at high altitude. The P loop of the
vectorcardiograms was increased in area and voltage
and was directed forward and inferiorly. An accentuated degree of right Â QRS deviation was present in

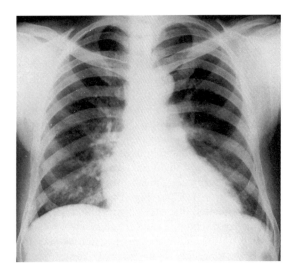

15.4 *Anteroposterior radiograph of the chest in a man of 47 years, a long-standing resident at 4330 m, who developed Monge's disease. There is increased size of the right ventricle, prominence of the pulmonary artery, and accentuation of the pulmonary vascular markings. There is also distinct enlargement of the left ventricle.*

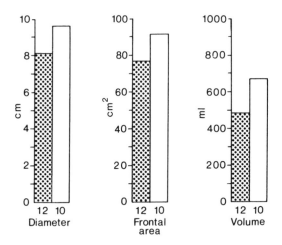

15.5 *Mean values per square metre of body surface area of the transverse diameter of the heart, frontal area, and heart volume in 10 patients with Monge's disease compared with 12 healthy highlanders.*

most patients, and the; mean value of Â QRS was + 152° compared with + 95° in healthy highlanders. The rS pattern in the right precordial leads and complexes of RS or rS type in the left precordial leads were common findings. Tall R waves were found over the left precordial leads in two of three patients in whom radiographic examination showed left cardiac enlargement. The horizontal QRS loop was orientated to the right and backward in most cases with counterclockwise rotation or a figure-of-eight configuration and enlarged final QRS vectors. Forward orientation and clockwise rotation were seen in only two cases. The vectorcardiographic pattern of biventricular hypertrophy was seen in one patient. Negative T waves over the right precordial leads were found in five patients and in most of them the negative T waves were peaked, deep, and symmetrical, reproducing the 'ischaemic' T wave pattern. As in the case of the radiological changes, the electrovectorcardiographic alterations slowly return to normal on descent to sea level.

HAEMATOLOGICAL VALUES

Patients with Monge's disease have higher haemoglobin and haematocrit values than those seen in healthy residents at high altitudes (Fig. 15.6(a),(b)). A value of 23 g/dl has been taken arbitrarily as the sole diagnostic criterion of chronic mountain sickness according to Carlos Monge-Cassinelli (1966), the son of the distinguished Peruvian physician. Thus, Hurtado (1942) gave, for eight cases of Monge's disease, a range of 22.9–27.2 g/dl for the haemoglobin level and 73–83%, for the haematocrit. The arbitrary value of 23 g/dl of haemoglobin certainly exceeds the figure corresponding to two standard deviations above the mean for healthy acclimatized people living between 4000 and 4400 m. However, it is overlapped by two standard deviations above the mean for people living about 4400 m (Monge-C 1966). This illustrates that there is some difficulty in distinguishing normal high-altitude physiology from the pathophysiology of 'Monge's disease'. The morphology of the circulating red cells is normal. There is no increase in the number of leucocytes in the blood, thus distinguishing the condition from polycythaemia vera. Hurtado (1942) gives a range of 3800–7200 × 10⁹/l. There is no abnormality in the differential count. Curiously, Monge's disease has never been regarded as primarily a haematological disease, although excessive polycythaemia is its main manifestation and the cause of its symptoms. The disease could in fact be regarded as an instance of a normal control mechanism gone awry (Winslow and Monge 1987).

PULMONARY HAEMODYNAMICS

In Monge's disease the degree of pulmonary arterial hypertension is higher than that observed in healthy

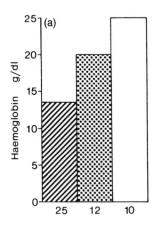 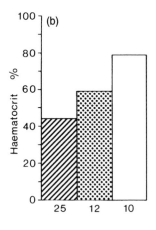

15.6 *Levels of (a) haemoglobin and (b) haematocrit in the subjects in Fig. 15.3. Both levels are higher in healthy highlanders than in sea-level residents, but higher still in patients with Monge's disease.*

highlanders (Peñaloza and Sime 1971; Peñaloza *et al.* 1971; see Fig. 15.7(a)). So too is the mean total pulmonary resistance (Fig. 15.7(b)). The cardiac index and pulmonary wedge pressure are not significantly different from those found in healthy highlanders.

ARTERIAL BLOOD GASES AND ACID–BASE EQUILIBRIUM

The arterial oxygen saturation in cases of Monge's disease is even lower than that found in normal, healthy residents at high altitudes (Hurtado 1942, 1955, 1960; Peñaloza and Sime 1971; Peñaloza *et al.* 1971; Fig. 15.8). This suggests that the increased

level of polycythaemia is a consequence of the increased hypoxic stimulus. There is also a higher arterial carbon dioxide tension than that normally present in the native population (Monge *et al.* 1964). The pH remains unaltered as the consequence of an elevation of plasma bicarbonate concentration.

BLOOD VOLUME

Hurtado (1942) found that in Monge's disease the total blood volume is elevated. He found the range in eight cases to be 149.6–211.9 ml/kg with a range of plasma volume of 27.7–46.8 ml/kg.

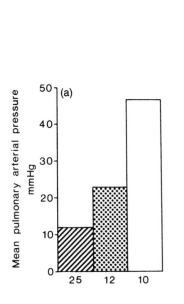 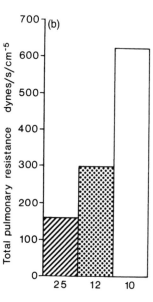

15.7 *(a) Mean pulmonary arterial pressure in the subjects in Fig. 15.3. There is slight pulmonary hypertension in healthy highlanders, but moderate elevation of pulmonary arterial pressure in patients with Monge's disease. (b) Total pulmonary vascular resistance in the subjects in Fig. 15.3. The resistance is higher in healthy highlanders than in sea-level residents, but it is higher still in patients with Monge's disease.*

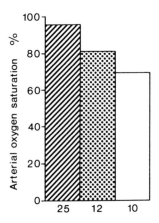

15.8 *Systemic arterial oxygen saturation in the subjects in Fig. 15.3. There is a fall in arterial oxygen saturation in healthy highlanders compared with sea-level residents, but the fall becomes even more pronounced in cases of chronic mountain sickness.*

ALVEOLAR HYPOVENTILATION

There are two ways in which even more inadequate oxygenation of blood in the pulmonary capillaries could develop even beyond that due to the lowered partial pressure of oxygen in the alveolar spaces inherent in life at high altitudes. One is decreased permeability in the alveolar capillary membrane; the other is deficient ventilation of the alveoli. There is no great diminution of vital capacity in Monge's disease to explain the further desaturation of systemic arterial blood. Hurtado found the range of vital capacity to be 2.24–4.46 litres in seven subjects. Hence the basis of Monge's disease appears to be alveolar hypoventilation. This leads to chronic alveolar hypoxia, exceeding that inherent in residence at high altitude. This in turn brings about pulmonary arteriolar muscularization by one of the mechanisms discussed in Chapter 10. An exaggeration of pulmonary arterial hypertension and increased blood viscosity follows. The haematological and psychological features of the condition are also secondary to hypoxaemia.

CONCEPT OF LOSS OF ACCLIMATIZATION

The alveolar hypoventilation has been ascribed to a loss of sensitivity of the respiratory centre to carbon dioxide (Hurtado 1960) or to an irreversible insensitivity of the peripheral chemoreceptors to hypoxia. This loss of respiratory drive is considered by the Peruvian school to represent a loss of acclimatization

to high altitude under the persistent stimulus of chronic hypoxia. Monge's disease is clearly a syndrome of alveolar hypoventilation (Fishman *et al.* 1957; Bergofsky 1967) occurring at high altitude (Severinghaus *et al.* 1966). It is possible that the disease corresponding to Monge's disease at sea level is the 'primary hypoventilation syndrome' (Richter *et al.* 1957; Rodman and Close 1959). In this condition there is a diminished ventilatory response to hypoxaemia and hypercapnia so that polycythaemia and cyanosis develop. We consider this concept of loss of acclimatization later in the chapter.

GEOGRAPHICAL PATHOLOGY

Monge's disease is classically associated with the Andes and is seen not infrequently at altitudes exceeding 4000 m on the Peruvian altiplano. However, it has now become clear that chronic mountain sickness is also to be found in the Himalaya. Haematological and electrocardiographic data on 27 cases of the syndrome in this region were reported and contrasted with those from 75 healthy native highlanders who acted as controls (Nath *et al.* 1983a). Mean values for haematocrit and haemoglobin for the subjects with chronic mountain sickness were 80% and 23 g/dl, while those for the controls were 43% and 17.9 g/dl respectively. As a result affected subjects had a plethoric appearance (Fig. 15.9). Mean Â QRS in the former was +118° and in the latter +76°. Cardiac catheterization was carried out in eight cases and showed an elevated pulmonary arterial pressure even after a recovery period of 4.2 days at sea level. The mean duration of stay at high altitude in these 27 cases was 7.02 years. The incidence of proteinuria was significantly higher in this group of cases of chronic mountain sickness and this prominent nephropathy led Nath *et al.* (1983a) to separate this variant of Monge's disease as the 'Phobrang type'. Chronic mountain sickness is also common in Tibet as described below.

The preponderance of reports of cases of Monge's disease in the Andes in the past has suggested that there may be predisposing factors peculiar to the region. Since mining is a major activity in the area of such towns as Cerro de Pasco, Morococha, and La Oroya, it has been thought possible that pollution of the air might predispose to chronic bronchitis and perhaps centrilobular emphysema, which could exaggerate the alveolar hypoxia of high altitude and lead to 'secondary Monge's disease' as discussed later. However, it has to be kept in mind that the villagers in the high-altitude desert environment of the Indus valley between the Himalaya and the

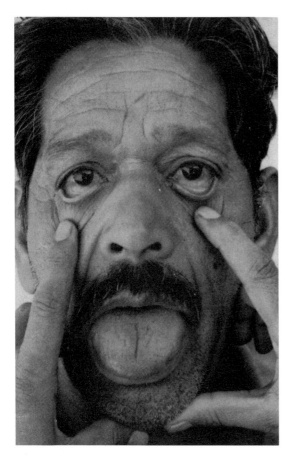

15.9 *A case of chronic mountain sickness of Phobrang type from the Himalaya. The patient has a plethoric appearance due to polycythaemia complicating exaggerated alveolar hypoxia.*

Karakorams commonly develop non-industrial silicosis on exposure to the dusty arid conditions (Chapter 2). What is more they are prone to chronic bronchitis on account of the smoky atmosphere of their houses due to the burning of animal excrement and the lack of ventilation (Chapter 2). In spite of this air pollution chronic mountain sickness is not characteristic of the region. It seems far more likely that the special factor operating in the Andes to cause a concentration of cases of Monge's disease there is the great altitude at which people live permanently. Although the Himalayan peaks are higher than those of the Andes, the permanent settlements of the Ladakhis and Sherpas are nowhere as high as those of the Quechua and Aymara Indians. The higher altitude would be associated with exaggera-

tion of physiological variables thought to underlie the syndrome as described below.

CHRONIC MOUNTAIN SICKNESS IN TIBET

The prevalence of chronic mountain sickness in a Tibetan hospital population was studied by Pei *et al.* (1989). The diagnosis was based on the symptoms, clinical examination, electrocardiogram, chest radiograph, and blood count. Twenty-four patients with the disease were admitted to the Workers' Hospital, Lhasa, during the 12 months following February 1986, giving a prevalence of 8.9% in the total hospital population. The opportunity was taken to compare the frequency, distribution of sex, race, and cigarette-smoking in the patients with Monge's disease with these factors in the general hospital population. The findings were striking. All 24 patients were male. This is probably related to the fact that menstruation in women prevents the build-up of significant polycythaemia. There was a strong association between race and chronic mountain sickness. No fewer than 23 patients were of Han origin, only one case occurring in a native Tibetan.

The investigation provided information on the length of time that is necessary for the development of Monge's disease. The average age of the Han patients was 48.6 years (± 10.0 SD) and the average length of stay at high altitude was 26.2 years (± 9.5 SD), although the shortest period necessary was only 9 years. The average haemoglobin level was 20.7 g/dl (± 2.0 SD) compared with 14.7 g/dl (± 2.0 SD) in Han males without chronic mountain sickness living at the same altitude. Tibetans appear to be less susceptible to the effects of hypoxia than the Quechua and Aymara natives of the Andes in whom Monge's disease is common. There was also an association between the development of chronic mountain sickness and the smoking of cigarettes. Since this habit in Tibet is almost entirely confined to the male population, it is necessary to eliminate the influence of sex before analysing the effects of cigarettes. The mechanism of the association is unknown, but it could be through the agency of the production of centrilobular emphysema which could interpose a dead space critically placed between the terminal bronchioles and the alveolar spaces, reducing alveolar ventilation. Once again this underlines the necessity for establishing the pathology of cases of Monge's disease reported in the literature. This association with smoking in the cases from Tibet suggests that they may be examples of 'secondary Monge's disease' as defined below. In Tibet there is a seasonal variation in the presentation of cases of chronic mountain sickness, most being admitted to hospital during the winter months.

The clinical features of chronic mountain sickness in Tibet proved to be very similar to those reported in highlanders from the Andes as described earlier in this chapter. The initial symptoms were attributable to polycythaemia and comprised headache, dizziness, fatigue, loss of memory, and a cyanotic appearance. Dyspnoea usually appeared gradually as the years went on and finally episodes of cardiac oedema occurred. A bleeding tendency was manifested by epistaxis, haemoptysis, purpura, haematemesis, and haematuria. The facial appearance was characteristic with cyanosis and fulness of the face, swelling of the eyelids, and congested conjunctivae. Cyanosis was universal and clubbing frequent. Half of the patients had been admitted with a raised venous pressure and oedema and clinical evidence of pulmonary hypertension. There was a tendency to systemic arterial hypertension. The chest radiograph showed cardiac enlargement and dilatation of central and peripheral pulmonary arteries. The electrocardiogram showed evidence of right atrial enlargement and clockwise rotation of the ventricles. Echocardiography revealed dilatation of the right ventricle.

Cardiorespiratory physiological studies were carried out in five patients with chronic mountain sickness in Tibet (Pei *et al.* 1989). Mean haemodynamic values were: systemic arterial pressure 150/104 mmHg; pulmonary arterial pressure 57/28 mmHg; wedge pressure 12 mmHg; cardiac index $4.01/min$ per m^2; pulmonary arterial resistance 4.7 mmHg/l per min. Oxygen inhalation caused a partial decrease in pulmonary arterial resistance. Arterial carbon dioxide tension averaged 33 mmHg in the five patients with chronic mountain sickness and 27 mmHg in normal residents, indicating a degree of alveolar hypoventilation in this disease. Arterial oxygen tension averaged 41 mmHg in patients and 52 mmHg in normal residents. Measurements of the alveolar-arterial difference in P_{o2} indicated an inhomogeneity of ventilation: perfusion ratios.

CLINICOPATHOLOGICAL TYPES

Arias-Stella *et al.* (1973) believed that there are three clinicopathological types of Monge's disease but their views are open to question. They thought there was a condition of 'chronic soroche' that occurs in people who have to move from sea level to live at high altitude and never adjust to this change. Apparently Monge-Medrano himself (1943) recognized that some examples of the syndrome to which

his name has been coupled were cases of chronic lack of adjustment to high altitude, but he did not give details of individual cases. It seems to us that such cases are examples of *failure to establish acclimatization* to high altitude and as such are more akin to the syndromes of subacute mountain sickness as described in Chapter 17 than to a *loss of acclimatization*, which Monge regarded as the basis of his disease.

Much more acceptable theoretically is 'secondary chronic mountain sickness' (Monge and Monge 1966) sometimes referred to as 'Monge's syndrome' (Arias-Stella *et al.* (1973). This is seen among people from sea level who have already acclimatized and have been living in good health at high altitude, or among natives of the Andes, in whom organic diseases develop and exaggerate the hypoxaemia. These are diseases that are themselves capable, even at sea level, of producing chronic hypoxia and associated pulmonary arterial remodelling. Such diseases include gross obesity (the Pickwickian syndrome), kyphoscoliosis, and pulmonary emphysema. Other conditions referred to as occurring in secondary Monge's disease by Arias-Stella *et al.* (1973) are neuromuscular disorders affecting the thoracic cage, pulmonary tuberculosis, and pneumoconiosis.

According to Arias-Stella and co-workers there is a third type of Monge's disease that occurs in persons who are native highlanders or who have acclimatized successfully to life at high altitude and then who subsequently develop the features of chronic mountain sickness, although no organic disease is found to explain their increased hypoxaemia. This is an attractive idea, but it should be noted that, as there have been no necropsy studies on unequivocal cases of primary Monge's disease, it is impossible at this time to prove or disprove that the condition occurs in the absence of demonstrable morbid anatomical change. Should such cases subsequently be proven to occur they are what Arias-Stella and his colleagues would call 'true Monge's disease'. Patients of this type have been accepted on clinical grounds by Monge-M (1928), Hurtado (1942), and Peñaloza and Sime (1971) but it should be noted that detailed pathological confirmation of absence of predisposing disease has not been forthcoming. The nature of 'true Monge's disease' as seen through the eyes of his son, Professor Monge-Cassinelli, is discussed below.

MORBID ANATOMY

A few years after Monge described the clinical syndrome that has come to bear his name, Hurtado

(1942) came to the conclusion that an understanding of the nature of the disease would be helped considerably by establishing its morbid anatomy. He said: 'The study of a greater number of cases and the anatomic investigation of the lungs and other organs after death will be necessary for the final understanding of the etiologic mechanism responsible for the hematologic alterations found in some cases of chronic mountain sickness. In this field, as in many others, the morphologic aspects have been unduly neglected in favour of the functional and chemical approximation.' Such data have been slow in coming and, in fact, it is salutary to realize that since Monge's disease was first described in 1928 there are only three reports of the histopathology in fatal cases of the condition (Fernan-Zegarra and Lazo-Taboada 1961; Reategui-López 1969; Arias-Stella *et al.* 1973). Furthermore, not one of them is a bona fide case of primary Monge's disease, since each had some condition like obesity, lordoscoliosis, or kyphoscoliosis that might on its own predispose to chronic alveolar hypoxia and hypoxic hypertensive pulmonary vascular disease. Hence all the cases so far described in the literature as illustrating the pathological features of the condition are in fact examples of 'secondary Monge's disease'.

Analysis of the macroscopic and histological features in these reports reveals that they are the result of pulmonary hypertension secondary to the alveolar hypoxia. Thus, all three reports refer to right ventricular hypertrophy and thickening of peripheral pulmonary arteries, thickening of the media being specified in two instances. An important point emerges from the most satisfactory report on a case of Monge's disease by Arias-Stella *et al.* (1973), although we may note that the patient reported also suffered from dorsal kyphoscoliosis, chronic bronchitis, and slight centrilobular emphysema. They note that the degree of right ventricular hypertrophy in their case is more severe than in normal cases at high altitude (Recavarren and Arias-Stella 1964). Similarly, the area of muscle in the media of the peripheral pulmonary arteries in their case exceeded that found in the muscularization of the normal pulmonary arterial tree at high altitude (Fig. 15.10(a)). Clearly such features are consistent with the greater elevation of pulmonary arterial pressure induced by an exaggeration of alveolar hypoxia over that normally experienced at the altitude in question. Arias-Stella *et al.* (1973) also reported the presence of fresh and partially organized thrombi (Fig. 15.10(b),(c)) in the pulmonary arteries and arterioles. This is consistent with the greater elevation of

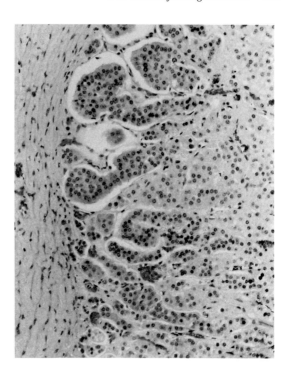

15.11 *Sections of the adrenal cortex from the same case of Monge's disease as illustrated in Fig. 15.10. It shows hyperplasia of the zona glomerulosa. HE, × 150.*

haematocrit induced by the worsening of the alveolar hypoxia. In passing we may note that their patient also had a colloid goitre and hyperplasia of the zona glomerulosa of the adrenal cortex (Fig. 15.11). The functional significance of these endocrine changes is discussed in Chapter 22.

THE NATURE OF MONGE'S DISEASE

Earlier in this chapter we pointed out the remarkable fact that there has never been a published account of the pathology of a case of Monge's disease occurring in the absence of conditions like pulmonary emphysema or kyphoscoliosis in themselves capable of enhanced alveolar hypoxia. The well-known paper on the pathology of chronic mountain sickness with its classification of subdivision into 'chronic soroche', secondary Monge's disease, and true Monge's disease was published in *Thorax* in 1973 (Arias-Stella *et al.* 1973). The essence of this classification was first presented by Arias-Stella (1971) at a symposium sponsored by the Ciba Foundation, *High Altitude Physiology: Cardiac and Respiratory Aspects*. He accepted that a case of primary Monge's disease had never come to

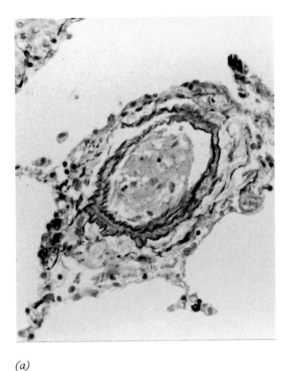

(a)

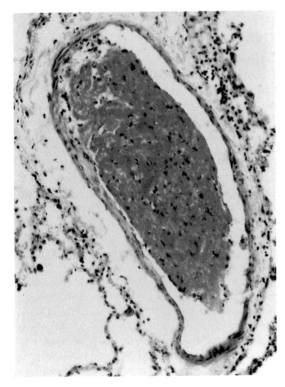

(b)

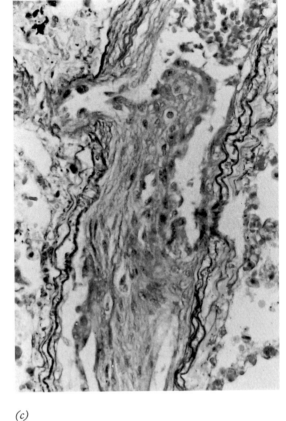

(c)

15.10 *(a) Transverse section of a muscularized pulmonary arteriole from a case of Monge's disease in a woman aged 48 years. There is a distinct media of circularly orientated smooth muscle bounded by internal and external elastic laminae. Although these changes are in essence precisely those found in the lungs of healthy highlanders, they are said to be quantitatively more severe in Monge's disease. Such morbid anatomical atomical changes are associated with the further elevation of pulmonary arterial pressure in this condition. Within the muscularized pulmonary arteriole is recent thrombus. EVG, × 375. (From the case reported by Arias-Stella et al. 1973).) (b), (c) Oblique and longitudinal sections of muscular pulmonary arteries from the same case. They contain recent and organizing thrombus, respectively. HE, × 177; EVG, × 375.*

post-mortem but he believed that such cases existed. One of us (D.H.) attending this meeting had the temerity to suggest that in the absence of any accepted pathology it was difficult to accept that there was a distinct disease entity of 'Monge's disease'. It was suggested rather that all chronic mountain sickness was due to impaired lung function at high altitude. This provoked Hurtado to say: 'I don't agree with the view that we are not justified in speaking of Monge's disease until we know its pathological anatomy. On such a vein we would be forced to eliminate most mental disease.' Nevertheless, as we point out earlier, Hurtado himself some 30 years before had also come to the conclusion that an understanding of the nature of the disease would be helped considerably by establishing its pathology (Hurtado 1942). By 1993 this has still not yet been established.

In this context it is enlightening to read the recent conclusions of Professor Carlos Monge-Cassinelli (Fig. 15.12) on the nature of the syndrome first reported by his father, Professor Carlos Monge-Medrano (Winslow and Monge 1987).

> We think there is no reason to believe that chronic mountain sickness is a 'disease' in the usual sense of the word. Rather it can be viewed as an accumulation of physiologic responses, each one of which is slightly off the mean for the population. For example, there is a normal variation in haemoglobin concentration at sea level and a range of hypoxic ventilatory response, just as there is a range in athletic ability, body size, strength and so on. If, under the added burden of hypoxia, an individual has a higher than normal haematocrit and a lower than normal ventilation rate, and is not in a highly conditioned, athletic state, perhaps the symptoms of chronic mountain sickness may appear.

They add:

> The authors do not share Monge-M's view, strictly, that chronic mountain sickness is a 'loss of acclimatization' because we are not convinced that most humans are well suited to life at high altitudes. In this sense, humans do not adapt to hypoxia in the way their genetically adapted animals do. Instead, well-conditioned, stoic strong humans live and reproduce at high altitudes, but we have yet to find one who would not prefer to live at sea level.

The integration of physiological variables that enable man to adjust to life at high altitude may break down with increasing age and this manifests itself as chronic mountain sickness. We believe that this process can be succinctly termed 'loss of acclimatization'. We think that the statement quoted above confuses two major biological adjustments to high altitude namely acclimatization in man and genetic adaptation in indigenous mountain mammals. One would not expect humans 'to adapt to hypoxia in the way that genetically adapted animals do'.

The integration of physiological variables surely constitutes acclimatization and its failure comprises a loss of acclimatization. This failure of integration may involve a wide range of factors but alveolar hypoventilation and consequent exaggeration of polycythaemia are of central importance. These disturbances enhance all the effects of chronic alveolar hypoxia inherent in a life in the mountains. They take time to develop so that the mean age of patients first diagnosed as having Monge's disease approaches 40 years. Increasing age is associated with

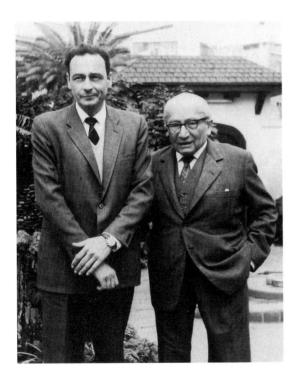

15.12 *Professor Carlos Monge-Medrano (right) with his son Professor Carlos Monge-Cassinelli, also a distinguished worker in the field of high-altitude medicine, in the garden of his home in Lima in July 1965.*

progressive hypoventilation in lowlanders and native highlanders. There is a correlation between ventilatory rate and age both in healthy highlanders and in cases of chronic mountain sickness (Sime *et al.* 1975). The relation is hyperbolic and Monge's disease represents the extreme situation in older people with a low ventilatory rate. Cases of the disease in other words are merely extreme examples of a normal trend, the results from such patients lying on the regression line obtained from data on control subjects. The same is true of correlations between haematocrit levels and ventilatory rate, cases of Monge's disease once again lying on the normal regression line, albeit at one extreme edge. Such findings lead Sime *et al.* (1975) to believe that chronic mountain sickness is in a sense a possible clinical manifestation of ageing at high altitude, being the result of an excessive polycythaemia secondary to the fall in ventilatory rate occurring with age. Patients with Monge's disease living at 4500 m and referred to in the literature are commonly in their forties, whereas 'controls' for these cases are in their twenties. For examples, in the report of Peñaloza *et al.* (1971) the mean age of the cases of Monge's disease was 38 years, whereas that of control subjects was 24 years. This important factor of age must not be overlooked, for chronic mountain sickness may evolve as a natural extension of what occurs in younger natives.

At sea level the ventilatory rate does not change with age from 16 to 69 years (Baldwin *et al.* 1948), but arterial oxygen tension diminishes linearly with age. This drop has been attributed to an increased inequality of the ventilation:perfusion ratio with age (Sorbini *et al.* 1968). At sea level the Pa_{O_2} falls on the flat part of the oxygen–haemoglobin dissociation curve, so that a moderate fall in Pa_{O_2} will not result in a noticeable polycythaemic response. However, at high altitude this fall in Pa_{O_2} occurs on the steep slope of the curve, so that significant polycythaemia results. As we have already noted in Chapter 5, the haematocrit rises as a function of age in addition to altitude (Whittembury and Monge-C 1972).

The degree of altitude at which the subject lives is also of importance, since the greater the elevation the younger the age at which alveolar hypoventilation may bring about the conditions consistent with the development of chronic mountain sickness. The physiological and pathological features of Monge's disease are but exaggerations of those found in healthy native highlanders of the Andes. However, this exaggeration is of great clinical importance for, whereas the healthy Quechua Indian can in no sense

be regarded as suffering from cor pulmonale, accentuation of his normal haematological and haemodynamic characteristics can lead to a potentially fatal condition.

It has not escaped the attention of some workers that the hypoventilation of sleep mimics the physiological basis of Monge's disease. At high altitude the shallowness of breathing during the hours of sleep induces severe hypoxaemia and appears to be a factor in the pathogenesis of what some authors term 'chronic mountain polycythaemia' (Kryger *et al.* 1978b). The combination of ambient hypoxia of high altitude and relative hypoventilation of sleep lowers Pa_{O_2} to the inflection point of the oxygen–haemoglobin dissociation curve, so that pronounced oxygen desaturation occurs.

MANAGEMENT OF MONGE'S DISEASE

The simple and effective treatment for Monge's disease is removal to a lower altitude. When a patient with the condition descends to sea level, his symptoms regress rapidly and there are immediate improvements in the haematological and haemodynamic disturbances. After a stay of 2 months at sea level the improvement is usually so pronounced that the abnormalities have returned virtually to normal (Table 15.1). Peñaloza *et al.* (1971) described the changes of that occurred in three patients with Monge's disease after 3, 11, and 60 days' sojourn at lower altitude. Cyanosis, the tendency to fatigue, and cerebral symptoms all improve rapidly. The heart decreases in size (Fig. 15.13(a),(b)) and the

Table 15.1 Clinical, haematological, and haemodynamic factors in a patient with Monge's disease at high altitude and after 2 months' residence at sea level (Peñaloza *et al.* 1971)

Factor	At high altitude (4375 m)	After 2 months at sea level
Heart rate (beats/min)	112	65
Haematocrit (%)	86.0	50.0
Haemoglobin (g/dl)	23.2	17.0
Arterial oxygen saturation (%)	66.6	98.0
Pulmonary arterial mean pressure (mmHg)	62	24

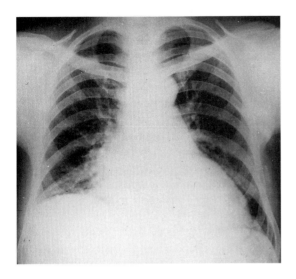
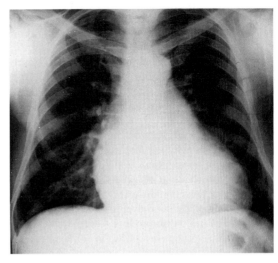

(a)   *(b)*

15.13 *(a) Anteroposterior radiograph of the chest in a man of 40 years with Monge's disease who resided at an altitude of 4330 m. There is cardiac enlargement and prominence of the pulmonary artery and vascular markings in the lung. (b) Anteroposterior radiograph of the chest from the patient in (a) after he had resided at sea level for 9 months. There is diminution in the size of the cardiac shadow.*

electrocardiographic indicators of right ventricular hypertrophy diminish. After residence at sea level for 2 months the heart rate, haematocrit, and haemoglobin level fall substantially; the arterial oxygen saturation increases and there is a sharp fall in the pulmonary arterial mean pressure (Table 15.1). There is a considerable decrease of circulating blood volume from a mean value of 175 to 120 ml/kg body weight (Hurtado 1942). This is largely due to lowering of the red cell volume. At the same time there is an increase in the plasma volume from just over 40 to 60 ml/kg body weight. This increase in plasma volume may be of aetiological significance in the development of high-altitude pulmonary oedema in native highlanders returning to the mountains after a period of residence at sea level, described in Chapters 13 and 33.

Patients who have had the disease relieved by residence at sea level not infrequently insist on returning to their mountain homes because of family reasons. When they do, symptomatology usually returns (Monge and Monge 1966).

PHLEBOTOMY

A distinction has to be made between normal and excessive high-altitude polycythaemia. Normal poly-

cythaemia is a well recognized feature of acclimatization to high altitude (Chapter 5). On the other hand, excessive polycythaemia carries with it disadvantages. As long ago as 1951 Newman *et al.* pointed out that, in polycythaemia rubrum vera, vital capacity and total lung volume are reduced and residual air is decreased, presumably because of the increased volume of blood in the chest. A reduction of haematocrit from 67.6 to 46% was achieved by repeated venesection in five subjects with the disease. They increased their maximal breathing capacity. In Monge's disease it would be anticipated that phlebotomy or haemodilution would lessen haematocrit and chest blood volume, and so increase the chest volume for gas exchange, increasing vital capacity and alveolar ventilation, with increase in lung elasticity. Cruz *et al.* (1979) reported the beneficial effects of phlebotomy on static lung function in all four native highlanders with chronic mountain sickness at La Oroya (3700 m). The results of phlebotomy and haemodilution on patients with chronic mountain sickness were reported by Winslow and Monge-C (1987). Improvement was assessed by enhancement of exercise testing. Over the 17-day period of study there was a striking fall in haematocrit and viscosity with a corresponding increased exercise performance. One subject reported that after reduction in haematocrit he slept much better and could concentrate on his work for the first time in years. In one subject a fall in haematocrit from 62 to 42% led to a fall in pulmonary arterial pressure from 40/30 to 23/15 mmHg. For details of the effects of phlebotomy or haemodilution in chronic mountain sickness, the reader is referred to Winslow and Monge-C (1987).

Oxygen is generally regarded as having no place in the treatment of Monge's disease, for it will achieve little more than a slight fall in pulmonary hypertension. However, Nath *et al.* (1983*b*) concluded that, as alveolar hypoventilation is the central problem in these cases, it should be overcome through wilful voluntary efforts at improving ventilation. They carried out a therapeutic trial in nine cases of chronic mountain sickness and two borderline cases in the Himalaya. This studied the somewhat exotic treatment of yogic deep-breathing exercises and acetazolamide, supported in seven subjects with oxygen inhalation. They reported a favourable response after a period of treatment lasting barely a month and agreed that further long-term and in-depth studies were required to evaluate the beneficial effects of deep breathing on chronic mountain sickness. Medroxyprogesterone acetate has been reported as an effective form of therapy in excessive polycythaemia of high altitude because of its stimulant effects on ventilation and tidal volume, and the resultant increase in arterial oxygen saturation (Kryger *et al.* 1978*a*). MPA led to a reduction of the haematocrit level from 60.1 to 52.1% after 10 weeks in 17 patients (Kryger *et al.* 1978*b*).

Monge's disease has to be sharply distinguished from the manifestations of failure to achieve initial acclimatization. In man these are the syndromes of infant and adult subacute mountain sickness (Chapter 17). In cattle the failure to achieve initial acclimatization is manifested by brisket disease (Chapter 16). In this next chapter we shall consider this condition in cattle where it will become clear that brisket disease is not a bovine form of Monge's disease.

References

Arias-Stella, J. (1971). Chronic mountain sickness: pathology and definition. In *High Altitude Physiology: Cardiac and Respiratory Aspects* Ciba Foundation Symposium (R. Porter and J. Knight, Eds). Edinburgh Churchill Livingstone p. 31 (See also the discussion on pp. 52–9

Arias-Stella, J., Krüger, H., and Recavarren, S. (1973). Pathology of chronic mountain sickness. *Thorax*, **28**, 701

Baldwin, F., Cournaud, A., and Richards, D.W. (1948). Pulmonary insufficiency. I. Physiological classification, clinical methods of analysis, standard values in normal subjects. *Medicine*, **27**, 243.

Bergofsky E.H. (1967). Cor pulmonale in the syndrome of alveolar hypoventilation. *Progress in Cardiovascular Diseases*, **9**, 414

Cruz, J.C., Diaz, C., Marticorena, E., and Hilario, V. (1979). Phlebotomy improves pulmonary gas exchange in chronic mountain sickness. *Respiration* **38**, 305

Fernan-Zegarra, L. and Lazo-Taboada, F. (1961). Mal de Montaña crónico. Consideraciones anatomopatológicas y referencias clinicas de un caso. *Revista Peruana de Patologia*, **6**, 49

Fishman, A.P., Turino, G.M., and Bergofsky, E.H. (1957). The syndrome of alveolar hypoventilation. *American Journal of Medicine*, **23**, 333

Hurtado, A. (1942). Chronic mountain sickness. *Journal of the American Medical Association*, **120**, 1278

Hurtado, A. (1955). Pathological aspects of life at high altitude. *Military Medicine*, **117**, 272

Hurtado, A. (1960). Some clinical aspects of life at high altitude. *Annals of Internal Medicine*, **53**, 247

Kryger, M., McCullough, R.E., Collins, D., Scoggin, C.H., Weil, J.V., and Grover, R.F. (1978*a*). Treatment of excessive polycythaemia of high altitude with respiratory stimulant drugs. *American Review of Respiratory Disease*, **117**, 455

Kryger, M., Weil, J., and Grover, R. (1978*b*). Chronic mountain polycythaemia: a disorder of the regulation of breathing during sleep? *Chest* (Suppl), **73**, 304

Monge-Cassinelli, C. (1966). Natural acclimatization to high altitudes: clinical conditions. In *Life at High Altitudes*, Scientific Publication No. 140. Washington; Pan American Health Organization, p. 46

Monge-Cassinelli, C., Lozano, R., and Carcelen, A. (1964). Renal excretion of bicarbonate in high altitude natives and in natives with chronic mountain sickness. *Journal of Clinical Investigation*, **43**, 2303

Monge-Medrano, C. (1928). La enfermedad de los Andes, sindromes eritremicos. *Anales de la Facultad de Medicina de Lima* **11**, 314

Monge-Medrano, C. (1943) Chronic mountain sickness. *Physiological Reviews*, **23**, 166

Monge-Medrano, C. and Monge-Cassinelli, C. (1966). High-altitude animal pathology. In *High Altitude Disease. Mechanism and Management.* Springfield, Illinois; Charles C. Thomas, p. 70

Nath, C.S., Kashyap, S.S., Grover, D.N., Durairaj, M., Kher, H.L., Narayanan, G.R., and Subramanian, A.R. (1983*a*). Clinical profile of chronic mountain sickness in the Himalayas. *Indian Heart Journal*, **35**, 288

Nath, C.S., Kashyap, S.S., and Subramanian, A.R. (1983*b*). Chronic mountain sickness — a therapeutic trial at high altitude. *Medical Journal of Armed Forces of India*, **39**, 131

Newman, W., Feltman, J.A., and Devlin, B. (1951). Pulmonary function studies in polycythemia vera. *American Journal of Cardiology*, **11**, 706

Pei, S.X., Chen, X.J., Si Ren, B.Z., Liu, Y.H., Cheng, X.S., Harris, E.M., Anand, I.S., and Harris, P.C. (1989). Chronic mountain sickness in Tibet. *Quarterly Journal of Medicine*, **NS 71**, 555

Peñaloza, D. and Sime F. (1971). Chronic cor pulmonale due to loss of altitude acclimatization (chronic mountain sickness). *American Journal of Medicine*, **50**, 728

Peñaloza, D., Sime F., and Ruiz, L. (1971). Cor pulmonale in chronic mountain sickness: present concept of Monge's disease. In *High Altitude Physiology: Cardiac and Respiratory Aspects*; Ciba Foundation Symposium (R. Porter and J. Knight, Eds). Edinburgh; Churchill Livingstone, p. 41

Reategui-López, L. (1969). Soroche crónico. Observaciones realisadas en la Cuzco en 30 casos. *Revista Peruana de Cardiologia*, **15**, 45

Recavarren, S. and Arias-Stella, J. (1964). Right ventricular hypertrophy in people born and living at high altitudes. *British Heart Journal*, **26**, 806

Richter, T., West, J.R., and Fishman, A.P. (1957). The syndrome of alveolar hypoventilation and diminished sensitivity of the respiratory center. *New England Journal of Medicine*, **256**, 1165

Rodman, T. and Close, H.P. (1959). The pulmonary hypoventilation syndrome. *American Journal of Medicine*, **26**, 808

Severinghaus, J.W., Bainton, C.R., and Carcelen, A. (1966). Respiratory insensitivity to hypoxia in chronically hypoxic man. *Respiration Physiology*, **1**, 308

Sime, F., Monge-Cassinelli, C., and Whittembury, J. (1975). Age as a cause of chronic mountain sickness. (Monge's disease). *International Journal of Biometeorology*, **19**, 93.

Sorbini, C.A., Grassi, V., Solinas, E., and Muiesan, G. (1968). Arterial oxygen tension in relation to age in healthy subjects. *Respiration*, **25**, 3

Whittembury, J. and Monge-Cassinelli, C. (1972). High altitude, haematocrit and age. *Nature (London)*, **238**, 278

Winslow, R.M. and Monge-Cassinelli, C. (1987). *Hypoxia, polycythemia, and chronic mountain sickness.* Baltimore and London; Johns Hopkins University Press

16

Brisket disease

In the previous chapter we have given an account of a disease directly attributable to hypobaric hypoxia that affects men of mean age of about 40 years after several years' residence at high altitude. Here we describe a disease of cattle that is also brought about by the effects of hypobaric hypoxia but with the important distinction that it involves calves on their first exposure to high altitude. The condition is of historical interest for it was first reported as long ago as 1915. It has more recently assumed a renewed theoretical interest in consideration of its relevance to Monge's disease (Chapter 15) and to infantile subacute mountain sickness (Chapter 17), which has become known to Western medical circles only during the last decade.

GEOGRAPHICAL LOCATION

The disease occurs in certain areas in the inter-mountain region of the USA, notably in Utah and Colorado (Hecht et al., 1959). For over a century it has been the custom of ranchers in this area to graze livestock during the summer months from July to October at altitudes ranging from 2500 to 3700 m (Hecht et al. 1962a). In Utah the disease is most prevalent in mountain ranges in two main regions. One comprises the southern slopes of the Uintah range and the other the western aspects of the Wasatch mountains (Hecht et al. 1959). The disease is generally regarded as being restricted to this region of the United States but Monge and Monge (1966) refer to the reports of Cuba-Caparó (1949, 1950) who described cases in lambs born in Peru. It should be noted, however, that these lambs showed prominent polycythaemia and an absence of oedema, neither of which are characteristic of brisket disease.

SPECIES INVOLVED

Apart from this isolated report of dubious validity from Peru, the disease has been described only in the European type of cattle (Bos taurus). It has been reported in Hereford cattle and also in the Holstein, Ayrshire, Angus, Shorthorn, Jersey, and Swiss breeds. The disease has not been seen in French Charolais cattle. As might be anticipated, species indigenous to high-altitude areas (Chapter 35) do not develop brisket disease. Thus Indian and African bovine species living respectively in the Himalaya and the highlands of Ethiopia tolerate high altitude well. The yak (B. grunniens) of the Himalaya and the Tibetan plateau is also resistant to the disease. Although the American buffalo is an animal of the plains, a herd of this species lives without difficulty at 3000 m in Utah (Hecht et al. 1962a).

CLINICAL FEATURES

In 1915 reports began to appear in the literature describing the occurence of a fatal disease in cattle characterized by systemic oedema (Newsom 1915; Glover and Newsom 1915, 1917, 1918). The oedema found in the condition is so severe that Hecht et al. (1962a) believe it unlikely that cases occuring before 1915 would have been overlooked and this leads them to consider whether it may have made its first appearance in 1915. According to Hecht et al. (1962a), the incidence of the disease in cattle has varied from herd to herd, from year to year, and from location to location. Brisket disease develops mostly in calves brought to high altitude for the first time but it may occur in young animals born in the highlands. The condition may occur in adult cattle, in which it tends to run a protracted course (Hecht et al. 1959); 1–5% of the animals in affected herds may be involved.

There is intense dyspnoea, so that the animal is unable to tolerate even mild exertion. Even if the animal survives grazing, the excitement of round-up may lead to death. The mucous membranes are cyanosed. The affected calf has a rough coat and its head is lowered with droopy ears (Hecht et al. 1962a). A foul-smelling diarrhoea, termed 'scours', is common. In the later stages of the disease there is oedema of the dependent parts of the trunk. It occurs particularly in the region between the forelegs and the neck, the 'brisket' of commerce, and hence the condition is commonly referred to as 'brisket

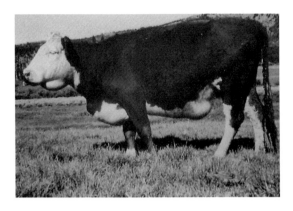

16.1 *Brisket disease. There is oedema between the forelegs and the neck (the 'brisket' of commerce) and associated oedema of the lower jaw.*

disease' (Fig.16.1). Associated oedema of the lower jaw may give the affected animal an appearance reminiscent of mumps. There is no oedema of the legs. Commonly the systemic oedema is accompanied by pleural effusions and ascites. The jugular veins are distended and there is commonly a pronounced systolic wave indicative of triscuspid incompetence. The breath sounds are vesicular. On auscultation of the heart there is accentuation of the second sound in the pulmonary area. There is commonly a loud, low-pitched systolic murmur in the apical region consistent with tricuspid incompetence. Frequently, there is a presystolic apical gallop. In summary, these are the features of congestive cardiac failure with tricuspid incompetence secondary to pulmonary arterial hypertension.

AETIOLOGICAL FACTORS

The important factor in the aetiology of the pulmonary hypertension is almost certainly the impact of the hypobaric hypoxia of high altitude on the pulmonary vasculature, comparable to but not identical with that described for the human lung in Chapter 10. As early as 1918, Glover and Newsom stated: 'We, therefore, have no hesitancy in concluding that the malady is due to failure of acclimatization at high altitudes.' Hecht *et al.* (1962*a*) and Reeves *et al.* (1960) also accept that influences inherent in high altitude bring about pulmonary arterial hypertension and right ventricular failure.

Other subsidiary factors may be the daily salt intake and the vegetation eaten by the grazing cattle. The areas in which the disease occurs are studded with small water pools and creeks and, in addition,

large troughs containing salt are spaced at irregular intervals. Affected cattle are likely to have ingested an excess of salt and it is conceivable that this may play some part in the development of the condition (Hecht *et al.* 1962*a*). The vegetation in the area of Utah in which the disease is found comprises salt grass, marsh marigolds, ranunculus, and groundsell but analysis of the flora has not revealed any toxic alkaloids (Hecht *et al.* 1959).

Cold exposure may be an additive stress to hypoxia in the causation of brisket disease (Bligh 1987). He reports that Chauca (1978) transported six calves from sea level to Huancayo (3300 m) in Peru. Here the animals were divided into a group kept outdoors in the cold, and another kept indoors at an ambient temperature of 20°C. Symptoms of brisket disease developed only in the outdoor animals. When these calves were moved indoors into a thermoneutral temperature, the disease disappeared. Bligh (1987) suggests that the addition of cold stress will increase the incidence or severity of brisket disease in cattle.

THE NORMAL BOVINE PULMONARY VASCULATURE

Cattle appear to be peculiarly susceptible to hypoxia because, as a family characteristic, they have such a muscular pulmonary vasculature with extremely thick-walled small pulmonary arteries and pulmonary arterioles with a naturally muscular medial coat. The ranges of medial thickness in different age groups at sea level have been found to be as follows: for fetuses, 21.1–24.5%; for calves 1 day to 3 months of age, 13.4%–22.6%; and for cattle over 1 year of age, 6.2–16.4% (Wagenvoort and Wagenvoort 1969; see Fig. 16.2).Earlier in a histological study of the pulmonary blood vessels in a wide range of species, Best and Heath (1961) pointed out that the percentage medial thickness of the bovine small pulmonary artery sometimes exceeds 20%, compared with 5% in man. The pulmonary arterioles normally show muscularization and the walls of the pulmonary veins show discontinuous muscular beading. Alexander (1962) confirmed our findings, noting that in cattle normal muscularization is found in pulmonary arterioles as small as 20 μm in diameter. He suggested that the muscle in the walls of the pulmonary veins was arranged in a spiral manner. Some years later we found that the pulmonary vasculature in two bulls and a cow from Cerro de Pasco (4330 m) in the Peruvian Andes was very muscular, but we were unable to conclude if this was an abnormal reaction

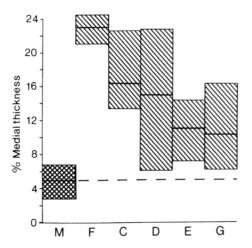

16.2 *The percentage medial thickness of pulmonary arteries in man and cattle. (Based on data from Heath and Best (1958) and Wagenvoort and Wagenvoort (1969.).) m, Adult human pulmonary arteries; f, fetal cattle; c, calves: 1 day to 3 months; d, calves: 9 months; e, calves: 1 year; g, cattle: more than 1 year. In each column the central bar is the mean value. The horizontal interrupted line is the mean value for the normal adult human lung.*

to hypobaric hypoxia because of the normal muscularity of the pulmonary blood vessels in cattle.

The implications of this innate muscularity of the pulmonary arterial tree on pulmonary haemodynamics in cattle are clear. Thus, the data of Will *et al.* (1962) and Reeves *et al.* (1962) show that, while the range of pulmonary arterial and wedge pressure in normal cattle is comparable to normal values in man, it tends to rise sharply on hypoxic stimulation. The muscular nature of bovine pulmonary arterioles renders them hyperreactive to the ambient hypobaric hypoxia of high altitude. Will *et al.* (1962) showed that, when 10 steers born at an altitude of 1100 m were taken up to 3050 m, six showed an elevation of pulmonary arterial pressure from 27 to 45 mmHg. The remaining four animals developed more severe pulmonary hypertension and in two instances the mean pressure exceeded 100 mmHg. In such steers there is no significant increase in cardiac output or blood volume and there is no elevation of pulmonary wedge pressure. It is thus clear that pulmonary hypertension is the result of increased pulmonary vascular resistance, and the relief afforded by oxygen administration confirms this.

Pulmonary arterial blood pressure in cattle increases with age at high altitude but not at sea level. The studies of Will *et al.* (1975) on 195 cattle confirm that, while hypoxia of high altitude elevates the pulmonary arterial pressure in all cattle, it takes weeks or months in newcomers to the mountain but years in native highland cattle. Such resistant and susceptible traits are probably genetically determined. Calves susceptible to the development of pulmonary hypertension die or are transported to low altitude before producing offspring. Hence cattle remaining at high altitude have a tendency to have a lower pulmonary arterial pressure. This would explain why less than 2% of the native cattle living in the mountains of Colorado develop brisket disease, whereas at the same altitudes up to 40% or more of the cattle native to low altitude develop the condition.

GENETIC FACTORS INFLUENCING THE DEVELOPMENT OF PULMONARY HYPERTENSION IN CATTLE AT HIGH ATTITUDE

Susceptibility or resistance to the development of pulmonary hypertension at high altitude in cattle is influenced by genetic factors. Weir *et al.* (1974) measured the pulmonary arterial pressure in 49 apparently healthy cattle kept at an elevation at 3000 m in Colorado. Two groups were selected from this herd for study. One consisted of the 15 animals with the lowest pulmonary arterial pressure; they were designated as 'resistant' to the development of pulmonary hypertension. A second group consisted of 10 animals with clinical evidence of brisket disease; they were regarded as 'susceptible' to pulmonary hypertension. Both groups were taken down to an altitude of 1500 m where the susceptible animals recovered. The animals within each group were bred and the first-generation offspring were studied at low and high altitudes. Pulmonary vascular resistance increased to a much greater extent in the offspring of the susceptible group at high altitude. This suggested that the susceptible and resistant groups were genetically different.

The second-generation offspring of the original susceptible and resistant groups were then studied similarly. After 2 weeks at 3400 m the mean pulmonary arterial pressure in the susceptible animals virtually doubled from 23 to 44 mmHg with a corresponding rise in pulmonary vascular resistance. On the other hand, the increase in pulmonary arterial pressure in the resistant animals from 28 to 32 mmHg was minimal. The difference increased still further after a further 2 weeks. These observations support the hypothesis that genetic factors are important in determining the magnitude of the tendency towards pulmonary hypertension in cattle at high altitude.

The mechanism of susceptibility is obscure. Pulmonary vascular hyperreactivity does not seem to be the distinguishing feature since prostaglandin $F_{2\alpha}$, a potent pulmonary vasoconstrictor, exerts the same effect in susceptible and resistant cattle. Cattle prone to develop pulmonary hypertension appeared to hypoventilate compared with the resistant cattle and hence could have been subjected to a more severe hypoxic stimulus (Weir *et al.* 1974). Further evidence to support this view comes from the fact that susceptible cattle had a significantly greater increase in haematocrit than did the resistant animals, implying a greater hypoxic stimulus to erythropoiesis in the former.

THE PULMONARY VASCULATURE IN BRISKET DISEASE

Alexander (1962) carried out post-mortem angiography on the lungs of calves that had died from brisket disease and found a 'tree-pruning effect' due to restriction of the peripheral pulmonary arterial tree due to vasoconstriction. He carried out histological studies on the pulmonary vasculature in 24 cases of the condition and found increased hypertrophy of the naturally muscular pulmonary arteries (Fig. 16.3) and pulmonary arterioles (Fig. 16.4) in most. There was no associated occlusive disease of the intima.

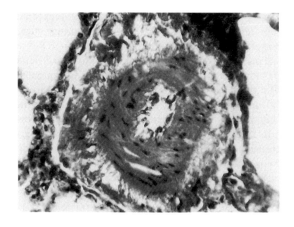

16.3 *Transverse section of small pulmonary artery from a calf suffering from brisket disease in the Wasatch mountains in Utah, USA. The medial coat is very thick and muscular.*

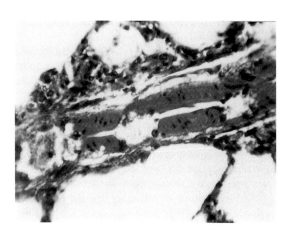

16.4 *Longitudinal section of pulmonary arteriole from the same calf as in the preceding figure. The arteriole has a thick muscular coat.*

He was also able to study the pulmonary blood vessels in 10 yearling Hereford steers that were taken to 3050 m. All developed pulmonary hypertension. In six it was moderate and there was no medial hypertrophy of the small pulmonary arteries. In the remaining four it was severe, and in three of them there was hypertrophy of the pulmonary arteries beyond normal muscularization.

REVERSIBILITY

In brisket disease right ventricular hypertrophy follows the pulmonary vascular changes of muscularity without intimal proliferation (Alexander and Jensen 1959; Hecht *et al.* 1959). The only intimal changes found are those of minor intimal mineralization and thrombotic changes. This being so, one would anticipate that the elevated pulmonary arterial pressure of brisket disease would be reversed on descent from high altitude with relief from hypoxic pulmonary vasoconstriction. This is precisely what is found. When calves with acute brisket disease are brought down from their summer grazing ranges in the mountains to Salt Lake City at an altitude of 1370 m, their clinical abnormalities disappear in 4–6 weeks (Kuida *et al.* 1963). At the same time there is a pronounced fall in their pulmonary arterial pressure. Thus, when haemodynamic studies were made on 14 calves that recovered from brisket disease, the mean pulmonary arterial pressure was found to have halved from 63 to 32 mmHg. Pulmonary vascular resistance, right atrial pressure, and pulmonary wedge pressure all fell on recovery at the lower altitude.

TRAINING EFFECT OF HIGH ALTITUDE ON CATTLE

There is some evidence that residence in mountainous regions may induce a beneficial exercise conditioning in cattle in contrast to the deleterious effects of brisket disease. Hays (1976) studied two groups of cattle, one kept in an alpine pasture (1700–2600 m) for 5 months, the other at 400 m. Subsequently both were subjected to treadmill exercise at a simulated altitude of 3500 m. After exercise the heart rates in the alpine cattle were 10 to 20 beats per minute slower than in the valley cattle. This was interpreted as indicating that the 5 months' residence in the alpine zone had exerted a training effect on the animals.

LEFT VENTRICULAR FUNCTION IN BRISKET DISEASE

Left ventricular function is impaired in brisket disease (Hecht *et al.* 1962*b*). Calves with the condition frequently show elevated pulmonary arterial wedge, and left atrial and left ventricular end diastolic pressures. Hecht and his colleagues consider a number of possible explanations for this. They reject the idea that in brisket disease the expansion of the left ventricle might be impaired by the confining restrictions of the pericardium or pericardial fluid. Arterial hypoxaemia is not a striking feature of brisket disease and in itself is unlikely to be a cause of left ventricular failure. No gross pulmonary disease leading to the development of bronchopulmonary anastomoses can be implicated as a cause of left ventricular enlargement. There is excessive fluid retention in brisket disease and it may be that interstitial oedema of the myocardium leads to impairment of left ventricular function. Finally, impairment and overstretching of myocardial fibres in the left ventricle due to anatomical continuity between the right and left ventricular muscle has been suggested.

MONGE'S DISEASE AND BRISKET DISEASE

It is clear from this and the preceding chapter that brisket disease is not a bovine form of Monge's disease. Human chronic mountain sickness is an affliction of men of around 40 years of age, depending on the elevation of their domicile, who have been living at high altitude for many years. In contrast, brisket disease is a condition of genetically predisposed young calves (Table 17.1). Monge's disease is essentially respiratory in nature, where the alveolar hypoventilation leads to an exaggeration of systemic arterial oxygen unsaturation, resulting in a greatly raised haematorcrit and moderate pulmonary hypertension that rarely leads to congestive cardiac failure. In contrast, the bovine disease is cardiovascular rather than respiratory in origin (Table 17.1). In brisket disease, arterial oxygen saturation is not greatly impaired, Hecht *et al.* (1959) quote a range of 78–94% with a mean value of 87%. As a result the haematorcrit is not raised, being in the range of 30–45%. Hypercapnia is not present. The basis of brisket disease is rather a hyperreactivity of the pulmonary arterial tree to hypobaric hypoxia, bringing about a much increased pulmonary vascular resistance leading to congestive cardiac failure (Table 17.1).

In summary, Monge's disease represents *a loss of long-established acclimatization* in contrast to brisket disease which is *a failure to achieve initial acclimatization*. This immediately raises the fascinating question as to whether there is a human counterpart of brisket disease. There is in fact such a condition and this missing link is to be found in Tibet. We consider it in Chapter 17.

PULMONARY ARTERIAL PRESSOR RESPONSE IN VARIOUS SPECIES AT HIGH ALTITUDE

Not all mammalian species respond in the same way as cattle to the hypoxia of high altitude. Tucker *et al.* (1975) found that there were great differences in the pulmonary arterial pressor response, as indicated by the percentage increase in right ventricular systolic pressure, in seven species exposed to a barometric pressure of 435 mmHg for periods ranging from 19 to 42 days (Fig. 16.5). Calves and pigs were very responsive to hypoxia but dogs, guinea-pigs, and sheep showed little or no response.

The lung structure and respiratory system of birds are considerably different from those of mammals. The greatest difference is the mechanism to maintain the distended state of the lungs. In the mammalian lung this is brought about by a subatmospheric pressure in the pleural cavity but in birds it is due to normal lung tissue adhesions in the rib cage. Hence the pulmonary circulation is independent of changes in the intrathoracic pressure (Burton *et al.* 1968). Nevertheless the chicken responds to high altitude by a consistent pulmonary arterial hypertension. It is quantitatively less than that found in cattle but the pressor response is twice that found in rabbits (Fig. 16.6). The right ventricular hypertrophy in healthy chickens at high altitude may lead to congestive cardiac failure (Olander *et al.* 1967). Burton *et al.*

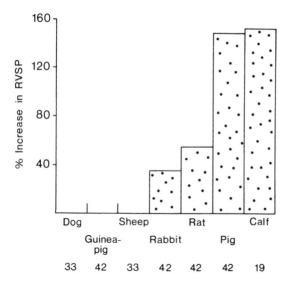

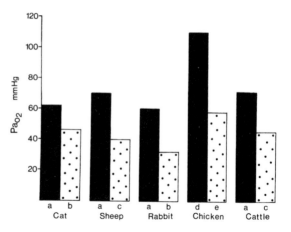

16.5 *The percentage increase in right ventricular systolic pressure in seven species exposed to a barometric pressure of 435 mmHg for periods ranging from 19 to 42 days (indicated in each instance at the foot of the column). (Based on data from Tucker* et al. *(1975).)*

16.7 *The effect of altitude on* Pa_{O_2} *in various animal species. The altitudes and sources of data are as in Fig. 16.6.*

sociated right ventricular hypertrophy. Inhalation of 95% oxygen and 5% carbon dioxide for 10 minutes had no effect on the pulmonary hypertension. Acute hypoxia produces pulmonary hypertension in sea-level chicken but this regresses within 2 days after return to sea level (Burton *et al.* 1968). These data are more consistent with the view that hypoxia exerts a direct effect on the vascular smooth muscle of the terminal portions of the pulmonary arterial tree than with the concept that intrathoracic and alveolar pressure may affect the patency of pulmonary blood vessels. The effect of altitude on Pa_{O_2} in various animal species is shown in Fig.16.7 for comparison with the pressor response seen in the same species.

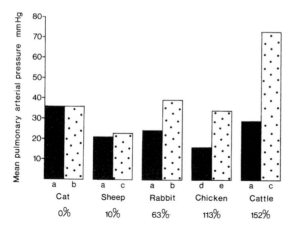

16.6 *The pressor response of the pulmonary arterial tree to hypoxia at high altitude in various animal species. Altitudes: a, 1585 m; b, 4315 m; c, 3870 m; d, 0 m; e, 3810 m. Data on cat and rabbit are systolic right ventricular blood pressures and from Reeves* et al. *(1963a). Data on cattle from Grover* et al. *(1963). Data on sheep from Reeves* et al. *(1963b). Data on chicken from Burton* et al. *(1968).*

References

Alexander, A.F. (1962). The bovine lung: normal vascular histology and vascular lesions in high mountain disease. *Medicina Thoracalis*, **19**, 528

Alexander, A.F. and Jensen, R. (1959). Gross cardiac changes in cattle with high mountain (brisket) disease and in experimental cattle maintained at high altitudes. *American Journal of Veterinary Research*, **20**, 680

Best, P.V. and Heath, D. (1961). Interpretation of the appearances of the small pulmonary blood vessels in animals. *Circulation Research*, **9**, 288

Bligh, J. (1987). The additive stresses of hypoxia and cold exposure: brisket disease in cattle. In *Hypoxia and Cold* (J.R., Sutton, C.S., Houston, and G. Coates Ed.). New York; Praeger, p. 178

(1968) found that White Leghorn chickens hatched and living at 3810 m had pulmonary arterial pressure about twice that found at sea level (34.2 mmHg as contrasted to 15.7 mmHg at sea level). There was as-

Burton, R.R., Besch, E.L., and Smith, A.H. (1968). Effect of chronic hypoxia on the pulmonary arterial blood pressure of the chicken. *American Journal of Physiology*, **214**, 1438

Chauca, D. (1978). Physiological Adaptation of Farm Animals to Natural Environments. Unpublished, Ph.D. thesis, University of Cambridge.

Cuba-Caparó, A. (1949). Policitemia de la Altura en corderos. *Revista De La Facultad de Medicina Veterinaria, Universidad Nacional Mayor De San Marcos*, **4**, 4

Cuba-Caparó, A. (1950). Policitemia y mal de montana en corderos. Unpublished D. Phil. thesis, Facultad de Medicina, Lima

Glover, G.H. and Newsom, I.E. (1915). Brisket disease (dropsy at high altitude). *Colorado Agricultural Experimental Station Bulletin*, **204**

Glover, G.H. and Newsom, I.E. (1917). Brisket disease. *Colorado Agricultural Experimental Station Bulletin*, **229**

Glover, G.H. and Newsom, I.E. (1918). Further studies on brisket disease. *Journal of Agricultural Research*, **15**, 409

Grover, R.F. Reeves, J.T., Will, D.H., and Blount, S.G. Jr. (1963). Pulmonary vasoconstriction in steers at high altitude. *Journal of Applied Physiology*, **18**, 567

Hays, F.L. (1976). Alp and valley cattle: exercise in cold, hot and high environments. *Pflügers Archiv*, **362**, 185

Heath, D. and Best, P.V. (1958). The tunica media of the arteries of the lung in pulmonary hypertension. *Journal of Pathology and Bacteriology*, **76**, 165

Hecht, H.H., Lange, R.L., Carnes, W.H., Kuida, H., and Blake, J.T. (1959). Brisket disease. I. General aspects of pulmonary hypertensive heart disease in cattle. *Transactions of the Association of American Physicians*, **72**, 157

Hecht, H.H. Kuida, H., Lange, R.L., Thorne, J.L., and Brown, A.M. (1962*a*). Brisket disease. II. Clinical features and hemodynamic observations in altitude-dependent right heart failure of cattle. *American Journal of Medicine*, **32**, 171

Hecht, H.H. Kuida, H., and Tsagaris, T.J. (1962*b*). Brisket disease. IV. Impairment of left ventricular function in a form of cor pulmonale. *Transactions of the Association of American Physicians*, **75**, 263

Kuida, H., Hecht, H.H., Lange, R.L., Brown, A.M., Tsagaris, T.J., and Thorne, J.L. (1963). Brisket

disease. III. Spontaneous remission of pulmonary hypertension and recovery from heart failure. *Journal of Clinical Investigation*, **42**, 589

Monge-M,C. and Monge-C,C. (1966). In *High Altitude Diseases. Mechanism and Management*. Springfield, Illinois; Charles C. Thomas, p.70

Newsom, I.E. (1915). Cardiac insufficiency at high altitude. *American Journal of Veterinary Medicine*, **10**, 890

Olander, H.J., Burton, R.R., and Adler, H.E. (1967). The pathophysiology of chronic hypoxia in chickens. *Avian Diseases*, **11**, 609

Reeves, J.T., Grover, R.F., Blount, S.G., Alexander, A.F., and Gill, D. (1960). Altitude as a stress to the pulmonary circulation of steers. *Clinical Research*, **8**, 138

Reeves, J.T., Grover, R.F., Will, D.H., and Alexander, A.F. (1962). Hemodynamics in normal cattle. *Circulation Research*, **10**, 166

Reeves, J.T., Grover, E.B., and Grover, R.F. (1963*a*). Circulatory responses to high altitude in the cat and rabbit. *Journal of Applied Physiology*, **18**, 575

Reeves, J.T., Grover, E.B., and Grover, R.F. (1963*b*). Pulmonary circulation and oxygen transport in lambs at high altitude. *Journal of Applied Physiology*, **18**, 560

Tucker, A., McMurty, I.F., Reeves, J.T., Alexander, A.F., Will, D.H., and Grover, R.F. (1975). Lung vascular smooth muscle as a determinant of pulmonary hypertension at high altitude. *American Journal of Physiology*, **228**, 762

Wagenvoort, C.A. and Wagenvoort, N. (1969). The pulmonary vasculature in normal cattle at sea level at different ages. *Pathologia Europeaea*, **4**, 265

Weir, E.K., Tucker, A., Reeves, J.T., Will, D.H., and Grover, R.F. (1974). The genetic factor influencing pulmonary hypertension in cattle at high altitude. *Cardiovascular Research*, **8**, 745

Will, D.H. Alexander, A.F., Reeves, J.T., and Grover, R.F. (1962). High-altitude-induced pulmonary hypertension in normal cattle. *Circulation Research*, **10**, 172

Will, D.H., Horrel, J.F., Reeves, J.T., and Alexander, A.F. (1975). Influence of altitude and age on pulmonary arterial pressure in cattle. *Proceedings of the Society for Experimental Biology and Medicine* **150**, 564

17

Infantile and adult subacute mountain sickness

We have already seen in this book that there are two well-known clinical syndromes associated with high altitude. The first is acute mountain sickness (Chapter 12) with its serious variants, high-altitude pulmonary oedema (Chapter 13) and cerebral mountain sickness (Chapter 14). This syndrome occurs within a few hours or days of arrival at high altitude. The second is chronic mountain sickness (Monge's disease), which develops gradually after a number of years' residence there (Chapter 15). In recent years it has become apparent that there are also two forms of subacute mountain sickness, which occur after an exposure of weeks or months to hypobaric hypoxia. One form occurs in infants and the other in young adults. Both reports have come from the Himalayan region. In both syndromes the symptoms begin on initial exposure to high altitude and appear to represent a failure to develop acclimatization. Infantile subacute mountain sickness appears to be the human counterpart of brisket disease in calves (Chapter 16).

INFANTILE SUBACUTE MOUNTAIN SICKNESS

During an expedition to Tibet in 1987 Professors Harris and Anand came across a new form of mountain sickness that is distinct from both the acute and chronic varieties (Heath 1989). This was familiar to their Chinese and Tibetan hosts but it was unknown to Western medicine, reference to it having been previously made only in the Chinese literature (Li 1983). The appearance of the disease seemed to be the consequence of demographic changes in the community. As a consequence of the policy of the Chinese government there has been extensive immigration of lowlanders of Han origin from lowland China to high altitude in Tibet. Thus the capital, Lhasa (3600 m), has come to have a mixed population of native Tibetan highlanders and Han lowlanders. In this way the authorities unwittingly set the scene for a great biological experiment at high altitude by admixing two biologically distinct populations. Since the new and often fatal disease affected infants and manifested itself over a period of weeks and months rather than days or years it came to be designated as 'subacute infantile mountain sickness' (Sui *et al.* 1988). Its relation to other forms of mountain sickness has proven to be of considerable theoretical interest. Since the nature of this disease has become apparent as the result of recent studies, the necessary steps have been taken to prevent new cases and the incidence of the disease has already decreased considerably.

CLINICAL FEATURES

The studies of Sui *et al.* (1988) were carried out on necropsy material from 15 infants and children at the People's Hospital, Lhasa, Tibet at an altitude of 3600 m. All were of Han origin except one who was Tibetan. Ten were male. Their ages ranged from 3 to 16 months the average being 9 months. Thirteen had been born at low altitude and had been brought subsequently to live at Lhasa. Two had been born at high altitude — a Tibetan boy (16 months) and a Han girl (14 months) — and had remained there since birth. The average duration spent at Lhasa by the entire group was 4.7 months and by the lowland infants was 2.1 months.

Most of the patients had been brought to hospital because of dyspnoea and cough. Other common symptoms were sleeplessness and irritability, cyanosis, oedema of the face, and oliguria. The salient features on clinical examination were tachypnoea, tachycardia, enlargement of the liver, and rales in the lungs. Many infants were febrile. The heart was often thought clinically to be enlarged and the chest radiograph characteristically showed cardiac enlargement. The haemoglobin was recorded in three cases and was not increased (11, 8, and 8 g/dl). The red cell count was recorded in five cases and was also not increased, ranging from 3.2 to 4.5×10^{12}/l. Subsequent data from the post-mortems on these infants suggested that the clinical features were the result of right ventricular enlargement and congestive heart failure secondary to pulmonary hypertension.

MORBID ANATOMY

The pathological examination of the heart and pulmonary vasculature in these 15 infants was quantitative to establish clearly the morbid anatomy and pulmonary vascular pathology of this disease. For these reasons it was deemed necessary to compare the findings at necropsy in affected patients with measurements from non-cardiopulmonary diseases in Lhasa. The control group consisted of 19 infants and young children of Tibetan origin. There were eight males and 11 females. Their ages ranged from 2 months to 3 years and the average age was 9.5 months (± 9.0 SD). All except three (aged 2, 2, and 3 years) were within the first year of life.

In infantile subacute mountain sickness the right ventricle shows severe hypertrophy with pronounced dilatation of the pulmonary trunk (Fig. 17.1). There is also some hypertrophy of the left ventricle.

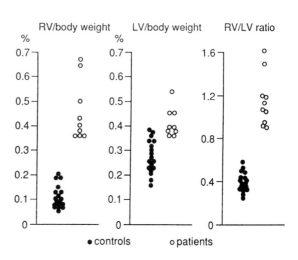

17.2 *Ratios of right ventricular and left ventricular weights to body weight and of right-to-left ventricular weight. Patients shown by open circles; controls by closed circles.*

Weighing of the individual cardiac ventricles and of the body confirmed increased RV/body weight, LV/body weight, and RV/LV ratios (Fig. 17.2).

PULMONARY VASCULAR DISEASE

The right ventricular hypertrophy in this condition is secondary to pulmonary vascular disease, which involves pulmonary arteries, arterioles, and venules. In normal Tibetan infants over the age of 4 months and up to the age of 2 years the small pulmonary arteries are thin-walled (Fig. 17.3) and the pulmonary arterioles have thin walls consisting of single elastic laminae (Fig. 17.3). In striking contrast, in infants with subacute mountain sickness both the pulmonary arteries (Fig. 17.4) and pulmonary arterioles (Fig. 17.5) are very muscular. The arteries show pronounced crenation of thickened elastic laminae around the hypertrophied media suggestive of vasoconstriction (Fig. 17.4). The adventitia is thick with undulating coarse strands of collagen. The arterioles have a thick media composed of circularly arranged smooth muscle cells sandwiched between distinct inner and outer elastic laminae (Fig. 17.5). The adventitia is greatly thickened by collagen fibres.

In one case of infantile subacute mountain sickness we saw a proliferation of spindle-shaped cells from the intima of the pulmonary arterioles (Fig. 17.6). These cells were elongated in the longitudinal axis of the vessel and gave a yellowish tinctorial reaction with Van Gieson's stain. Although electron

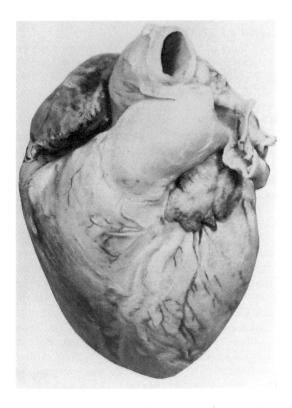

17.1 *Heart of a Tibetan infant aged 16 months with infantile subacute mountain sickness who failed to acclimatize to the hypobaric hypoxia of high altitude at Llasa (3600 m) and died in congestive cardiac failure. There is severe right ventricular hypertrophy and dilatation of the pulmonary trunk.*

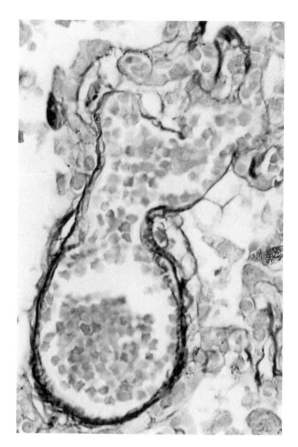

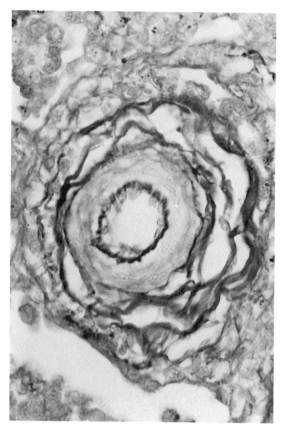

17.3 *Thin-walled pulmonary artery from a child of 2 years, dying in Lhasa from causes other than those associated with hypobaric hypoxia. In one arc there is a very thin media bounded by inner and outer elastic laminae. Much of the circumference of the artery is formed by a thickened and blurred elastic lamina. The arteriole arising from this vessel is distended and has a wall composed of a single elastic lamina. E VG, × 1000.*

17.4 *Transverse section of a small pulmonary artery from a Tibetan infant of 11 months with subacute mountain sickness. There is severe medial hypertrophy and fibrous thickening of the adventitia but no intimal proliferation. E VG, × 1000.*

microscopy was not carried out on the lung, it was thought on histological grounds that the proliferated cells were muscle cells. In this case there was also intimal proliferation in the pulmonary veins and venules (Fig. 17.7). This led to prominent cellular masses protruding into the lumen and producing significant venous obstruction. Scattered throughout the lung were focal collections of haemosiderin-laden macrophages.

THE NATURE OF INFANTILE SUBACUTE MOUNTAIN SICKNESS

The presence of severe hypertrophy and dilatation of the right ventricle with dilatation of the pulmonary

trunk in the absence of pulmonary stenosis in this disease leaves little doubt that the patients die from the results of severe pulmonary arterial hypertension. The histopathological findings demonstrate that the basis for the elevation of pulmonary arterial pressure is pulmonary vascular disease rather than pathological changes in the lung parenchyma. The vascular disease is largely muscular in nature, comprising medial hypertrophy of the small pulmonary arteries and muscularization of the pulmonary arterioles.

In Table 17.1 a comparison is made between the features of Monge's disease in Andean highlanders, brisket disease in cattle, and infantile subacute mountain sickness in Han infants in Tibet. It is clear that the disease of Chinese infants in Lhasa is the human counterpart of brisket disease in cattle. Like

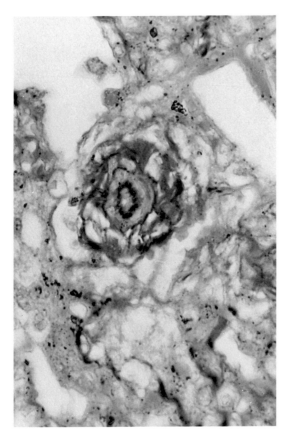

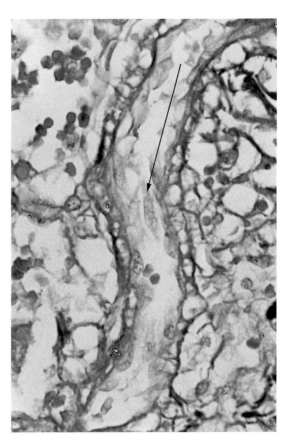

17.5 *Transverse section of muscularized pulmonary arteriole from the same case as in Fig. 17.4. There is a very thick muscular media sandwiched between the elastic laminae, the inner of which is particularly thick. E VG, × 1000.*

17.6 *Longitudinal section of a pulmonary arteriole from a male infant of 16 months, of the Han race, who died from subacute infantile mountain sickness at Lhasa (3600 m). Elongated smooth muscle cells line the vessel and some have migrated into the lumen. E VG, × 1000.*

the bovine disease it appears to represent a failure to achieve an initial acclimatization to the hypobaric hypoxia of high altitude. The disease is clearly distinguished from both acute and chronic mountain sickness. Chronic mountain sickness afflicts adults, usually in middle age, after they have been resident at high altitude for at least several years. It is characterized by severe polycythaemia, while patients with infantile subacute mountain sickness have a normal or even reduced red cell count and haemoglobin content. Acute mountain sickness, on the other hand, manifests itself within a few hours or days of arrival at high altitude and is uncommon in infants, perhaps because they do not undertake the exercise that seems to be a strong factor in its causation.

PULMONARY ENDOCRINE CELLS

In one case of infantile subacute mountain sickness occurring in a male infant of 16 months of the Han race we were able to study the pulmonary endocrine cells (Heath *et al.* 1989). Gastrin-releasing peptide (analogous to the bombesin of amphibian skin) and calcitonin were readily identified by the use of antisera but leucine-enkephalin and serotonin could not be detected. Labelled cells were conspicuous in being aggregated into irregular, enlarged clusters of up to 20 cells in the case of calcitonin (Fig. 17.8) and from two to eight cells in the case of bombesin (Fig. 17.9). The clusters of pulmonary endocrine cells were disorganized so that they did not resemble those seen in the lungs of normal human infants. The pulmonary endocrine cells were confined to

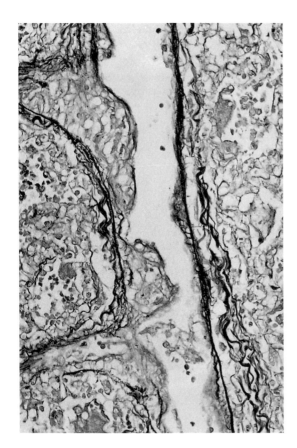

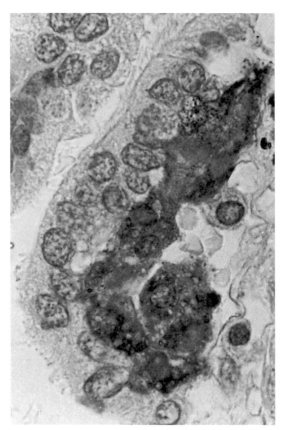

17.7 *Longitudinal section of pulmonary vein from the same case. There is a prominent proliferation of cells from the intima considered to be myofibroblasts. E VG, × 375.*

17.8 *A large cluster of calcitonin-containing pulmonary endocrine cells in a bronchiole in a case of infantile subacute mountain sickness in a male Han infant of 16 months. Peroxidase–anti-peroxidase anti-calcitonin, × 1500.*

bronchioles. In addition to the enhanced size of the clusters, the numbers of clusters and solitary immunoreactive cells were increased. Quantitative studies revealed 98 bombesin-containing cells and 31 immunoreactive for calcitonin per cm^2 of sectional area of lung.

In this infant there was considerable migration of vascular smooth muscle cells into the intima and lumen of both pulmonary arterioles (Fig. 17.6) and pulmonary veins (Fig. 17.7). There was no increase in neuroendocrine cells in the lungs of eight other cases of subacute infantile mountain sickness that were examined. This suggests that the increase in number of peptide-rich cells may be stimulated by free migration of vascular smooth muscle cells from the media into the intima and lumen of pulmonary blood vessels. The same association is found in plexogenic pulmonary arteriopathy where the heightened

levels of bombesin-containing pulmonary endocrine cells are found in the presence of cellular plexiform lesions but are at their greatest in the pre-plexiform stage when migration of vascular smooth muscle cells is most active (Heath *et al.* 1990). In contrast, increased numbers of pulmonary endocrine cells immunoreactive for bombesin are not found in mestizos and Aymaras of the Bolivian Andes in whom there is but limited migration of vascular smooth muscle cells to form a layer of longitudinal muscle in the intima (Williams *et al.* 1993; Chapter 10, this volume).

A REFLECTION FROM HISTORY

The rarity of infantile subacute mountain sickness in native Tibetan highland infants implies that the resident population in Lhasa enjoys the same genetic

Table 17.1 Comparison between Monge's disease in Andean highlanders, brisket disease in cattle, and infantile subacute mountain sickness in Han infants in Tibet

Criterion	Monge's disease	Brisket disease	Infantile subacute mountain sickness
Age of subject	Middle-aged men	Calves	Infants
Nature of exposure to high altitude	After prolonged exposure	On acute exposure	On subacute exposure
Acclimatization status	Loss of established acclimatization	Failure of initial acclimatization	Failure of initial acclimatization
Basic mechanism	Alveolar hypoventilation	Hyperreactivity of muscular pulmonary vasculature	Hyperreactivity of muscular pulmonary vasculature
Form of syndrome	Respiratory	Cardiovascular	Cardiovascular
Unsaturation of systemic arterial blood	Pronounced	Slight	Slight
Hypercapnia	Pronounced	Absent	Absent
Haematocrit	Greatly raised	Normal	Normal
Polycythaemia	Pronounced	None	None
Pulmonary arterial hypertension	Moderate	Severe	Severe
Right ventricular failure	Rare	Very common	Very common

protection against the effect of hypobaric hypoxia as is evident in the Quechua and Aymara populations of the Andes. This has an interesting parallel in history. Soon after their arrival in the Andes, the Spaniards expanded the ancient silver-mining city of Potosi at an altitude of 4000 m. According to Monge (1948), the historian Antonio de la Calancha described how, in the early years, no infant born of Spanish immigrants in that city survived. Mothers learned to descend to the neighbouring valleys to give birth and the child would not be brought up to Potosi until it was more than 1 year old. The first Spanish infant to live was born on Christmas Eve in the year 1598, 53 years after the founding of the city. The disease which we describe is no less fatal. It is not uncommon at the moderate elevation of Lhasa and may, therefore, be found to be of importance in other mountainous areas of the world.

ADULT SUBACUTE MOUNTAIN SICKNESS

In 1988 40 young, healthy Indian soldiers of mean age 22.2 ± 1.8 yr developed clinical features of severe congestive heart failure while serving at extreme altitudes between 5800 and 6700 m in the Western Himalaya (Anand *et al.* 1990; Anand and Chandrashekhar 1992). All of them were Garhwalis,

an ethnic group belonging to a sub-mountainous area bordering Nepal. A planned programme of acclimatization took place over 6 weeks and was followed by the soldiers being sent to high snow-bound posts where no local inhabitants or permanent settlements existed. Access to these isolated posts was only by lightweight helicopters due to the difficult weather conditions including nocturnal temperatures varying between –20°C and –40°C. The soldiers' daily duties largely comprised patrol duties involving walking several kilometres up and down the slopes to carry supplies.

Subacute mountain sickness in these young soldiers started after they had lived at extreme altitude for 10.8 ± 5.9 weeks. The illness (Fig. 17.10) was characterized by gross anasarca and severe shortness of breath. After a total stay of 18 ± 5.5 weeks at these elevations the patients were airlifted to Chandigarh (300 m). Here 21 of the soldiers were investigated within 3 days of leaving extreme altitude. Most of them started developing spontaneous diuresis on descent.

The soldiers showed features of congestive cardiac failure and polycythaemia. Most had papilloedema. A right ventricular third heart sound was heard in 10 subjects and the murmur of tricuspid incompetence in two. None of the patients had crepitations in the

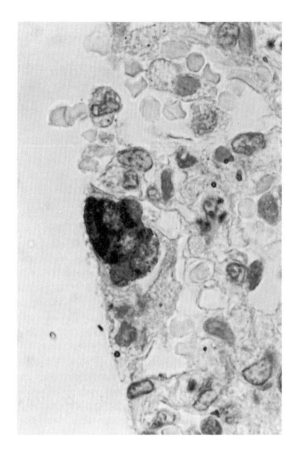

17.9 *A cluster of bombesin-containing pulmonary endocrine cells in a bronchiole from the same case as in the preceding figure. Peroxidase–anti-peroxidase-anti-bombesin, × 1500.*

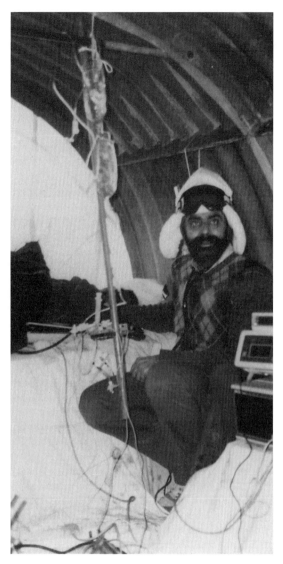

17.10 *Professor Inder Anand carrying out a Swan Ganz catheterization on a young Indian soldier who had developed adult subacute mountain sickness at 4800 m in the Himalaya.*

lungs. Both the total body water (642.6 ± 49./2 ml/kg) and the total body exchangeable sodium (54.6 ± 1.8 μmol/kg) were significantly increased (Anand and Chandrashekhar 1992). All the features of congestive heart failure cleared spontaneously within 2 weeks at sea level unaided by drugs. The electrocardiogram showed right-axis deviation with T wave inversion in chest leads and right ventricular hypertrophy in all patients. Radiographs of the chest showed cardiomegaly in all with evidence of venous congestion. Pleural effusions were found in three subjects. Echocardiography revealed right ventricular dilatation in all. There was mild pulmonary arterial hypertension on cardiac catheterization (26 ± 4.5 mmHg) which was not responsive to oxygen inhalation. Nine patients had mild systemic hypertension, the mean systolic pressure for the group being 136 ±

16 mmHg and the diastolic 89 ± 15.6 mmHg. When the haemodynamic studies were repeated 3 or 4 months later, all the abnormalities had reverted to normal.

Anand and Chandrashekhar (1992) are of the opinion that it was unlikely that in the affected soldiers hypoxic pulmonary vasoconstriction resulted in significantly higher resting pulmonary arterial pressure than that recorded on return to sea level.

However, even mild exercise at sea level in the soldiers with adult subacute mountain sickness increased pulmonary arterial pressure to nearly 40 mmHg. Since the soldiers were engaged in strenuous physical activity for most of the day, they could have developed high pulmonary arterial blood pressure.

Anand and Chandrashekhar (1992) believe that the pulmonary vasoconstrictive effects of cold and the effects of polycythaemia could exaggerate the influence of hypoxia and exercise on the pulmonary arterial pressure. The degree of right ventricular hypertrophy with strain, especially the degree of right axis deviation, observed on the ECG of the soldiers, was much greater than that found in the native highlander (Chapter 19). The considerable right ventricular hypertrophy and dilatation seen on echocardiography further suggests that the modest elevation of pulmonary arterial pressure seen in these patients at sea level may not reflect the actual afterload faced by the right ventricle at altitude. It seems possible, therefore, that pulmonary hypertension may contribute appreciably to the congestive heart failure.

The difficulty of assessing the nature of this syndrome of subacute mountain sickness in young Indian soldiers lies in the fact that so far there has been no fatal case to yield tissue to establish the pathology of the condition. In particular we do not know if there is pulmonary vascular pathology in this syndrome and, if so, its nature. In Chapter 9, where we considered disorders of blood coagulation at high altitude, we referred to the syndrome described by Singh (1973) in young Indian soldiers in Ladakh who developed pulmonary hypertension after a stay of 5 months at elevations between 3660 and 5490 m. There are differences between the syndrome described by Anand and Chandrashekhar (1992) and the disease reported by Singh (1973) in that in the latter the pulmonary hypertension was often severe and irreversible at sea level. The disease described by Singh (1973) proved to have a basis in thrombotic, occlusive hypertensive pulmonary vascular disease and this pulmonary vascular pathology will have to be excluded before the new syndrome of adult subacute mountain sickness can be regarded as a new distinct entity.

Eight of the 40 soldiers at high altitude described by Anand *et al.* (1990) had symptoms suggestive of left ventricular failure at high altitude. Two had low cardiac output at sea level and the resting pulmonary wedge pressure was elevated in seven suggesting some degree of left ventricular dysfunction even on return to sea level. Anand and Chandrashekhar (1992) found that, although the average resting cardiac output at admission was normal, it increased significantly at recovery and the patients could generate the same stroke volume at lower filling pressures, indicating an improvement in left ventricular function. It is quite possible, therefore, that there is an element of myocardial dysfunction at high altitude that might contribute to the congestive heart failure.

HORMONES IN ADULT SUBACUTE MOUNTAIN SICKNESS

In the soldiers with adult subacute mountain sickness there was a 20% increase in total body water and 23% increase in total body sodium. Anand and his colleagues measured body fluid compartments, renal blood flow, and plasma hormones in normal asymptomatic soldiers stationed for about 10 weeks at an extreme altitude of 6000 m (Anand and Chandrashekhar 1992). There was a significant increase in all the body compartments. Total body water rose by 18%, plasma volume by 34%, blood volume by 115%, and total body exchangeable sodium by 14%. Effective renal plasma flow was reduced by 55%. Plasma noradrenaline rose by 180% while plasma adrenaline was unaffected. Plasma renin activity did not change but serum aldosterone rose by 107%. Plasma cortisol levels rose 2.5 times and growth hormone was increased by 16 times normal. Erythropoietin levels increased by 18%. Atrial natriuretic peptide levels were within normal limits. These changes in the body fluid compartments in normal healthy subjects exposed to heavy physical activity at extreme altitude are very similar to those seen in patients with severe untreated congestive heart failure due to cardiomyopathy (Anand *et al.* 1989). The degree of reduction in renal blood flow was also similar. In contrast, the hormone response was somewhat different from that seen in congestive heart failure. In particular, in severe untreated congestive heart failure due to cardiomyopathy levels of noradrenaline, renin, aldosterone, and atrial natriuretic peptide were disproportionately raised (Anand and Chandrashekhar 1992). These findings raise the possibility that the salt and water accumulation seen in normal subjects at high altitude and in soldiers with adult subacute mountain sickness could have resulted from mechanisms acting to reduce renal blood flow independent of pulmonary arterial hypertension. However, the exact sequence of events leading to fluid retention in the patients at high altitude remains to be determined.

References

Anand, I.S. and Chandrashekhar, Y. (1992). Subacute mountain sickness syndromes: role of pulmonary hypertension. In *Hypoxia and Mountain Medicine* J.R. Sutton, G. Coates and C.S. Houston, Ed.). Oxford; Pergamon Press, p. 241

Anand, I.S., Ferrari, R., Kalra, G.S., Wahi, P.A., Poole-Wilson, P.A., and Harris, P. (1989). Edema of cardiac origin: studies of body water and sodium, renal function, haemodynamic indexes, and plasma hormones in untreated congestive cardiac failure. *Circulation*, **80**, 299

Anand, I.S. Malhotra, R.M., Chandrashekhar, Y., Bali, H.K., Chauhan, S.S., Bhandari, R.K., and Wahi, P.I. (1990). Adult subacute mountain sickness — a syndrome of congestive heart failure in man at very high altitude. *Lancet*, **335**, 561

Heath, D. (1989). Missing link from Tibet. *Thorax*, **44**, 981

Heath, D., Harris, P., Sui, G.J., Liu, Y.H., Gosney, J., Harris, E., and Anand, I.S. (1989). Pulmonary blood vessels and endocrine cells in subacute infantile mountain sickness. *Respiratory Medicine*, **83**, 77

Heath, D., Yacoub, M., Gosney, J.R., Madden, B., Caslin, A.W., and Smith, P. (1990). Pulmonary endocrine cells in hypertensive pulmonary vascular disease. *Histopathology*, **16**, 21

Li, J.B.(1983). In (People's Hospital of Tibetan Autonomous Region, Ed.).*High Altitude Medicine*. Lhasa; Tibetan People's Publisher, p. 288

Monge-M, C. (1948). Quotation from de la Calancha, A. (1639), *Crónica Moralizada de la Orden de San Augustin*, Vol. 1, In *Acclimatization in the Andes*. Baltimore; Johns Hopkins Press, p. 36

Singh, I. (1973). Pulmonary hypertension in new arrivals at high altitude. World Health Organization meeting on Primary Pulmonary Hypertension, Geneva, October

Singh, I., Khanna, P.K., Lal, M., Hoon, R.S., and Rao, B.D.P. (1965). High altitude pulmonary hypertension. *Lancet*, **ii**, 146

Sui, G.J., Liu, Y.H., Cheng, X.S., Anand, I.S., Harris, E., Harris, P., and Heath, D. (1988). Subacute infantile mountain sickness. *Journal of Pathology*, **155**, 161

Williams, D., Heath, D., Gosney, J., and Rios-Dalenz, J. (1993). Pulmonary endocrine cells of Aymara Indians from the Bolivian Andes. *Thorax*, **48**, 52

18

Systemic circulation

The cardiovascular system influences the supply of oxygen to the tissues at high altitude by changes in the cardiac output and by alterations in the distribution of blood flow in the body.

CARDIAC OUTPUT

Resting stroke volume and cardiac output start to fall immediately upon the arrival of lowlanders at high altitude. They fall until about the third day and then show a secondary decline at about the tenth day according to Hoon *et al.* (1977). These workers estimated stroke volume and cardiac output in 50 healthy lowlanders by non-invasive plethysmography, and then airlifted them to 3660 m so that serial estimations could be carried out until the tenth day of exposure to high altitude, and for up to 5 days after return to sea level. At high altitude the mean stroke volume was 63 ml, this representing a reduction of 19.4% of sea-level values. At sea level the mean cardiac output was 4.92 l/min and on arrival in the mountains this value fell by 19.5%. By the third day of exposure to high altitude the reduction in cardiac output was 24.8% and by the tenth day a maximum decline of 26.2% was found. On return to sea level the cardiac output returned to normal.

The reduction in stroke volume is not fully compensated by tachycardia and this is why the overall effect of the chronic hypoxia of high altitude is to reduce cardiac output. Earlier work in the Andes (Sime *et al.* 1974) had also showed a reduction of 10% in stroke index at rest during the first hour of ascent to 2380 m, but a further reduction of up to 20% by the fifth day of exposure. Alexander *et al.* (1967) had also reported earlier a decrease in cardiac output during exercise after 10 days at 3100 m compared with sea level. The decrease was caused by a fall in stroke volume. Some investigations, however, have suggested to the contrary that, on acute exposure to high altitude, the stroke volume does not alter (Stenberg *et al.* 1966) and, coupled with the characteristic tachycardia, this has been reported as resulting in an increased cardiac output that does not persist for more than a few days (Klausen 1966; Vogel and Harris 1967).

In healthy Andean residents the cardiac output has been reported as normal rather than diminished (Peñaloza *et al.* 1963). The resting cardiac output of the lowlander resident on a long-term basis in the mountains is also normal. However, return to sea level for only 10 days results in a pronounced augmentation in the stroke volume of such long-term residents (Hartley 1971). There had been one earlier report (Rotta *et al.* 1956) that highlanders, like those ascending to high altitude, have a diminished stroke volume and cardiac output.

Exposure to high altitude prevents maximal cardiovascular performance. Pronounced reduction in maximum cardiac output is more apparent in sojourners than in native highlanders (Pugh 1964a; Hartley *et al.* 1967). There is also a reduction in maximal heart rate that is related to both the altitude and the duration of exposure to it. Thus, while the reduction is maximal heart rate is seen inconsistently at 4300 m, it occurs regularly at 5800 m (Hartley 1971). In Operation Everest II maximal heart rates decreased from 160 ± 7 at sea level to 137 ± 4 at a simulated altitude of 6100 m, 123 ± 6 at 7620 m, and 118 ± 3 at 8848 m (Reeves *et al.* 1987). On exercise at high altitude, cardiac output increases disproportionately about 20% beyond that caused by the same work load at sea level (Lenfant and Sullivan 1971)

MECHANISMS OF EFFECTS OF HIGH ALTITUDE ON CARDIAC OUTPUT

During the initial phase of exposure to high altitude the predominant factor that works in the direction of increasing cardiac output is tachycardia, and this appears to be an expression of increased sympathetic activity, which is reflected by a rise in the level of plasma and urinary catecholamines (Cunningham *et al.* 1965). The cause of the reduction in stroke volume and cardiac output is more controversial. A reduced venous return to the heart due to redistribution of blood as discussed below is a possibility. More likely, however, is a direct depressing action of hypoxia on the myocardium (Alexander *et al.* 1967). The contractility of the myocardium of goats exposed to reduced barometric pressure is depressed and contributes significantly to the reduction in stroke volume. Tucker *et al.* (1976) could demonstrate this depression of myocardial contractility only by removal of chemical blockage of the beta sympathetic drive referred to above. This suggests that the hypoxic myocardial depression of high altitude may be partially or even completely overcome by increased sympathetic stimulation. In contrast, a two-dimensional echocardiography study during Operation Everest II (Suarez *et al.* 1987) suggested that cardiac contractile function appeared to be unimpaired.

Left ventricular function in newcomers to high altitude was studied by non-invasive methods on normal volunteers airlifted or taken by road to 3660 m (Balasubramanian *et al.* 1978). A significant reduction of all indices of left ventricular function was observed from the second day of induction to high altitude, despite increased urinary catecholamine excretion. On return to sea level all the

values returned to normal by the third day. Permanent residents of high altitude had normal left ventricular function and temporary residents a moderate depression. These findings confirm that left ventricular dysfunction occurs on exposure to the hypoxia of high altitude.

REDISTRIBUTION OF BLOOD FLOW

The diminished cardiac output characteristic of high altitude is advantageous in the sense that the work load of the heart is not increased (Lenfant and Sullivan 1971). The smaller systemic flow of blood is redistributed so that vital organs and muscles are able to function efficiently in the face of chronic hypoxia. Fig. 18.1 derived from data of Finch and Lenfant (1972), expresses diagrammatically the fact that the proportion of the total cardiac output received by an organ does not equate with the proportions of the total oxygen being transported. Some tissues such as the skin have modest requirements of oxygen compared with organs like the heart and this is evidenced by the low extraction rate of oxygen

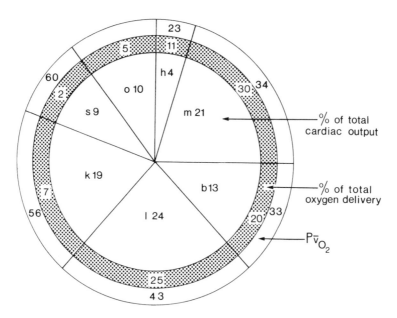

18.1 *Distribution of blood flow and oxygen to the various tissues of the body. The inner circle represents the total cardiac output, and the segments into which it has been divided represent the percentage of the total output received by each organ. The figure indicated in the surrounding ring is the percentage of the total oxygen delivery being received by the corresponding organ. The figure in the outermost ring is the value for venous oxygen tension, indicating the extraction rate of oxygen from the blood in that organ. Thus the heart, h, receives 4% of the cardiac output and 11% of the available oxygen, while the oxygen saturation of blood in the coronary veins is only 23% indicating a high extraction rate of oxygen. In contrast the skin, s, receives 9% of the cardiac output, but only 2% of the available oxygen, the venous oxygen tension being 60%, indicating a low extraction rate of oxygen. h, heart; m, muscle, b, brain; l, liver, k, kidneys; s, skin; o, other tissue. (Based on data from Finch and Lenfant (1972).*

(Fig. 18.1). At high altitude there is a redistribution of blood away from such areas to increase the oxygen reservoir for the remainder of the body. This decrease in the cutaneous circulation, both in indigenous natives and in long-standing sojourners, has been studied by Martineaud *et al.* (1969). This change is most pronounced when the temperature of the skin is initially high and the flow increased. As will be seen, the fraction of the total blood carried in the skin is small but its redistribution under such conditions of chronic hypoxia is probably of importance.

In the same way there is a decreased renal flow at high altitude both in highlanders (Becker *et al.* 1957) and in sojourners (Pauli *et al.* 1968). However, there is a close relation between packed cell volume and the decrease in renal plasma flow (Lozano and Monge-M 1965), so in effect there is a normal amount of oxygen being transported to the kidneys, the fall in renal flow being matched by the increased arterial oxygen content. Renal function remains unimpaired, with increased filtration rate to perform its role in acclimatization at high altitude.

The effect of high altitude on the coronary arterial flow is somewhat surprising when one observes from Fig. 18.1 that the extraction of oxygen from blood in the coronary blood vessels is very considerable (see Chapter 19), so that there would appear to be but little physiological reserve for any decrease in coronary arterial flow. Nevertheless, the coronary arterial flow is decreased at high altitude (Grover *et al.* 1970). This is in line with the general decrease in cardiac output at high altitude referred to above. As noted in the following chapter, it seems likely that during prolonged residence at high altitude increased myocardial vascularization counteracts the effects of diminished coronary arterial flow, thus avoiding the dangers of myocardial ischaemia and its sequelae.

PLASMA AND BLOOD VOLUME

On initial ascent to high altitude there is commonly a diuresis in those not developing acute mountain sickness with a contraction of plasma volume (Chapter 12). The possible role of the carotid bodies in the control of sodium homeostasis in this early exposure to high-altitude hypoxia is considered at the end of the chapter. Vigorous exercise during the ascent will expand the plasma volume (Milledge *et al.* 1983) by stimulation of the renin–aldosterone system. Sufferers from acute mountain sickness will also show a lowered output of urine and expansion of plasma volume. Over the following weeks the reduction in plasma volume is sustained. There was a

21% reduction in plasma volume after 18 weeks at altitudes above 4000 m in four members of the 1960–61 Himalayan Scientific Expedition (Pugh 1964*b*). During the following 2–3 months the plasma volume returned towards control levels. Native highlanders of Cerro de Pasco (4330 m) were still found to have a plasma volume only two–thirds that of a group of lowlanders from Lima. They had 27% less plasma volume in a blood volume that was 14% greater.

A characteristic feature of native highlanders and long-standing residents at high altitude is an increased blood volume brought about by increased red cell mass on the background of a diminished plasma volume (Sanchez *et al.* 1970) (Fig. 18.2). The total blood volume increases from about 80 ml/kg body weight at sea level to some 100 ml/kg body weight (Fig. 18.2; Hurtado 1964). The total blood volume is some 40% above this in patients with chronic mountain sickness (Chapter 15, this volume; Hurtado, 1964). Merino (1950) found that after only 1–3 weeks' residence at high altitude there

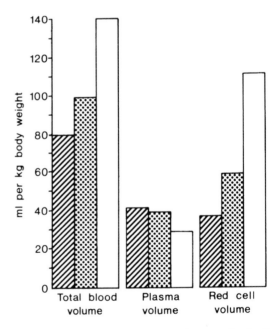

18.2 *Total blood volume, plasma volume, and red cell volume in subjects living at sea level (hatched column), at 4540 m (stippled column), and in patients with Monge's disease (open column). At high altitude there is an increase in total blood volume and red cell volume. These changes are exaggerated in Monge's disease. (Based on data from Hurtado (1964).)*

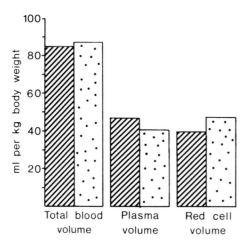

18.3 *Total blood volume, plasma volume, and red cell volume in subjects at sea level (hatched column) and after residence at 4540 m for 1–3 weeks (light stippling). After such a short period the changes illustrated in Fig. 18.2 are already taking place. (Based on data from Merino (1950).)*

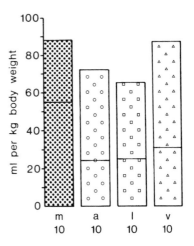

18.4 *Red cell volume (below the line) and plasma volume (above the line) in 10 men (m), 10 alpacas (a), 10 llamas (l), and 10 vicuñas (v). At high altitude the ratio of plasma to red cell volume is disproportionately high in indigenous camelids compared with highlanders. (Based on data from Reynafarje (1966).)*

was already a detectable increase in red cell volume and a decrease in plasma volume (Fig. 18.3).

The reversible nature of the changes in blood volume are indicated by data on the red cell and plasma volume from natives of Huancayo (3260 m) who first ascended to Morococha (4540 m) and then descended to Lima (150 m) (Monge-M and Monge-C 1966). On the ascent there was a definite increase in total blood volume due to increased red cell mass. On subsequent descent to sea level total blood volume and red cell mass fell progressively over 8 weeks. The ratio of plasma to red cell volume in camelids indigenous to high altitude is much higher than in the highlander (Fig. 18.4). Thus in man the ratio is 0.6, in the alpaca 1.9, in the llama 1.6, and in the vicuña 1.8.

Regulation of plasma volume

A wide variety of factors influence plasma volume and an account of these has been given by Ward *et al.* (1989). Atrial natriuretic peptide (ANP) (Chapter 12) is released in response to stretching of the right atrium. Such stretching results from an increase in pressure within the right atrium, which may be brought about shifts of blood from the periphery or an increase in plasma volume. ANP causes the kidney to excrete sodium and water. Apart from this central mechanism there are many other factors which affect plasma volume. These include hydra-

tion and rehydration. The tone of the venous capacitance vessels and vessels in the skin (Chapter 25) exert an influence. Peripheral vasoconstriction shifts blood from the periphery to the centre raising right atrial pressure and stretching the right atrium. Another important factor is posture. Lying down or lower body immersion will cause a shift of blood volume to the centre. Conversely, the upright position tends to shift volume away from the centre to the lower body reducing right atrial pressure and inhibiting ANP release. Sodium intake will cause water retention and increase plasma volume but an increase in ANP secretion will compensate for this. Stimulation of the renin– angiotensin–aldosterone system causes sodium retention in the same way.

Exercise may exert an important effect on plasma volume and lead to peripheral systemic oedema as we consider now.

PERIPHERAL OEDEMA

On a mountaineering expedition to Mt Kinabalu (4100 m) in Borneo all six members of the party developed pronounced peripheral oedema (Sheridan and Sheridan 1970). The climbers, one woman and five man aged 22–30 years, spent sequentially 2 days at 3500 m, 3 days at 3800 m, and 5 days at 4000 m. On the sixth day of the climb all members of the party showed oedema which was most obvious on the face, back of hands, and ankles. Measurements of ankle circumference showed that oedema increased until the tenth day. Descent to 1550 m was made in less than 5 hours and during that time there was a dramatic loss of oedema in all members of the party. Frequent halts had to be made because of the diuresis.

Seven years later Hackett and Rennie (1977) observed the same peripheral oedema in 10 hikers at Pheriche (4240 m) on the approach route to Mt Everest. Seven of the cases occurred in women, the mean age being 45 years. In the majority the oedema was facial and especially periorbital (Fig. 18.5). Oedema of the hands was also common and in two

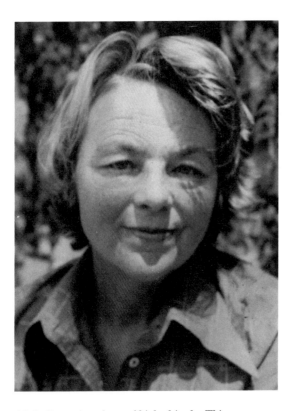

18.5 *Systemic oedema of high altitude. This woman developed facial and periorbital oedema while on a trekking holiday in the Himalaya to altitudes approaching 4500 m. Outlines of goggles on her face left pits in the oedematous tissues. The facial oedema persisted for the entire 4 weeks that she was in the Himalaya, but disappeared immediately on her descent to Kathmandu (1200 m). (We are grateful to Mr W. Butt for the photograph and to Mrs Enid Ellison for allowing us to publish it.)*

instances there was severe oedema of the legs. There was no relationship between the oedema and the menstrual cycle or the taking of oral contraceptives. Two of the worst cases were postmenopausal and not on replacement therapy. It is of interest that five of the seven women, and all three men, affected by peripheral oedema also had loud pulmonary rales. One woman had anasarca in addition. One of the two women without rales had been treated with diuretics for dyspnoea. Two of the affected subjects had retinal haemorrhages and two had papilloedema. The peripheral oedema was not associated with increased proteinuria.

It is apparent from these reports that peripheral oedema is common in newcomers at high altitude, but it is not so clear whether the oedema is related to hypoxia or exercise as noted above. Williams *et al.* (1979) have studied the effect of exercise involved in seven consecutive days of hill-walking on fluid homeostasis at an altitude of only up to 1100 m in the Welsh hills. In five subjects they found a fall in packed cell volume, reaching a maximum of 11% by the fifth day, and a retention of sodium. After an initial loss of water on the first day there was a modest retention reaching a cumulative maximum on the fifth day. It was calculated that by the end of the hill-walk there was an average increase of 22% in plasma volume, an increase of 17% in interstitial fluid, and a decrease of 8% in intracellular fluid volume. These changes were associated in all five subjects with facial oedema. Pitting oedema of the lower leg was present in some subjects and was pronounced in one. These workers consider that on prolonged exercise of this type there is an increase in the capacity of the vascular space, presumably the capillary beds of working muscles and possibly the venous beds, and it is this which underlies the increase in plasma volume. They believe that the increase in extracellular fluid indicated by their study explains the dependent and periorbital oedema noted after the strenuous exercise involved in hill-walking or mountain-climbing. Hence at high altitude the effects of exercise and hypoxia on fluid retention and fluids shifts may be additive. Their results give support to the impression that exercise on ascent to mountainous areas is a factor in the genesis of high-altitude pulmonary oedema.

SYSTEMIC BLOOD PRESSURE IN NATIVE HIGHLANDERS IN THE ANDES

Early observations by Peruvian physicians like Monge that native highlanders in the Andes had lower systemic blood pressures than mestizos living on the coast were confirmed by Marticorena *et al.* (1967). They found that even with increasing age the systolic pressure in the Quechuas was lower than that found in two groups of normal subjects in the USA (Master *et al.* 1950; Comstock 1957) whose blood pressures corresponded rather to those of the sea-level residents of Peru. Peñaloza (1971) refers to the thesis of Chávez (1965), who found that the levels of systemic blood pressure in 300 subjects born and living in La Oroya (3750 m) were less than those in lowlanders.

During the period 1967–73, surveys of systemic blood pressure were carried out in Peru by Ruiz and Peñaloza (1977) on three communities in the 4100–4360 m altitude range (Milpo, Colquijirca, and Cercepuquio), as contrasted with two communities at sea level (Puente Piedra and Infantas). This investigation was sizable, comprising 3055 subjects at high altitude and 4359 subjects at sea level. The prevalence of systolic and diastolic hypertension, expressed as the age-adjusted rate per thousand of population, was determined in the five communities. The upper limit of normal systolic blood pressure was taken to be 160 mmHg and the upper limit of normal diastolic blood pressure was taken to be 95 mmHg. The prevalence of systemic systolic hypertension in males was at least 12 times greater at sea level than at high altitude and the difference was even more pronounced in females (Fig. 18.6). Systemic diastolic hypertension was also commoner at sea level, but the differences were less striking than for systolic pressure (Fig. 18.7). At sea level, systemic hypertension tends to be more frequent in females and systolic hypertension is commoner than diastolic. At high altitude, systemic hypertension is more frequent in men and diastolic hypertension is commoner (Ruiz and Peñaloza 1977).

SYSTEMIC BLOOD PRESSURE IN LOWLANDERS AT HIGH ALTITUDE

Permanent residence at moderately increased altitude appears to maintain a slightly lower systemic blood pressure in Caucasians as well as in native highlanders of the Andes. Thus, in the USA, Appleton (1967) studied 2782 high school students living at 1220, 1980 and 2350 m. The mean systolic pressure in the residents at the highest of these three altitudes was 119 mmHg, compared with 124 mmHg in those from the lowest elevation. Permanent residence at these elevations had, however, little effect on the level of diastolic blood pressure.

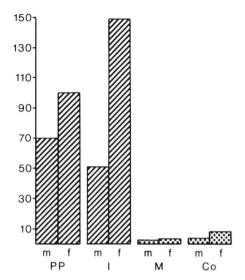

18.6 *Prevalence of systemic systolic hypertension (>160 mmHg) in two communities at sea level (hatched columns) and in two communities at high altitude (stippled columns) in Peru. Prevalence expressed as age-adjusted rate per thousand of population. PP, Puente Piedra; I, Infantas; M, Milpo (4100 m); Co, Colquijirca (4260 m). (Based on data from Ruiz and Peñaloza (1977).)*

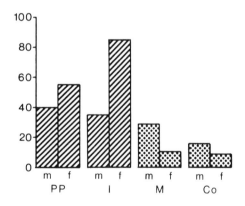

18.7 *Prevalence of systemic diastolic hypertension (>95 mmHg) in the four communities referred to in Fig. 18.6. (Based on data from Ruiz and Peñaloza (1977).)*

Prolonged residence at substantial high altitude induces a more pronounced diminution in systemic blood pressure. Rotta *et al.* (1956) found that, after residence at 4500 m for 1 year, both systolic and diastolic pressures were diminished. After several years' residence in the mountains not inconsiderable decrements in systemic pressure may be recorded. Marticorena *et al.* (1969) studied 100 men who had been born at sea level but who lived at 3750 m in the Peruvian Andes for 2 to 15 years. None was Peruvian and the majority came from the USA, Canada, and Britain. Blood pressure measurements were obtained from records of annual physical examinations. A decrease of 10 mmHg or more in systemic systolic pressure was observed in 56% of the subjects and in diastolic pressure in 46% of them. Furthermore, the longer the residence at high altitude, the greater was the decrease in systolic pressure. Indeed the systolic pressure at the final examination was lower than that of healthy native highlanders living at the same altitude. Peñaloza (1971) also refers to the changes in systemic blood pressure found in men from sea level between the ages of 25 and 66 years residing at La Oroya (3750 m) for periods ranging from 2 to 15 years. These are summarized in Fig. 18.8.

Peñaloza (1971) reported that some patients with established systemic hypertension living at this same mining town in the Andes for the same lengthy period showed some amelioration of their condition. However, there was no improvement in four patients in whom the diastolic pressure exceeded 95 mmHg.

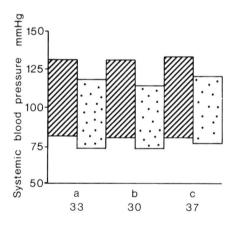

18.8 *Initial and final systemic blood pressure in 100 sea-level subjects residing at an altitude of 3750 m for periods ranging from 2 to 15 years. a, Residence at high altitude from 2 to 5 years (33 subjects); b, residence at high altitude from 6 to 9 years (30 subjects); c, residence at high altitude from 10 to 15 years (37 subjects). Hatched column, initial systemic blood pressures; lightly stippled column, final systemic blood pressures. (From data in Peñaloza (1971).)*

This suggests that, when the basis for the hypertension is vasoconstrictive and muscular, the chronic hypobaric hypoxia exerts a beneficial vasodilating effect. In cases with organic lesions in the arteries, the dilating effect of hypoxia is less effective. The major effects in the amelioration of the systemic hypertension appear to be environmental rather than genetic, for the fall in blood pressure occurs in Caucasians as well as native highlanders. Almost certainly the major factor in hypobaric hypoxia. The fall in blood pressure in residents at high altitude is greater in the systolic than the diastolic component. Peñaloza (1971) believes that, whereas hypoxia lowers the pressure by a relaxing effect on arterial muscle, it may counteract its effect on the diastolic pressure by inducing polycythaemia which raises blood viscosity and peripheral vascular resistance. There appears to be some supporting evidence for the idea of a relation between the levels of polycythaemia and systemic diastolic blood pressure in the fact that in women below the age of 40 years at high altitude there is some diminution of systemic diastolic pressure, and this may be related to the lower degree of polycythaemia brought about by menstrual loss. In contrast, in cases of Monge's disease (Chapter 15) there is a severe degree of polycythaemia and diastolic hypertension in the systemic circulation. Halhuber *et al.* (1985) found that mild hypertensives who ascended to and lived at up to 3000 m had few symptoms and both systolic and diastolic pressure fell. No cases of cerebrovascular accident or cardiac failure were noted in 593 patients. The improvement was continued for 4–8 months after returning to lower levels.

SYSTEMIC BLOOD PRESSURE IN THE HIMALAYA

Systemic hypertension is rare in the native highlanders of much of the Himalaya just as it is in the Quechuas of the Andes. Puri *et al.* (1986) determined systemic blood pressure in 3103 healthy natives residing at altitudes between 3000 and 4410 m in Himachal Pradesh. They found the prevalence of systemic hypertension in this highland group to be 2.4% as compared with 3.6% in a rural population of Haryana (Gupta *et al.* 1978). This low prevalence is comparable with that of 1.7% found in Aymara Indians of the Bolivian altiplano (Murillo *et al.* 1980) and that of 1.9% found elsewhere in the Himalaya (Dasgupta *et al.* 1982). Baker (1978) reported that only 4.0% of 70 ethnic Tibetans had a systemic blood pressure exceeding 165/90 mmHg in North Bhutan.

However, there are anecdotal reports that in low-landers ascending into the Karakorams of 'Little Tibet' in Ladakh the systemic blood pressure may become elevated. Norboo (1986), a physician at Leh (3500 m), the capital of Ladakh, speaking at a symposium on 'Aspects of hypoxia', in Liverpool said that in his experience most lowlanders visiting his area had a slight rise in systemic blood pressure that remained for about a week. Forster (1986), speaking at the same meeting, reported that astronomers and supporting staff working on the British infrared telescope on the summit of the volcano Mauna Kea (4200 m) in Hawaii for 5 days, showed an increase in their systemic blood pressure. This persisted for the 5 days that they were working on the summit, but it was reversed immediately on their descent to sea level. Harris (1986), at the same symposium, said that he had been made aware that systemic hypertension was a problem in Tibet and also in soldiers of the Indian army stationed in Ladakh. He had personally measured the systemic blood pressure in troops who had been stationed in the mountains for 6 months or more and found it to be raised. One possible factor in the elevation of systemic blood pressure in subjects ascending to high altitude may be an increased secretion of noradrenaline (Chapter 22).

Norboo (1986) thought that systemic hypertension was to be found in about a fifth of the population living in the mountainous regions of Ladakh. He related this to the high intake of salt in the diet in butter and the local tea. Apparently as many as 30 cups of very salty tea may be imbibed in the course of a day. There is an interesting link here with the work in rats relating high altitude, sodium metabolism, and the carotid bodies by Honig *et al.* (1985) described below. Sun (1986) also reported a high prevalence of systemic hypertension among indigenous Tibetans. He found that the increase in blood pressure was related to age. Its frequency was greater in the urban population around Lhasa than in rural communities. He also relates the prevalence of systemic hypertension to the very high intake of salt, which Ward *et al.*, (1989) estimate to be as much as 1 kilogram per month. They believe that in the Bhutanese and Sherpa varieties of 'Tibetan tea' neither the salt nor the yak butter content appears by taste to be as high. It has been reported that Tibetans living at 2080 m have a low systemic blood pressure up to the age of 40 years, but compared with Peruvian highlanders living at 3750 m their systolic pressure rises after this age (Fig. 18.9; Sehgal *et al.* 1968)

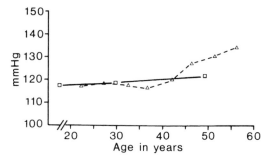

18.9 *Systemic systolic blood pressure in Quechuas living at 3750 m (continuous line) and Tibetans living at 2080 m (dotted line). Note the rise in blood pressure in the Tibetans at the age of 45 years. (Based on data from Sehgal* et al. *(1968).)*

SYSTEMIC BLOOD PRESSURE IN ETHIOPIAN HIGHLANDERS

Clegg *et al.* (1976) found that systemic blood pressures were greater among highland Ethiopians than in lowlanders, but attributed this to different factors from those considered above. They thought that socio-economic factors were of importance, those of higher status having generally higher pressures than those of low status and exhibiting significant rises of diastolic pressure with age. They also suggested that the prevalence of infectious disease at lower altitudes may be a factor in lowering systemic blood pressure. Maddocks and Vines (1966) had previously demonstrated that in a New Guinean population more severe malarial, infection was associated with lowered systemic blood pressure, especially systolic.

SYSTEMIC BLOOD PRESSURE AND SODIUM METABOLISM

As noted earlier in this chapter, on early exposure to the hypobaric hypoxia of high altitude there is a contraction of plasma volume. The regulation of sodium and water excretion is controlled by the interaction of several hormones, particularly by aldosterone and atrial natriuretic hormone as we describe in Chapters 12 and 22. Honig (1989) has suggested that the carotid bodies are involved in the resetting of sodium homeostasis on exposure to high altitude. Experiments on rats demonstrate that the reduction in plasma volume that accompanies acclimatization to hypobaric hypoxia can be attained by two mechanisms: a reduction in dietary intake of salt and water and their increased excretion by the kidneys (Honig 1989).

Sodium homeostasis and the peripheral chemoreceptors appear to influence the level of systemic blood pressure in rats subjected to simulated high altitude (Honig *et al.* 1985). Spontaneously hypertensive rats (SHR) of the Okamoto–Aoki strain are useful for such experiments because they have a naturally high appetite for salt thus rendering changes in intake to be detected readily. It was noted that, when SHR rats are exposed to a simulated altitude of 4000 m and are allowed access to food and water without additional salt, there is a clear natriuretic response within the first 2 days. When they are allowed unrestricted access to hypertonic saline, they voluntarily suppress their intake of sodium. At the same time there is a decrease in urinary sodium excretion to parallel the reduced salt intake (Behm *et al.* 1984). On exposure to this simulated high altitude of 4000 m the rats showed a fall in their systolic blood pressure of 30–40 mmHg over a period of 3–5 days (Honig *et al.* 1985). It remained at this lower level for the following 15–17 days while the animals were subjected to hypobaric hypoxia. On return to sea-level conditions the systemic blood pressure returned within 1 or 2 days to the original level.

When young SHR rats from their fifth to eighteenth week of age are reared at a simulated altitude of 4000 m without access to hypertonic saline, they do not develop systemic hypertension (Behm *et al.* 1986; see Fig. 18.10). These effects of hypobaric hypoxia are attenuated but not abolished by the addition of salt (Fig. 18.11).

Such animal experiments confirm that sodium homeostasis is involved in the adjustment of systemic arterial blood pressure to the hypobaric hypoxia of high altitude. The hypoxic environment appears to induce a natriuresis and a fall in systolic systemic blood pressure in adult animals, and a low sodium intake prevents the development of systemic hypertension in the young. It is obvious that the establishment of a lower sodium content of the body in the hypoxic environment can be achieved by either a diminished salt intake or an increased sodium excretion. In animals this depends to a great extent on the species and strain, whether they are herbivores or carnivores, for example, or the situation, for example, whether salt is available or not.

There is much evidence to suggest that the peripheral arterial chemoreceptors may be involved in the control of sodium homeostasis in the hypobaric hypoxia of high altitude (Honig *et al.* 1985; Heath and Smith 1992). The carotid bodies are the only sensors able to inform the brain of the occurrence of hypoxia. Honig *et al.* (1985) speculate that even the

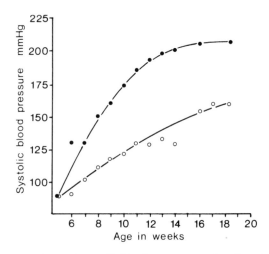

18.10 *Systemic systolic blood pressure as a function of age in spontaneously hypertensive rats without free access to additional salt, growing in hypobaric hypoxia (open circles) or normoxia (filled circles). (After Behm et al. (1986).)*

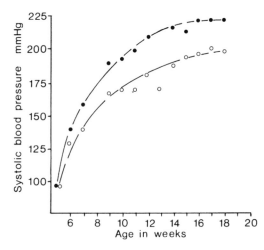

18.11 *Systemic systolic blood pressure as a function of age in SHR rats with free access to salt, growing in hypobaric hypoxia (open circles) and normoxia (filled circles). The hypoxia still exerts an ameliorating effect on the level of systemic pressure, but it is diminished in the presence of excess sodium. (After Behm et al. (1986).)*

inhibition of voluntary sodium intake in rats at simulated high altitude may in some unexplained way result from stimulation of the arterial chemoreceptors. The increased natriuresis of hypobaric hypoxia results from an inhibition of renal tubular sodium reabsorption. This appears to be independent of altered renal haemodynamics, but instead seems to be a specific and reflex effect arising from stimulation by hypoxia of the carotid bodies and other peripheral arterial chemoreceptors. Section of the renal nerves abolishes the responses of the vascular bed of the kidney evoked by stimulation of the carotid body, but fails to prevent the simultaneously occurring inhibition of renal tubular sodium reabsorption and natriuresis. This indicates that hormones mediate the natriuretic effects of arterial chemoreceptor stimulation. This could be through reduced secretion of aldosterone (Chapter 22), which has an antinatriuretic effect, through increased output of atrial natriuretic peptide (Chapters 12 and 22), or due to enhanced secretion of glucocorticoids having a natriuretic action. Stimulation of the carotid bodies appears to change the balance between natriuretic and antinatriuretic hormones. This might be effected from a natriuretic substance emanating from chemoreceptor tissue itself.

The resetting of sodium and water homeostasis at high altitude may be of importance in the process of early acclimatization to high altitude as well as to a lowering of systemic blood pressure. On early exposure to hypobaric hypoxia there is a contraction of extracellular and plasma volume that leads to the well-recognized phenomenon of 'haemoconcentration', which is considered to improve the transport of oxgyen to the tissues (Chapter 5). Since the osmotic pressure of the extracellular fluid is precisely controlled, the reduced volume can only be achieved by a negative sodium balance. This is achieved by the mechanisms described above. Honig *et al.* (1985) speculate that even the normal activity of the carotid body at sea level may help to control sodium balance by suppressing plasma aldosterone and by facilitating renal sodium excretion. We have seen earlier (Chapter 7) that native highlanders of the Andes show enlarged carotid bodies with histological and ultrastructural alterations in the glomic tissue. The relationship of this enlargement and the structural changes in the glomic tissue to sodium homeostasis is not yet known.

It has been reported that rats acclimatized to high altitude may have a lower sodium concentration in their erythrocytes. This may also apply to vascular smooth muscle cells where enhanced intracellular sodium may result in exaggerated reactivity to vasoconstrictive humoral agents, probably mediated by calcium ions (Honig *et al.* 1985).

References

Alexander, J.K., Hartley, H., Modelski, M., and Grover, R.F. (1967). Reduction of stroke volume during exercise in man following ascent to 3,100 m altitude. *Journal of Applied Physiology*, **23**, 849

Appleton, F. (1967). Possible influence of altitude on blood pressure. *Circulation*, **36**. (Suppl. 11), 55

Baker, P.T. (1978). The adaptive fitness of high altitude populations. In *The Biology of High Altitude Peoples* (P.T. Baker Ed.). Cambridge; Cambridge University Press, p. 317

Balasubramanian, V., Mathew, O.P., Tiwari, S.C., Behl, A., Sharma, S.C., and Hoon, R.S. (1978). Alterations in left ventricular, function in normal man on exposure to high altitude (3,658 m). *British Heart Journal*, **40**, 276

Becker, F.E., Schilling, J.A., and Harvey, R.B. (1957). Renal function in man acclimatized to high altitude. *Journal of Applied Physiology*, **10**, 79

Behm, R., Honig, A. Griethe, M., Schmidt, M., and Schneider, P. (1984). Sustained suppression of voluntary sodium intake of spontaneously hypertensive rat (SHR) in hypobaric hypoxia. *Biomedica Biochimica Acta*, **43**, 975

Behm, R., Habeck, J.O., Huckstorf, C., and Honig, A. (1986). Blood pressure adjustment, left ventricular weight and carotid body size in young spontaneously hypertensive rats growing up in hypoxia. *Biomedica Biochimica Acta*, **45**, 787

Chávez, A. (1965). Presión arterial en altura. Br. Thesis Universidad Nacional Mayor de San Marcos Facultad de Medicina, Lima

Clegg, E.J., Jeffries, D.J., and Harrison, G.A. (1976). Determinants of blood pressure at high and low altitudes in Ethiopia. *Proceedings of the Royal Society*, London, **194**, 63

Comstock, G. (1957). An epidemiologic study of blood pressure levels in a biracial community in the Southern Unites States. *American Journal of Hygiene*, **65**, 271

Cunningham, W.I., Becker, F.J., and Kreuzer, F. (1965). Catecholamines in plasma and urine at high altitude. *Journal of Applied Physiology*, **20**. 607

Dasgupta, D.J., Prasher, B.S., Vaidya, N.K., Ahluwolia, S.K., Sharma, P.D., Puri, D.S., and Mehrotra, A.N. (1982). Blood pressure in a community at high altitude (3,000 m) at Pooh (North India). *Journal of Epidemiology and Community Health*, **36**, 251

Finch, C.A. and Lenfant, C. (1972). Oxygen transport in man. *New England Journal of Medicine,* **286,** 407

Forster, P. (1986). Telescopes in high places. In *Aspects of Hypoxia* (D. Heath, Ed.). Liverpool; Liverpool University Press, pp. 224–5

Grover, R.F., Lufschanowski, R., and Alexander, J.K. (1970). Decreased coronary blood flow in man following ascent to high altitude. In *Hypoxia, High Altitude and the Heart,* Vol. 5, Advances in Cardiology. (J.H.K. Vogel, Ed.). Basel; Karger, p. 32

Gupta, S.P., Siwach, S.B., and Moda, V.K. (1978). Epidemiology of hypertension based on total community survey in the rural population of Haryana. *Indian Heart Journal,* **30,** 315

Hackett, P. and Rennie, D. (1977). Acute mountain sickness. *Lancet,* **i,** 491

Halhuber, M.J., Humpeler, R., Inama, A.K., and Jungmann, H. (1985). Does altitude cause exhaustion of the heart and circulatory system? Indications and contraindications for cardiac patients in altitudes. In *High Altitude Deterioration* (R.J. Rivolier, P. Cerretelli, J. Foray, and P. Segantini, Ed.). Basel; Karger, p. 192

Harris, P. (1986). Discussion. In *Aspects of Hypoxia* (D. Heath, Ed.). Liverpool; Liverpool University Press, pp. 128 and 129

Hartley, H. (1971). Effects of high-altitude environment on the cardiovascular system of man. *Journal of the American Medical Association,* **215,** 241

Hartley, H. Alexander, J.K., Modelski, M., and Grover, R.F. (1967). Subnormal cardiac output at rest and during exercise in residents at 3,100 m altitude. *Journal of Applied Physiology,* **23,** 839

Heath, D. and Smith, P. (1992). The carotid bodies and sodium metabolism. In *Diseases of the Human Carotid Body.* London; Springer-Verlag, p. 127

Honig, A. (1989). Peripheral arterial chemoreceptors and reflex control of sodium and water homeostasis. *American Journal of Physiology,* **257,** R1282

Honig, A., Behm, R., and Habeck, J.O. (1985). Sodium metabolism in high-altitude hypoxia, primary systemic hypertension and the peripheral arterial chemoreceptors. *Acta Physiologica Polonica,* **36,** 21

Hoon, R.S., Balasubramanian, V., Mathew, O.P., Tiwari, S.C., Sharma, S.C., and Chadha, K.S. (1977). Effect of high-altitude exposure for 10 days on stroke volume and cardiac output. *American Journal of Physiology: Respiratory, Environmental and Exercise Physiology,* **42,** 722

Hurtado, A. (1964). Some physiologic and clinical aspects of life at high altitudes. In *Aging of the Lung* (L. Cander and J.H. Moyer Eds). New York; Grune and Stratton, p. 257

Klausen, K. (1966). Cardiac output in man at rest and work during and after acclimatization to 3,800 m. *Journal of Applied Physiology,* **21,** 609

Lenfant, C. and Sullivan, K. (1971). Adaptation to high altitude. *New England Journal of Medicine,* **284,** 1298

Lozano, R. and Monge-M.C. (1965). Renal function in high altitude natives with chronic mountain sickness. *Journal of Applied Physiology,* **20,** 1026

Maddocks, I. and Vines, A.P. (1966). The influence of chronic infections on blood pressure in New Guinea males. *Lancet,* **ii,** 262

Marticorena, E., Severino, J., and Chávez, A. (1967). Presión arterial sistemica en el nativo de altura. *Archivos Instituto de Biologia Andina (Lima),* **2,** 18

Marticorena, E., Ruiz, L., Severino, J., Galvez, J., and Peñaloza, D. (1969). Systemic blood pressure in white men born at sea level. Changes after long residence at high altitudes. *American Journal of Cardiology,* **23,** 364

Martineaud, J.P., Durand, J., Coudert, J., and Seroussi, S. (1969). La circulation cutanée au cours de l'adaptation á l'altitude. *Pflügers Archiv, European Journal of Physiology,* **310,** 264

Master, A., Dublin, L., and Marks, H. (1950). The normal blood pressure range and its clinical implications. *Journal of the American Medical Association,* **143,** 1464

Merino, C.F. (1950). Studies on blood formation and destruction in the polycythemia of high altitude. *Blood,* **5,** 1

Milledge, J.S., Catley, D.M., Williams, E.S., Withey, W.R., and Minty, B.D. (1983). Effect of prolonged exercise at altitude on the renin-aldosterone system. *Journal of Applied Physiology, (Respiratory, Environmental, and Exercise Physiology),* **55,** 413

Monge-M, C. and Monge-C, C. (1966). In *High-Altitude Diseases. Mechanism and Management.* Springfield, Illinois; Charles C. Thomas, p. 62

Murillo, F., Barton, S.A., Palomino, H., Lenart, V., and Schull, W.J. (1980). The Aymara of Western

Bolivia : health and disease. *Bulletin of the Pan American Health Organization*, **14**, 52

Norboo, T. (1986). Discussions. In *Aspects of Hypoxia* (D. Heath, Ed.). Liverpool; Liverpool University Press, pp. 75 and 129

Pauli, H.G., Truniger, B., Larsen, J.K., and Mulhausen, R.O. (1968). Renal function during prolonged exposure to hypoxia and carbon monoxide. I. Glomerular filtration and plasma flow. Scandinavian *Journal of Clinical and Laboratory Investigations*, **22** (Suppl. 103), 55

Peñaloza, D. (1971). In *High Altitude Physiology. Cardiac and Respiratory Aspects*, Ciba Foundation Symposium (R. Porter and J. Knight, Eds). Edinburgh; Churchill Livingstone, p. 169

Peñaloza, D., Sime, F., Banchero, N., Gamboa, R., Cruz, J., and Marticorena, E. (1963). Pulmonary hypertension in healthy man born and living at high altitudes. *American Journal of Cardiology*, **11**, 150

Pugh, L.G.C.E. (1964*a*). Cardiac output in muscular exercise at 5,800 m (19,000 feet). *Journal of Applied Physiology*, **19**, 441

Pugh, L.G.C.E. (1964*b*). Blood volume and haemoglobin concentration at altitudes above 18,000 ft (5,500 m). *Journal of Physiology*, **170**, 344

Puri, D.S., Pal, L.S., Gupta, B.P., Swami, H.M., and Dasgupta, D.J. (1986). Distribution of blood pressure and hypertension in healthy subjects residing at high altitude in the Himalayas. *Journal of the Association of Physicians of India*, **34**, 477

Reeves, J.T., Groves, B.M., Sutton, J.T., Wagner, P.D., Cymerman, A., Malconian, M.K., Rock, P.B., Young, D.M., and Houston, C.S. (1987), Operation Everest II: Preservation of cardiac function at extreme altitude. *Journal of Applied Physiology*, **63**, 531

Reynafarje, C. (1966). Physiological patterns: hematological aspects. In *Life at High Altitudes*, Scientific Publication No. 140. Washington; Pan American Health Organization, p. 32

Rotta, A., Cánepa, A., Hurtado, A., Velasquez, T., and Chávez, R. (1956). Pulmonary circulation at sea level and at high altitudes. *Journal of Applied Physiology*, **9**, 328

Ruiz, L. and Peñaloza, D. (1977). Altitude and hypertension. *Mayo Clinic Proceedings*, **52**, 442

Sanchez, C., Merino, C., and Figallo, M. (1970). Simultaneous measurement of plasma volume and cell mass in polycythemia of high altitude. *Journal of Applied Physiology*, **28**, 775

Sehgal, A., Krishan, I., Malhotra, R., and Gupta, H. (1968). Observations on the blood pressure of Tibetans. *Circulation*, **37**, 36

Sheridan, J.W. and Sheridan, R. (1970). Tropical high-altitude peripheral oedema. *Lancet*, **i**, 242

Sime, F.D., Peñaloza, D., Ruiz, L., Gonzales, N., Covarrubias, E., and Postigo, R. (1974). Hypoxemia, pulmonary hypertension, and low cardiac output in newcomers at low altitude. *Journal of Applied Physiology*, **36**, 561

Stenberg, J., Ekblom, B., and Messin, R. (1966).Hemodynamic response to work at stimulated altitude, 4,000 m. *Journal of Applied Physiology*, **21**, 1589

Suarez, J.M., Alexander, J.K., and Houston, C.S. (1987). Enhanced left ventricular systolic performance at high altitude during Operation Everest II. *American Journal of Cardiology*, **60**, 137

Sun, S.F. (1986). Epidemiology of hypertension in the Tibetan plateau. *Human Biology*, **58**, 507

Tucker, C.E., James, W.E., Berry, M.A., Johnstone, C.J., and Grover, R.F. (1976). Depressed myocardial function in the goat at high altitude. *Journal of Applied Physiology*, **41**, 356

Vogel, J.A. and Harris, C.W. (1967). Cardiopulmonary responses of resting man during early exposure to high altitude. *Journal of Applied Physiology*, **22**, 1124

Ward, M.P., Milledge, J.S., and West, J.B. (1989) In *High Altitude Medicine and Physiology*. London; Chapman and Hall Medical, pp. 163

Williams, E.S., Ward, M.P., Milledge, J.S., Withey, W.R. Older, M.W.J., and Forsling, M.L. (1979). Effect of the exercise of seven consecutive days hill-walking on fluid homeostasis. *Clinical Science*, **56**, 305

19

Heart and coronary circulation

Heart muscle is heavily dependent on an adequate supply of oxygen. Extraction of the gas from the coronary arterial supply is high so that the oxygen saturation of the blood in the coronary sinus is less than 25% (see Fig. 18.1). This contrasts with the oxygen saturation of mixed venous blood that is in the region of 70%. Thus about three-quarters of the content of oxygen is removed from the blood during its passage through the myocardium. The oxygen tension of coronary sinus blood is in the region of 15–20 mmHg and that of myocardial tissue cannot be higher. Allowing for the diffusion gradient to the mitochondria, the partial pressure of oxygen in the vicinity of the myocardial respiratory chain must be very low. However, oxidative phosphorylation can proceed in cardiac mitochondria at the remarkably low level of 0.5 mmHg (Tenney and Ou; 1969 Chapter 6, this volume). Furthermore, the diffusion gradient for oxygen is enhanced by the richness of the blood capillary network diminishing the length of the diffusion pathway and by the transport function of myoglobin in the cytoplasm (Chapter 6). The increased uptake of oxygen by the heart that accompanies physical exercise is accomplished by an augmented coronary blood flow, so that the oxygen saturation of the coronary sinus blood does not change (Harris *et al.* 1964). Thus, under normal circumstances the supply of oxygen to the myocardium during exercise is well provided for. This is accomplished without the production of lactate and, in fact, the lactate:pyruvate ratio in the blood of the coronary sinus is actually lower than that in the arterial blood (Harris *et al.* 1964).

MYOCARDIAL RESPONSE TO ACUTE HYPOXIA

When the oxygen tension of coronary arterial blood is suddenly and severely reduced, a number of metabolic mechanisms come into play (Harris 1981). The reduced supply of oxygen limits the function of the respiratory chain and this in turn leads to a reduction of entry into the other end of the chain. This results in a build-up of the reduced form of coenzymes and flavoproteins. This limits the oxidative decarboxylation of pyruvate and the β-oxidation of fatty acyl coenzyme (see Fig. 6.11), so that the concentrations of pyruvate and fatty acyl coenzyme increase. The uptake of fatty acid by the myocardium becomes diminished, since the pathways involved in fatty acid catabolism have no alternative way of disposing of hydrogen (Harris 1981). Glycolysis on the other hand can continue by means of the production of lactate from pyruvate, which forms a mechanism for the disposal of hydrogen (Harris 1981; see Fig. 6.11).

Just as severe hypoxia limits the entry of hydrogen into the respiratory chain, so does it curtail the entry of adenosine diphosphate (ADP) so that the rate of oxidative phosphorylation falls (see Fig. 6.9). This leads to an increase in the concentration of ADP and a decrease in that of adenosine triphosphate (ATP). This in turn has an important influence on glycolysis (Harris 1981). ADP releases the inhibition of the conversion of fructose-6-phosphate to fructose-1,6-diphosphate. Thus, phosphofructokinase is disinhibited and glycolysis is stimulated. Hence, acute hypoxia diminishes the uptake of free fatty acid but augments the uptake of glucose and thus the metabolic response to acute, severe hypoxia is determined by changes in substrate and cofactor concentrations and the modification of enzyme activities.

MITOCHONDRIAL ENZYMES

Over a longer period of exposure to hypoxia it might be anticipated that such changes in emphasis of the importance of different metabolic pathways might be determined by changes in enzyme concentrations. There are, however, few data on this subject and it is still not clear that such changes occur in the myocardium as an acclimatization to chronic hypoxia. Tenney and Ou (1969) reported an increase in the activity of succinate dehydrogenase in the hearts of cattle reared at high altitude. Barrie and Harris (1976) found that, in guinea-pigs subjected experimentally to an atmospheric pressure of 400 mmHg for 14 days, there was a slight increase in the activity of succinate dehydrogenase in myocardial homogenates when compared with that from control animals receiving the same diet. The effect was more obvious in the right ventricle and did not reach a level of significance in the left ventricle. After 28 days' exposure of the animals to hypobaric hypoxia, however, the activity of the enzyme was slightly lower than in the corresponding ventricles of the controls. These authors went on to study a range of enzymes partly or wholly associated with mitochondrial activity in the same guinea-pigs exposed to an atmospheric pressure of 400 mmHg for 28 days. The activity of all was slightly lower than in the corresponding ventricles of the controls. Barrie and Harris (1976) found it difficult to distinguish between the effects of hypertrophy and chronic hypoxia on the level of activity of glycolytic enzymes in the myocardium.

MYOCARDIAL RESPONSE TO CHRONIC HYPOXIA

There is a similarity between the work of hypertrophy and chronic hypoxia on the protein synthetic mechanisms of the heart,which suggests that in both cases the stimulus to an increased protein synthesis is a deficiency of high-energy phosphate groups (Meerson 1971–72, 1975). In the case of hypertrophy this is due to an increased hydrolysis of ATP and in the instance of hypoxia it is due to a decreased oxidative phosphorylation. The cell is able to respond only to the deficit of ATP and cannot distinguish the different courses of events that have given rise to the deficit. At high altitude there are, of course, adequate explanations for the development of right ventricular hypertrophy other than the direct effects of chronic hypoxia on protein synthesis. Thus constriction and muscularization of the peripheral portions of the pulmonary arterial tree are of prime importance (Chapter 10). Meerson (1971–72, 1975) studied rats subjected to a simulated altitude of 7000 m for 6 hours each day for 40 days. By the tenth day the weight of the right ventricle had increased by 80% and that of the left ventricle by 28%. There was an increased incorporation of radioactive amino acids into myocardial protein, indicating an increased protein synthesis. The maximal metabolic changes occurred at about 20 days. The right ventricle was affected more than the left and the increase in labelling of mitochondrial protein was greater than that of nuclear protein.

CORONARY BLOOD FLOW AT HIGH ALTITUDE

After 10 days at an altitude of 3100 m the newcomer from sea level experiences a diminution of the coronary blood flow by some 32% (Grover *et al.* 1976). At the same time there is an increase in extraction of oxygen from coronary arterial blood by some 28% maintaining delivery of oxygen to the myocardium. Although these authors found a decrease in the oxygen saturation of coronary sinus blood, there was no change in the oxygen tension, implying a decrease in the affinity of haemoglobin for oxygen. Such observations are consistent with the view that coronary blood flow is regulated to maintain constant myocardial tissue oxygen tension. The lack of any fall in oxygen tension in coronary sinus blood implies that myocardial hypoxia does not develop.

The coronary blood flow is also diminished in people living permanently at high altitude. Moret (1971) measured coronary flow in two groups of native highlanders living at La Paz (3800 m) and Cerro de Pasco (4330 m) and contrasted his findings with those in subjects living at sea level. The coronary blood flow was diminished by some 30%, the value falling from a mean of 72 ml/min per 100 g of left ventricle at sea level to 55 ml/min per 100 g in La Paz, and 49 ml/min per 100 g in Cerro de Pasco. Coronary vascular resistance was also found to be elevated at high altitude. Hence the magnitude of the decrease in coronary flow in highlanders is very similar to that found in newcomers to high altitude by Grover *et al.* (1976). The oxygen supply to the myocardium was reduced by about one-third at high altitude. The average oxygen uptake by the myocardium was 8.7 ml/min per 100 g at sea level, 7.1 ml/min per 100 g at 3800 m, and 6.8 ml/min per 100 g at 4330 m. Despite the low oxygen uptake, the external work of the heart was not reduced. The oxygen tension of the coronary sinus blood was 20 mmHg at sea level and 17 mmHg at 3800 and 4330 m, so that, by this criterion, no significant degree of tissue hypoxia was occurring in the myocardium at high altitude.

The coronary blood flow in four patients with Monge's disease (Chapter 15) was found to be higher (63 ml/min per 100 g) than in healthy highlanders (Moret 1971). This may be an expression of increased left ventricular work in this condition. As a result of the higher haematocrit in this syndrome, the supply of oxygen to the myocardium is higher, since the desaturation of blood in the coronary sinus is within normal limits.

In the studies of Moret (1971–72), measurements were made of the arteriovenous differences of glucose, lactate, pyruvate, and free fatty acids. The arterial concentration of glucose was slightly lower at high altitude and the myocardial uptake tended to decrease.

The arterial concentrations of lactate and pyruvate were increased at high altitude and the uptake of each tended to increase. That of free fatty acids was similar at high and low altitudes, while the myocardial uptake tended to decrease at high altitude.

INCIDENCE OF CORONARY ARTERY DISEASE AT HIGH ALTITUDE

Since diminished coronary flow in those living at high altitude appears to be balanced by increased extraction of oxygen from coronary arterial blood, with resulting maintenance of myocardial tissue oxygen tension, it is perhaps not surprising that highlanders show little clinical evidence of myocardial ischaemia. Reliable necropsy data are difficult to come by in such isolated areas as the Andes. However, those available suggest that both coronary artery disease and myocardial infarction are decidedly uncommon at high altitude. Arias-Stella and Topilsky (1971) refer to a study of Ramos *et al.* (1967) who found not a single case of myocardial infarction or significant coronary artery disease in a consecutive series of 300 necropsies carried out at 4330 m. Epidemiological studies at Milpo (4100 m) have revealed that angina of effort and electrocardiographic evidence of myocardial ischaemia are less common than at sea level (Ruiz *et al.* 1969). It has to be kept in mind in assessing the low prevalence of coronary artery disease at high altitude that the native highlanders are low-risk subjects anyway. They tend to have low levels of cholesterol, total lipids, triglycerides, and lipoproteins in their blood (Peñaloza 1971). We have already noted the rarity at high altitude of such predisposing diseases as systemic hypertension (Chapter 18) and obesity (Chapter 3). Native highlanders tend to be active physically, and they are not subjected to the same stresses as the dweller in a modern urban environment in a developed country. Peñaloza (1971) believes that the predominant blood group O of the Quecha Indians (Chapter 3) tends to be associated with lesser susceptibility to ischaemic heart disease.

There is some evidence that there is a progressive decline in mortality from coronary arterial disease in Caucasians with increasing altitude of residence. Thus, Mortimer *et al.* (1977) carried out epidemiological studies in New Mexico, where inhabited areas range from 900 to 2200 m. They compared age-adjusted mortality rates for coronary heart disease for White men and women for the years 1957–70 in five sets of counties, grouped by altitude in 300 m increments. The results showed a serial decline in mortality from the lowest to the highest

altitude for males but not for females. Compared with the situation at an altitude of 914 m, the mortality rates were at 98% at 1220m, 90% at 1525 m, 86% at 1830 m, and 72% at 2135 m.

Mortimer and co-workers thought it possible that adjustment to living at high altitude by the low-landers was incomplete, so that ordinary daily activities demanded greater exercise than when undertaken at lower altitudes. The increased physical activity was thought to be beneficial in avoiding coronary thrombosis.

INCREASED VASCULARIZATION OF THE MYOCARDIUM AT HIGH ALTITUDE

A more intense vascularization of the myocardium of highlanders has been reported by Arias-Stella and Topilsky (1971). At necropsy they injected neoprene latex into the coronary arterial tree in highlanders (4330 m) and in 10 lowlanders of comparable age. The number of secondary branches from both main coronary arteries was counted on the casts obtained. At sea level the mean number was 56.4, but at high altitude it was 79.6. Standard photographs were taken of each specimen at identical distances and magnifications, so that the areas occupied by ramifications of the smaller coronary arterial branches could be compared. In the specimens from sea level the range of area occupied by the ramifications was 33–52%, but in the hearts from high altitude it was 55–58%. Further evidence to support the concept that highlanders have a more abundant coronary vasculature than sea-level subjects comes from the work of Carmelino (1970). He demonstrated by stereoangiography of hearts from subjects at sea level and at Puno (3500 m) that at high altitude the distribution of branches is predominantly from the right coronary artery. His work also revealed a statistically significant greater number of coronary arterial branches of the first order, together with a greater number of intercoronary anastomoses.

The increased vascularization of the myocardium extends down to capillary level. We have already noted in Chapter 6 that one of the features of acclimatization at tissue level is increased capillary density. So it appears to be in the myocardium, for Valdivia (1962) found an increased number of blood capillaries per myocardial fibre in guinea-pigs kept in decompression chambers compared with those at sea level. A larger capillary area was found in the hearts of puppies born at 6000 m (Becker *et al.* 1955). It is not certain whether this increased number of coronary blood vessels, both of arterial and capillary dimensions, is perfused at rest, but it seems likely that the increased vascular network represents a greater coronary reserve and may explain in part at least the infrequency of myocardial infarction at high altitude. On the other hand, Clark and Smith (1978) found no increase in capillary density in the myocardium of rats subjected to simulated high altitude. They believe that the myocardium contains an optimal capillary density and that hypoxia should not be expected to act as a stimulus for capillary proliferation, provided an adequate pressure gradient of oxygen exists between capillaries and the centre of the myofibres. Certainly the increased extraction of oxygen from coronary arterial blood reported by Grover et al. (1976) may balance the diminished coronary blood flow at high altitude and maintain a constant myocardial tissue oxygen tension. They find it difficult to reconcile an increased vascularity of the heart with a diminished coronary blood flow. It is possible that their inability to demonstrate increased vascularization of the myocardium is a reflection of the fact that their experiment lasted only 34 days. It seems to us that this is an inadequate amount of time to allow a significant proliferation of capillaries. It is not to be compared to the age of the native highlanders studied by Arias-Stella and Topilsky (1971). We believe there are dangers in too readily applying the results of very short-term experiments employing simulated high altitude to the long-term problems of natural altitude.

THE ELECTROCARDIOGRAM AT HIGH ALTITUDE

There have been several studies of the changes in the electrocardiogram associated with high altitude and it has to be kept in mind that they have been carried out on unlike groups of subjects under different circumstances. Thus the early studies of Peñaloza and Echevarria (1957) and Penaloza (1958) were mainly concerned with changes induced by passive transport of subjects from sea level to 4330 m and the further modifications during prolonged residence at those heights. Another group of investigations on the effect of simulated high altitude has been carried out in decompression chambers, particularly at centres of aviation medicine because of the importance of the findings in relation to airmen. Forster (1983, 1986) studied the electrocardiographic changes shown by commuters and shift-workers manning the UK infrared telescope on the summit of the Hawaiian volcano, Mauna Kea. These changes occurred during tours of duty lasting 5 days at an altitude of 4200 m. Jackson and Davies (1960) carried out a study of the electrocardiogram of the mountaineer at high altitude climbing under

the stress of acute hypoxia and load-bearing at an extreme elevation of 5800 m on Ama Dablam in the Himalaya. Milledge (1963) carried out a similar study on Makalu at 7320 m. All these studies are concerned with electrocardiographic changes in lowlanders being acutely exposed to high altitude. Extensive studies on the electrocardiograms of native highlanders in the newborn, in infants, children, adolescents, and adults have been made by Peñaloza et al. (1959, 1961).

Electrocardiograms in lowlanders on acute exposure to high altitude

Right-axis deviation

Forster (1983, 1986), studying astronomers and supporting staff, found that on repeated ascent for 5 successive days to an altitude of 4200 m there was a progressive right-axis shift of the QRS complex vector at high altitude. At sea level the mean QRS axis was 58.1° (SD 15.5). On the first day at 4200 m, the QRS axis was rotated to 63.9° (SD 21.0). After five days the mean QRS axis was 65° (SD 20.9). Jackson and Davies (1960) had also found right-axis deviation in the standard limb leads in a group of 12 mountaineers. Six of them were Europeans normally resident at sea level and one was a Nepalese subject of Indian descent living at 1330 m. The other five subjects in this group were Sherpas whose home was at 3660 m. Jackson and Davies (1960) found that in their high-altitude climbers an extreme degree of right-axis deviation developed and was proportional to the altitude reached. This change occurred both in Europeans and Sherpas. They considered the possible explanations for these electrocardiographic changes in high altitude. They thought that the clockwise rotation of a vertical heart around its longitudinal axis may be related to the hyperventilation that characterizes residence in the mountains and that is associated with a lower position of the diaphragm. The normal lead III at high altitude resembles that on full inspiration at sea level. However, the changes are not dissimilar to those occurring with pulmonary embolism or pneumothorax. Since right-axis shift may develop irrespective of whether the pneumothorax is on the right or left side, it is probably related to acute right ventricular overload. Hence all the changes in the QRS complex referred to so far may reflect the increased right ventricular work necessitated by pulmonary vasoconstriction induced by hypoxia, as described in Chapter 10. Milledge (1963) also found right-axis deviation and agrees with the interpretation that this is due to right ventricular overload. He found that, initially on exposure to high altitude, the administration of oxygen caused reversal of the right-axis deviation. Subsequent inhalations of oxygen did not produce this effect. This is clearly related to the nature of the elevated pulmonary vascular resistance, as described in Chapters 10 and 34. Initially due entirely to hypoxic pulmonary vasoconstriction, it is subsequently based on the less easily reversible factors of polycythaemia and muscularization of the terminal portions of the pulmonary arterial tree.

T-wave inversion in the right precordial leads

Forster (1983, 1986) found that, at sea level, inversion of the T wave in lead VI was observed in a quarter of the astronomers and their supporting staff. Within hours of arrival at 4200 m, T-wave inversion was seen in half of them. Furthermore, this change persisted at high altitude. The European and Sherpa climbers reported by Jackson and Davies (1960) also shared in showing lowering or inversion of the T wave in right chest leads. These changes tended to increase in extent if the stay at high altitude was prolonged for some weeks. The lower position of the heart is not responsible for such changes, since deep inspiration causes T in VI to become more upright than the reverse. Almost certainly these changes in the right precordial leads are in keeping with the increased load on the right ventricular myocardium.

T-wave changes in the left precordial leads

Significantly, these changes occurred in all the European but in none of the Sherpa climbers. They comprised lowering of the T wave in the left precordial leads. There was some associated depression of the ST segment in the two oldest members of the European party, who were 44 and 53 years of age. These changes over the left ventricle have a different significance from those over the right ventricle (Fig. 19.1). They very likely indicate ischaemia of the left myocardium under the hypoxic conditions of life at high altitude. The fact that they occur in lowlanders but not in native highlanders is in keeping with the view, advanced earlier in this chapter, that the blood supply to the myocardium is better in the highlander. The superior vascularization of the heart muscle described there is the basis for the absence of inversion of the T waves.

Tachycardia

Electrocardiograms (ECGs) taken on climbers acutely exposed to very high altitudes confirm the very rapid heart rates that occur on exercise under such conditions. Jackson (1975) recorded an ECG

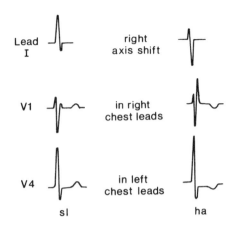

19.1 *Principal changes that occur in the electrocardiogram of those acutely exposed to high altitude. Complexes as seen at sea level, sl, are contrasted with those that occur at high altitude, ha. At high altitude there is right-axis deviation with a prominent S wave in lead I, consistent with acute right ventricular overload and right ventricular hypertrophy. There is also T-wave inversion in the right precordial leads, which is also in keeping with the increased load on the right ventricular myocardium. This change and right-axis deviation has been reported in European and Sherpa climbers. At high altitude there is lowering of the T wave in the left precordial leads, possibly indicative of ischaemia of the left myocardium; this has been found in European but not in Sherpa climbers. (After Jackson (1975).)*

on a fit 25-year-old man climbing between 5180 and 5800 m in the Sierra Nevada de Santa Marta and it shows a heart rate of 208 beats/min (Fig. 19.2).

Changes in rhythm

Changes in rhythm are surprisingly uncommon on acute exposure to high altitude (Jackson 1975), apart from ventricular extrasystoles, one of which is shown in Fig. 19.2. Atrial ectopic beats also occur (Jackson 1975). On Mauna Kea, Forster (1983, 1986) found in a 45-year-old engineer multifocal ventricular extrasystoles occurring in a bigeminal pattern, following a standard exercise test (Fig. 19.3). He experienced no discomfort, other than awareness of this irregular pulse rhythm. A 37-year-old technician showed unifocal ventricular extrasystoles in a bigeminal pattern following exercise at 4200 m. Subsequently, both men underwent submaximal exercise tests on a bicycle-ergometer, with continuous

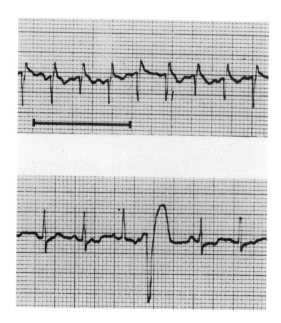

19.2 *Electrocardiograms recorded on magnetic tape during climbing at altitudes between 5200 and 5800 m. The upper trace is from a fit young man of 25 years and shows a sinus tachycardia of 208/min. The lower trace is from a man of 37 years and shows sinus tachycardia with a ventricular ectopic beat. Scale bar, 1 s. (After Jackson (1975).)*

ECG monitoring at sea level. No ECG abnormalities were noted, other than occasional extrasystoles in the older man. Both subjects continued to work at high altitude on the volcano without ill effects.

Electrocardiographic changes associated with right ventricular hypertrophy

Eventually one would anticipate the electrocardiographic changes of right ventricular hypertrophy with dominant R waves in the right chest leads, but this has not been reported in visiting mountaineers (Jackson and Davies 1960). In contrast, electrocardiographic evidence of right ventricular hypertrophy is forthcoming in native highlanders both in childhood and in adult life, as will be seen later in this chapter (Peñaloza *et al.* 1959, 1961).

Other changes

Jackson and Davies (1960) found no changes in the amplitude of the P waves, and no changes in the P–R, QRS, and Q–T intervals in Europeans or Sherpas. These findings were confirmed by Milledge (1963). It is of interest that the electrocardiograms of mountaineers who have climbed as high as 7440 m often show very little evidence of the severe physiological stress they are under (Milledge 1963; Jackson 1975). Jackson (1968) suggests that the electrocardiographic changes at high altitude are not unlike those seen in hypokalaemia.

A study of the ECG of 19 lowlanders climbing to extreme altitude was included in the American Medical Research Expedition to Everest (Karliner *et al.* 1985). Traces were obtained at sea level, 5400 m, 6300 m, and again at sea level. Most of the changes found were attributable to pulmonary hypertension. The amplitude of the P wave in lead II increased by over 40% from sea level to 6300 m consistent with right atrial enlargement. There was right-axis deviation of the QRS axis. There were abnormalities of right bundle branch condition at the highest altitude in three subjects and changes consistent with right ventricular hypertrophy in three others. Seven subjects developed flattened T waves and four showed T-wave inversion. All the changes returned to normal in tracings obtained at sea level after the expedition.

Electrocardiograms in native highlanders

Extensive studies of the influence of high altitudes on the electrical activity of the heart in native highlanders have been made by Peñaloza and co-workers in Lima. They carried out electrocardiographic and vectorcardiographic observations in the newborn, in infants, and in children (Peñaloza *et al.* 1959) and during adolescence and adulthood (Peñaloza *et al.* 1961).

In newborn, infants, and children

The electrocardiograms of 540 normal children were studied by Peñaloza *et al.* (1959), 350 of them at sea level and 190 at 4540 m. A comparative study was made in five age groups, ranging from newborn to 14 years of age. In the newborn the electrical activity of the heart was similar at sea level and at high altitude. In both environments the newborn shows normally a right ventricular preponderance. At sea level this decreases rapidly and is replaced by a physiological left ventricular preponderance. However, at high altitudes the right ventricular preponderance remains throughout infancy and childhood, manifesting itself as an accentuated right Â QRS deviation and a tall R wave in lead VI. According to Peñaloza *et al.* (1959) another important characteristic of the ventricular activation process is an increased magnitude of the terminal QRS vectors. This finding, and not a special position of the heart, determines both the tall late R wave in lead aVR and the deep or pre-

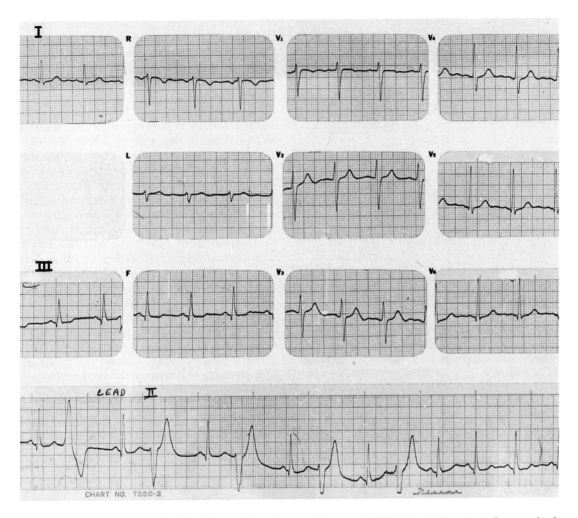

19.3 *Electrocardiogram from a healthy 45-year-old engineer working on the UK infrared telescope at the summit of the Hawaiian volcano, Mauna Kea (4200m). The trace shows multifocal ventricular extrasystoles occurring in a bigeminal pattern. These abnormalities followed a standard exercise test of 30 steps on to a 15-in (38 cm) high platform in 1 min.*

dominant S waves found in the standard limb leads and in the left precordial leads. The positive T waves in the right precordial leads are also related to right ventricular overload.

There is a delay in the normal evolution of the ventricular activation process that occurs at sea level, so there is an absence of transitional patterns that are seen frequently at low altitude between 3 months and 3 years of age. However, when highland children are taken down to sea level, the ventricular activation process is accelerated and vectors corresponding to left ventricular activation increase in magnitude and transitional patterns are seen. The

morbid anatomical basis for these electrocardiographic findings is apparent in Chapter 10, where we described the persistence from birth of mild pulmonary hypertension and muscularization of the terminal portions of the pulmonary arterial tree. The associated increase in pulmonary vascular resistance leads to persistent right ventricular hypertrophy from birth. This persistence of a heavy right ventricle causes the T wave, which becomes negative within a few hours to days after birth at both sea level and at high altitude, to become positive again in highland infants. At sea level Â QRS is generally orientated to the left by the age of 4 months, but at high altitude pronounced right Â QRS deviation remains throughout infancy and childhood.

Peñaloza *et al.* (1959) believe the characteristic features of the electrocardiogram in normal children at high altitude are reminiscent of those found in pulmonary stenosis with a right ventricular systolic pressure similar to that in the systemic circulation, as occurs in some cases of pure pulmonary stenosis and in cases with an overriding aorta. In both there is pronounced right Â QRS deviation, a tall R wave in lead VI, and positive T waves in the right precordial leads. There are, however, differences and for details of these the reader is referred to the paper by Peñaloza *et al.* (1959).

In adolescence and adult life

Electrocardiograms and vectorcardiograms were studied by Peñaloza *et al.* (1961) in 550 normal subjects, 300 of them at sea level and 250 at 4540 m. Comparative studies were made in three age groups. The electrocardiograms of adolescents and adults who live permanently at high altitude are not similar to those of subjects of comparable age who live at sea level. In the adult highlander, right ventricular preponderance is less than in children at the same altitudes, but the physiological left ventricular prepoderance seen at sea level does not occur even in the older adults. As in the case of the children, this electrical right ventricular preponderance is explained by the morbid anatomical events outlined in Chapter 10. Whereas electrocardiographic and vectorcardiographic patterns are almost stereotyped in infancy and childhood at high altitudes, they are highly variable in adult inhabitants of the same altitude (Fig. 19.4). Five principal QRS patterns are described by Peñaloza *et al.* (1961) as occurring in adult highlanders according to the spatial SA QRS orientation. They do not represent different types of ventricular activation. Instead they appear to be varieties of an activation process, which has two main characteristics. These are a delay in the pattern of development of the QRS changes that normally occur with ageing and increasing magnitude of the terminal QRS vectors. For details of the principal electrocardiographic patterns seen, the reader is referred to Peñaloza *et al.* (1961).

Differences in electrocardiographic findings in natives of the Andes and Tibet

Jackson (1975) makes the interesting point that in two Himalayan population surveys at about 3660 m there was a surprising lack of electrocardiographic evidence of right ventricular hypertrophy. The average of the mean frontal QRS axis of 117 adults in Sola Khumbu and Lunana differed by less than 10° from the average of 74 healthy adults from Edinburgh. In the Andes, however, the average axis of 200 adults at 4660 m and at sea level differed by 70° (Peñaloza *et al.* 1961). A possible explanation for this difference put forward by Jackson is that the Tibetans have lived at these heights for so many thousands of years that they have outbred the reactivity of the pulmonary arteries to hypoxia and that the Andeans may in genetic time be relative newcomers to the environment (Jackson 1975). This problem of the different biological status of the Sherpa and the Quechua is enlarged upon in Chapter 36.

Electrocardiograms during sleep at extreme altitudes

Heart rate and rhythm are disturbed during sleep at extreme altitudes. These effects were monitored in eight normal young men during a simulated ascent of Mt Everest in a hypobaric chamber over a period of 40 days (Malconian *et al.* 1990). Recordings were made for 1 hour before sleep, during sleep, and for 1 hour after awakening in all subjects at sea level, in seven subjects at 5490 m, in six at 6100 m, and in four at 7620 m.

Periods of sinus bradycardia occurred during sleep in all subjects at the three levels of high altitude, with a mean rate of 41 ± 0.5 beats/minute compared to a rate of 44 ± 2 beats/minute at sea level.

Cyclical variations in the heart rate, presumably due to periodic breathing, were found in 14 of 17 studies at high altitude but not at sea level. The cycles consisted of bradycardia (40 beats/minute) for 13 seconds followed by tachycardia (120 beats/minute) for 5 seconds. Simultaneous records of ventilation and the ECG were made in five other normal subjects at the Barcroft Laboratory at the White Mountain Research Station (3810 m) in California. These studies confirmed that bradycardia occurred during apnoea and that tachycardia was found with hyperpnoea. Variations in heart rate with periodic breathing were also found by Karliner *et al.* (1985) during the American Medical Research Expedition to Mt Everest when recordings were made on eight subjects at 6300 m.

Arrhythmias were found to occur in all eight subjects studied as part of the Operation Everest II (Malconian *et al.* 1990). These took various forms. There were periods of transient bradycardia with heart rates as low as 20 beats/minute. These were frequently associated with escape rhythms and occasional blocked P waves without preceding PR

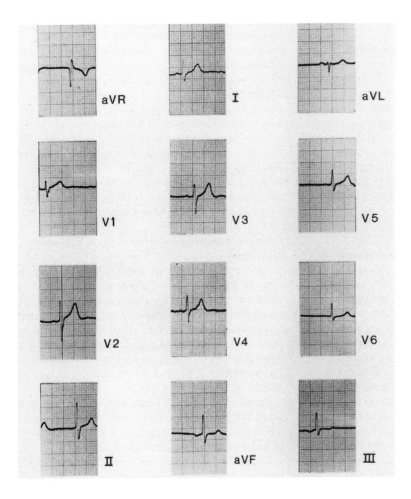

19.4 *Electrocardiogram in a male Indian resident, 23 years of age, of La Paz, Bolivia (3800 m). It demonstrates that the ECG of native highlanders may show little or no abnormality. It shows a normal axis deviation. The R wave in precordial lead VI is of greater magnitude than the S wave and there is a small secondary r wave in this lead. In a young man of this age these findings could be indicative of early right ventricular hypertrophy.*

prolongations. Occasional atrial and ventricular premature beats were found. The bradyarrhythmias were benign and no sustained arrhythmias were found. In conclusion, the ECG during sleep at high altitude shows cyclical variations in heart rate related to periodic breathing (Chapter 28) and bradyarrhythmias. These variations are likely to have a basis in vagal overaction since similar arrhythmias associated with the sleep apnoea syndrome at sea level are eliminated by atropine.

References

Arias-Stella, J. and Topilsky, M. (1971). Anatomy of the coronary circulation at high altitude. In *High Altitude Physiology: Cardiac and Respiratory Aspects* (R. Porter and J. Knight, Ed.). Edinburgh; Churchill Livingstone, p. 149

Barrie, S.E. and Harris, P. (1976). Effects of chronic hypoxia and dietary restriction on myocardial enzyme activities. *American Journal of Physiology*, **231**, 1308

Becker, E.L., Cooper, R.G., and Hataway, G.D. (1955). Capillary, vascularization in puppies born at a simulated altitude of 20,000 feet. *Journal of Applied Physiology*, **8**, 166

Carmelino, M. (1970). Unpublished B.S. thesis. Universidad Peruana Cayetano Heredia, Lima

Clark, D.R. and Smith, P. (1978). Capillary density and muscle fibre size in the hearts of rats subjected to simulated high altitude. *Cardiovascular Research*, **12**, 578

Forster, P.J.G. (1983). *Work at High Altitude. A Clinical and Physiological Study at the United Kingdom Infrared Telescope, Mauna Kea, Hawaii.* Edinburgh; Royal Observatory

Forster, P. (1986). Telescopes in high places. In *Aspects of Hypoxia* (D. Heath, Ed.). Liverpool; Liverpool University Press, pp. 225–226

Grover, R.F., Lufschanowski, R., and Alexander, J.K. (1976). Alterations in the coronary circulation of man following ascent to 3,100 m altitude. *Journal of Applied Physiology*, **41**, 832

Harris, P. (1981). Myocardial metabolism. In *Man at High Altitude* 2nd edn. Edinburgh; Churchill Livingstone, p. 196

Harris, P., Howel-Jones, J., Bateman, M., Chlouverakis, C., and Gloster, J. (1964). Metabolism of the myocardium at rest and during exercise in patients with rheumatic heart disease. *Clinical Science*, **26**, 145

Jackson, F. (1968). The heart at high altitude. *British Heart Journal*, **30**, 291

Jackson, F.S. (1975). Hypoxia and the heart. In *Mountain Medicine and Physiology*, Proceedings of a Symposium sponsored by the Alpine Club, February 1975 (E.S. Williams, M.P. Ward, and C. Clarke, Ed.), p. 99

Jackson, F. and Davies, H. (1960). The electrocardiogram of the mountaineer at high altitude. *British Heart Journal*, **22**, 671

Karliner, J.S., Sarnquist, F.F., Graber, D.J., Peters, R.M., and West, J.B. (1985). The electrocardiogram at extreme altitude: experience on Mt. Everest. *American Heart Journal*, **109**, 505

Malconian, M., Hultgren, H., Nitta, M., Anholm, J., Houston, C., and Fails, H. (1990). The sleep electrocardiogram at extreme altitudes (Operation Everest II). *American Journal of Cardiology*, **65**, 1014

Meerson, F.Z. (1971–72). Role of the synthesis of nucleic acids and proteins in the adaptation of the organism to altitude hypoxia. *Cardiology*, **56**, 173

Meerson, F.Z. (1975). Role of synthesis of nucleic acids and protein in adaptation to the external environment. *Physiological Reviews*, **55**, 70

Milledge, J.S. (1963). Electrocardiographic changes at high altitude. *British Heart Journal*, **25**, 291

Moret, P.R. (1971). Coronary blood flow and myocardial metabolism in man at high altitude. In *High Altitude Physiology: Cardiac and Respiratory Aspects*, Ciba Foundation Symposium (R. Porter and J. Knight, Ed.). Edinburgh; Churchill Livingstone, p. 131

Moret, P.R. (1971–72). Myocardial metabolic changes in chronic hypoxia. *Cardiology*, **56**, 161

Mortimer, E.A., Monson, R.R., and McMahon, B. (1977). Reduction in mortality from coronary heart disease in men residing at high altitude. *New England Journal of Medicine*, **296**, 581

Peñaloza, D. (1958). *Electrocardiographic changes observed during the first month of residence at high altitude* Report No. 58–90, August 1958, School of Aviation Medicine. US Air Force, Randolph Base, Texas

Peñaloza, D. (1971). In *High Altitude Physiology: Cardiac and Respiratory Aspects*, Ciba Foundation Symposium (R. Porter and J. Knight, Ed). Edinburgh; Churchill Livingstone, p. 156

Peñaloza, D. and Echevarria, M. (1957). Electrocardiographic observations on ten subjects at sea level and during one year of residence at high altitudes. *American Heart Journal*, **54**, 811

Peñaloza, D., Gamboa, R., Dyer, J., Echevarria, M., and Marticorena, E. (1959). The influence of high altitudes on the electrical activity of the heart. I. Electrocardiographic and vectorcardiographic observations in the newborn, infants and children. *American Heart Journal*, **59**, 111

Peñaloza, D., Gamboa, R., Marticorena, E., Echevarria, M., Dyer, J., and Gutierrez, E. (1961). The influence of high altitudes on the electrical activity of the heart. Electrocardiographic and vectorcardiographic observations in adolescence and adulthood. *American Heart Journal*, **61**, 101

Ramos, A., Krüger, H., Muro, M., and Arias-Stella, J. (1967). Patologia del hombre nativo de las grandes alturas. Investigacion de las causas de muerte en 300 autopsias. *Boletin de la Oficina Sanitoria Panamericano*, **62**, 496

Ruiz, L., Figueroa, M., Horna, C., and Peñaloza, D. (1969). Prevalencia de la hipertension arterial y cardiopatia isquemica en los grandes alturas. *Archives del Instituto de Cardiologia de Mexico*, **39**, 476

Tenney, S.M. and Ou, L.C. (1969). In *Biomedicine Problems of High Terrestrial Elevations* (A.H. Hegnauer, Ed.). US Army Research Institute of Environmental Medicine, p. 160

Valdivia, E. (1962). Total capillary bed of the myocardium in chronic hypoxia. *Federation Proceedings: Federation of American Societies for Experimental Biology*, **21**, 221

20

Renal function and electrolytes

The kidney is able to maintain adequate tubular function at high altitude in the face of considerable reduction of plasma flow, greatly increased blood viscosity, and pronounced hypoxaemia. Up to an altitude of 5800 m, which we define as the beginning of extreme altitude (Chapter 32), the kidney concentrates urine normally and is able to eliminate a water load as well as it does at sea level. At extreme altitude, however, the renal compensation for respiratory alkalosis becomes slow and incomplete so that the blood bicarbonate is very little further reduced and the blood pH becomes very alkaline as the blood carbon dioxide tension is reduced by extreme hyperventilation (Chapter 32). Ward *et al.* (1989) believe that this should be regarded as a feature of acclimatization rather than of renal failure, for the alkaline pH of the blood results in a shift of the oxygen–haemoglobin dissociation curve to the left that benefits oxygen transport at extreme altitude. However, even at lower altitudes there is characteristically proteinuria.

PROTEINURIA

There is an increased excretion of protein in the urine in native highlanders (Fig. 20.1). Rennie *et al.* (1971*b*) found that, although this increase barely exceeded physiological levels, it was unequivocal. They studied young male residents of Yauricocha (4640 m) who had lived in the town for at least 2 years, and found that the proteinuria was associated with normal creatinine clearance rates, suggesting to them that it was independent of glomerular filtration rate. A slightly older group of men from San Cristobel (4710 m) was found to have a depression of creatinine clearance associated with their proteinuria and this was considered to be related to their higher degree of polycythaemia. In native highlanders it has proved impossible to demonstrate any deficiency in oxygen uptake by the kidney (Rennie *et al.* 1971*a*). Hence, proteinuria in highlanders is not directly and obviously related to a deprivation of oxygen in the kidney.

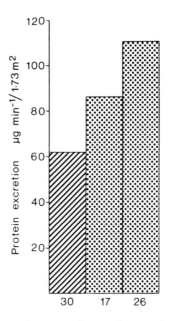

20.1 *Mean urinary protein excretion rates in 30 lowlanders at 160 m (hatched column), in 17 native highlanders at 4640 m (stippled column), and in 26 native highlanders at 4710 m (stippled column). Protein excretion is increased in highlanders. (From data of Rennie* et al. *(1971b).)*

Proteinuria is also found in climbers undergoing acclimatization. The protein concentration in early-morning urine specimens collected from 13 climbers undergoing acclimatization was found to correlate significantly with the altitude when adjusted for urine-concentration effects (Rennie and Joseph 1970). There is a time lag of about a day between exposure to high altitude and the onset of proteinuria. This recalls the similar delay before the onset of acute mountain sickness that is described in Chapter 12. Pines (1978) reported the occurrence of proteinuria in seven climbers who spent 6 weeks in the mountain areas of Ruwenzori (5110 m), Kilimanjaro (5960 m), and Mt Kenya (5200 m) in

East Africa. The mean protein urine concentration in morning specimens as determined by reagent strips was over 100 mg/dl after climbs during the first 12 days. In subsequent climbs it fell to 15 mg/dl. The highest concentrations (100–300 mg/dl) were found in five climbers with peripheral oedema and three of them had obvious acute mountain sickness. The proteinuria was a response to altitude and not to exercise, for it was not provoked by the most strenuous and exhausting part of the trip below 3000 m. Pines (1978) also found proteinuria in eight climbers on Nanda Devi (7820 m) in the Himalaya. Its characteristics were the same in the climbers in East Africa, in that it occurred during the earlier climbs on acute exposure to high altitude, diminished with repeated ascents, and was most pronounced in climbers who developed acute mountain sickness. We have, ourselves, noted the association of proteinuria with the onset of acute mountain sickness during expeditions to the Andes. Bradwell and Delamere (1982) found that there was a significant correlation between the height attained and both the concentration and excretion rate of urinary albumin in normal subjects after rapid ascent. They found that the increase in albumin excretion rate was virtually abolished in subjects treated with acetazolamide, although a subsequent study showed no significant effect of acetazolamide on the proteinuria (Winterborn *et al.* 1987).

Origin of proteinuria at high altitude

The site of the renal protein leak on ascent to high altitude was studied by Winterborn *et al.* (1987) who note that two hypotheses have been advanced as to its cause. First, the active tubular reabsorption of protein might be inhibited by hypoxia. This explanation would be supported by the appearance in the urine of low-molecular-weight proteins such as α_1-microglobulin that are normally reabsorbed completely in the proximal tubule. Second, an increase in capillary permeability secondary to hypoxia might lead to a greater filtered load of protein exceeding the reabsorptive capacity of the renal tubule.

Winterborn *et al.* (1987) determined the site of the renal protein leak by using intravenous lysine, which acts as a powerful but transient inhibitor of renal tubular protein reabsorption (Mogensen and Solling 1977), offering a means of distinguishing between tubal and glomerular proteinuria in normal man. Urinary protein excretion was measured before and after the intravenous infusion of lysine in 14 normal subjects after 4–6 days' acclimatization at 4850 m. Urinary albumin excretion before lysine

was elevated in 11 subjects, but α_1-microglobulin was detected in only four. After lysine, a large increase in albumin excretion occurred in all subjects. Taken together with the absence of α_1-microglobulin before lysine, this suggests that increased glomerular capillary permeability is the major cause of proteinuria after acclimatization to high altitude. The alteration in glomerular permeability with hypoxia could be mediated by a direct effect on the glomerular epithelial cells or by local hormonal effects on renal blood flow. It is not known what ultrastructural changes occur in the renal glomeruli of those ascending rapidly to high altitude, but enlargement of the glomeruli is known to develop in children living permanently at high altitude. The increase in the permeability of the glomerular capillaries with the leakage of protein at high altitude is reminiscent of the leakage of protein from the pulmonary capillaries in high-altitude pulmonary oedema (Chapter 13). The frequent association of proteinuria with the onset of acute mountain sickness is noteworthy.

RENAL GLOMERULI IN HIGHLANDERS

Patients with cyanotic congenital heart disease, in whom the hypoxaemia is due to the developmental anomaly rather than exposure to high altitude, also develop proteinuria. Its degree correlates with the length and severity of systemic oxygen unsaturation (Rennie *et al.* 1971*b*). It was noted that such patients had enlarged renal glomeruli (Meeson and Litton 1953; Spear 1960) and this stimulated Naeye (1965) to study the histology of the kidney in 15 children who died in Leadville, Colorado (3100 m) and compare it with that of 80 sea-level children. He determined by planimetry the areas of 20–40 glomeruli and thus the mean glomerular area for each case. He found that, at birth, children at high altitude have renal glomeruli of normal size, but disproportionate enlargement occurs in childhood compared to subjects at sea level. Naeye (1965) determined what he called the 'parenchymal cell density' in individual glomeruli by dividing the number of parenchymal cells by total glomerular area. This proved to be the same in native highlanders as in lowlanders. Hence the glomerular enlargement found at high altitude appears to be due to a proliferation of normal glomerular elements. This is precisely what is found in patients with cyanotic congenital heart disease (Naeye 1965). It seems likely that this enlargement of the glomeruli of native highlanders is related to the sustained increased glomerular capillary permeability described above.

RENAL FUNCTION

When renal haemodynamics are studied in native highlanders and patients with Monge's disease they show a normal total renal blood flow, a reduction of plasma flow because of the raised haematocrit, but a lesser fall in glomerular filtration rate (Fig. 20.2). Hence there is an elevated filtration fraction in the highlanders, which becomes even more pronounced on the development of chronic mountain sickness (Fig. 20.2). In this way glomerular filtration rate is not reduced to levels that would prove of clinical significance. The findings of Becker *et al.* (1957) were subsequently confirmed by Lozano and Monge-M (1965). Monge-C *et al.* (1969) found that there was a positive correlation between filtration fraction and haematocrit (Fig. 20.2). They thought that the increased filtration fraction can be explained by increased resistance at the level of the efferent arteriole and that this resistance could be the result of high blood viscosity due to the elevated haematocrit. Renal tubular function is maintained at an adequate level at high altitude in the presence of considerable reduction of plasma flow, greatly increased blood viscosity, and pronounced hypoxaemia.

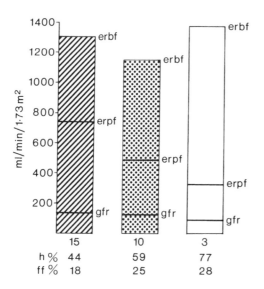

20.2 *Effective renal blood flow (erbf), effective renal plasma flow (erpf), and glomerular filtration rate (grf) in 15 lowlanders (hatched column), in 10 healthy highlanders (stippled column), and in 3 subjects with Monge's disease (open column). The studies were carried out at an altitude of 4500 m. For each group the values for haematocrit (h%) and filtration fraction (ff%) are shown at the foot of the column. (Based on data from Monge-C* et al. *(1969).)*

HYDRATION AND ANTIDIURETIC HORMONE

Initial exposure to high altitude may lead to the passing of copious urine, the so-called 'Hohendiuresis' of alpine climbers. If hypobaric hypoxia is tolerated well, there may be a diuresis that lasts for days (Burrill *et al.* 1945). This polyuria of mild hypoxia brings about a contraction of extracellular and plasma volume producing the 'haemo-concentration' characteristic of early days at high altitude. Such diuresis is typical of those who tolerate rapid ascent to high altitude well. In contrast, subjects likely to develop subsequently acute mountain sickness become oliguric during the first 4 hours of their exposure to the hypobaric hypoxia of the mountain environment (Singh *et al.* 1969). Trekkers with acute mountain sickness gained weight, whereas those free of the condition lost weight by the time that they reached 4243 m (Hackett *et al.* 1982).

Diuresis is influenced by antidiuretic hormone, ADH, which is secreted by the posterior lobe of the pituitary, the neurohypophysis, which is part of the brain (Chapter 22). It regulates water reabsorption in the distal renal tubules and collecting ducts. In the absence of ADH, also called vasopressin and pitressin, the nephron is virtually impermeable to water and the urine is voluminous and very dilute. In the presence of ADH, the tubule is freely permeable to water and comes into osmotic equilibrium with the extracellular fluid through outward movement of water.

However, the relationship between plasma concentration of ADH and hypoxia is not at all clear. Breathing 10% oxygen for 4 hours has no effect on levels of ADH in blood samples taken at intervals from 3 minutes to 4 hours of hypoxia (Forsling and Milledge 1977). In a further experiment when subjects were taken to a simulated altitude of 4000 m for 16 hours there was no significant change in plasma concentration of ADH until the subjects became nauseated when levels rose markedly (Forsling and Milledge 1980). Claybaugh *et al.* (1982) found that exposure to comparable simulated altitudes led to an increase in urinary ADH after 8–12 hours of hypoxia with a subsequent return to sea-level values. In two subjects with acute mountain sickness there was a rise in urinary excretion of ADH at 2–4 hours of hypoxia. In summary, acute hypoxia appears to have little effect on ADH secretion but the onset of acute mountain sickness is associated with a rise in ADH (Eversman *et al.* 1978).

So far as chronic exposure to hypobaric hypoxia is concerned, Singh *et al.* (1974) measured levels of antidiuretic hormone amongst a range of hormones in a group of subjects with a history of high-altitude pulmonary oedema. Once again, in those subjects who did not develop acute mountain sickness there was no change in ADH levels. In those who did, there was some elevation of ADH concentration, which was not statistically significant and which occurred after only a few days. Harber *et al.* (1981) found that not only was there no significant change in urinary ADH concentration on going to altitudes up to 5400 m but, furthermore, there was no relationship with acute mountain sickness. Even in a fatal case of high-altitude cerebral oedema there was no significant rise in ADH (Hackett *et al.* 1978). There were higher concentrations only in two cases of high-altitude pulmonary oedema. The conclusion from all these data must be that hypoxia *per se* has no significant effect on ADH concentration. High values may be associated with some but not all cases of acute mountain sickness.

There is controversy as to the state of hydration of the body once this initial stage of acute exposure to high altitude is passed. A significant part of the early weight loss at high altitude is due to dehydration. At extreme altitude climbers may become dehydrated due to the greatly increased pulmonary ventilation induced by elevation and exercise, coupled with the low humidity of the ambient air (Pugh 1962). Bulstrode (1975) reports that he lost 6 kg in body weight in rapidly climbing and descending Mt Kenya (5200 m) and regained it within 24 hours of descent. He concluded that this remarkable loss of weight was due to fluid loss. Consolazio *et al.* (1968) observed a negative water balance in troops after 4 weeks' exposure to conditions at 4300 m. In other studies Consolazio *et al.* (1972) and Krzywicki *et al.* (1969) have attributed much of the loss of body weight at high altitude to absolute dehydration with decrease in plasma volume. Consolazio *et al.* (1972) believed that at the same time intracellular water falls on acute exposure to altitude so that, according to this view, total body water falls.

Other investigators have found that the decrease in plasma volume referred to above is associated with an increase in intracellular water and redistribution of body fluids. The net result of this is that normal body hydration is maintained (Surks *et al.* 1966; Hannon *et al.* 1969, 1972). Hannon *et al.* (1976) found little evidence of a net loss of body water during a stay of 1 week at 4300 m of eight young women. Rather there appeared to be renal water conservation, probably in response to respiratory water loss. The analysis of carcasses of laboratory animals shows little or no change in body water content on exposure to high altitude (Schnakenberg *et al.* 1971).

SODIUM

On exposure to high altitude the sodium balance is positive during the first 2 days but then becomes negative (Ullman 1953; Slater *et al.* 1969*a,b*). The natriuresis is due to decreased reabsorption of sodium ions in the renal tubules, which is associated with diminished secretion of aldosterone (Chapter 22). This is itself related to plasma renin activity. Renin is a proteolytic enzyme that is synthesized, stored, and secreted mainly by the granular cells in the walls of the distal part of the afferent glomerular arterioles forming part of the juxtaglomerular apparatus in the kidney. A few renin-secreting cells are also found in the walls of the efferent arterioles within the kidney. Another component of the juxtaglomerular apparatus is the macula densa, which is a group of specialized tubular epithelial cells lining that part of the distal convoluted tubule adjacent to the glomerular-arteriolar axis. This is probably a sensor mechanism that regulates the release of renin in response to a low concentration of sodium ions in the tubule. Renin releases angiotensin I, an inactive decapeptide, from angiotensinogen, an α_2-globulin in plasma and tissue fluids. Angiotensin I is converted to the octapeptide angiotensin II by angiotensin-converting enzymes that are widely distributed in the tissues, but particularly concentrated in the endothelial cells of the pulmonary blood capillaries. It is angiotensin II that is mainly responsible for stimulating the secretion of aldosterone by the adrenal cortex (Chapter 22) encouraging sodium retention. Thus, renin regulates a system whose effects such as the regulation of sodium levels are mediated by angiotensin II and aldosterone. The effect of high altitude on plasma renin activity has been studied by various groups but the results have been conflicting. Some have reported a rise (Slater *et al.* 1969*a*; Frayser *et al.* 1975) and others a fall (Hogan *et al.* 1973; Keynes *et al.* 1982). However, it is significant that at high altitude there appears to be a reduced response of aldosterone to renin.

Systemic oedema has been associated with ascent into high altitude since the first report by Sheridan and Sheridan in 1970. However, Williams *et al.* (1979) demonstrated that oedema of the face and ankles may be the result of exercise *per se*. They found that the degree and type of exercise associated with trekking may in itself result in appreciable sodium retention with expansion of the extracellular fluid volume at the expense of the intracellular fluid volume. This was found to be due to activation of the renin–angiotensin–aldosterone axis (Milledge *et al.* 1982). When the *combined* effects of high altitude and exercise were studied, great rises in renin activity, up to eight times those of control levels, were found (Milledge *et al.*, 1983). They reported, however, that the much increased levels of renin induced by exercise at high altitude did *not* result in equivalent high levels of angiotensin II and aldosterone. Thus, in many subjects ascending mountains there appears to be blunted response of aldsterone to renin. This has been attributed to a deficiency of converting enzyme brought about by hypobaric hypoxia (Leuenberger *et al.* 1978). Milledge speculates that, in subjects prone to acute mountain sickness, converting enzyme activity does *not* fall in response to hypobaric hypoxia so that they have raised levels of angiotensis II and aldosterone. This would result in considerable sodium retention and an increase in extracellular fluid volume, together with an increased pressor response in both pulmonary and systemic circulations.

POTASSIUM

There is a tendency for the body to conserve potassium on acute exposure to high altitude, especially during the first 3 days (Hannon *et al.* 1972; Janowski *et al.* 1969). A positive potassium balance over a 5-day period of exposure to 3500 m was observed by Slater *et al.* (1969*b*). There have been reports of a rise in plasma potassium (Slater *et al.* 1969*b*; Epstein and Saruta 1973; Frayser *et al.* 1975). Sutton *et al.* (1977) found no change in plasma potassium concentration in four men exposed to a simulated altitude of 4760 m for 2 days but, like other observers, they found a decrease in urinary potassium excretion. The loss of sodium and retention of potassium naturally causes the ratio of sodium to potassium to increase at high altitude in both urine and saliva. These changes in electrolyte excretion are related to the fall in aldosterone secretion that occurs during the early stages of exposure to high altitude (Ayres *et al.* 1961; Williams 1966; Janowski *et al.* 1969; Hannon *et al.* 1972). The fall in aldosterone secretion is itself probably related to the increased blood volume that occurs on exposure to high altitude (Williams 1966; Chapters 18 and 22, this volume).

ZINC

During an expedition to Kanchenjunga (8600 m) in 1975, plasma and urinary concentrations of various electrolytes were measured in 11 climbers (Rupp *et al.* 1982). Both the plasma zinc level and the urinary zinc output showed what the authors termed 'an astonishing increase'. Plasma zinc concentration rose immediately by 230% from 10.9 mmol/l, and remained at that level until the end of the expedition. Urinary zinc output increased steadily from 14.8 to 183.4 mmol/day, a 12-fold increase. Rupp *et al.* (1982) speculated that these high levels might have been due to the local food in the Himalaya or the tinned food, which might have contained zinc released from the cans themselves.

MAGNESIUM

The content of magnesium in both erythrocytes and leucocytes is said to be significantly higher in normal and healthy residents at high altitude, but has been reported to be reduced in patients with high-altitude pulmonary oedema (Chohan 1984).

URINARY PURINES

Metabolic processes involving ATP are affected by hypobaric hypoxia. It has been thought that the degree of breakdown of tissue nucleotides caused by exercise or hypoxia can be quantitatively related to the level of hypoxanthine and xanthine (Harkness *et al.* 1982). An alternative view is that elevated levels of serum hypoxanthine are associated with impaired renal excretion (Forster *et al.* 1987). Forster *et al.* (1986) studied changes in serum and urinary purines at high altitude in 20 lowlanders, aged 20–47 years, during a 15-day trek to 4850 m in the Himalaya. Ten of them took acetazolamide in a dose of 500 mg/day. They found that serum urate, xanthine, and total purines were not significantly different at the two altitudes or between the treatment groups, and 24-hour urate, xanthine, and total purine excretion were not altered. However, serum hypoxanthine levels were significantly raised (37 ± 11 μmol/l) at 4850 m compared with 20 ± 6.6 μmol/l at 3000 m. In subjects taking acetazolamide, the corresponding levels were 46.4 ± 14.7 μmol/l, contrasted to 32 ± 13 μmol/l. These increases were associated with significant decreases in hypoxanthine clearance.

References

Ayres, P.J., Hurter, R.C., Williams, E.S., and Rundo, J. (1961). Aldosterone excretion and potassium retention in subjects living at high altitude. *Nature* (London), **191**, 78

Becker, E.L., Schilling, J.A., and Harvey, R.B. (1957). Renal function in man acclimatized to high altitude. *Journal of Applied Physiology*, **10**, 79

Bradwell, A.R. and Delamere, J.P. (1982). The effect of acetazolamide on the proteinuria of altitude. *Aviation, Space, and Environmental Medicine*, **53**, 40

Bulstrode, C.J.K. (1975). A preliminary study into factors predisposing mountaineers to high altitude pulmonary oedema. *Journal of the Royal Naval Medical Service*, **61**, 101

Burrill, M.W., Freeman, S., and Ivy, A.C. (1945). Sodium, potassium and chloride excretion of human subjects exposed to simulated altitude of 18 000 feet. *Journal of Biological Chemistry*, **157**, 297

Chohan, I.S. (1984). Blood coagulation changes at high altitude. *Defence Science Journal*, **34**, 361

Claybaugh, J.R., Wade, C.E., Sato, A.K., Cucinell, S.A., Lane, J.C., and Maher, J.T. (1982). Antidiuretic hormone responses to eucapnic and hypocapnic hypoxia in humans. *Journal of Applied Physiology (Respiratory, Environmental and Exercise Physiology)*, **53**, 815

Consolazio, C.F., Matoush, L.O., Johnson, H.L., and Daws, T.A., (1968). Protein and water balances of young adults during prolonged exposure to high altitudes (4300 meters). *American Journal of Clinical Nutrition*, **21**, 154

Consolazio, C.F., Johnson, H.L., Krzywicki, H.J., and Daws, T.A. (1972). Metabolic aspects of acute altitude exposure (4300 meters) in adequately nourished humans. *American Journal of Clinical Nutrition*, **25**, 23

Epstein, M. and Saruta, T. (1973). Effect of simulated high altitude on renin–aldsterone and Na homeostasis in normal man. *Journal of Applied Physiology*, **33**, 204

Eversman, T., Gottsman, M., Uhlich, E., Ulbrecht, G., von Werder, K., and Scriba, P.C. (1978). Increased secretion of growth hormone, prolactin, antidiuretic hormone and cortisol induced by the stress of motion sickness. *Aviation, Space, and Environmental Medicine*, **49**, 53

Forsling, M.L. and Milledge, J.S. (1977). Effect of hypoxia on vasopressin release in man. *Journal of Physiology*, **267**, 22

Forsling, M.L., and Milledge, J.S. (1980). The effect of simulated altitude (4000 m) on plasma cortisol and vasopressin concentration in man. *Proceedings of the International Union of Physiological Sciences*, **14**, 414

Forster, P.J.G., Nuki, G., Rylance, H.J., and Wallace, R.C., (1986). Effect of high altitude and acetazolamide on human serum and urine purines. *Advances in Experimental Medicine and Biology*, **195**, 601

Forster, P.J.G., Rylance, H.J., Wallace, R.C., and Nuki, G. (1987). Changes in serum and urinary purines at high altitude. *Postgraduate Medical Journal*, **63**, 193

Frayser, R., Rennie, I.D., Grey, G.W., and Houston, C.S. (1975). Hormonal and electrolyte response to exposure to 17 500 ft. *Journal of Applied Physiology*, **38**, 636

Hackett, P.H., Forsling, M.L., Milledge, J., and Rennie, D. (1978). Release of vasopressin in man at altitude. *Hormone and Metabolic Research*, **10**, 571

Hackett, P.H., Rennie, D., Hofmeister, S.E., Grover, R.F., Grover, E.B., and Reeves, J.T. (1982). Fluid retention and relative hypoventilation in acute mountain sickness. *Respiration*, **43**, 321

Hannon, J.P., Chinn, K.S.K., and Shields, J.L. (1969). Effects of acute high altitude exposure on body fluids. *Federation Proceedings: Federation of American Societies for Experimental Biology*, **28**, 1178

Hannon, J.P., Chinn, K.S.K., and Shields, J.L. (1972). Alterations in serum and extracellular electrolytes during high altitude exposure. *Journal of Applied Physiology*, **31**, 266

Hannon, J.P., Klain, G.J., Sudman, D.M., and Sullivan, F.J. (1976). Nutritional aspects of high-altitude exposure in women. *American Journal of Clinical Nutrition*, **29**, 604

Harber, M.J., Williams, J.D., and Morton, J.J. (1981). Antidiuretic hormone excretion at high altitude. *Aviation, Space, and Environmental Medicine*, **52**, 38

Harkness, R.A., Whitelaw, A.E.L., and Simmonds, R.J. (1982). Intrapartum hypoxia: the association between neurological assessment of damage and abnormal excretion of ATP metabolites. *Journal of Clinical Pathology*, **35**, 999

Hogan, R.P., Kotchen, T.A., Boyd, A.E., and Hartley, L.W. (1973). Effect of altitude on renin–aldosterone system and metabolism of water and electrolytes. *Journal of Applied Physiology*, **35**, 385

Janowski, A.H., Whitten, B.W., Shields, J.L., and Hannon, J.P. (1969). Electrolyte patterns and regulation in man during acute exposure to high altitude. *Federation Proceedings: Federation of American Societies for Experimental Biology*, **28**, 1185

Keynes, J.R., Smith, G.W., Slater, J.D.H., Brown, M.M., Brown, S.E., Payne, N.N., Jowett, T.P., and Monge-C, (1982). Renin and aldosterone at high altitude in man. *Journal of Endocrinology*, **92**, 131

Krzywicki, H.J., Consolazio, C.F., Matoush, L.O., Johnson, H.L., and Barnhart, R.A. (1969). Body composition changes during exposure to altitude. *Federation Proceedings: Federation of American Societies for Experimental Biology*, **28**, 1190

Lozano, R. and Monge-M, C. (1965). Renal function in high-altitude natives and in natives with chronic mountain sickness. *Journal of Applied Physiology*, **20**, 1026

Leuenberger, P.J., Stalcup, C.A., Mellins, R.B., Greenbaum, L.M., and Turino, G.M. (1978). Decrease in angiotensin I conversion by acute hypoxia in dogs. *Proceedings of the Society for Experimental Biology and Medicine*, **158**, 586

Meeson, H. and Litton, M.A. (1953). Morphology of the kidney in morbus caeruleus. *Archives of Pathology*, **56**, 480

Milledge, J.S., Bryson, E.I., Catley, D.M., Hesp, R., Luff, N., Minty, B.D., Older, M.W., Payne, N.N., Ward, M.P., and Withey, W.R. (1982). Sodium balance, fluid homeostasis and the renin–aldosterone system during the prolonged exercise of hill walking. *Clinical Science*, **62**, 595

Milledge, J.S., Catley, D.M., Williams, E.S., Withey, W.R., and Minty, B.D. (1983). Effect of prolonged exercise on the renin–aldosterone system. *Journal of Applied Physiology: Respiratory, Environmental and Exercise Physiology*, **55**, 413

Mogensen, C.E. and Solling, K. (1977). Studies on renal tubular protein reabsorption; partial and near complete inhibition of certain amino acids. *Scandinavian Journal of Clinical and Laboratory Investigation*, **37**, 477

Monge-C, C., Lozano, R., Marchena, C., Whittembury, J., and Torres, C. (1969). Kidney function in the high altitude native. *Federation Proceedings: Federation of American Societies for Experimental Biology*, **28**, 1199

Naeye, R.L. (1965). Children at high altitude: pulmonary and renal abnormalities. *Circulation Research*, **16**, 33

Pines, A. (1978). High-altitude acclimatization and proteinuria in East Africa. *British Journal of Diseases of the Chest*, **72**, 196

Pugh, L.G.C.E. (1962). Physiological and medical aspects of Himalayan, Scientific and Mountaineering Expedition 1960–61. *British Medical Journal*, **ii**, 621

Rennie, I.D.B. and Joseph, B.J. (1970). Urinary protein excretion in climbers at high altitudes. *Lancet*, **i**, 1247

Rennie, I.D.B., Lozano, R., Monge-C, C., Sime, F., and Whittembury, J. (1971a). Renal oxygenation in male Peruvian natives living permanently at high altitudes. *Journal of Applied Physiology*, **30**, 450

Rennie, D., Marticorena, E., Monge-C, C., and Sirotzky, L. (1971b). Urinary protein excretion in high-altitude residents. *Journal of Applied Physiology*, **31**, 257

Rupp, C., Zink, R.A., and Brendel, W. (1982). Electrolyte changes in the blood and urine of high altitude climbers. In *High Altitude Physiology and Medicine*. New York; Springer-Verlag, p. 183

Schnakenberg, D.D., Krabill, L.F., and Weiser, P.C. (1971). The anorexic effect of high altitude on weight gain, nitrogen retention and body composition of rats. *Journal of Nutrition*, **101**, 789

Sheridan, J.W. and Sheridan, R. (1970). Tropical high altitude peripheral oedema. *Lancet*, **i**, 242

Singh, I., Khanna, P.K., Srivastava, M.C., Lal, M., Roy, S.B., and Subramanyam, C.S.V. (1969). Acute mountain sickness. *New England Journal of Medicine*, **280**, 175

Singh, I., Malhotra, M.S., Khanna, P.K., Nanda, R.B., Purshottam, T., Upadhyay, T.D., Radhakrishnan, U., and Brahmachan, H.D. (1974). Changes in plasma cortisol, blood antidiuretic hormone and urinary catecholamines in high-altitude pulmonary oedema. *International Journal of Biometeorology*, **18**, 211

Slater, J.D.H., Tuffley, R.E., Williams, E.S., Beresford, C.H., Sonksen, P.H., Edwards, R.H.T, Ekins, R.P., and McLaughlin, M., (1969a). Control of aldosterone secretion during acclimatization to hypoxia in man. *Clinical Science*, **37**, 327

Slater, J.D.H., Tuffley, R.E., Williams, E.S., Edwards, R.H.T., Ekins, R.P., Sonksen, P.H., Beresford, C.H., and McLaughlin, M., (1969*b*). Potassium retention during the respiratory alkalosis of mild hypoxia in man: its relationship to aldosterone secretion and other metabolic changes. *Clinical Science*, **37**, 311

Spear, G.S. (1960). Glomerular alterations in cyanotic congenital heart disease. *Bulletin of Johns Hopkins Hospital*, **106**, 347

Surks, M.I., Chinn, K.S.K., and Matoush, L.O. (1966). Alterations in body composition in man after acute exposure to high altitude. *Journal of Applied Physiology*, **21**, 1741

Sutton, J.R., Viol, G.W., Gray, G.W., McFadden, M., and Keane, P.M. (1977). Renin, aldosterone, electrolyte and cortisol responses to hypoxic decompression. *Journal of Applied Physiology*, **43**, 421

Ullman, E.A. (1953). Renal water and cation excretion at moderate altitude. *Journal of Physiology*, **120**, 58

Ward, M.P., Milledge, J.S., and West, J.B. (1989). The endocrine and renal systems. In *High Altitude Medicine and Physiology*. London; Chapman and Hall Medical, p. 293

Williams, E.S. (1966). Electrolyte regulation during the adaptation of humans to life at high altitude. *Proceedings of the Royal Society*, **B165**, 266

Williams, E.S., Ward, M.P., Milledge, J.S., Withey, W.R. Older, M.W.J., and Forsling, M.L. (1979). Effect of the exercise of seven consecutive days hill-walking on fluid homeostasis. *Clinical Science*, **56**, 305

Winterborn, M.H., Bradwell, A.R., Chesner, I.M., and Jones, G.T., (1987). The origin of proteinuria at high altitude. *Postgraduate Medical Journal*, **63**, 179

21

Body weight and alimentary system

Most newcomers to high altitude above 4000 m lose weight, sometimes to a considerable extent. The mean loss of body weight was 0.4 kg in 10 climbers who flew to Kathmandu (1300 m) and then after 2 days climbed from Gorka to Rupina La (4850 m) over 10 days, stopping there for a further 6 days until a rapid descent to Kathmandu (Bradwell *et al.* 1986). At extreme altitude weight loss is even more pronounced. As part of the American Medical Research Expedition to Everest in 1981, Boyer and Blume (1984) measured the loss of body weight that occurred in Caucasian members of the group. During the approach march to, and residence at, 5400 m for the first week the mean loss was 1.9 kg. This involved a walking distance of 260 km, with a rise of 5000 m. On further ascent to an extreme altitude of 6300 m, for some for more than 1 week and for others for less, there was a further loss of 4.0 kg. A prolonged stay at extreme altitude may lead to emaciation. The causes of loss of body weight at high altitude are complex and differ in their relevant importance according to the stage of the ascent and the altitudes reached.

DEHYDRATION

Some of the initial loss of body weight that is common on exposure to moderate altitude is brought about by dehydration. Mild hypoxia induces polyuria and, in those who acclimatize well, there may be diuresis that lasts for days. With increasing elevation there is progressive dehydration due to the increased pulmonary ventilation induced by both hypobaric hypoxia and exercise, coupled with the low humidity of the ambient air (Pugh 1962). Consolazio *et al.* (1968) observed a negative water balance in troops after 4 weeks of exposure to conditions at 4300 m.

In further studies, Consolazio *et al.* (1972) and Krzywicki *et al.* (1969) attributed much of the loss of body weight at high altitude to absolute dehydration, with decrease in plasma volume (Jain *et al.* 1980). Consolazio *et al.* (1972) believe that intracellular water falls on acute exposure to altitude, while

extracellular water remains constant. Total body water, therefore, falls according to this view. Bulstrode (1975) lost 6 kg in body weight in rapidly ascending and descending Mt Kenya, and regained it within 24 hours of descent. He concluded that these remarkable changes were due to fluid loss and replenishment. However, in the early stages of an ascent into the mountains there is commonly an increase in body weight due to retention of water and sodium, with oliguria and acute mountain sickness (Chapter 12). Subsequent loss of weight at high altitude depends on energy imbalance at high altitude so that energy output due to basal metabolism and on exercise is not matched by energy intake due to food.

BASAL METABOLIC RATE

On exposure to an altitude of 3350 m there is an increase in basal metabolic rate of about 12% for a week, which subsequently falls for 2 weeks only to rise again after a period of 3 weeks at high altitude (Nair 1971*a,b*; see Fig. 21.1). The initial elevation of basal metabolic rate was ascribed by Nair *et al.* (1971*a*) to the stress of acute exposure to hypobaric hypoxia with associated sympathetic activity and stimulation of the adrenal cortex (Chapter 22). The subsequent fall of the basal metabolic rate in the following 2 weeks in the absence of the additional factor of cold has been considered to be brought about by a diminution of thyroid activity. Beckwith *et al.* (1966) and Consolazio *et al.* (1966) have also reported that in newcomers to high altitude there is a decline in heat production after an initial rise.

An attempt has been made to distinguish the effects of hypoxia and cold on the basal metabolic rate of newcomers to high altitude (Nair *et al.* 1971*a,b*). Twenty healthy subjects between the ages of 22 and 28 years were studied at sea level at room temperatures of 25°C to 28°C and were then flown to an altitude of 3350 m where they were restudied. There, half of them (group A in Fig. 21.1) had their basal metabolic rate measured daily while they were kept for 3 weeks in warm clothing in a building, the

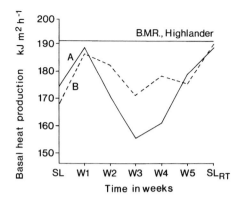

21.1 *Basal heat production (kJ/m²/h) in two groups of lowlanders studied at sea level (SL) and at 3350 m (for up to 6 weeks, WI, W2, etc.). A, Half of the 20 subjects exposed to hypoxia and warmth for 3 weeks and then to hypoxia and cold, both periods of time at 3350 m. B, The other half of the 20 subjects exposed first to hypoxia and cold for 3 weeks and then to hypoxia and warmth, both periods of time at 3350 m. SL_{RT}, Return to sea level. The level of basal metabolic rate in the native highlander of the Andes is also shown.*

temperature of which was maintained in the range of 25°C to 29°C. During this period the stimulus presumed to be operating was hypoxia alone. Subsequently, they were exposed to the combined stimuli of cold and hypoxia for 3 weeks being kept in a tent for 6 hours a day, clothed in cotton shirts and pants and exposed to a cold temperature range of 6°C to 11°C. The other half (group B in Fig. 21.1) were subjected to the same two environments in reverse order. During the same investigation the basal metabolic rate of five native highlanders between the age of 21 and 29 years were studied.

In the group initially exposed to cold the secondary fall in metabolic rate referred to above did not take place to anything like the same extent. This may be because the cold stimulates thyroid activity. Once the cold stimulus was withdrawn, however, there was no fall in basal heat production and these subjects maintained a metabolic rate approaching that of the highlander (Fig. 21.1). Hence simultaneous exposure to hypoxia and cold appears to achieve a faster elevation of basal metabolism and a more rapid acclimatization.

As acclimatization progresses there is a lessening of suppression of thyroid activity with an increase in basal metabolic rate (Fig. 21.1). It should be noted that the rise in basal metabolic rate occurs only 2 weeks after the simultaneous stimulus of cold so

either there is a time lag in the response to thyroid hormone, or the rise in basal metabolic rate is not directly attributable to it. Basal heat production is significantly raised after sustained exposure to hypoxia at high altitude (Fig. 21.1) and probably should be regarded as a feature of acclimatization (Nair *et al.* 1971*a*). Other authors have reported no change or a slight increase in basal metabolism at high altitude (Houston and Riley 1947; Stickney and Van Liere 1953; Grover 1963).

Basal metabolism in the five highlanders studied by Nair *et al.* (1971*a*) was found to be somewhat elevated compared to that of lowlanders (Fig. 21.1). Studies on miners at 4540 m have supported the concept of elevation of basal metabolism to be part of long-term acclimatization (Picón-Reátegui 1961).

ANOREXIA AND HYPOPHAGIA
It is likely that the basis for much of the initial loss of weight at high altitude is the anorexia and hypophagia induced by the headache and nausea of acute mountain sickness. An investigation of the restriction of diet at high altitude was carried out by Hannon *et al.* (1976) who studied the intake of nutrients by eight female students, ranging in age from 18 to 23 years, over a period of 4 days at 140 m and over a subsequent period of 7 days at 4300 m. Hyphophagia was most pronounced during the first 3 days of exposure to high altitude, where there was a transient decrease in the consumption of a wide range of nutrients including protein, carbohydrate, fat, sodium, calcium, phosphorous, vitamin A, thiamine, and niacin. There was a more sustained decrease in the consumption of potassium and ascorbic acid. The degree of anorexia and hypophagia was related to the severity of acute mountain sickness. During the first 3 days at 4300 m, the consumption of calories was reduced by as much as 40%. A reduction of calorie intake of this magnitude is roughly comparable to that reported for soldiers at the same altitude by Surks *et al.* (1966), Johnson *et al.* (1969), and Whitten *et al.* (1968).

The hypophagia observed in man can be induced experimentally in animals. We subjected six young male guinea-pigs to a simulated altitude of 5000 m for 14 days and contrasted their food intake with that of six controls of the same mean body weight (Gloster *et al.* 1974). The total weight of food consumed by the test animals was only 63% of that eaten by the controls. In another experiments we studied three groups of rats. A test group was exposed to a subatmospheric pressure of 400 mmHg for 14 days (Gloster *et al.* 1972). Two groups of

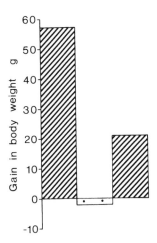

21.2 *Effect of hypobaric conditions and food intake on whole body weight in rats. The gain in body weight of a group of free-fed rats over a period of 14 days at sea level is indicated by the first hatched column. When rats were exposed to a barometric pressure of 400 mmHg, simulating an altitude of 5000 m for the same length of time, they actually lost weight (lightly stippled column). However, failure to gain weight normally was also shown by a third group of rats (second hatched column) kept at sea-level barometric pressure but given a restricted diet equivalent in amount to that eaten by the hypoxic test rats.*

controls were studied. A free-fed control group was allowed an unlimited amount of food. A food-restricted group was given each day the same amount of food eaten by the test animals in the previous 24 h. The body weights of the three groups of adult rats over the course of the experiment are shown in Fig. 21.2. It will be noted that, as in man, there is a fall in body weight in the hypoxic rats. However, the food-restricted control rats kept at sea-level barometric pressure also failed to gain weight normally. In the hypoxic group there was a gradual recovery in body weight, although the initial starting weight was not regained by the end of the experiment.

Such experimental studies suggest that the anorexia and hypophagia of high altitude can account entirely for the loss of body weight. The loss of appetite is not due entirely to the nausea of high altitude. The diet of the local inhabitants of the Himalaya and Andes may not be immediately attractive to the newcomer at high altitude. Furthermore, men involved in climbing or scientific expeditions at high altitude commonly engage in more prolonged

and vigorous exercise than is customary in their more sedentary occupations at sea level.

LOSS OF BODY FAT

The diminished intake of food is inadequate to maintain the level of energy required to sustain activity at high altitude. The deficit has to be made up by body tissues and as a result loss of body weight occurs. In the women studied by Hannon *et al.* (1976), the loss of weight after 7 days at 4300 m was 1.76% of total body weight. In soldiers stopping for 12 days at the same altitude, the loss of weight reported was 3.49% (Surks *et al.* 1966) and 5.0% (Krzywicki *et al.* 1969). It seems likely that the initial weight loss is primarily due to loss of stored body fat (Surks *et al.* 1966). In Caucasian members of the American Research Expedition to Everest in 1981, loss of 1.8% of total body fat accounted for 70.5% of the mean weight loss of 1.9 kg during the approach march to the Everest Base Camp at 5400 m (Boyer and Blume 1984). However, a further loss of 1.5% of total body fat accounted for only 27.2% of the greater mean weight loss of 4.0 kg during residence above 5400 m (Boyer and Blume 1984). Clearly the loss of body weight at extreme altitude is due increasingly to a cause other than loss of stored body fat. Weight loss during the approach march was closely correlated with the initial body fat measured in Kathmandu.

MALABSORPTION OF FAT AND XYLOSE

In the studies of Hannon *et al.* (1976) it was noted that, on acute exposure to high altitude, carbohydrate is chosen in preference to fat in food intake. The same distaste for fat was also remarked upon by Ward (1975) in climbers. He notes that a craving for sweet foods like pineapple cubes commonly develops. This distaste for fatty food is associated with malabsorption of fat at high altitude, which appears to contribute to the weight loss. Over 40 years ago, Pugh (1954) noted the greasy stools of climbers at high altitude and postulated that malabsorption of fat was responsible. This was confirmed in three members of the American Medical Research Expedition to Everest in 1981, at extreme altitude. At sea level, fat intake was 128 g/day, with 79.3% fat absorption. At 6300 m the fat intake was 79 g/day, with 40.8% fat absorption. In others, fat absorption decreased by 48.5% (Boyer and Blume 1984).

At the same time there was a decrease of 24% in xylose absorption, as reflected in urine excretion, at 6300 m as contrasted to sea level (Boyer and Blume

1984). The same malabsorption of xylose from the small intestine had been associated with hypoxaemia *per se* some years before by Milledge (1972). He expressed the opinion that loss of body weight is associated directly with hypoxaemia and he noted that children with cyanotic congenital heart disease are stunted and underweight.

Patients with severe emphysema and hypoxaemia also may lose weight. Milledge (1972) studied the absorption of xylose from the small intestine in 16 patients with varying degrees of arterial oxygen desaturation due to either congenital heart anomalies or chronic lung disease. There was a significant correlation between xylose absorption and systemic arterial oxygen saturation. In nine cases, hypoxia was relieved by the administration of oxygen by surgery, and repeat testing in such instances showed a mean increase of 11.7% in xylose absorption. Absorption of the pentose sugar appears to depend on the intraluminal concentration and can be influenced by the effect of steatorrhoea from small bowel pathology (Finlay *et al.* 1964). Thus, in view of the poor fat absorption at high altitude, the effect on xylose absorption may be secondary.

PROTEIN CATABOLISM

With sustained sojourn at extreme altitude over 5500 m, the main cause of loss of body weight becomes catabolism of muscle protein. Perhaps the changeover occurs at an elevation where haemoglobin oxygen saturation becomes low enough to lead to significant malabsorption through the small intestine. Boyer and Blume (1984) found that in climbers sojourning above 5400 m there was a significant proportionate decrease in arm and leg circumferences of, respectively, 1.5 and 2.9 cm. Some years earlier, Ward (1975) referred to the severe wasting of muscle that occurs at extreme altitudes due to protein breakdown. He commented on the emaciated appearance of the members of the 1953 Everest expedition who ascended to 7920 m. During the Himalayan expedition of 1960–61, all members of the party lost weight at the rate of 0.45–1.36 kg/week at 5790 m. By the end of the expedition, weight losses ranged from 6.4 to 9.0 kg (Pugh 1962). Negative nitrogen balance was reported in men acutely exposed to 4300 m for 8 days (Surks *et al.* 1966) and 28 days (Consolazio *et al.* 1968). Guilland and Klepping (1985) found a reduction of 35–57% in total calorie intake in four acclimatized climbers between 26 and 42 years of age at extreme altitudes above 6000 m. They showed a progressive loss of weight due to a reduction in body fat and

protein. Ward *et al.* (1989) do not subscribe to the view that at high altitude there is a distinct initial phase of loss of body fat followed by wasting due to loss of protein.

Sherpas maintain body weight and limb circumference at extreme altitude. They probably work less and eat more on expeditions than at home. The maintenance of their limb circumferences indicates that they are not catabolizing protein.

EFFECT OF ACETAZOLAMIDE

It has been reported that acetazolamide may help to maintain muscle mass and exercise performance at high altitude (Bradwell *et al.* 1986). The effects of the drug were studied in 11 acclimatized subjects at 4850 m, 10 other climbers given only a placebo acting as controls. Exercise performance at 85% maximum heart rate fell by 45% in the controls, but by only 37% in the group given acetazolamide. Weight loss was also greater in the placebo group. During the expedition, anterior quadriceps muscle thickness fell by 12.9% in the control group and 8.5% in the acetazolamide group, while biceps muscle thickness fell respectively by 8.6% and 2.3%. Measurements of skin-fold thickness indicated a loss of 18% of total body fat in the placebo group and 5% in the acetazolamide group by the end of the expedition. Calorie (energy) intake was similar in the two groups. The climbers taking acetazolamide had fewer symptoms of acute mountain sickness. Bradwell *et al.* (1986) conclude that this drug is beneficial to acclimatized climbers at extreme altitude in slowing loss of muscle mass and body weight and helping to maintain exercise performance.

ANAEMIA AT HIGH ALTITUDE

The acute and pronounced decrease in the intake of nutrients by lowlanders on ascent to high altitude is brief and does not constitute a lasting nutritional problem. This is not the case, however, in native highlanders in whom chronic dietary deficiencies may occur, interfering in the maintenance of natural acclimatization. A case of special interest is iron-deficiency anaemia.

Haemoglobin has a role in acclimatization to hypobaric hypoxia (Chapter 5) and iron is required for its formation. Evidence as to the need for additional iron to support increased erythropoiesis at high altitude is conflicting (Hornbein 1962). Female newcomers to altitude have significantly higher haemoglobin levels when given supplemental iron (Hannon *et al.* 1966). Malnutrition in native highlanders may have important repercussions on haemoglobin formation and hence on acclimatization to hypobaric hypoxia. Beard *et al.* (1986) studied this problem over a period of 8 months in 23 children of pre-school age admitted to the protein malnutrition wards, in hospitals in La Paz (3800 m). Sixteen of them had marasmic kwashiorkor and five died within a few weeks of treatment. They also studied 24 healthy highland children of the same age as controls. The malnourished children presented with a mean haemoglobin level of 9.7 ± 2.7 g/dl, this being more than two standard deviations below the value of 14.5 ± 1.4 g/dl for the control high-altitude group. Serum iron in the malnourished children was 35 ± 22 μg/dl and in the controls was 72 ± 26 μg/dl. Serum and erythrocyte folate concentrations were 44% and 82% respectively of control values. This anaemia proved to have a significant effect on acclimatization to high altitude, for there were significant decrements in arterial oxygenation in the malnourished children. Their mean Pa_{O_2} was 52 ± 6 mmHg compared with 62 ± 4 mmHg in the controls. There was a progressive 40% increase in red cell 2,3-DPG concentration, from 4.7 ± 1.0 to 5.5 ± 1.5 μmol/ml cells. There was thus a rightward displacement of the oxygen-haemoglobin dissociation curve, the P_{50} rising from 26.0 ± 1 mmHg in the controls to 28.2 ± 1.2 in the malnourished children. Furthermore, this reduction of 40% in haemoglobin levels proved to be very resistant to improvement during 10 weeks of protein feeding.

In the later stages of recovery, iron and folate availability to the bone marrow may be involved in the perpetuation of the anaemia. Nutrition in native highlanders is commonly inadequate over a much wider range than iron deficiency. This is more an expression of the poor socio-economic conditions of isolated mountain communities throughout the world than of any specific effect at high altitude. Thus, Picón-Reátegui (1978) notes that in the Andes the diet of the highlander is poor in both fat and protein.

MINERAL AND VITAMIN CONTENT OF THE DIET

The range of daily intake of some minerals and vitamins in five communities in the Peruvian Andes, as determined by Collazos *et al.* (1954) and Gursky (1969) and as presented by Picón-Reátegui (1978) are shown in Table 21.1. Also shown in the same table are the daily need of these nutrients as estimated by the National Academy of Sciences of the United States (NAS/NRC 1974).

Picón-Reátegui (1978) gives some interesting examples of local geographical and social factors that may influence the adequacy of intake of minerals and vitamins. Thus vitamin C intake is intimately related to the availability of fresh potatoes, which are consumed in large quantities from April to August, thus ensuring an adequate intake of ascorbic acid, estimated to be 20.5 mg per 100 g of potato. After the seasonal harvest the consumption of the fresh tubers is replaced by the dehydrated form of potatoes, *chuño* which contains a very much lower ascorbic acid content of only 1.7 mg per portion. Water boils at a lower temperature at high altitude and this may preserve the content of ascorbic acid in native foods during the process of cooking. This effect of the lower boiling point in mountains may also protect the thiamine content of cooked food.

It will be noted from Table 21.1 that considerable variation in the vitamin A content of the food of native highlanders has been reported by various observers. Not only that, in some instances the intake of vitamin A reported has been totally inadequate. The variation in intake is probably related to the availability of such foods as liver. In spite of these estimates of a low vitamin A intake, there have been no reports of clinically detectable hypovitaminosis A.

There is high absorption of calcium from the food ingested by the Quechuas. This may be related to the increased levels of ultraviolet radiation at high altitude (Chapter 2) that may increase the availability of vitamin D. Calcium absorption may also be aided by the low fat content of the Quechua diet.

BODY COMPOSITION OF HIGHLANDERS

Bharadwaj *et al.*(1973) studied the body composition of 30 young Tamil soldiers from sea level using anthropometric techniques and compared these results with those from 45 Ladakhis at Leh (3660 m). No significant difference in body fat, water, and cell solids could be detected. Bone mineral was significantly greater in the Ladakhis and this was thought to be due to their wider bi-iliac, wrist, knee, and ankle widths. These authors speculate that this increased width may be associated with a larger volume of bone marrow. Earlier studies by Siri *et al.* (1954) and Picón-Reátegui *et al.* (1961) had also indicated that there is no difference in body fat and cell solids between highlanders and sea-level residents.

GASTRIC ULCERS AND HAEMORRHAGE AT HIGH ALTITUDE

The incidence of gastric and duodenal ulcers in patients attending the Obrero hospital in La Oroya

Table 21.1 Mineral and vitamin contents of the diet in high-altitude communities in Peru (Chacan, Vicos, Chillihua, Nuñoa, Sincata). (After Collazos *et al.* 1954; Gursky 1969)

	Calcium (mg)	Phosphorus (mg)	Iron (mg)	Vitamin A retinol equivalents	Thiamine (mg)	Riboflavin (mg)	Niacin (mg)	Ascorbic acid (mg)
Range of intake	76–870	761–1706	12.1–31.8	1.4–2203.5	1.44–4.16	0.69–1.92	13.06–29.62	10.9–76.9
Daily need*	800	800	10		1.37	1.65	18.1	45

*Based on dietary allowances recommended by National Academy of Sciences/National Research Council, USA (NAS/NRC 1974).

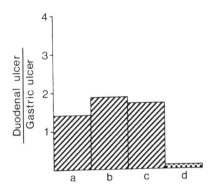

21.3 *Ratio of duodenal to gastric ulcer at low and high altitude. The data shown in the first three hatched columns are derived from studies at low altitude: a, from USA; b, from Europe; c, from Peru. The data in the fourth stippled column, d, are derived from high altitude in Peru. It is seen that gastric ulcer is much commoner than duodenal ulcer at high altitude in the Andes. (Sources: a, Feldman and Weinberg (1951); b, Knutsen and Selvaag (1947); c, Garrido-Klinge and Peña (1959), (Lima, 150 m); d, Garrido-Klinge and Peña (1959) (La Oroya, 3750 m).)*

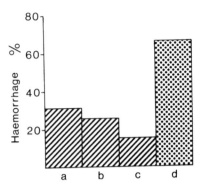

21.4 *Incidence of haemorrhage in cases of peptic ulcer diagnosed at low and high altitude. The data shown in the first three (hatched) columns are derived from studies at low altitude, those in a and b coming from the USA and those in c coming from Peru. The data in the fourth (stippled) column, d, are derived from high altitude in Peru. It is seen that the incidence of haemorrhage as a presenting symptom of peptic ulcer is greater at high altitude (Sources: a, Bockus (1944); (b, Ivy et al. (1950); c, Garrido-Klinge and Peña (1959) (Lima, 150 m); d, Garrido-Klinge and Peña (1959) (La Oroya, 3750 m).)*

at 3750 m in the Peruvian Andes was studied by Garrido-Klinge and Peña (1959). They found that the proportion of gastric ulcers is greater at high altitude than at sea level (Fig. 21.3). Furthermore, the incidence of haemorrhage from them is considerably greater than at low altitude (Fig. 21.4). Finally, the age of onset of gastric ulceration in the native highlander is usually early, no fewer than 48% of the cases being in the third decade. It is possible that spontaneous haemorrhages in the gastric mucosa, similar to those in the mouth (Chapter 9), may account for the high prevalence of haemorrhages reported in patients with peptic ulcer at high altitude.

The native populations of mountainous areas have dietary habits that may be of some importance in the aetiology of the increased prevalence of gastric ulceration. In the Andes the diet is composed largely of cereals, insufficiently cooked on account of the low barometric pressure, and many of the population are unable to chew it adequately due to loss of teeth as a result of inadequate dental care from childhood (Garrido-Klinge and Peña 1959). The Quechua Indians are very fond of potent spices and flavourings on their food, and an inferior rough alcohol is consumed by many in considerable quantity. Many are addicted to the chewing of coca leaves, from which cocaine is obtained. It will be seen from this imposing list that this native population is chronically exposed to a wide variety of potent gastric irritants, so that both dietary and vascular factors could operate in bringing about this increased prevalence of gastric ulceration.

Steele (1971) also refers to indigestion being common among the Sherpas and he also relates this to their disposition to drink large quantities of rough, home-brewed spirit, *arak*. Three of these native highlanders accompanying a party climbing Mt Everest had to be brought down, as they were suffering from acute peptic ulceration with severe epigastric pain, nausea, and vomiting. One Sherpa had a brisk haematemesis of about 1 litre after a heavy drinking bout (Steele 1971). Vargas (1967) has also reported that at high altitude gastric ulcers are commoner than the duodenal variety, but he found the ratio to be much lower at 2.5:1 than the ratio (20:1) reported by Garrido-Klinge and Peña (1959). He confirmed that the most frequent complication of peptic ulcer at high altitude is haemorrhage, which is much commoner than at sea level. Garrido-Klinge and Peña (1959) did not find high levels of acidity in the cases they reported.

In contrast, the prevalence of duodenal ulcer is not increased at high altitude, so that overall peptic ulceration is not commoner in high mountainous areas. Thus, Garrido-Klinge and Peña (1959) found that the incidence of peptic ulceration in a group of 17 500 labourers, chiefly miners, born and living in the Andes at altitudes between 3050 and 4880 m was 0.4% of the insured population or 1.85% of patients admitted to hospital. These figures are similar to those found in other countries according to the medical literature. Vargas (1967) also found that the incidence of peptic ulcer in the native highlander of Peru is no different from that in sea-level residents. Singh *et al.* (1977) found that the incidence of peptic ulcer in Indian soldiers stationed over a prolonged period at high altitude in the Himalaya was actually lower than at sea level. The morbidity rate from peptic ulcer among 20 000 soldiers stationed between altitudes of 3690 and 5550 m was 1.3 per 1000, whereas among 130 700 soldiers on the plains it was 1.75 per 1000.

SERUM GASTRIN AND GASTRIC ACID SECRETION

In view of the prevalence of symptoms related to gastric ulcer at high altitude Jo *et al.* (1987) studied the levels of serum gastrin and gastric acid secretion in a group of native highlanders and compared these with findings in a group of lowlanders. They studied 16 highlanders, in the age range of 21–40 years born and living between 3000 and 4200 m with at least 6 years' residence at La Oroya (3730 m) and 16 lowlanders between 24 and 28 years of age, living on the coast at Lima. They found the basal concentration of gastrin in the highlanders was significantly higher (38.9 ± 6.1 pg/ml, mean $\pm$ SEM) than in the coastal dwellers (23.8 ± 3.1 pg/ml). The basal free gastric acid output was similar in the highlanders (2.4 ± 0.71 mEq HCl/hour) and lowlanders (2.9 ± 0.51 mEq HCl/hour). After histamine stimulation the highlanders showed a lower free acid secretion (8.0 ± 1.00 mEq HCl/hour) in comparison to lowlanders (14.0 ± 1.44 mEq HCl/hour; $p = 0.01$). This diminished acid secretion in response to histamine stimulation may be related to a lower sensitivity of parietal cells produced by hypoxia (Jo *et al.* 1987). The hypergastrinaemia may reflect a compensatory increase in G cell activity in order to maintain adequate gastric function at basal state and after food intake. The earlier studies of Singh *et al.* (1977) also showed that gastric acidity diminished on arrival at high altitude and remained low during the remainder of the stay in mountainous areas. Gastric motility was not altered. Pepsin activity was low for 1

week after arrival at high altitude but reverted subsequently to sea-level values.

SIGMOID VOLVULUS

Sigmoid volvulus causing intestinal obstruction is said to be common in the Andes. Asbun *et al.* (1992) reviewed 230 consecutive cases of volvulus, apart from those associated with Chagas' disease, treated in a hospital in La Paz, Bolivia. They found that sigmoid volvulus accounted for 79% of all cases of intestinal obstruction, an extremely high figure when contrasted with corresponding data from the United States. It is not clear why volvulus of the sigmoid colon should be so common at high altitude. Asbun *et al.* (1992) believe the intraluminal gas volume is related inversely to the diminished barometric pressure at high altitude. They postulate that such gases as carbon dioxide and methane generated in the lumen of the bowels may contribute to chronic distension of the sigmoid colon. If this segment of the gut is disproportionately long compared with its mesenteric base, its chronic distension would set up the right conditions to allow torsion of the loop.

DISTURBANCE OF MINERALIZATION OF ENAMEL AT HIGH ALTITUDE

Dental fluorosis is a clinical condition typified by white flecks, white or brown patches, or even pitting of the surface enamel that characteristically affects many or all of the teeth (Fig. 21.5). It is due to hypoplasia of enamel caused by high levels of fluoride present during the time of amelogenesis when the ameloblasts are extremely sensitive to a wide range of environmental disturbances such as childhood exanthematous diseases and avitaminosis D. Because most environmental enamel hypoplasias are due to episodic events, they manifest as limited bands of defects in groups of teeth chronologically related by stage of development. The results of a high intake of fluoride are somewhat different. Being continuous throughout the whole period of the development of the teeth, its effect is typically widespread. In general the defects are not seen at water levels of 1–1.5 parts per million (ppm) fluoride, but there is an increase in severity as the fluoride concentration rises. However, there is marked individual variation and certain teeth such as premolars and upper incisors appear to be more susceptible than others. The structural changes affect the enamel prisms. They are not specific for fluoride and exactly similar changes are found in other hypoplasias. There is accompanying hypocalcification. This effect

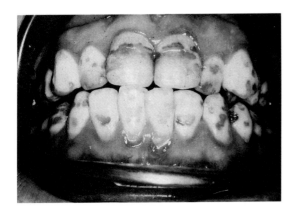

21.5 *Dental fluorosis.*

of fluoride on matrix formation and its ability to calcify is different from the anticaries effect of high fluoride ingestion that continues after the teeth have formed and is related to the formation of fluorapatite, in place of hydroxapatite, in the crystals of the enamel prisms.

It was discovered that the renal clearance of fluoride was pH-dependent, being depressed by acidosis and enhanced by alkalosis (Whitford *et al.* 1976). Residence at high altitude is characterized by respiratory alkalosis (Chapter 4). It was thought initially, therefore, that, because of their alkaline urine, highlanders and prolonged sojourners at high altitude would excrete relatively more fluoride than lowlanders and thus be less susceptible to dental fluorosis (Angmar-Månsson and Whitford 1990). For a given level of fluoride, the prevalence and severity of dental fluorosis would be lower at high altitude. In fact, experimental work on rats subjected to simulated high altitude by Whitford *et al.* (1983) showed just the reverse. Unexpectedly, the fluoride concentrations and fluoride-to-phosphorus molar ratios of the femur distal epiphyses averaged 60% higher in the rats of the high-altitude group compared to controls. Plasma, liver, and heart concentrations of fluoride were also higher by about the same percentage. The explanation for these higher tissue fluoride levels is not yet apparent. Further experimental work by Angmar-Månsson *et al.* (1984) confirmed that chronic hypobaric hypoxia is associated with a significant increase in fluoride retention.

A striking finding in rats subjected to simulated high altitude is the extremely disturbed mineralization pattern of the incisor enamel. The enamel is uniformly bleached to the colour of chalk and it may be crazed or fractured so that the underlying dentin

is often exposed (Angmar-Månsson and Whitford 1990). A significant fact is that disrupted mineralization may occur at simulated high altitude in rats not exposed to substantial fluoride intake. This raises the possibility that disturbances in enamel mineralization induced by the hypobaric hypoxia of high altitude alone could be mistaken for fluorosis.

Some clinical studies have suggested that populations living at high altitude may be more susceptible to dental fluorosis than those in the lowlands for a given concentration of fluoride in drinking water (Manji *et al.* 1986). Studies were made in Kenya of children aged 11–15 years from three low-fluoride zones (<0.5 ppm in drinking water) situated at sea level, 1500, and 2400 m and from two higher-fluoride zones, (0.5–1.0 ppm in drinking water). In the low-fluoride zones. 36% of the children at sea level had dental fluorosis, as compared with 78% at 1500 m and 100% at 2400 m. In the higher-fluoride zones 71% had dental fluorosis at sea level, compared with 94% at 1500 m.

However, Angmar-Månsson and Whitford (1990) question the validity of the diagnosis of dental fluorosis in some of these studies at high altitude. Thus, they refer to an epidemiological study of the prevalence of fluorosis, part of which was conducted in mountainous regions (Leatherwood *et al.* 1965), and believe that the diagnosis of dental fluorosis may have been confounded by the effect of hypobaric hypoxia on amelogenesis. Leatherwood and his colleagues (1965) found that water fluoride levels ranged from non-detectable to a low 0.8 ppm and yet what was diagnosed as dental fluorosis affected nearly half of the subjects. If enamel defects caused by hypobaric hypoxia were wrongly attributed to fluoride, it could lead to unnecessary or even harmful actions such as adjustment of water fluoride levels or fluoride intake from other sources below those that would be optimal for the control of dental caries. Angmar-Månsson and Whitford (1990) also question the validity of the diagnosis of dental fluorosis in the study of Manji *et al.* (1986) referred to above. They note that in the two areas of 1500 m the teeth of 78–94% of the children were said to be affected by dental fluorosis regardless of the concentration of fluoride in the drinking water. Manji *et al.* (1986) suggested that certain physiological changes may occur in man living at high altitude whereby the effects of fluoride on mineralizing tissues become exacerbated. However, the lack of a fluoride dose–response effect on the occurrence of the enamel defects suggests that another variable was chiefly responsible for the findings. There would appear to be indications for further research into the effects of high altitude on amelogenesis. In particular, the role of acid–base status needs further consideration.

DECOMPRESSION TOOTHACHE

During World War II it was noted that some air crew personnel complained of dental pain when flying at high altitudes and when entering low-pressure chambers (Harvey 1943; Joseph *et al.* 1943). This barodentalgia was attributed by Coons (1943) to nitrogen bubbles in the dental pulp. Some dental authorities (Stones 1966), however, think it likely that in most cases of this type there is some pathological condition in a vital pulp.

This may be secondary to caries or to a filling that has not previously given rise to symptoms. Orban and Ritchey (1945) investigated 250 cases of decompression toothaches and studied histological sections of 75 of the teeth involved. They found oedematous pulps in 16, acute pulpitis in 17, chronic pulpitis in 15, non-vital pulps in 7, and normal pulps in 3. Seventeen cases were regarded as unclassifiable. They consider that teeth with normal pulps do not give rise to pain during decompression whether they are intact, carious, or filled.

SPLANCHNIC BLOOD FLOW AND LIVER METABOLISM

Studies on Amerindians of the Bolivian altiplano living at 4000 m by Capderou *et al.* (1977) show that splanchnic blood flow and liver metabolism are not modified by the lifelong exposure to hypoxia. They found that splanchnic blood flow fell within normal sea-level values of 1.42–1.70/l min the mean value being 1.55 l/min. Estimates expressed per square metre body surface area, to take into account the smaller stature of the highlander, were almost normal. Blood pressure in the hepatic vein of highlanders (10 mmHg) is similar to that in lowlanders. Splanchnic arteriovenous oxygen difference shows no abnormality. The uptake of indocyanine green, a sensitive and specific test of liver function, was found to be normal in highlanders by Capderou *et al.* (1977). This confirmed the previous finding of Berendsohn (1962) that hepatic function is essentially normal in Peruvian highlanders living at 4540 m. Ramsoe *et al.* (1970) found that hepatic function was normal in newcomers to the mountain environment during the first week at 3500 m.

In sea-level man there is a fall in splanchnic blood flow as part of the response of the circulation to physical exercise to provide a better perfusion and oxygen supply of the exercising muscles. The lactate produced by the exercising muscles is largely removed by increased liver gluconeogenesis. Native highlanders are capable of hard, efficient physical work at high altitude and in carrying this out produce a much lower arterial lactate than sea-level man. This could clearly arise from a lower production of lactate by the muscles or an increased conversion into glycogen in the liver. Capderou *et al.* (1977) tentatively conclude that lactate produced by exercising muscles in highlanders is utilized for liver gluconeogenesis, as demonstrated in lowlanders.

References

Angmar-Månsson, B. and Whitford, G.M. (1990). Environmental and physiological factors affecting dental fluorosis. *Journal of Dental Research*, **69**, 706

Angmar-Månsson, B., Whitford, G.M., Allison, N.B., Devine, J.A., and Maher, J.I. (1984). Effects of simulated altitude on fluoride retention and enamel quality. *Caries Research*, **18**, 165A

Asbun, H.J., Castellanos, H., Balderrama, B., Ochoa, J., Arismendi, R., Teran, H., and Asbun, J. (1992). Sigmoid volvulus in the high altitude of the Andes. Review of 230 cases. *Diseases of the Colon and Rectum*, **35**, 350

Beard, J.L., Gomez, I.H., and Haas, J.D. (1986). Functional anemia of complicated protein–energy malnutrition at high altitude. *American Journal of Clinical Nutrition*, **44**, 181

Beckwith, H.J., Sarks, M.I., and Chidsey, C.A. (1966). Basal metabolism, thyroid and sympathetic activity in man at high altitude. *Federation Proceedings: Federation of American Societies for Experimental Biology*, **25**, 399

Berendsohn, S. (1962). Hepatic function at high altitudes. *Archives of Internal Medicine*, **109**, 56

Bharadwaj, H. Singh, A.P., and Malhotra, M.S. (1973). Body composition of the high-altitude natives of Ladakh. A comparison with sea level residents. *Human Biology*, **45**, 423

Bockus, H.L. (1944). *Gastroenterology*. Philadelphia; Saunders

Boyer, S.J. and Blume, F.D. (1984). Weight loss and changes in body composition at high altitude. *Journal of Applied Physiology*, **57**, 1580

Bradwell, A.R., Dykes, P.W., Coote, J.P., Forster, P.J.E., Milles, J.J., Chesner, I., and Richardson, N.V. (1986). Effect of acetazolamide on exercise performance and muscle mass at high altitude. *Lancet*, **i**, 1001

Bulstrode, C.J.K. (1975). A preliminary study into factors predisposing mountaineers to high altitude pulmonary oedema. *Journal of the Royal Naval Medical Service*, **61**, 101

Capderou, A., Pollanski, J., Mensch-Dechene, J., Drouet, L., Antezana, G., Zetter, M., and Lockhart, A. (1977). Splanchnic blood flow O_2 consumption, removal of lactate, and output of glucose in highlanders. *Journal of Applied Physiology: Respiratory, Environmental and Exercise Physiology*, **43**, 204

Collazos, C., White, H.C., Huenemann, R.I., Reh, E., White, P.L., Castellanos, A., Benites, R., Bravo, Y., Loo, A., Moscoso, I., Carceres, C., and Dieseldorff, A. (1954). Dietary surveys in Peru. III Chacan and Vicos. Rural communities in the Peruvian Andes. *Journal of the American Dietetic Association*, **30**, 1222

Consolazio, C.F., Matoush, L.O., and Nelson, R.A. (1966). Energy metabolism in maximum and sub-maximum performance of high altitude. *Federation Proceedings: Federation of American Societies for Experimental Biology*, **25**, 1380

Consolazio, C.F., Matoush, L.O., Johnson, H.L., and Daws, T.A., (1968). Protein and water balances of young adults during prolonged exposure to high altitude. *American Journal of Clinical Nutrition*, **21**, 154

Consolazio, C.F., Johnson, H.L., Krzywicki, H.J., and Daws, T.A., (1972). Metabolic aspects of acute altitude exposure (4,300 meters) in adequately nourished humans. *American Journal of Clinical Nutrition*, **25**, 23

Coons, D.S. (1943). Aeronautical dentistry. *Journal of the Canadian Dental Association*, **9**, 320

Feldman, M. and Weinberg, T. (1951). Healing of peptic ulcer. *American Journal of Digestive Diseases*, **18**, 295

Finlay, J.M., Hogarth, J., and Wrightman, K.J.R. (1964). A clinical evaluation of the D-xylose tolerance test. *Annals of Internal Medicine*, **61**, 411

Garrido-Klinge, G. and Peña, L. (1959). The gastro-duodenal ulcer in high altitudes/Peruvian Andes. *Gastroenterology*, **37**, 390

Gloster, J., Heath, D., and Harris, P. (1972). The influence of diet on the effects of reduced atmospheric pressure in the rat. *Experimental Physiology and Biochemistry*, **2**, 177

Gloster, J., Hasleton, P.S., Harris, P., and Heath, D. (1974). Effects of chronic hypoxia and diet on the weight and lipid content of viscera in the guinea-pig. *Experimental Physiology and Biochemistry*, **4**, 251

Grover, R.F. (1963). Basal oxygen uptake of man at high altitude. *Journal of Applied Physiology*, **18**, 909

Guilland, J.C. and Klepping, J. (1985). Nutritional alterations at high altitude in man. *European Journal of Applied Physiology*, **54**, 517

Gursky, M.J. (1969). Dietary survey of three Peruvian highland communities. Master's thesis in anthropology. Pennsylvania State University

Hannon, J.P., Shields, J.L., and Harris, C.W. (1966). High altitude acclimatization of women. In *The Effects of Altitude on Physical Performance*. Chicago; The Athletic Institute, p. 37

Hannon, J.P., Klain, G.J., Sudman, D.M., and Sullivan, F.J., (1976). Nutritional aspects of high-altitude exposure in women. *American Journal of Clinical Nutrition*, **29**, 604

Harvey, W. (1943). Tooth temperature with reference to dental pain while flying. *British Dental Journal*, **75**, 221

Hornbein, T.E. (1962). Evaluation of iron stores as limiting high altitude polycythaemia. *Journal of Applied Physiology*, **17**, 243

Houston, C.S. and Riley, R.L. (1947). Respiratory and circulation changes during acclimatization to altitude. *American Journal of Physiology*, **149**, 565

Ivy, A.C., Grossman, M.I., and Backrach, W.H. (1950). *Peptic Ulcer*. New York; Blakiston

Jain, S.C., Bardham, J., Swamy, Y.V., Krishna, B., and Nayar, H.S. (1980). Body fluid compartments in humans during acute high altitude exposure. *Aviation, Space, and Environmental Medicine*, **51**, 234

Jo, N., Garcia, O., Jara, F., Garmendia, F., Nago, A., Garcia, R., Hidalgo, H., and Flores, L. (1987). Serum gastrin and gastric acid secretion at high altitude. *Hormone and Metabolic Research*, **19**, 182

Johnson, H.L., Consolazio, C.F., Matoush, L.O., and Krzywicki, H.J. (1969). Nitrogen and mineral metabolism at altitude. *Federation Proceedings: Federation of American Societies for Experimental Biology*, **28**, 1195

Joseph, T.V., Gell, C.F., Carr, R.M., and Shelesnyak, M.C. (1943). Toothache and the aviator: study of tooth pain provoked by simulated high altitude runs in low pressure chamber. *United States Naval Medical Bulletin*, **41**, 643

Knutsen, B. and Selvaag, O. (1947). The incidence of the peptic ulcer: an investigation of the population of the town of Dramen. *Acta Medica Scandinavica*, **196**, 341

Krzywicki, H.J., Consolazio, C.F., Matoush, L.O., Johnson, H.L., and Barnhart, R.A. (1969). Body composition changes during exposure to altitude. *Federation Proceedings: Federation of American Societies for Experimental Biology*, **28**, 1190

Leatherwood, E.C., Burnett, G.W., Chandravej- jsmarn, R., and Siskikaya, P. (1965). Dental caries and dental fluorosis in Thailand. *American Journal of Public Health*, **55**, 1792

Manji, F., Baelum, V., and Fejerskov, O. (1986). Fluoride, altitude and dental fluorosis. *Caries Research*, **20**, 473

Milledge, J.S. (1972). Arterial oxygen desaturation and intestinal absorption of xylose. *British Medical Journal*, **iii**, 557

Nair, C.S., Malhotra, M.S., and Gopinath, P.M. (1971*a*). Effect of altitude and cold acclimatization on the basal metabolism in man. *Aerospace Medicine*, **42**, 1056

Nair, C.S., Malhotra, M.S., Gopinath, P.M., and Mathew, L., (1971*b*). Effect of acclimatization to altitude and cold on basal heart rate, blood pressure, respiration and breath-holding in man. *Aerospace Medicine*, **42**, 851

NAS/NRC (1974). *Recommended Dietary Allowances*, a report of the Food and Nutrition Board, National Research Council. Washington, DC; National Academy of Sciences

Orban, B. and Ritchey, B.T. (1945). Toothache under conditions simulating high altitude flight. *Journal of the American Dental Association*, **32**, 145

Picón-Reátegui, E. (1961). Basal metabolic rate and body composition at high altitude. *Journal of Applied Physiology*, **16**, 431

Picón-Reátequi, E. (1978). The food and nutrition of high-altitude populations. In *The Biology of High-Altitude Peoples* (P.M. Baker, Ed.). Cambridge; Cambridge University Press, p. 219

Picón-Reategui, E., Lozano, R., and Valdivieso, J. (1961). Body composition at sea level and high altitudes. *Journal of Applied Physiology*, **16**, 589

Pugh, L.G.C. (1954). Himalayan rations with special reference to the 1953 expedition to Mount Everest. *Proceedings of the Nutrition Society*, **13**, 60

Pugh, L.G.C.E. (1962). Physiological and medical aspects of Himalayan, Scientific and Mountain-eering Expedition 1960–61. *British Medical Journal*, **ii**, 621

Ramsoe, K., Jarnum, S., Preisig, R., Tauber, J., Tygstrup, N., and Westergaard, H. (1970). Liver function and blood flow at high altitude. *Journal of Applied Physiology*, **28**, 725

Singh, I., Chohan, I.S., Lal, M., Khanna, P.K., Srivastava, M.C., Nanda, R.B., Lambda, J.S., and Malhotra, M.S. (1977). Effects on high altitude stay on the incidence of common diseases in man. *International Journal of Biometeorology*, **21**, 93

Siri, W.E., Reynafarje, C., Berlin, N.I., and Lawrence, J.H., (1954). Body water at sea level and at altitude. *Journal of Applied Physiology*, **7**, 333

Steele, P. (1971). Medicine on Mount Everest 1971. *Lancet*, **ii**, 32

Stickney, J.C. and Van Liere, E.J. (1953). Acclimatization to oxygen tension. *Physiological Reviews*, **33**, 13

Stones, H.H. (1966). Bacteriology, inflammation, necrosis and gangrene of the pulp. In *Oral and Dental Disease*, 5th edn (E.D. Farmer and F.E. Lawton, Eds). Edinburgh; Churchill Livingstone, p. 376

Surks, M.I., Chinn, K.S.K., and Matoush, L.O. (1966). Alterations in body composition in man after acute exposure to high altitude. *Journal of Applied Physiology*, **21**, 1741

Vargas, A.C. (1967). Peptic ulcer in the native Peruvian. *Proceedings of the Third World Congress of Gastroenterology*. Tokyo; Nankodo

Ward, M. (1975). *Mountain Medicine. A Clinical Study of Cold and High Altitude*. London; Crosby Lockwood Staples

Ward, M.P., Milledge, J.S., and West, J.B. (1989). *High Altitude Medicine and Physiology*. London; Chapman and Hall Medical, p. 286

Whitford, G.M., Pashley, D.H., and Stringer, G.I. (1976). Fluoride renal clearance: a pH dependent event. *American Journal of Physiology*, **230**, 527

Whitford, G.M., Allison, N.B., Devine, J.A., Maher, J.T., and Angmar-Månsson, B. (1983). Fluoride metabolism at simulated altitude. *Journal of Dental Research*, **62**, 262 (Abstract No. 840)

Whitten, B.K., Hannon, J.P., Klain, G.J., and Chinn, K.S.K., (1968). Effect of high altitude (14,000 ft) on nitrogenous components of human serum. *Metabolism*, **17**, 360

22

Endocrines

The environment of high altitude has pronounced effects on most of the endocrine glands, which may be manifested clinically or may require for their detection estimates of hormone levels in blood or other body fluids. Clinical and pharmacological investigations of lowlanders ascending to altitude have been supported by animal studies in decompression chambers and these have included histological examination of the endocrine organs concerned. The major factor that affects the endocrine system at high altitude is almost certainly hypoxia but other factors such as exercise and cold may be implicated. The 'leader of the endocrine orchestra', the pituitary gland, is affected by the high-altitude environment and, since the alterations on its different cell populations have specific effects on the individual endocrine glands, we will start our survey with it.

PITUITARY

The pituitary gland has two lobes that are concerned with very dissimilar aspects of life at high altitude. The anterior lobe consists of the pars distalis, pars tuberalis, and pars intermedia, and secretes a number of glycoprotein and peptide hormones, among which are those responsible for the control of the thyroid, the adrenal cortex, and the gonads.

The posterior lobe is part of the brain and is termed the neurohypophysis. It secretes antidiuretic hormone (ADH). Diuresis characteristically develops in climbers exposed to mild but persistent hypoxia and early reports suggested that this was associated with a diminution of circulating ADH (Silvette 1943). A possible mechanism for this supposed decrease in the hormone might be inhibitory impulses originating from receptors in the right atrium when it is distended by the increased blood volume resulting from exposure to high altitude (Chapters 18 and 20; Henry *et al.* 1956; Henry and Pearce 1956). In contrast, the onset of acute mountain sickness is associated with oliguria. Early reports suggested that this was linked with a sudden discharge of ADH (Brun *et al.* 1945; Noble and Taylor 1953). However, as we discuss at greater length in

Chapter 20, later studies showed that the relationship between plasma concentration of ADH and hypoxia is not at all clear.

Studies of the morphology of the pituitary gland in hypoxia are largely confined to laboratory animals exposed to simulated high altitude in decompression chambers. Such experiments have demonstrated lighter pituitary glands in hypoxic animals compared with eupoxic controls (Gordon *et al.* 1943; Gosney 1984a). The apparent decrease in size usually becomes much less pronounced when expressed as a ratio of body weight, but may still indicate the presence of changes in the structure of the gland not revealed by merely weighing it (Gosney 1986a). Thus, when Wistar albino rats were exposed for 28 days to a barometric pressure of 380 mmHg to simulate an altitude of 5500 m, the mean weight of their pituitaries was 7.6 ± 1.1 mg, in contrast to the mean weight of 11.8 ± 0.4 mg in the controls ($p<0.001$) (Gosney 1984a). Since the body weight of the hypoxic rats was also less than that of the controls, the difference in the weights of the pituitaries became statistically insignificant when expressed in terms of the weight of the whole animal. However, morphometric studies on coronal sections of the glands demonstrated that the smaller size of the hypoxic pituitaries was a consequence of a small pars distalis. The pars intermedia and pars nervosa were unaffected. The mean volume of the pars distalis was assessed morphometrically and was unequivocally smaller in the hypoxic rats ($4.40 ± 0.3$ mm^3 compared with $6.19 ± 0.4$ mm^3 in the controls, $p<0.001$). There was no difference in the number of cells per unit volume of the pars distalis, but the smaller volume of this part of the pituitary gland meant that the overall size of the cell population within it was diminished. Clearly one or more of the component subpopulations of the pituitary gland had become smaller, and throughout this chapter we shall discover which they were and the implications of this for the life of man at high altitude.

THYROID AND PITUITARY THYROTROPHS

The thyroid gland is one of the main regulators of oxygen consumption and hence one would expect its function at high altitude to be modified. Most studies have been carried out on animals acutely exposed to hypoxia in decompression chambers and much less is known about thyroid function in man exposed to chronic hypoxia at natural high altitude. In general, human studies have suggested increased function (Mordes *et al.* 1983; Sawhney and Malhotra 1991*a*), whereas those on animals have indicated decreased function (Surks 1966*a*). There are two complicating factors in the study of the effect of high altitude on thyroid function under natural conditions. The first is that mountain ranges are often deficient in iodine, as we discuss below. The second is that a cold environment affects thyroid function both in man (Williams 1974) and laboratory animals. These variables are much easier to control in experimental animals than in man.

Gosney (1986*b*), working in our laboratory, found that the thyroids of 10 male Wistar albino rats exposed for 28 days to a barometric pressure of 380 mmHg, simulating an altitude of 5500 m, were smaller than those of matched controls (mean weight 11.8 ± 0.9 mg in comparison with 17.1 ± 1.6 mg for the control group; $p < 0.001$). The smaller size of the thyroids was associated with an appearance typical of decreased activity. The thyroid of the normal rat is somewhat heterogeneous, with a tendency for active follicles to be located at the centre of the lobe, while those at the periphery are usually larger and appear less active. In the hypoxic rats, however, inactive follicles containing a large amount of colloid were present throughout the gland. Working in our laboratory, Gradwell (1978) had previously made a similar histological study on rats exposed to the same degree of hypobaric hypoxia for the same period (Figs 22.1 and 22.2). He found that compared with those of sea-level controls the thyroid glands of the test animals showed a statistically significant decrease in the amount of follicular epithelium without any significant change in the mean diameter of the follicles, but with an increase in colloid (Figs 22.3). Gordon *et al.* (1943) and Surks (1966*a*) had earlier reported similar appearances that are consistent with reduced thyroid activity.

From a physiological standpoint, the results of experiments of more than 3 days' duration uniformly show a reduction in thyroid function, which occurs both in animals born and bred at high altitudes, such as free-living gophers (Tryon *et al.* 1968) and

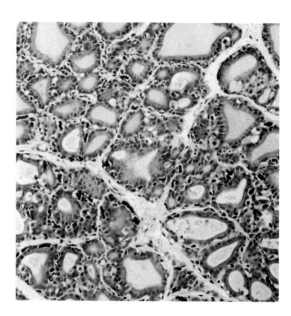

22.1 *Section of thyroid of control rat at sea level. The small follicles are lined by cuboidal epithelium. HE, × 150.*

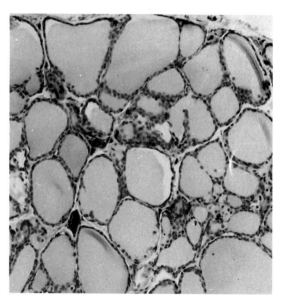

22.2 *Section of thyroid from a rat exposed to a simulated altitude of 5500 m for 4 weeks. The follicles are enlarged and lined by flattened epithelium. HE, × 150.*

experimental rats, and in animals developing in a normal environment and then exposed to low barometric pressure (Gordon *et al.* 1943; Surks 1966a; Martin *et al.* 1971; Galton 1972).

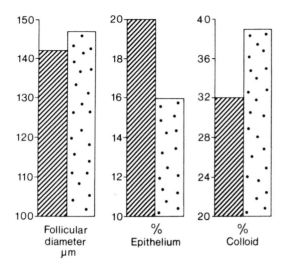

22.3 *Mean follicular diameter, mean percentage content of epithelium, and mean percentage of colloid in rats at sea level (hatched column) and after being subjected to a simulated altitude of 5500 m for 4 weeks (stippled column). (Based on data from Gradwell (1978).)*

It seems unlikely that the changes produced could be accounted for by a primary effect of hypoxia on the thyroid itself and it is suggested by Gosney (1986a) that they result from a primary inhibitory effect on the hypothalamic–pituitary unit, with inhibition of thyroid-stimulating hormone (TSH). He found that, in rats subjected to a simulated altitude of 5500 m, the pituitary thyrotrophs were solitary in the main, with very few of the clusters that characterize the normal pituitary. Cell counts revealed that in the hypoxic pituitary they accounted for only 0.41 ± 0.21% of the total population instead of the normal 1.34 ± 0.37%. This smaller proportion is certainly suggestive of a decrease in pituitary TSH. In surgical or pharmacological thyroidectomy the thyrotrophs become very large and vacuolate, the so-called 'thyroidectomy cells', and they are depleted of TSH and fail to label with antisera to it. The thyrotrophs of the hypoxic pituitary are neither enlarged nor vacuolate. Much earlier, Surks (1969) had claimed that injections of TSH had restored thyroid function to normal in intact hypoxic rats.

It has been suggested that this well-established depression of thyroid function in animals at high altitude may have some significance in acclimatization. Martin *et al.* (1972) studied what they called 'myocardial resistance' of rats made hyperthyroid by the injection of thyroxine, or hypothyroid by injection of propyl thiouracil. Using the method of McGrath and Bullard (1968), they suspended strips of right ventricular muscle in deoxygenated Krebs–Ringer solution and measured the percentage of normal contractile strength remaining after 200 anoxic contractions. This percentage was raised by exposure to altitude or by drug-induced hypothyroidism and was abolished by exogenous thyroxine. This so-called 'myocardial anoxic resistance' may be a feature of acclimatization. Certainly thyroxine inhibits enzymes that catalyse anaerobic metabolism and thus increases cardiac dependence on aerobic processes. The hypothyroid state has the opposite effect. Glycogen stores in cardiac muscle are augmented in hypothyroidism and appear to be important in surviving hypoxic stress. The hypothyroid state appears to have no influence on inducing polycythaemia.

In contrast, there is evidence that thyroid activity is increased in man at high altitude. Moncloa *et al.* (1966) transported 10 young men from sea level to a height of 4300 m and studied thyroid function for 14 days. The 24-hour thyroidal ^{131}I uptake rose significantly from 34.4% to 51.4% but basal metabolic rate was unchanged. Tetraiodothyronine (T_4) and triiodothyronine (T_3) are iodinated amino acids that increase heat production by uncoupling oxidative phosphorylation. T_4 is a prohormone and is converted in the tissues to T_3, the active hormone thyroxine. T_3 binds to nuclear receptors of cells sensitive to it. It influences transcription of DNA and thus cellular metabolism. The iodinated amino acids are essential for normal physical and mental development and in the metabolism of protein, carbohydrate, and fat.

Surks (1966b) found elevated levels of free thyroxine and thyroglobulin in subjects during the first 2 weeks at an altitude of 4300 m. Kotchen *et al.* (1973) also reported free and bound T_4 to be elevated in subjects exposed to a simulated altitude of 3650 m. TSH was found to be unchanged suggesting that there was no increased pituitary activity. Rastogi *et al.* (1977) found that levels of free and bound thyroxine returned towards control values during the third week at high altitude. This is consistent with the reports, noted in Chapter 21, that the basal metabolic rate is elevated during the first week at high altitude, falls for about 2 weeks, and then rises again after 3 weeks in the mountains. This correlates with levels of free T_4 (Stock *et al.* 1978a). It has been reported that at very high altitudes above 5500 m basal metabolic rate may remain elevated for months (Gill and Pugh 1964).

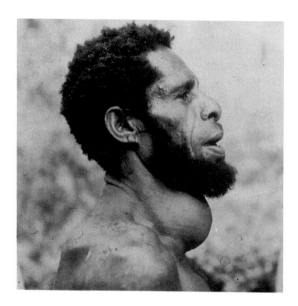

22.4 *Goitre in a native of the highlands of New Guinea.*

In a more recent study Sawhney and Malhotra (1991*a*) were able to confirm the persistent elevation of T_4 and T_3 during a brief stay at high altitude, previously reported by Mordes *et al.* (1983) in subjects who were airlifted to 3500 m. In contrast Wright (1979) observed a decline in T_3 during ascent to high altitude in the eastern Himalaya. In this group the trekkers had experienced much physical exertion.

COLLOID GOITRE IN MOUNTAINOUS AREAS

Enlargement of the thyroid gland due to colloidal adenomatous hyperplasia is the result of increased levels of TSH brought about by some block in the output of thyroid hormone. Three distinct mechanisms lead to the same histopathological changes (Robbins 1967). These are a deficiency of iodine, ingestion of goitrogenic foods or compounds that block thyroglobulin synthesis, and genetic defects involving enzymes vital to the elaboration of thyroid hormones. A deficiency of iodine is characteristic of some but not all mountain regions of the world. The lack of exogenous iodine leads to the formation of inadequate amounts of thyroid hormone and excessive TSH stimulation from the pituitary. Endemic goitre (Figs 22.4 and 22.5) is common where iodine intake falls below 100 μg/per day.

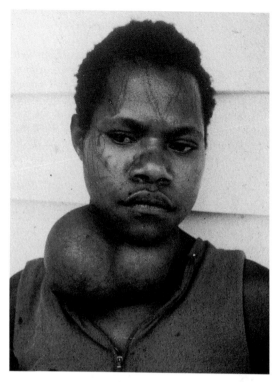

22.5 *Goitre in a girl from the highlands of New Guinea.*

There is not a universal distribution of the disease throughout the population at risk and this may be because the other two factors referred to above operate unevenly in the community. Thus some members of the group at risk may ingest goitrogenic substances such as turnips or cabbage, which contain antithyroid compounds. Other may have hereditary defects in the synthesis or transport of thyroid hormone. Ward (1975) refers to this patchy distribution of goitre in the population of the mountainous areas of northern Greece and he points out that Malamos *et al.* (1965) suggested that the goitres may be genetically determined. The classical studies of McCarrison (1906, 1908) suggested that pollution of drinking water with human and animal excreta brought about the development of goitres in iodine-deficient areas. Work in the same valley of the Karakoram mountains over 60 years later (Chapman *et al.* 1972) did not substantiate any correlation between bacterial contamination of water supply and prevalence of goitre. The diet in the mountains that is both rich in calcium and poor in iodine may be important (Hellwig 1934). For many years goitre has been known as 'Derbyshire neck', indicating the high prevalence of goitres in a limestone area.

While goitre is common in mountainous regions it is seen more frequently at moderate than at extreme high altitude. Thus, whereas goitre is characteristic of the population of the Himalaya, it is seen far less commonly in the Andes where highlanders frequently live at higher altitudes exceeding 4000 m. Both Moncloa (1966) and Fierro-Benitez *et al.* (1969) report that there is a lower prevalence of goitre at altitudes exceeding 3000 m in Peru. Norboo (1986) points out that the people of Ladakh live in the Indus valley with two mountain ranges nearby, the transHimalayan ranges in the south and the Karakorams in the north. There is a much higher prevalence of goitre in the Karakorams, where 15% of the female population have a goitre, in comparison with that of the Himalaya. Gosney (1986*a*) believes this difference is explained by the fact that in the more moderate altitude of the Karakorams there is relatively little suppression of the pituitary–thyroid axis, so that iodine is required. As this is not available, a goitre develops. Furthermore, we have already seen that hypoxia reduces the number of thyrotrophs in the pituitary, so that at more extreme altitude there are fewer thyrotrophs to produce TSH to produce a goitre.

Ward (1970) found that the prevalence of goitre in the general population at high altitude at Dhankuta in Nepal was no less than 32%. Ibbertson *et al.* (1972) found that 92% of Sherpas living in the Sola Khumbu region of north-east Nepal had a palpable goitre, which was visibly enlarged in 63%. Thirty per cent were clinically hypothyroid and 75% had less than normal levels of protein-bound iodine in the blood. Classical myxoedema was present in 5.9% of the population, deaf mutism in a further 4.7%, and isolated deafness in a further 3.1%. McCarrison (1906) found an incidence of goitre of 65% in the Gilgit area of Kashmir and later in 1972 Chapman *et al.* found an even higher incidence of 74%. Clearly, the treatment of such a common and disfiguring disease is an important medical problem. In the native highlanders of the Himalaya, enormous goitres may compress the recurrent laryngeal nerves and cause gross cosmetic disfigurement. Surgical treatment under such conditions is very difficult, for the goitres are often so vascular as to produce severe haemorrhage from dilated veins and arteries, and their size leads to grossly distorted anatomy making operation difficult. In isolated mountainous areas such as Nepal, the necessary excellent theatre facili-

ties and blood transfusion services are hard to come by. Radioiodine is easy to administer, but the strict precautions in its use would be difficult to enforce in an uneducated population. Traditional treatment by thyroid extract offers a better proposition. Ward (1970) reports that, in Dhankuta, 18 patients were treated with thyroid extract in a dose of 60 mg daily, increased by 60 mg weekly until a top dose of 300 mg daily was attained and sustained for 3–6 months. In the first 6 weeks of such treatment there were startling reductions in the size of the goitres. Such treatment must, of course, be followed up either by an adequate intake of iodine to prevent recurrence or by surgical excision.

Endemic goitre has been known to occur in the mountainous Huon peninsula of eastern New Guinea for many years (Figs 22.4 and 22.5). A study in 1964 indicated that the inhabitants of the area suffered from a severe iodine deficiency and trials were undertaken to determine whether or not the injection of iodized oil (iodized oil fluid injection B.P.) would correct that deficiency. Studies were also made to determine what effect injections given in the previous years had had. The results showed that, whereas the urinary iodine and [130]I uptake in New Guineans who had received iodized oil in 1957 were similar in untreated persons, yet a single injection of 4 ml iodized oil, containing 2.15 g iodine, appeared substantially to correct iodine deficiency for 4–5 years (Buttfield and Hetzel, 1967). There was also a significant regression of goitre in all but one of a group of 61 persons with easily visible goitres, within 3 months of their receiving an injection. No case of thyrotoxicosis or iodism was seen in the group of more than 2000 subjects who were given injections. The injection of iodized oil is particularly recommended for the correction of iodine deficiency in children and in women of child-bearing age whenever the efficacy of other measures is uncertain (Buttfield and Hetzel 1967). The method is relatively inexpensive and well suited to mass prophylaxis for a population with a low standard of living. Iodized salt should be made freely available to such mountain populations, but it is obvious that this is a far less reliable method of administration of iodine than by injection.

ADRENAL CORTEX AND PITUITARY CORTICOTROPHS

There is a considerable volume of evidence for increased adrenocortical activity in man and animals exposed to hypoxia, including hypobaric hypoxia, and this seems to be the result of increased synthesis

Table 22.1 Weights of pituitary and adrenal glands and percentage of pituitary corticotrophs in five lowlanders and five native highlanders

Racial type	Age (years)	Cause of death	Pituitary weight (g)	Corticotrophs (%)	Adrenal weight (g)
From Liverpool (sea level)					
Caucasian	21	Congenital heart disease	0.55	19.5	11.1
Caucasian	37	Epilepsy	0.50	21.3	10.8
Caucasian	39	Chronic pyelonephritis	0.50	18.7	9.9
Caucasian	37	Pneumonia	0.55	19.6	10.5
Caucasian	38	Coronary artery thrombosis	0.45	17.9	9.5
Mean (SD)	34 (7.5)		0.51 (0.04)	19.4 (1.26)	10.4 (0.66)
From La Paz (3600 m)					
Aymara	42	Gastric lymphoma	0.60	24.9	18.1
Aymara	28	Cerebellar gloma	0.40	25.6	14.3
Mestizo	32	Chronic pyelonephritis	0.40	27.1	14.7
Aymara	40	Peritonitis	0.75	28.3	15.9
Mestizo	29	Tuberculosis	1.20	21.9	14.5
Mean (SD)	34 (6.4)		0.67 (0.52)	25.6 (2.44)	15.3 (1.64)

and secretion of adrenocorticotrophic hormone by the corticotrophs of the pituitary. We carried out a study of the weight of the pituitary and adrenal glands from five Aymara and mestizo subjects born and living in La Paz (3600 m) and compared these with findings in five White lowlanders born and living in Liverpool at sea level (Gosney *et al.* 1991). The mean age of both groups was 34 years. In the same investigation, sections of pituitary glands were cut through the gland in the horizontal plane in order to obtain the best representation of the component cell populations. The sections were stained with haematoxylin and eosin and immunolabelled for adrenocorticotrophic hormone reactivity using the peroxidase–antiperoxidase technique. The results are shown in Table 22.1.

It transpired that the adrenals of the five lifelong residents at La Paz were significantly larger than those in age-matched controls from sea level (15.3 versus 10.4 g; $p < 0.001$), and appeared hyperplastic. The pituitary glands of the highlanders were not

significantly different in size from those of the controls (0.67 versus 0.51 g) but contained larger populations of corticotrophs expressed in terms of the total cell populations of their anterior lobes (25.6% versus 19.4%; $p < 0.001$). In conjunction with other studies of this endocrine axis in man and animals exposed to a hypoxic environment, these data suggest that greater amounts of adrenocorticotrophic hormone (ACTH) are required to maintain normal adrenocortical function under such circumstances, probably as a result of hypoxic inhibition of adrenocortical sensitivity to stimulation.

Pituitary corticotrophs were labelled uniformly with a dense granularity in both control and highland groups and were polygonal in shape (Fig. 22.6). In all subjects, they were most numerous in the area between the fibrous cores, the so-called mucoid wedge, but were found throughout the pars distalis except for the areas in the lateral part of the gland where somatotrophs are concentrated. In most subjects, there was some extension of corticotrophs into

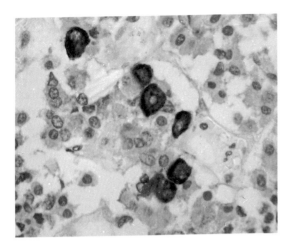

22.6 *Corticotrophs in the pars distalis of the pituitary gland of one of the subjects from Liverpool. Their distribution, separated by non-corticotrophs, is typical. Peroxidase–antiperoxidase, anti-ACTH, × 600.*

the anterior neurohypophysis. Although most often single, small groups of corticotrophs were commonplace and occasional large sheets were seen, especially in the pituitaries from highlanders (Fig. 22.7), giving the impression that these glands contained a larger proportion of corticotrophs than those of the control subjects.

Histological examination of the adrenals of the highlander revealed that the enlargement was due to an increase in the size of the cortex with, in all cases, incipient nodularity (Fig. 22.8). Many of these nodular areas elevated and distorted the capsule. Expansion of the zona reticularis with effacement of the zona fasciculata as seen in 'exhausted' adrenal glands was not a notable feature. Although present to some degree in most subjects of both groups, the increased size of the glands of the highlanders was predominantly due to expansion of lipid-rich tissue (Fig. 22.8). The cortical expansion was basically diffuse with a subtle focal nodularity superimposed. The same structural changes in both organs have been reported in laboratory animals exposed to simulated high altitude in decompression chambers. In Wistar albino rats thus treated there is proliferation of pituitary corticotrophs (Gosney 1984*a*) and an increase in the weight of the adrenals (Gosney 1985*b*).

Such histological changes in the pituitary and adrenal glands in man and animals are consistent with the stimulation of both organs that takes place on ascent to high altitude. It has to be kept in mind that there may be other factors that are involved in

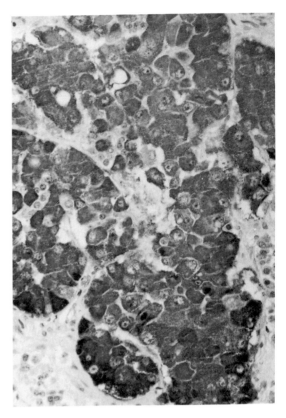

22.7 *A large confluent sheet of corticotrophs from the pars distalis of the pituitary of one of the highlanders from La Paz. Peroxidase–antiperoxidase, anti-ACTH, × 375.*

rapid ascent to great elevations, such as cold and increased intensity of solar or ultraviolet radiation. Halhuber and Gabl (1964) studied the relation of adrenocortical activity to time of exposure to high altitude and as a marker of this employed the level of excretion of 17-hydroxycorticosteroids (17-OHCS). They kept five male students aged 20–25 years under observation for 4 weeks at 2000 m. Adrenocortical activity increased sharply during the first week at high altitude, decreased during the second, varied during the third, and returned to sea-level values during the fourth. Klein (1964) studied men on exposure to the much greater elevation of 6200 m in the Andes and he also found a distinct rise in 17-OHCS on ascent. In this study, however, plasma corticosteroids were still elevated by some 60%, even after 5 weeks' sojourn at high altitude. There have been many confirmatory reports in the literature of a rapid and reversible rise in plasma cor-

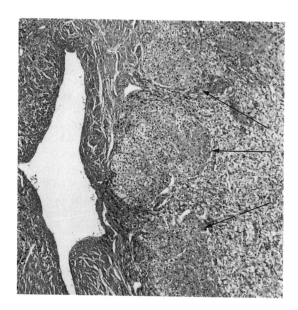

22.8 *Corticomedullary region of a hyperplastic adrenal gland from a subject from La Paz showing nodules of cortical tissue* (arrowheads) *impinging on the medulla. HE, × 60.*

tisol levels and urinary excretion of 17-OHCS in men and women rapidly transported to altitudes exceeding 4000 m (Mackinnon *et al.* 1963; Moncloa *et al.* 1965; Sutton *et al.* 1977). Abnormally high levels of 17-OHCS in the urine occur in climbers on exposure to extreme altitude exceeding 8000 m (Siri *et al.* 1969). Arias-Stella *et al.* (1973) reported that at necropsy on a woman of 48 years with Monge's disease there was hyperplasia of the adrenal cortex and the development of a nodular goitre.

In addition to the acute reaction of the pituitary–adrenal axis to acute exposure to high altitude, there is evidence that increased activity of these tissues accompanied by morphological changes in them persists after this initial period of stress and beyond the point when the organism has adjusted to the new environment and reached homeostatic equilibrium. Our own studies in La Paz referred to above provide histological support for this. Moncloa *et al.* (1961) and Moncloa and Pretell (1964) investigated the function of the hypothalamic–pituitary–adrenocortical axis in lifelong residents of Morococha and Cerro de Pasco, communities in the Peruvian Andes located at altitudes greater than 4000 m. In comparison with controls resident at sea level, the highlanders showed no differences in urinary excretion of glucocorticoid metabolites, cortisol metabolism,

or the response of the axis to suppression with dexamethasone (Moncloa *et al.* 1961). However, although both groups responded equally to doses of ACTH sufficient to stimulate maximally the adrenal cortex, the response of the highlanders to smaller doses was significantly less than subjects at sea level (Moncloa and Pretell 1964). This finding indicated that, although the capacity of the adrenal cortices for secretion was the same for both groups, those of the highlanders showed a relative insensitivity; more ACTH was required for the same level of response. Hypoxia appears to have an inhibitory effect on the response of the adrenal cortex to ACTH such that, in order to maintain a normal output of glucocorticoids, levels of ACTH are tonically elevated. This could lead to morphological changes described: an increase in the number of pituitary corticotrophs and enlargement of the adrenal cortex.

Although we believe that the increased proportion of corticotrophs in the pituitaries of the highlanders indicates increased function, it could be argued that they are, in fact, inactive, storing rather than secreting their content of ACTH. Although the latter possibility cannot be entirely excluded in the absence of complementary functional data, this could be explained only in terms of increased adrenocortical function developing as the primary event and leading to hypothalamic–pituitary inhibition. This would not be in keeping with the known facts about the effects of hypoxia on this endocrine axis, nor with the changes in pituitary corticotrophs described here, which is quite unlike that seen in primary adrenocortical hyperplasia characterized by accumulation of homogeneous material, Crooke's hyaline, in the cytoplasm.

ALDOSTERONE

One of the characteristic features of life at high altitude is the loss of control of hydration of the body with incipient oedema and retention of sodium. Such overhydration may account for some of the symptomatology of acute mountain sickness (Chapter 12), and for those ascending into high altitude there is the risk of developing pulmonary and cerebral oedema. The hormone that acts directly on the renal tubules is aldosterone, which promotes the reabsorption of sodium. It would be anticipated that in the environment of high altitude there would be adjustments to the levels of aldosterone and alterations in the activity of the renin–aldosterone system from which it arises. Such is indeed the case so that there is a characteristic fall in the levels of aldosterone in those ascending to high altitude.

Renin is released from the juxtaglomerular cells of the body in response to the stimuli of exercise and probably hypoxia. The mechanism common to these stimuli is sympathetic activation, and both circulating catecholamines and direct sympathetic nervous stimulation result in release of renin from these cells (Ward *et al.* 1989). Renin, which has no biological activity, acts on an α protein, angiotensinogen, circulating in the blood. This is split to form a decapeptide, angiotensin I, which is also biologically inactive. This is converted into the active octapeptide, angiotensin II, by angiotensin-converting enzyme on the luminal aspect of the endothelial cells lining the pulmonary capillaries. Angiotensin II is a powerful vasopressor and also acts on the cells of the adrenal cortex to release aldosterone. Aldosterone acts on the distal renal tubules to promote the reabsorption of sodium.

Both Ayres *et al.* (1961) and Williams (1961, 1966) found that ascent to high altitude caused a rise in the sodium:potassium ratio in saliva. This increased sodium loss indicated a fall of aldosterone activity at high altitude. At the same time there was a rise in total body potassium and a fall in urine aldosterone secretion. The hormone normally stimulates potassium excretion and hence its suppressed activity at altitude leads to potassium retention. Williams related the fall in aldosterone to the increased blood volume that occurs in acclimatization to altitude. This leads to stimulation of the stretch receptors in the right atrium, which is known to depress aldosterone secretion (Anderson *et al.* 1959). Jung *et al.* (1971) found that the fall in blood aldosterone is more prominent in older subjects than in the young.

The reduction in aldosterone secretion is very notable in climbers. Aldosterone excretion in urine over a period of 24 hours was measured by Pines *et al.* (1977) in five climbers during an ascent of a 7500 m mountain in the Hindu Kush. Expressed in units of $\mu g/24$ h, normal excretion at sea level was found to be 13.40. This fell to a level of 2.52 in the climbers at 5400 m and to 1.01 at 6600 m. Two of the climbers developed episodes of peripheral oedema at 6600 m and in them the level fell to 0.49. The sustained, vigorous exercise undertaken by climbers and trekkers itself stimulates the release of renin (Williams *et al.* 1979). During such exercise there is an expansion of interstitial fluid volume at the expense of intracellular volume with a small increase in plasma volume. Milledge *et al.* (1983*a*, *b*) confirmed these effects in subjects undertaking hill walking for 5 consecutive days. Bärtsch *et al.* (1991)

found that an exercise level corresponding to the efforts of mountaineering elicits hormonal changes favouring enhanced renal sodium and water retention in subjects susceptible to acute mountain sickness. Thus, 30 minutes of exercise on a bicycle ergometer at 4560 m led to a significantly greater increase of aldosterone and antidiuretic hormone plasma levels in mountaineers subsequently developing acute mountain sickness than in those who stayed well during a stay of 3 days at this altitude.

There have been many papers confirming the suppression of aldosterone at high altitude (Tuffley *et al.* 1970; Hogan *et al.* 1973; Pines *et al.* 1977; Sutton *et al.* 1977; Keynes *et al.* 1982). Milledge *et al.* (1983*b*) studied the time course of the effect of altitude over a 6-week stay at or above 4500 m. After initial suppression aldosterone concentration rose to control values after 12–20 days. Histological changes are associated with the suppression of aldosterone secretion. In contrast to the hyperplasia of the zona reticularis of the adrenal cortex, with increased levels of plasma cortisol, is the demonstration of a reduction in the width of the zona glomerulosa in dogs, rabbits, and rats kept at 1520–4260 m for five months (Hartroft *et al.* 1969). This glomerular zone of the adrenal cortex is the source of aldosterone and hence such histological appearances are compatible with the reported diminution in the secretion of this hormone at high altitude.

There appears to be variation in the secretion of aldosterone throughout the day. Sutton *et al.* (1977) found that in four men during 2 days at a simulated altitude of 4760 m, aldosterone was significantly lower in the morning at 09.00 h, whereas plasma cortisol was higher at most times throughout the day during exposure to hypobaric hypoxia compared with control values at sea level. Concentrations of serum and plasma aldosterone at low altitude are normally at their highest in the morning, which thus becomes the best time to determine any variations in response to high altitude. Under basal conditions, plasma aldosterone and cortisol concentrations are closely linked throughout the day (Takeda *et al.* 1984). This normal circadian relationship between the two hormones is disrupted by the hypobaric hypoxia of high altitude. It has been appreciated for many years that the reduced P_{O_2} is implicated in the decrease in aldosterone secretion (Moncloa *et al.* 1970). McLean *et al.* (1989) used saliva aldosterone concentration as an index of aldosterone secretion because frequent collection and processing of blood is inconvenient during an expedition. Few *et al.* (1984) had already shown that aldosterone concentration in saliva correlates closely with that in plasma. The use of saliva for this purpose by McLean *et al.* (1989) allowed them to investigate the temporal pattern of aldosterone secretion during an expedition to Mt Kenya. By this means they were able to demonstrate the reduction or complete absence of the marked rise in aldosterone that normally occurs in the first few hours after rising. These long periods of extremely low aldosterone levels had not been encountered by workers using traditional assays on blood samples.

Aldosterone concentrations at high altitude appear to depend on the duration of exposure. Okazaki *et al.* (1984) reported significant increases in aldosterone on arrival at a simulated altitude of 6000 m and these rose still further during a stay for 2 hours at that elevation. This increased level appeared to be due to increased ACTH because concentrations of serum cortisol were also elevated significantly. After longer periods of exposure to hypobaric bypoxia there are significant decreases in both blood and urinary aldosterone (Jung *et al.* 1971; Hogan *et al.* 1973; Maher *et al.* 1975; Milledge *et al.* 1983*a,b*; Maresh *et al.* 1985). The mechanisms of this subsequent decrease in aldosterone have not been elucidated.

There is no general agreement as to the level of plasma renin activity at high altitude. Some authors report a rise (Tuffley *et al.* 1970), others a fall (Hogan *et al.* 1973; Keynes *et al.* 1982), and some no change (Sutton *et al.* 1977). There appears to be a reduced response of aldosterone to renin. When the aldosterone:plasma renin activity ratio is calculated, it is found that for a given concentration of aldosterone plasma renin activity is higher at altitude than at sea level (Frayser *et al.* 1975). This led Milledge *et al.* (1983*b*) to suggest that hypobaric hypoxia decreased the rate of conversion of angiotensin I to angiotensin II.

ATRIAL NATRIURETIC PEPTIDE

Atrial natriuretic peptide (ANP) may be regarded as an endogenous antagonist to the renin–angiotensin–aldosterone system. Thus it brings about vasodilatation rather than vasoconstriction. It increases renal blood flow and glomerular filtration rate. It diminishes the production of aldosterone and antidiuretic hormone. These two opposing systems allow fine-tuning of blood volume and systemic pressure by the body (Johnston *et al.* 1989). Increases in ANP have been reported at high altitude (Tunny *et al.* 1989). We consider this peptide and its possible role in acute mountain sickness in

Chapter 12. Ramirez *et al.* (1988) speculate that atrial natriuretic hormone may mediate the inhibition of ACTH-stimulated aldosterone secretion brought about by hypoxaemia.

Elevated plasma atrial natriuretic peptide and vasopressin in high-altitude pulmonary oedema were reported in five male skiers with the disease at 3000 m by Cosby *et al.* (1988). Five healthy age-matched controls with similar physical activity at the same altitude served as controls. Mean plasma ANP immunoreactivity averaged 17.6 ± 5.6 pmol/l in patients with high-altitude pulmonary oedema compared with 6.8 ± 0.7 pmol/l in the controls. Elevated ANP levels normalized to 7.5 ± 1.9 pmol/l at 1600 m. Plasma arginine vasopressin levels were 1.8 ± 0.37 pmol/l in the subjects with lung oedema compared with 0.92 ± 0.29 pmol/l in the controls. The arginine vasopressin levels decreased to 1.29 ± 0.37 pmol/l on recovery at 1600 m.

This rise of ANP in high-altitude pulmonary oedema seems to be related to the increased pressure in the right atrium, an important source of the peptide. This increased tension in the walls of the right atrium is secondary to the increased pulmonary arterial pressure that is a central cause of the lung oedema (Chapter 13). As well as being a marker for an increase in right atrial pressure, the ANP probably exerts a vasodilatory effect on the pulmonary arterial tree, ameliorating the pulmonary hypertension (Cosby *et al.* 1988). Atrial natriuretic peptide increases vascular permeability and this may play a role in the causation of the high-altitude pulmonary oedema. The fact that ANP may suppress both plasma renin activity and aldosterone release provides a possible explanation for the normal plasma values of renin and aldosterone found in the patients of Cosby *et al.* (1988) with lung oedema. Hypoxia is known to be a potent stimulus for arginine vasopression release and its finding by Cosby *et al.* (1988) in their patients with lung oedema may be secondary to their diminished arterial oxygen tension.

ADRENAL MEDULLA

Chronic hypoxia induces histological changes in the medulla of the adrenal gland just as it does in the cortex. In the medullary tissue in the normal rat, loosely arranged phaeochromocytes in ill-defined aggregates are separated by wide sinusoidal spaces. In contrast, adrenal medullary cells of rats subjected to simulated high altitude are arranged in almost spherical, well-circumscribed clusters over which the sinusoidal lining cells appear to be stretched

(Gosney 1985*b*). This adrenal medullary hyperplasia underlines the physiological evidence of increased medullary activity in this species by Klain (1972), who found a transitory rise in catecholamine turnover in rats on their exposure to an altitude of 4300 m. Urinary noradrenaline excretion increased in men taken from sea level to 3850 m and, during 2 weeks' stay there, noradrenaline excretion doubled (Pace *et al.* 1964). Myles (1972) found that catecholamines were increased at simulated altitudes of 5500 and 7300 m. Cunningham *et al.* (1965) found evidence of increased adrenal medullary activity in men exposed acutely to natural high altitude at 4560 m on the Monte Rosa in the Alps.

Some workers have claimed that the level of catecholamines in the urine is related to the incidence of acute mountain sickness. Hoon *et al.* (1976) exposed 47 subjects to an altitude of 3660 m and 29 of them developed acute mountain sickness. Those with symptoms showed an immediate rise of 30% above the mean sea-level value of 44.7 μg/24 h in their urinary catecholamines. On subsequent days the excretion showed a steady and sustained increase until the tenth day of exposure. On the other hand, the asymptomatic group showed only an insignificant increase in catecholamine excretion on arrival at high altitude or subsequently at any stage during their stay in the mountains. On return to sea level the symptomatic group showed a sudden decline in catecholamine excretion and reached initial control values on the fourth day. It has been proposed that hypersecretion of catecholamines may increase systemic vascular resistance, leading to an extensive shift of blood to the pulmonary circulation, increasing the likelihood of the development of acute mountain sickness and even high-altitude pulmonary oedema. A similar investigation was undertaken on 58 subjects who were taken to high altitude slowly (Hoon *et al.* 1977). Twenty-five lowlanders ascended from 1800 to 3658 m in 50 hours and the remainder in 6 hours. None of them developed acute mountain sickness and their urinary catecholamine excretion remained normal during 10 days' stay at high altitude.

Mazzeo *et al.* (1991) found that there was a dissociation between the secretion of adrenaline from the adrenal medulla and the neural release of noradrenaline during exercise for men with exposure to high altitude. Adrenaline secretion appears early during such exposure, where it may augment glycogenolysis and lactate production during exercise, thereby influencing substrate mobilization and utilization. With improved oxygenation, which accompanies ventilatory acclimatization and erythropoiesis, adrenaline secretion subsides. Neural spillover of noradrenaline appears to increase later than adrenaline release and could be responsible for the increased systemic arterial pressure and resistance found in the recently acclimatized resident at high altitude (Chapter 18).

ENDOCRINE TESTIS

As will be seen in the following chapter, the hypobaric hypoxia of high altitude has an effect on spermatogenesis, bringing about structural damage to the seminiferous tubules and having a deleterious effect on the fertility of both man and animals living in high mountainous regions. Here we are concerned with the effects of hypoxia on the endocrine testis. When male rats are exposed to a barometric pressure of 380 mmHg in a decompression chamber, simulating an altitude of 5500 m, their testes become lighter and smaller. The mean testicular weight for ten hypoxic animals was 1.220 ± 0.108 g compared with 1.553 ± 0.049 g for the controls ($p<0.005$) (Gosney 1984*b*). Corresponding volumes were 1.556 ± 0.097 ml compared with 2.009 ± 0.179 ml ($p<0.005$) (Gosney 1984*b*). The proportion of the testis occupied by Leydig cells, the major source of androgens in the male, was 3.28 ± 0.25% compared with 4.70 ± 0.24% for the controls ($p<0.001$). The loss of Leydig cells is in excess of that explicable by the smaller testicular size alone. It has been shown that, in male subjects with chronic hypoxia due to longstanding chronic bronchitis and emphysema, there is a similar diminution in Leydig cell volume (Gosney 1985*a*; see Figs 22.9 and 22.10). Semple *et al.* (1980) have shown that such patients have a low level of serum testosterone.

The changes in the Leydig cells in the rats referred to above were accompanied by a decrease in pituitary gonadotrophs containing luteinizing hormone (LH). They comprised only 4.4 ± 1.2% of the total population of the pars distalis in comparison with 9.6 ± 1.6% for controls ($p<0.001$) (Gosney 1984*b*). No change was found in the proportion of gonadotrophs containing follicle-stimulating hormone (FSH) or lactotrophs containing prolactin (PRL).

These findings in experimental animals have obvious testosterone relevance to man. Sawhney *et al.* (1985) studied levels of testosterone, LH, FSH, and PRL in lowlanders after ascent to 3500 m. On the first day at high altitude levels of testosterone and LH began to fall. By the end of the week these hormones had fallen significantly, but prolactin levels were elevated. After a week on return to sea

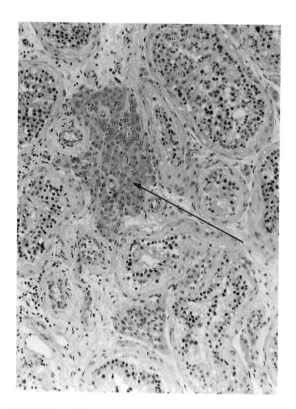

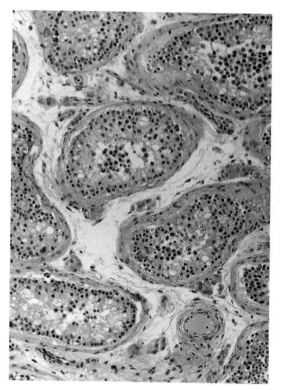

22.9 *Normal human testis from a 62-year-old man. Clusters of Leydig cells (arrow) are abundant between the seminiferous tubules. HE,* × *150.*

22.10 *Testis from a 62-year-old man with a 15-year history of chronic bronchitis and emphysema with frequent episodes of hypoxia. Leydig cells are infrequent and identified with difficulty. HE,* × *150.*

level these values had returned to control levels. Bangham and Hackett (1978) found reduced levels of LH after 10 days in residents at high altitude but no changes in FSH or PRL. In an earlier study by Guerra-Garcia (1971), the 24-h urinary testosterone excretion was measured in 10 normal men between the age of 19 and 25 years who were exposed to an altitude of 4250 m. Expressed in units of μg per 24-hour period, the mean value of testosterone was 99.8 ± 14.3 at sea level and this fell to 39.1 ± 7.1 by the third day at high altitude. By the seventh day of exposure the mean daily excretion rate of testosterone had recovered to 144 ± 23. Native highlanders show a similar urinary excretion of testosterone of 96.5 ± 10.16. Guerra-Garcia (1971) found that, although there was a diminished excretion of testosterone on acute exposure to the hypoxia of high altitude, the androgen-producing Leydig cells maintain their normal response to an adequate stimulus. The suggestion made above that the fall in excretion of urinary testosterone is due to a diminished plasma level of LH is confirmed by the fall in

plasma LH found by Sobrevilla and Midgley (1968) to occur in men exposed for 28 days to the hypoxic environment of Cerro de Pasco (4330 m).

The origin of the effects of hypoxia on the endocrine testis may be the hypothalamus. Hypobaric hypoxia may adversely affect the pulsatile release of gonadotrophin-releasing hormone (GnRH) into the hypothalamo-hypophyseal portal system. This may lead to subnormal levels of LH and, if combined with an effect on pituitary gonadotrophs as described above, may depress further the synthesis and release of this pituitary hormone (Gosney 1986a). This diminution in the level of LH would in time lead to atrophy of its target cell, the Leydig cell. This finally would result in reduced output of testosterone.

INSULIN AND OTHER GLUCOREGULATORY HORMONES

There is general agreement that levels of glucose in the blood increase on ascent to high altitude.

Williams (1975) reported that, after an effortless ascent to 3500 m by airlift, five men showed increases in blood glucose to values between 115 and 135 mg/dl. Earlier, Forbes (1936) found that fasting blood sugars decreased as men went sea level to 3660 m but then increased at higher altitudes. In Indian soldiers studied by Singh *et al.* (1977) the blood sugar was found to be raised 2 weeks after arrival at high altitude and persisted for 10 months before falling again so that by 2 years the blood glucose level was significantly lower than the initial values at sea level. Native highlanders have been reported to show reduced blood sugars (Picón-Reátegui *et al.* 1970).

In one investigation Sawhney *et al.* (1986) found that fasting blood glucose levels were not significantly altered on acute ascent to high altitude. They found that in seven sea-level residents in Delhi (226 m) fasting blood glucose levels ranged between 63.6 and 85.3 mg/dl, with a mean value of 72.38. When these subjects were airlifted to 3500 m in the Himalaya and kept there for 2 weeks, the basal blood glucose level remained at 77.00 mg/dl. The fasting blood sugar in a comparable number of native highlanders was 71.86 mg/dl. In a subsequent investigation (Sawhney *et al.* 1991) they studied blood glucose levels and glucoregulatory hormones in 15 men, euglycaemic at sea level, at low altitude, and on ascent to altitudes of 3500 and 5080 m. They compared their findings with those from 17 acclimatized lowlanders and from 17 native highlanders. They found that mean fasting glucose levels (4.60 mmol/l) rose sharply by the third day at 3500 m (5.54 mmol/l) but by the seventh day had fallen back to sea-level values and were sustained at that level for the remainder of time spent at that altitude. There was a further increase in blood glucose again on further ascent to 5080 m. However, blood glucose levels fell to normal by day 41 at high altitude.

The increased blood glucose concentration immediately on arrival at high altitude may be the result of increased hepatic glycogenolysis and glucose release due to activation of the sympathetic nerves and of the adrenal medulla and cortex. Sawhney *et al.* (1991) believe that hypoxia may exert a direct effect on glucose metabolism by increasing the rate-limiting enzymes such as pyruvate kinase and pyruvate phosphotransferase. Increased adrenal secretion of cortisol referred to earlier in this chapter may be involved in the hyperglycaemia of early arrival at high altitude through inhibition of peripheral glucose utilization, overproduction of glucose by the liver, or increased gluconeogenesis.

Williams (1975) found that, in five men passively transported to 3500 m, the average blood insulin concentration rose. In one subject the mean insulin concentration in microunits per ml (μU/ml) of blood serum rose from 19.00 over 4 days before ascent, to 21.25 over 4 days at 3500 m, and then fell to 14.40 over 5 days on return to sea level. Each laboratory establishes its own expected range of values for this hormone but it may be taken that mean fasting levels for individuals at sea level lie below 20 μU/ml. Sawhney *et al.* (1986) found the greatest difference in plasma levels of insulin in μU/ml to occur at 18.00 hours, when the mean value of 10 subjects at sea level of 9.67 μU/ml rose to 24.52 after 15 days at 3500 m by 10 sojourners, compared with 21.92 in 11 native highlanders. In their later investigation Sawhney *et al.* (1991) found that insulin concentrations at sea level varied between 1.5 and 15 μU/ml with a mean of 9.3 μU/ml. By the third day at an altitude of 3500 m they showed a significant increase (12.74 μU/ml). The maximum increase was found at the seventh day (14.69 μU/ml). Thereafter plasma insulin concentrations returned to sea-level values and were unaltered during the remainder of the stay at 3500 m. On arrival at 5080 m there was a further slight rise (11.95 μU/ml). By day 41 at high altitude the insulin values were not significantly different from those found at sea level. The incidence of diabetes mellitus was found to be lower in soldiers stationed at high altitude in the Himalaya than in men stationed on the plains of India (Singh *et al.* 1977).

The literature reveals disagreement as to whether or not there is a true loss of glucose tolerance at high altitude. Decreased (Janoski *et al.* 1969), increased (Forbes *et al.* 1936), and unaltered glucose tolerance have been reported in subjects taken to high altitude. Some authors have reported that both oral and intravenous glucose tolerance tests have shown that glucose utilization is increased in native highlanders (Picón-Reátegui *et al.* 1970). Glucose loading increases both blood glucose and insulin levels at altitude just as it does at sea level but the rise in both is less than at sea level (Stock *et al.* 1978*b*). Studies employing the infusion of ^{14}C glucose have revealed that this is also the case in recent arrivals at high altitude (Johnson *et al.* 1974). Associated with the reduced levels of blood sugar is a low glycogen content of the liver (Blume and Pace 1967; Johnson *et al.* 1974). Such a reduction in the liver glycogen store would represent one reason why glucose tolerance tests do not produce as large an elevation in blood glucose levels at high altitude as at sea level.

Glycogen synthesis would be stimulated by reduced stores and this would rapidly remove the excess glucose from the blood. In contrast to this, Sawhney *et al.* (1986) reported decreased glucose tolerance at high altitude as had previously been reported by Janoski *et al.*(1969). They considered that the decreased glucose tolerance they found was not due to high dietary intake of carbohydrate.

As we note above, the altered relationship between glucose and insulin levels immediately on arrival at high altitude appears to be due to some extent to increased secretion of adrenal hormones. In contrast, in acclimatized lowlanders and native highlanders glucose concentrations were found to be higher for the prevailing insulin concentration (Sawhney *et al.* 1991). Earlier Sawhney *et al.* (1986) had commented that at high altitude hyperglycaemia occurs in the face of hyperinsulinism. This might suggest a simultaneous and disproportionate rise of a hormone antagonistic to insulin modifying its effect on glucose metabolism. It has been thought that plasma growth hormone may be involved.

PLASMA GROWTH HORMONE

Plasma growth hormone did not show any appreciable changes on arrival of lowlanders at high altitude (Sawhney *et al.* 1991). Hence the hyperglycaemia and hyperinsulinaemia during the first few days and weeks at high altitude is not due to increased pituitary secretion of growth hormone (GH). However, concentrations of GH were found to be elevated in the acclimatized and in native highlanders. Longer elevation of GH limits glucose transport into the cells and produces an insulin-resistant state. GH does not stimulate insulin secretion directly but the hyperglycaemia produced by GH stimulates pancreatic secretion of insulin.

Elevation of levels of growth hormone occurs in association with many forms of stress, including physical exercise and heat (Schalch 1967). Pituitary secretion of GH undergoes cyclic variation over the 24-hour period (Takahashi *et al.* 1968). Sawhney and Malhotra (1991*b*) studied the circadian rhythmicity of growth hormone at high altitude in man. They investigated the plasma concentrations of GH at different timings of the day in a group of healthy sea-level residents in Delhi (226 m) and in native highlanders in the western Himalaya. Studies were carried out every 6 hours from 06.00. In both groups growth hormone levels were lowest at 06.00 hours and highest at midnight. Native highlanders have higher circulatory levels of GH compared to lowlanders. This elevation is evident at all periods of the day. Hence the circadian rhythmicity of the hormone is well maintained in highlanders albeit at a higher level. It is not clear at present if these increased levels are due to increased pituitary secretion of the hormone or a delay in its clearance rate.

References

Anderson, C.H., McCally, M., and Farrel, G.L. (1959). The effects of atrial stretch on aldosterone secretion. *Endocrinology*, **64**, 202

Arias-Stella, J., Krüger, H., and Recavarren, S. (1973). On the pathology of chronic mountain sickness. *Pathologia et Microbiologia*, **39**, 283

Ayres, P.J., Hunter, R.C., Williams, E.S., and Rundo, J. (1961). Aldosterone excretion and potassium retention in subjects living at high altitude. *Nature, London*, **191**, 78

Bangham, C.R.M. and Hackett., P.H. (1978). Effects of high altitude on endocrine function in the Sherpas of Nepal. *Journal of Endocrinology*, **79**, 147

Bärtsch, P., Maggiorini, M, Schobersberger, W., Shaw, S., Rascher, W., Girard, J., Weidmann, P., and Oelz, O. (1991). Enhanced exercise-induced rise of aldosterone and vasopressin preceding mountain sickness. *Journal of Applied Physiology*, **71**, 136

Blume, F.D. and Pace, N. (1967). Effect of translocation to 3,800 m altitude on glycolysis in mice. *Journal of Applied Physiology*, **23**, 75

Brun, C., Knudsen, E.O.E., and Raaschon, F. (1945). On cause of post-syncopal oligura. *Acta Medica Scandinavica*, **122**, 486

Buttfield, I.H. and Hetzel, B.S. (1967). Endemic goitre in eastern New Guinea. With special reference to the use of iodized oil in prophylaxis and treatment. *Bulletin of the World Health Organization*, **36**, 243

Chapman, J.A., Grant, I.S., Taylor, G., Mahamud, K., Sardar-Ul-Mulk, and Shadid, M.A. (1972). Endemic goitre in the Gilgit Agency, West Pakistan. *Philosophical Transactions of the Royal Society*, **B263**, 459

Cosby, R.L., Sophocles, A.M., Durr, J.A., Perrinjaquet, L., Yee, B., and Schrier, R.W. (1988). Elevated plasma atrial natriuretic factor and vasopressin in high-altitude pulmonary oedema. *Annals of Internal Medicine*, **109**, 796

Cunningham, W.L., Becker, E.J., and Kreuzer, F. (1965). Catecholamines in urine and plasma at high altitude. *Journal of Applied Physiology*, **20**, 607

Few, J.D., Chaudry, S., and James V.H.T. (1984). The direct determination of aldosterone in human saliva. *Journal of Steroid Biochemistry*, **21**, 87

Fierro-Benitez, R., Penafiel, W., DeGroot, L.J., and Ramirez, I. (1969). Endemic goitre and endemic cretinism in the Andean region. *New England Journal of Medicine*, **280**, 296

Forbes, W.H. (1936). Blood sugar and glucose tolerance at high altitudes. *American Journal of Physiology*, **116**, 309

Frayser, R., Rennie, I.D., Gray, G.W., and Houston, C.W. (1975). Hormonal and electrolyte response to exposure to 17,500 ft. *Journal of Applied Physiology*, **38**, 636

Galton, V.A. (1972). Some effects of altitude on thyroid function. *Endocrinology*, **92**, 1393

Gill, M.B., and Pugh, L.G.C.E. (1964). Basal metabolism and respiration in men living at 5800 m (19,000 feet). *Journal of Applied Physiology*, **19**, 949

Gordon, A.S., Tornetta, F.J., d'Angelo, S.A., and Charipper, H.A. (1943). Effects of low atmospheric pressures on activity of the thyroid, reproductive system and anterior lobe of the pituitary in the rat. *Endocrinology*, **33**, 366

Gosney, J.R. (1984*a*). The effects of hypobaric hypoxia on the corticotroph population of the adenohypophysis of the male rat. *Journal of Pathology*, **142**, 163

Gosney, J.R. (1984*b*). Effects of hypobaric hypoxia on the Leydig cell population of the testis of the rat. *Journal of Endocrinology*, **103**, 59

Gosney, J.R. (1985*a*). Histopathology of endocrine organs in hypoxia. MD thesis, University of Liverpool

Gosney, J.R. (1985*b*). Adrenal corticomedullary hyperplasia in hypobaric hypoxia. *Journal of Pathology*, **146**, 59

Gosney, J.R. (1986*a*). Histopathology of the endocrine glands in hypoxia. In *Aspects of Hypoxia*, (D. Heath, Ed.). Liverpool; Liverpool University Press, p. 132

Gosney, J.R. (1986*b*). Morphological changes in the pituitary and thyroid of the rat in hypobaric hypoxia. *Journal of Endocrinology*, **109**, 119

Gosney, J., Heath, D., Williams, D., and Rios-Dalenz, J. (1991). Morphological changes in the pituitary–adrenocortical axis in natives of La Paz. *International Journal of Biometeorology*, **35**, 1

Gradwell, E. (1978). Histological changes in the thyroid gland in rats on acclimatization to simulated high altitude. *Journal of Pathology*, **125**, 33

Guerra-Garcia, R. (1971). Testosterone metabolism in men exposed to high altitude. *Acta Endocrinologica Panama*, **2**, 55

Halhuber, M.J. and Gabl, F. (1964). 17-OHCS excretion and blood eosinophils at an high altitude of 2000 m. In *The Physiological Effects of High Altitude* (W.H. Weihe, Ed.). Oxford; Pergamon Press, p. 131

Hartroft, P.M., Bischoff, M.B., and Bucci, T.J. (1969). Effects of chronic exposure to high altitude on the juxta-glomerular complex and adrenal cortex of dogs, rabbits and cats. *Federation Proceedings: Federation of American Societies of Experimental Biology*, **28**, 1234

Hellwig, C.A. (1934). Experimental colloid goiter. *Endocrinology*, **18**, 197

Henry, J.P., Gauer, O.H., and Reeves, J.L. (1956). Evidence of atrial location of receptors in influencing urine flow. *Circulation Research*, **4**, 85

Henry, J.P. and Pearce, J.W. (1956). Possible role of cardiac atrial stretch receptors in induction of changes in urine flow. *Journal of Physiology*, **131**, 572

Hogan, R.P., Kotchen, T.A., Boyd, A.E., and Hartley, L.H. (1973). Effects of altitude on renin–aldosterone system and metabolism of water and electrolytes. *Journal of Applied Physiology*, **35**, 385

Hoon, R.S., Sharma, S.C., Balasubramanian, V., Chadha, K.S., and Mathew, O.P. (1976). Urinary catecholamine excretion on acute induction to high altitude (3658 m). *Journal of Applied Physiology*, **41**, 631

Hoon, R.S., Sharma, S.C., Balasubramanian, V., and Chadha, K.S. (1977). Urinary catecholamine excretion in induction to high altitude (3658 m) by air and road. *American Journal of Physiology: Respiratory, Environmental and Exercise Physiology*, **42**, 728

Ibbertson, H.K., Tair, J.M., Pearl, M., Lim, T., McKinnon, J.R., and Gill, M.B. (1972). Himalayan cretinism. *Advances in Experimental Medical Biology*, **30**, 51

Janoski, A.H., Johnson, H.L., and Sanbar, S.S. (1969). Carbohydrate metabolism in men at high altitude. *Federation Proceedings: Federation of American Societies of Experimental Biology*, **28**, 593

Johnson, H.L., Consolazio, C.F., Burk, R.F., and Daws, T.A. (1974). Glucose ^{14}C-UL metabolism in man after abrupt altitude exposure (4,300 m). *Aerospace Medicine*, **45**, 849

Johnston C.I., Hodsman, P.G., Kohzuki, M., Casley, D.J., Fabris, B., and Phillips, P.A. (1989). Interaction between atrial natriuretic peptide and the renin angiotensin aldosterone system. Endogenous antagonists. *American Journal of Medicine*, **87**, 6B(1), 24S

Jung, R.C., Dill, D.B., Horton, R., and Horvath, S.M. (1971). Effect of age on plasma aldosterone levels and hemoconcentration at altitude. *Journal of Applied Physiology*, **31**, 593

Keynes, R.J., Smith, G.W., Slater, J.D.H., Brown, M.M., Brown, S.E., Payne, N.N., Jowett, T.P., and Monge, C.C. (1982). Renin and aldosterone at high altitude in man. *Journal of Endocrinology*, **92**, 131

Klain, G.J. (1972). Acute high altitude stress and enzyme activities in the rat adrenal medulla. *Endocrinology*, **91**, 1447

Klein, K. (1964). Contribution to discussion after paper by Halhuber and Gabl (above). In *The Physiological Effects of High Altitude* (W.H. Weihe, Ed.). Oxford; Pergamon Press, p. 136

Kotchen, T.A., Mougey, E.H., Hogan, R.P., Boyd, A.E., Pennington, L.L., and Mason, J.W. (1973). Thyroid responses to simulated altitude. *Journal of Applied Physiology*, **34**, 165

Mackinnon, P.C.B., Monk-Jones, M.E., and Fotherby, K. (1963). A study of various indices of adrenocortical activity during 23 days at high altitude. *Journal of Endocrinology*, **26**, 555

Maher, J.T., Jones, L.B., Hartley, L.H., Williams, G.H., and Rose, L.I. (1975). Aldosterone dynamics during graded exercise at sea level and high altitude. *Journal of Applied Physiology*, **39**, 18

Malamos, B., Miras, C., Kostamis, P., Mantzos, J., Kralios, A.C., Rigopoulos, G., Zerefos, N., and Koutras, D.S. (1965). In *Current Topics in Thyroid Research* (C.Cassano and M. Andreoli, Ed.). New York; Academic Press

Maresh, C.M., Noble, B.J., Robertson, K.I., and Harvey, J.S. (1985). Aldosterone, cortisol, and electrolyte responses to hypobaric hypoxia in moderate-altitude natives. *Aviation, Space and Environmental Medicine*, **56**, 1078

Martin, L.G., Westernberger, G.E., and Bullard, R.W. (1971). Thyroidal changes in the rat during acclimatization to simulated high altitude. *American Journal of Physiology*, **221**, 1057

Martin, L.G., Westernberger, G.E., Hippensteele, J.E., and Bullard, R.W. (1972). Thyroidal influence on myocardial changes induced by simulated high altitudes. *American Journal of Physiology*, **222**, 1599

Mazzeo, R.S., Bender, P.R., Brooks, G.A., Butterfield, G.E., Groves, B.M., Sutton, J.R., Wolfel, E.E., and Reeves, J.T. (1991). Arterial catecholamine responses during exercise with acute and chronic high-altitude exposure. *American Journal of Physiology (Endocrinology, Metabolism)*, **261**, E419

McCarrison, R. (1906). Observations on endemic goitre in the Chitral and Gilgit Valleys. *Lancet*, **i**, 1110

McCarrison, R. (1908). Observations on endemic cretinism in the Chitral and Gilgit Valleys. *Lancet*, **ii**, 1275

McGrath, J.J. and Bullard, R.W. (1968). Altered myocardial performance in response to anoxia after high altitude exposure. *Journal of Applied Physiology*, **25**, 761

McLean, C.J., Booth, C.W., Tattersall, T., and Few, J.D. (1989). The effect of high altitude on saliva aldosterone and glucocorticoid concentrations. *European Journal of Applied Physiology*, **58**, 341

Milledge, J.S., Catley, D.M., Blume, F.D., and West, J.B. (1983*a*). Renin, angiotensin-converting enzyme and aldosterone in humans on Mount Everest. *Journal of Applied Physiology*, **55**, 1109

Milledge, J.S., Catley, D.M., Ward, M.P., Williams, E.S., and Clarke, C.R.A. (1983*b*). Renin–aldosterone and angiotensin-converting enzyme during prolonged altitude exposure. *Journal of Applied Physiology*, **55**, 699

Moncloa, F. (1966). Physiological patterns: endocrine factors. In *Life at High Altitudes*, Scientific Publication No. 140. Washington, DC; Pan American Health Organization, p. 36

Moncloa, F. and Pretell, E. (1964). Cortisol secretion rate, ACTH, and methopyrapone tests in high altitude native residents. *Journal of Clinical Endocrinology*, **24**, 915

Moncloa, F., Pretell, E., and Correa, J. (1961). Studies on urinary steroids of men born and living at high altitude. *Proceedings of the Society for Experimental Biology and Medicine*, **108**, 336

Moncloa, F., Donayre, J., Sobrevilla, L.A., and Guerra-Garcia, R. (1965). Endocrine studies at high altitude: II Adrenal cortical function in sea level natives exposed to high altitude (4300 meters) for two weeks. *Journal of Clinical Endocrinology and Metabolism*, **25**, 1640

Moncloa, F., Guerra-Garcia, R., Subauste, C., Sobrevilla, L.A., and Donayre, J. (1966). Endocrine studies at high altitude. I. Thyroid function in sea level natives exposed for two weeks to an altitude of 4300 meters. *Journal of Clinical Endocrinology and Metabolism*, **26**, 1237

Moncloa, F., Velasco, I., and Beteta, L. (1970). Physical exercise, acid base balance, and adrenal function in newcomers to high altitude. *Journal of Applied Physiology*, **28**, 151

Mordes, J.P., Blume, F.D., Boyer, S., Zheng, M.R., and Braverman, L.E. (1983). High altitude pituitary thyroid dysfunction on Mount Everest. *New England Journal of Medicine*, **308**, 1135

Myles, W.S. (1972). The excretion of 17-hydroxy-corticosteroids by rats during exposure to altitude. *International Journal of Biometeorology*, **16**, 367.

Noble, R.L. and Taylor, N.B.G. (1953). Antidiuretic substances in human urine after haemorrhage, fainting, dehydration and acceleration. *Journal of Physiology*, **122**, 220

Norboo, T. (1986). Discussion. In *Aspects of Hypoxia* (D.Heath, Ed.). Liverpool; Liverpool University Press, p. 162

Okazaki, S., Tamura, Y., Hatano, T., and Matsui, N. (1984). Hormonal disturbance of fluid–electrolyte metabolism under altitude exposure in man. *Aviation, Space, and Environmental Medicine*, **55**, 200

Pace, N., Grisnold, R.L., and Grunbaum, B.W. (1964). Increase in urinary norepinephrine excretion during 14 days sojourn at 3800 meters elevation. *Federation Proceedings: Federation of American Societies for Experimental Biology*, **23**, 521

Picón-Reátegui, E., Buskirk, E.R., and Baker, P.T. (1970). Blood glucose in high altitude natives and during acclimatization to altitude. *Journal of Applied Physiology*, **29**, 560

Pines, A., Slater, J.D.H., and Jowett, J.P. (1977). The kidney and aldosterone in acclimatization at altitude. *British Journal of Diseases of the Chest*, **71**, 203

Ramirez, G., Bittle, P.A., Hammond, A., Ayers, C.W., Dietz, J.R., and Colice, G.L. (1988). Regulation of aldosterone secretion during hypoxemia at sea level and moderately high altitude. *Journal of Clinical Endocrinology and Metabolism*, **67**, 1162

Rastogi, G.K., Malhotra, M.S., Srivastava, M.C., Sawhney, R.C., Dua, G.L., Sridharan, K., Hoon, R.S., and Singh, I. (1977). Study of the pituitary–thyroid functions at high altitude in man. *Journal of Clinical Endocrinology and Metabolism*, **44**, 447

Robbins, S.L. (1967). The endocrine system. In *Pathology*, 3rd edn. Philadelphia; Saunders, p. 1202

Sawhney, R.C. and Malhotra, A.S. (1991*a*). Thyroid function in sojourners and acclimatised lowlanders at high altitude in man. *Hormone and Metabolic Research*, **23**, 81

Sawhney, R.C. and Malhotra, A.S. (1991*b*). Circadian rhythmicity of growth hormone at high altitude in man. *Indian Journal of Physiology and Pharmacology*, **35**, 55

Sawhney, R.C., Chabra, P.C., Malhotra, A.S., Singh, T., Riav, S.S., and Rai, R.M. (1985). Hormone profiles at high altitude in man. *Andrologia*, **17**, 178

Sawhney, R.C., Malhotra, A.S., Singh, T., Rai, R.M., and Sinha, K.C. (1986). Insulin secretion at high altitude in man. *International Journal of Biometeorology*, **30**, 231

Sawhney, R.C., Malhotra, A.S., and Singh, T. (1991). Glucoregulatory hormones in man at high altitude. *European Journal of Applied Physiology*, **62**, 286

Schalch, D.S. (1967). The influence of physical stress and exercise on growth hormone and insulin secretion in man. *Journal of Laboratory and Clinical Medicine*, **69**, 256

Semple, P.d'A., Beastall, G.H., Watson, W.S., and Hume, R. (1980). Serum testosterone depression associated with hypoxia in respiratory failure. *Clinical Science*, **58**, 105

Silvette, H. (1943). Some effects of low barometric pressure on kidney function in the white rat. *American Journal of Physiology*, **140**, 374

Singh, I., Chohan, I.S., Lal, M., Khanna, P.K. Srivastava, M.C., Nanda, R.B., Lamba, J.S., and Malhotra, M.S. (1977). Effects of high altitude stay on the incidence of common diseases in man. *International Journal of Biometeorology*, **21**, 93

Siri, W.E., Cleveland, A.S., and Blanche, P. (1969). Adrenal gland activity in Mount Everest climbers. *Federation Proceedings: Federation of American Societies for Experimental Biology*, **28**, 1251

Sobrevilla, L.A. and Midgley, A.R. (1968). In *Gonadotropins* (E. Rosemberg, Ed.). Los Altos, California; Geron-X, p. 367

Stock, M.J., Norgan, N.G., Ferro-Luzzi, A., and Evans, E. (1978*a*). Effect of altitude on dietary-induced thermogenesis at rest and during light exercise in man. *Journal of Applied Physiology: Respiratory, Environmental and Exercise Physiology*, **45**, 345

Stock, M.J., Chapman, C., Stirling, J.L., and Campbell, I.T. (1978*b*). Effects of exercise, altitude, and food on blood hormone and metabolic levels. *Journal of Applied Physiology: Respiratory, Environmental and Exercise Physiology*, **45**, 350

Surks, M.I. (1966*a*). Effect of hypoxia and high altitude on thyroidal iodine metabolism in the rat. *Endocrinology*, **78**, 307

Surks, M.I. (1966*b*). Elevated PBI, free thyroxine, and plasma protein concentration in man at high altitude. *Journal of Applied Physiology*, **21**, 1185

Surks, M.I. (1969). Effect of thyrotropin metabolism during hypoxia. *American Journal of Physiology*, **216**, 436

Sutton, J.R., Viol, G.W., Gray, G.W., McFadden, M., and Keane, P.M. (1977). Renin, aldosterone, electrolyte, and cortisol responses to hypoxic decompression. *Journal of Applied Physiology*, **43**, 421

Takahashi, Y., Kipuis, D.M., and Daughaday, W.H. (1968). Growth hormone secretion during sleep. *Journal of Clinical Investigation*, **47**, 2079

Takeda, R., Mryamori, C., Ikeda, M., Koshida, H., Takeda, Y., Yashuhara, S., Morise, T., and Takimoto, H. (1984). Circadian rhythm of plasma aldosterone and time dependent alterations of aldosterone regulators. *Journal of Steroid Biochemistry*, **20**, 321

Tryon, C.A., Kodric, W.E., and Cunningham, H.N. (1968). Measurement of relative thyroid activity in free-ranging rodents along an altitudinal transect. *Nature (London)*, **218**, 278

Tuffley, R.E., Rubenstein, D., Slater, J.D.H., and Williams, E.S. (1970). Serum renin activity during exposure to hypoxia. *Journal of Endocrinology*, **48**, 497

Tunny, T.J., van Gelder, J., Gordon, R.D., Klemm, S.A., Hamlet, S.M., Finn, W.L., Carney, G.M., and Brand-Maher, C. (1989). Effects of altitude on atrial natriuretic peptide: the bicentennial Mount Everest expedition. *Clinical and Experimental Pharmacology and Physiology*, **16**, 287

Ward, J.P. (1970). The medical treatment of large group III goitres with thyroid extract. *British Journal of Surgery*, **57**, 587

Ward, M. (1975). Mountain medicine. *A Clinical Study of Cold and High Altitude*. London; Crosby Lockwood Staples

Ward, M.P., Milledge, J.S., and West, J.B. (1989). The endocrine and renal systems. In *High Altitude Medicine and Physiology*. London; Chapman and Hall Medical, p. 293

Williams, E.S. (1961). Salivary electrolyte composition at high altitude. *Clinical Science*, **21**, 37

Williams, E.S. (1966). Electrolyte regulation during the adaptation of humans to life at high altitudes. *Proceedings of the Royal Society*, **B165**, 266

Williams, E.S. (1975). Mountaineering and the endocrine system. In *Mountain Medicine and Physiology* (C. Clarke, M. Ward, and E. Williams, Ed.). London; Alpine Club, p. 38

Williams, E.S., Ward, M.P., Milledge, J.S., Withey, W.R., Older, M.W.J., and Forsling, M.L. (1979). Effect of the exercise of seven consecutive days hill-walking on fluid homeostasis. *Clinical Science*, **56**, 305

Williams, R.H. (1974). The thyroid gland. In *Textbook of Endocrinology*, 5th edn. Philadelphia; Saunders, p. 126

Wright, A.D. (1979). Birmingham Medical Research Expeditionary Society 1977 expedition. Thyroid function and acute mountain sickness. *Postgraduate Medical Journal*, **55**, 483

23

Fertility and pregnancy

Data from population censuses in Bolivia, Ecuador, and Peru make it clear that the birth rate is diminished at high altitude (James 1966). The problem of infertility at high altitude applies to veterinary as well as human medicine and has proven to be of economic importance in Peru. In the early part of this century many ewes were slaughtered on the tacit assumption that they were infertile. However, in a series of papers, Monge-M and San Martin (1942, 1944, 1945) established that the responsibility for the infertility was with the males. At sea level one or two rams were used to serve 100 ewes, but at high altitude five to seven males were required. Mature spermatozoa are not affected by hypobaric hypoxia (Monge-M and Monge-C 1966) and the practical implication of this is that normal healthy rams can be kept at sea level and their semen sent to high altitude for the artificial insemination of acclimatized ewes. When the rams themselves are taken to high altitude, however, their semen shows abnormalities. Monge-M and San Martin (1942) studied the semen of rams transported to an altitude of 3260 m and found that after 50 days of exposure to the mountain environment there was azoospermia and severe oligospermia, with an increase of abnormal forms and low motility. Only one of these animals showed reversibility of these changes after living at high altitude for 5 months.

CHANGES IN SEMEN OF MEN AT HIGH ALTITUDE

The effects of acute exposure to high altitude on the semen of lowlanders were reported by Donayre (1966). He investigated 10 men at sea level and after 8 and 13 days of exposure to an altitude of 4330 m. There was a pronounced decrease in the sperm count, dropping from a mean of 216.2×10^6/ml to 98.2×10^6/ml (Fig. 23.1). At the same time there was an increase in abnormal forms from 0 to 39.3% (Fig. 23.2) and a decrease in motile forms (Fig. 23.2). The levels of fructose increased (Fig. 23.3) probably due to lack of utilization by the non-motile spermatozoa (Donayre 1966). At the same time the

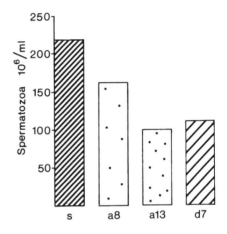

23.1 *Number of spermatozoa in millions per ml in the semen of 10 men at sea level (s), after 8 (a8) and 13 (a13) days of exposure to an altitude of 4330 m, and 7 days (d7) after return to sea level. Acute exposure to high altitude produces a pronounced decrease in the number of sperms, but this effect is reversible after return to sea level. (After Donayre (1966).)*

citric acid level in the semen fell and this was associated with elevation of the pH of the seminal fluid to slight alkalinity. After return to sea level for 7 days all these deleterious effects were undergoing reversal (Fig. 23.1–23.3). It is clear from this study that acute exposure to the hypoxia of high altitude brings about mild and reversible damage to the seminiferous epithelium.

Subsequent studies were carried out by Donayre (1968) on the semen of nine young healthy lowlanders who were taken to 4270 m for 4 weeks after a 5-week control period at sea level. The sperm count fell gradually to the penultimate day of the exposure period and continued to decline for 15 days after descent to sea level. Motile cells decreased from control values of 85.8% to 53.4% at the end of the experimental period, although the percentage of live cells was normal. A return to sea level restored motility after 15 days. The incidence of abnormal

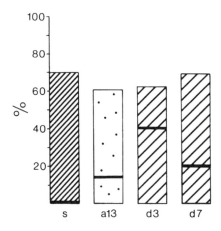

23.2 *Percentage of motile spermatozoa in semen of 10 men at sea level (s), after 13 (a13) days of exposure to an altitude of 4330 m, and 3 (d3) and 7 (d7) days after descent to sea level. On acute exposure to high altitude there is a reversible fall in the number of motile forms. In each column the horizontal bar indicates the percentage of abnormal forms. This percentage rises to a maximal level 3 days after descent to sea level and then begins to reverse. It is, however, still elevated 7 days after the descent. (After Donayre (1966).)*

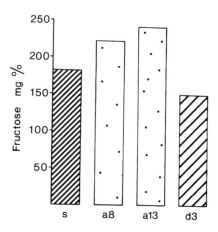

23.3 *Fructose content of semen in mg%, of 10 men at sea level (s), after 8 (a8) and 13 (a13) days of exposure to an altitude of 4330 m, and 3 days (d3) after descent to sea level. On acute exposure to high altitude the fructose content of the semen rises and falls on return to sea level. (After Donayre (1966).)*

forms increased from a control level of 15.5% to 31.6% and this high incidence was maintained after return to the coast. Initially, alterations of the neck and middle piece occurred with the formation of tapering forms. Later, structural alterations occurred in the head.

Hence it appears that the hypoxia of high altitude induces morphological changes in the spermatozoa, while the continuing fall in the sperm count suggests gradual damage at an early stage of the spermatogenic cycle. The rapidity with which these changes occur suggests that there is an effect on epididymal sperm. The alterations in morphology of the sperms brought about by chronic hypoxia are similar to those induced by viral infections or allergic reactions (MacLeod 1965), suggesting that the testis has a limited variability of response. It is clear from these studies that hypoxia has profound effects on spermatogenesis.

HISTOLOGICAL CHANGES IN THE TESTES

The testicles of male rats transported to 4500 m were found to be devoid of germinal epithelium, with Sertoli cells replacing spermatogonia (Mori-Chavez 1936; Monge-M and Mori-Chavez 1942).

Leydig cells were increased noticeably in number. Similar lesions were also found in rabbits. Guerra-Garcia (1959) showed that the exposure of guinea-pigs born and bred at sea level to an altitude of 4330 m for 2 weeks produces profound alterations in the epithelium of the seminiferous tubules with a marked decrease of all cellular types.

Working with simulated altitudes of 7620 m, Altland (1949) found severe destruction of the germinal epithelium of albino rats. This began on the third day of exposure and had led to considerable damage by the fourteenth day. There was no amelioration of the damage during the course of the experiment, but recovery took place 1 month after its termination. Simulated altitudes of 5790 m led to pronounced degeneration of the germinal cells of guinea-pigs after 60 days (Shettles 1947). The occurrence of acellular areas and the sloughing of cells in the seminiferous tubules of rats exposed to intermittent low pressure equivalent to elevations of 6500 m has been reported by Altland and Highman (1968). According to Monge-M and Mori-Chavez (1942), cats and rabbits show various degrees of destruction of the germinal epithelium 6 months and 15 days, respectively, after natural exposure to an altitude of 4510 m.

THE OVARY

We are not aware of any data on ovarian morphology in native highlanders. In rats exposed to simulated high altitude the ovary has been reported as diminished in weight in some series (Gordon *et al.* 1943) but not in others (Moore and Price 1948). Very little is known about changes in the endocrinology of the ovarian–pituitary axis at high altitude.

MENARCHE

Menarche occurs after the major part of the adolescent growth spurt has passed, so that it provides a rough indicator of the age at which adolescence is well under way rather than of the age at which this stage of development begins (Pawson 1976). Since a girl's first few menstrual cycles are usually anovular, age at menarche is not a satisfactory measure of reproductive maturity but only a rough guide to this. There is a considerable range in the age of menarche in various high-altitude populations (Table 23.1). Thus Greksa (1990) found that, in European and Aymara girls born and living in La Paz, Bolivia (3600 m), the median age of menarche was delayed by only 0.8 years so that the age of menarche in European girls was 13.1 years. Greksa (1990) is of the opinion that studies of bodily and sexual maturation at high altitude may be confused because of differences in the nutritional and health status of the groups being compared. For this reason his studies focused on children of upper socio-economic status who were healthy and well-nourished. In such children the effects of hypobaric hypoxia in delaying menarche were not great. In contrast to these findings, Kapoor and Kapoor (1986) found evidence of retardation in sexual maturity in native Bhotia women of the central Himalaya so that menarche was delayed to 15.6 years. Confirmation of this trend was found in girls of the Bundi highlands of New Guinea with an age of menarche at 18.0 years and in Sherpas of the Nepalese Himalaya at an age of 18.2 years (Table 23.1). In the Peruvian Andes, Moncloa, quoted by Donayre (1966), reported that at Cerro de Pasco (4330 m) only 38% of girls aged 13 years had arrived at menarche, compared with 73% in a comparable age group at sea level. Greksa (1990) found that the median age of menarche of European migrants to La Paz was 13.8 years, some 0.7 years older than that found in European girls born and raised at high altitude. The median age of menarche in European girls born and living in Santa Cruz (400 m) was 12.3 years, a value falling within the range of 12.2 and 13.4 years found in urban European girls. It is apparent that the delaying effect of high altitude is a composite of the effect of hypobaric hypoxia and socio-economic status. It is very difficult to determine any difference in median age of menarche in areas like Bolivia where intermingling of Spanish and native Aymara blood is profound and it is difficult to distinguish between mestizos and Aymaras.

FERTILITY

We have already seen that the reduction in fertility at high altitude is in large part due to damage to the germinal epithelium and to alterations in spermatozoa. However, it is also contributed to by the female

Table 23.1 Age of menarche in various high-altitude populations

Area	Mean age at menarche (years)	Reference
La Paz Europeans born and living at high altitude	13.1	Greksa (1990)
La Paz Aymaras born and living at high altitude	13.4	Greksa (1990)
Andes	13.6	Frisancho (1978)
Himalaya	14.1–18.4	Beall (1983) Malik and Hauspie (1986)
Tien Shan mountains	14.4	Frisancho (1978)
Ethiopia	14.5	Pawson (1976)
India (Himalayan Bhotias in Uttar Pradesh)	15.6	Kapoor and Kapoor (1986)
Nepal	16.8	Weitz *et al.* (1978)
New guinea (Bundi Highlands)	18.0	Malcolm (1970)
Nepal Highland Sherpas	18.2	Pawson (1974)

and some of the factors concerned were defined in an investigation by Laurenson *et al.* (1985). They elicited the mean age of menarche, of first marriage, and of childbirth and the number of live births born during the reproductive life span (the so-called 'completed fertility rate'). Two populations were studied. One was at high altitude (3800 m) in central Nepal and was composed of native highlanders originating from western Tibet. The other was from a lower altitude of 2600 m. It transpired that, although there was no significant difference in reported menarchial ages between the two groups, the age at first marriage and that of the first childbirth were both later in highlanders. As a result the completed fertility rate was significantly lower in the highlanders (Table 23.2). There was increased birth-spacing in highlanders (4.35 years) compared with that in lowlanders (2.62 years). Longer post-partum amenorrhoea and breast feeding did not account for the increased average pregnancy gap. There was an absence of venereal disease at high altitude.

PREGNANCY AT HIGH ALTITUDE

Pregnant women at sea level hyperventilate (Hytten and Thomson 1965). The increased ventilation raises systemic arterial oxygen tension but it does not normally affect arterial saturation levels, which are already nearly maximal. At high altitude, the hyperventilation of pregnant women exaggerates that induced by the hypobaric hypoxia (Hellegers *et al.* 1961; Moore *et al.* 1982*a*). At high altitude this heightening of ventilation does raise arterial oxygen saturation (Moore *et al.* 1982*a*). Birthweight is reduced in mountainous areas and in pregnancies complicated by maternal congenital heart disease, severe anaemia, and smoking (Moore *et al.* 1986), suggesting that reduced maternal oxygen transport can exaggerate fetal hypoxia and limit fetal growth. At high altitude, women who ventilate more and who have higher levels of oxygen in their arterial blood produce infants of heavier birth weight (Moore *et al.* 1982*b*).

To test the hypothesis that increased ventilatory responsiveness to hypoxia with pregnancy raises maternal ventilation and arterial oxygenation and leads to an increase in birth weight, Moore *et al.* (1986) studied Quechua women at Cerro de Pasco (4330 m) while pregnant and again post-partum. Above 4000 m, arterial oxygen tension and saturation are located on the steep part of the oxygen–haemoglobin dissociation curve and thus the increase in ventilation with pregnancy would be expected to have a greater effect on arterial oxygenation than at lower elevations. Twenty-one pregnant (36 weeks gestation) women from Cerro de Pasco (4330 m) were studied. Fifteen were studied 13 weeks post-partum (Table 23.3). While breathing room air, ventilation was 2.4 ± 0.7 l/min (25%) higher in the pregnant compared to non-pregnant women. With pregnancy the partial pressure of oxygen in the alveolar spaces was higher and that of carbon dioxide was lower than when the women were non-pregnant. Vital capacity did not change. Infant birth weight was positively correlated with the increase in maternal hypoxic ventilatory response associated with pregnancy and tended also to be associated with the rise in ventilation and fall in alveolar carbon dioxide tension. The rise in ventilation with pregnancy had, in turn, a large effect on maternal oxygenation, increasing oxygen levels in the arterial blood. Although ventilating responsiveness to hypoxia is blunted or absent after years of residence at high altitude (Chapter 4), it returns during pregnancy according to Moore *et al.* (1986) converting the ventilatory response to one within a normal range for women at low altitude. Opportunities for high-altitude treks continue to expand but they are not appropriate for pregnant lowlanders. Prolonged exposure of pregnant women to altitudes above 4500 m has not been studied and caution should be exercised (Barry and Bia 1989).

UMBILICAL ARTERIAL OXYGEN TENSION

While the hyperventilation of pregnancy helps to improve the oxygenation of maternal blood at high altitude, there is an additional factor that appears to maintain oxygen tension in the umbilical vessels at levels more appropriate to the lowlands. Most of the information we have on this subject comes from studies on ewes. It has been established for many years that even at sea level the umbilical arterial oxygen saturation in the fetus is low (Huggett 1927; Eastman 1930). This is an expression of the resistance offered to the diffusion of oxygen by the tissue barrier of the placenta and to its intrinsic oxygen utilization. At sea level the umbilical arterial oxygen tension is barely 20 mmHg, which corresponds to an atmospheric oxygen tension of about 60 mmHg which would be found at an elevation of 7500 m. Hence even at sea level the fetus is hypoxaemic and lives under physiological conditions, which in some areas resemble those experienced by the native highlander. This being so, one might anticipate that, during pregnancy at high altitude where oxygen tension in the systemic arteries and hence maternal

Table 23.2 Mean ages of menarche, first marriage, and first childbirth and completed fertility rate (total no. of births) for high- and low- altitude women (after Laurenson *et al.* 1985)

| Altitude (m) | Age (years) of | | | | | | | | | Completed Fertility rate (total no. of births) | | |
| | Menarche | | | First marriage | | | First childbirth | | | | | |
	n	Mean	SD	n	Mean	SD	n	Mean	SD	n	Mean	SD
3800	30	16.7	1.4	37	24.1	8.6	37	26.2	5.9	43	3.2	2.3
2600	42	16.2	1.7	35	19.6	5.5	30	21.9	2.9	41	4.9	3.7

Table 23.3 Ventilation in Quechua women during and after pregnancy at 4300 m. (From Moore *et al.* 1986, by courtesy of the American Physiological Society)

Parameters	*n*	During pregnancy	Post-partum
Tidal volume (l)	15	0.63 ± 0.02	0.53 ± 0.03
Respiratory frequency (breaths per min.)	15	$19 \quad \pm 1$	$19 \quad \pm 1$
Forced vital capacity (l)	15	3.51 ± 0.10	3.46 ± 0.90
Arterial O_2 saturation (%)	15	$87.4 \quad \pm 0.4$	$83.4 \quad \pm 1.0$
Arterial O_2 content (ml O_2/100 ml whole blood)	14	$15.6 \quad \pm 0.4$	$15.9 \quad \pm 0.4$
End-tidal P_{o2} (mmHg)	15	$65.3 \quad \pm 1.0$	$57.8 \quad \pm 1.2$
End-tidal P_{co2} (mmHg)	15	$26.1 \quad \pm 0.9$	$31.3 \quad \pm 0.8$
Cardiac output (1 min)	12	5.84 ± 0.12	5.17 ± 0.53

capillaries is low, even more pronounced hypoxaemia might be suffered by the fetus, perhaps endangering its very survival.

This interesting problem has been studied by Metcalfe *et al.* (1962) who investigated 21 pregnant ewes carrying fetuses ranging from 52 to 135 days in gestational age at Morococha (4540 m) in the Peruvian Andes where they had been bred and pastured. They determined the oxygen and carbon dioxide contents and tensions in the maternal arterial, uterine venous, umbilical arterial, and umbilical venous bloods. Their studies confirmed that at high altitude there is a distinct reduction in the oxygen tension in the uterine and maternal placental capillaries. Thus, while oxygen tension in the maternal uterine capillaries at sea level is 63 mmHg (Barcroft *et al.* 1940; Kaiser and Cummings 1957), at an altitude of 4540 m it is 41.3 mmHg (Metcalfe *et al.* 1962). The effective carbon dioxide tension in uterine capillaries is lowered by 11 mmHg, from a range of 35–36 mmHg to that of 24–25 mmHg.

However, despite the lowered oxygen tension in the maternal uterine and placental capillaries, the oxygen tension in the umbilical vein is similar to that reported for fetuses carried by ewes at sea level. Thus the oxygen tension in the umbilical vein at sea level is in the range 21.3–27.5 mmHg, with an average value of 24.9 mmHg (Kaiser and Cummings 1957). At 4540 m its range is 14.2– 28.1 mmHg, with an average value as high as 22.0 mmHg, virtually the same level as that seen at sea level (Metcalfe *et al.* 1962). The oxygen tension in the umbilical arteries at sea level is in the range 11.6–15.4 mmHg, with an average value of 13.4 mmHg (Kaiser and Cummings 1957). At 4540 m its range is 10.4–

14.8 mmHg, with an average value of 12.5 mmHg (Metcalfe *et al.* 1962). Once again this value is not much different from that found at sea level. These results demonstrate that, despite the lowered transplacental gradient in oxygen tension, the rate at which oxygen reaches the fetal blood per kilogram of tissue supplied is the same at high altitude as at sea level. The presumption is that at high altitude the placenta is modified in some way to decrease the resistance to the diffusion of oxygen across the placental barrier.

PLACENTAL WEIGHT

Krüger and Arias-Stella (1970) studied birth weights and placentae resulting from 118 pregnancies at Lima (150 m) and 84 pregnancies at Rio Pallanga (4600 m). They found that the placenta was 12% heavier in the highlanders (Fig. 23.4). There was no significant difference in weight in relation to the sex of the newborn infant. However, the placental weight in the primiparous at high altitude was 23% higher, whereas in multiparous pregnancies it was only 9% higher. These characteristic changes in fetal and placental weight at high altitude are also found in animals. Thus, Prystowsky (1960), in observations of the placenta in sheep living at altitudes between 4570 and 4880 m, reported that the placentae appeared to be much larger and the fetuses slightly smaller, for a given gestational age, than those of sea-level sheep.

A 'placental coefficient' was defined as the weight of the placenta related to the weight of the newborn infant (Krüger and Arias-Stella 1970). In cases from Lima this coefficient was 0.144, but in those from Rio Pallanga it was 0.192, a highly significant

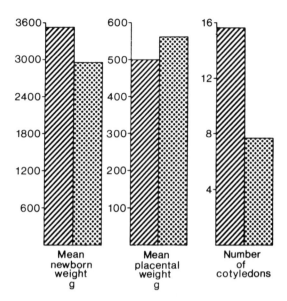

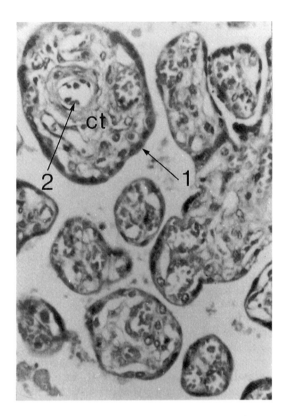

23.4 *Mean birth weight, mean placental weight, and number of placental cotyledons in 118 pregnancies at sea level and in 84 pregnancies at 4600 m. Data from sea level indicated by hatched columns and from high altitude by stippled columns. (After Krüger and Arias-Stella (1970).)*

23.5 *Histological section of placenta from a native Amerindian woman from Santa Cruz (400 m), Bolivia. The barrier between maternal and fetal vascular beds consist of trophoblast (arrow 1), villous connective tissues (ct), and fetal capillary endothelium (arrow 2). Masson trichrome stain, × 350.*

difference. The upper limit of normal for this coefficient at sea level is given as 0.180 by Little (1960). The increased weight of the placenta is not readily explicable since there is no concomitant increase in placental volume. It is clearly of importance to establish the histological structure of the placenta to see if this is modified at high altitude to help improve the oxygenation of the fetal highlander.

DIFFUSING CAPACITY OF THE PLACENTA

It is possible to calculate the diffusing capacity of the placenta of the highlander by morphometric study of histological sections of the organ (Mayhew *et al.* 1984; Jackson *et al.* 1985). In the placentae of lowlanders the main resistance to the diffusion of oxygen to fetal blood is the 'villous membrane'. This is the barrier between maternal and fetal vascular beds and consists of trophoblast, villous connective tissue, and fetal capillary endothelium (Fig. 23.5). Transfer of oxygen between mother and fetus depends on the physical dimensions of the villous membrane. Diffusing capacity through this barrier can be monitored effectively by estimating the

surface areas of the villi and of the fetal capillaries and also by measuring the harmonic mean thickness (see Chapter 4) of the villous membrane. Blood space volumes and plasma diffusion distances have a negligible effect on diffusing capacity (Mayhew *et al.* 1986).

Mayhew (1986) reported studies of birth weight and various aspects of the placenta in 68 individuals, comprising high- and low-altitude groups. The former group comprised 16 native Amerindians (Quechua or Aymara) and 28 non-Indians (mestizos and Europeans) who were delivered at La Paz (3600 m), all having been born and brought up at altitudes above 3000 m. The lowland group consisted of 10 Amerindians and 14 non-Indians whose pregnancy and delivery were at Santa Cruz (400 m). He found that altitude appeared to exert a significant influence on villous surface area and villous membrane thickness as well as on birth weight. It did not appear to influence fetal capillary surface area or the absolute diffusing capacity of the villous membrane. Mayhew and co-workers were unable to demonstrate any change in placental weight at high altitude. Placentae from highlanders were different from those of lowlanders in terms of their microscopical dimensions. The combined surface area of terminal and intermediate villi was 6.7–7.0 m^2 in the lowlanders, but only 5.2–6.3 m^2 in the highlanders. The harmonic mean thickness of the villous membrane was 4.9–5.6 μm at low altitude, but was significantly less (4.5 μm) in the highland group. These differences in the dimensions of the villous membrane were sufficient to maintain highland diffusing capacities at but not in excess of lowland levels. Put succinctly, babies born at high altitude are small and the placentae have smaller villous areas, the individual villi being thinner; there are conflicting data as to whether the placentae are heavier or not.

Villous growth is substantially reduced at high altitude in both the native Indian and the non-Indian population. Thus as well as surface area the total volume and length of villi decline (Jackson *et al.* 1987). The volume proportions of the villi in terms of trophoblast, connective tissue, and fetal capillaries remain constant, so that differences due to altitude are not due to failure of villi to mature (Jackson *et al.* 1987). Highland villi differ from their lowland counterparts in several ways. On average they possess a thinner barrier due to closer approximation of capillaries to overlying trophoblast (Jackson *et al.* 1988). In consequence, the villous core is more irregular in outline and its surface (that of the inner aspect of the trophoblast) exceeds in area that of the outer aspect of the trophoblast. Peripheralization of capillaries and obtrusion into the trophoblastic epithelium is sufficient to account for the differences observed. The thinning of the villous membrane would appear to compensate for the reduced villous surface area in the placenta found at high altitude.

It was reported over 20 years ago that reversible thinning of trophoblast occurs when human placental tissue is cultured at lower than normal oxygen tensions (Tominaga and Page 1966; MacLennan *et al.* 1972). The studies of Tominaga and Page have been criticized by Burton *et al.* (1989) on the grounds that they gave no indication as to the number of organs examined and, furthermore, did not describe the methods by which the placentae were sampled. Significant regional differences in villous anatomy and thickness of the villous membrane exist within human placentae. For such reasons Burton *et al.* (1989) carried out a stereological re-examination of the effects of varying oxygen tensions on human placental villi maintained in organ cultures. Villi from 10 normal mature placentae was cultured under hypoxic (6% O$_2$) and hyperoxic (40% O$_2$) conditions for 6 or 12 hours. Control tissue (zero time in culture) was also taken. Pieces of tissue were fixed by immersion and embedded in resin for semi-thin sectioning. Systematically sampled microscopical fields were analysed stereologically to estimate harmonic and arithmetic mean thicknesses for the trophoblast and for the villous membrane and to assess the volumetric composition and mean diameter of villi. Trophoblastic and villous membrane thicknesses were influenced significantly by oxygen tension, being smaller in hypoxia and greater in hyperoxic media. No significant differences in the composition of villi were detected but villi tended to be greater in diameter during hyperoxia. There is a disparity between the estimate of villous membrane thickness made by Tominaga and Page (1966) and by Burton *et al.* (1989). The former did not describe how they estimated villous membrane thickness but it is likely that they measured the minimum distance. Thus for control samples they arrived at a figure of 4.4 μm whereas Burton *et al.* (1989) found it to be 7.4 μm.

Further sterological analysis of tissue sections was undertaken by Mayhew (1991) to estimate partial and total conductances of the human placental oxygen diffusion pathway. Analyses were undertaken for neonates and term placentae from populations living at low (400 m) and high (3600 m) altitude in Bolivia. At both altitudes the partial conductance on the maternal side of the oxygen pathway scaled to birth weight in a similar fashion, but this similarity did not extend to conductances on the fetal side. Beyond a limiting weight of roughly 3 kg, the highland fetus was disadvantaged in terms of its placental oxygen diffusive conductance and trophoblast volume. His findings suggest that the structural adjustments seen at high altitude are more successful on the maternal rather than the fetal side of the placenta.

BIRTH WEIGHT AT HIGH ALTITUDE

It is well established that at high altitude birth weight is low (Frisancho 1970; Haas *et al.* 1980). Krüger and Arias-Stella (1970) studied birth weights resulting from 118 pregnancies at Lima (150 m) and 84 pregnancies at Rio Pallanga (4600 m). They found that fetuses at high altitude had a mean weight some 16% below those from Lima (see Fig. 23.4). The difference was more pronounced in female newborns and in multiparous pregnancies. In the study in Bolivia referred to above, Mayhew *et al.* (1984) also found that the average birth weights at high altitude were 280– 300 g less than in the lowland controls. There was a significant ethnic difference in birth weight, the Amerindian newborns being on average 190–210 g heavier than non-Indians. Ulstein *et al.* (1988) analysed 4600 single live births in the Patan Hospital, Kathmandu and found the median birth weight for females was 2900 g while that for males was 3010 g. Compared with Norwegian newborns the birth weight of Nepali babies was lower for all gestational ages while this difference increased with length of gestation. Yip (1987) studied birth records from the US birth files from all White infants born in the United States from 1978 to 1981 as compiled by the National Center for Health Statistics. A total of 12 798 462 individual records was included in the analysis of the relationship between low birth weight and altitude. He confirmed that altitude is a strong predictor of low birth weight especially that related to intra-uterine growth retardation.

Lichty *et al.* (1957) found that low birth weight was characteristic in high-altitude areas of Colorado. The fact that highland regions of the state are inhabited by ethnic populations similar to those residing at low altitude suggests that the low birth rate of high altitude is related to the hypobaric hypoxia of high altitude rather than to any ethnic or socio-economic differences. These authors were particularly interested in low birth weight at high altitude in Colorado in relation to the problem of prematurity. Defining prematurity as a birth weight of less than 2500 g, they found its prevalence to be 30.8% for high-altitude areas of the state (above 3050 m) compared with an average of 10.4% for the state as a whole. However, the neonatal mortality was not proportionally high. This led them to suggest that the lower limit of birth weight of 2500 g was not applicable to high-altitude communities for distinguishing between premature and full-term births. In other words, babies weighing less than 2500 g at birth are not premature, just lighter. McCullough *et al.* (1977) and Unger *et al.* (1988) subsequently both confirmed that in Colorado there is a progressive decrease in birth weight with increasing altitude. They found that low birth weight was not an adverse factor among full-term infants born at higher altitudes.

In the study of 1977 McCullough *et al.* found that the mortality rate among *premature* babies at altitudes between 2740 and 3100 m was almost double that found at altitudes between 1140 and 2130 m. However, the later study by Unger *et al.* (1988) did not confirm this. In fact, the mortality risk for low-birth-weight infants was actually decreased at high as compared with low altitudes. However, these results have to be seen in the context that in the decade between the two investigations there was an overall reduction of 46% in infant mortality rate throughout the state of Colorado. This improvement may reflect an improvement of prenatal care and access to it. There may be a greater detection of complications of pregnancy and prompt referral to larger, better equipped hospitals. An improvement of affluence is thus likely to account for this fall in infant mortality rate in Colorado.

Birth weight is reduced in pregnancies marked by maternal hypoxaemia stemming from cyanotic cardiac or pulmonary disease. It may be that the same phenomenon occurs at high altitude. Moore *et al.* (1982*b*) found that there was a relation between maternal arterial oxygen content and infant birth weight in high-altitude residents in Leadville, Colorado (3100 m). In a later study in Quechua women in the Andes, Moore *et al.* (1986) were unable to confirm this direct relationship. Nevertheless, in general, babies with higher birth weights were born to mothers with greater increases in hypoxic ventilatory responsiveness, suggesting that increased maternal oxygenation may have resulted in less retardation of fetal growth.

HYPOXAEMIA IN THE HUMAN FETUS AT HIGH ALTITUDE

As pointed out earlier, even at sea level the umbilical arterial oxygen tension is less than 20 mmHg and corresponds to an atmospheric oxygen tension of about 60 mmHg which would be found at an elevation of 7500 m. Even so, there is some evidence that the fetus at high altitude experiences a greater degree of hypoxic stress. The human fetus is capable of producing erythropoietin by the eleventh week of gestation and responds to intrauterine hypoxia with increases in haemoglobin concentration, haematocrit, and in the level of HbF. Ballew and Haas (1986) studied the levels of haematocrit, haemoglobin concentration, and proportion of HbF in cord blood from 105 newborns at La Paz (3600 m) and 46 newborns from Santa Cruz (400 m) in Bolivia. They found that there was an increase from low to high altitude of haematocrit (50.6 to 53.5%), of haemoglobin concentration (15.5 to 17.1 g/dl), and of the proportion of HbF (56.5 to 64.4%). It seems likely that HbF is the most sensitive indicator of fetal hypoxia. There is always a negative correlation between gestational age and the proportion of HbF in cord blood, but at high altitude there is a delay in the switch from HbF to HbA production.

References

Altland, P.D. (1949). Effect of discontinuous exposure to 25,000 feet simulated altitude on growth and reproduction of the albino rat. *Journal of Experimental Zoology*, **110**, 1

Altland, P.D. and Highman, B. (1968). Sex organ changes and breeding performance of male rats exposed to altitude: effect of exercise and training. *Journal of Reproduction and Fertility*, **15**, 215

Ballew, C. and Haas, J.D. (1986). Hematologic evidence of fetal hypoxia among newborn infants at high altitude in Bolivia. *American Journal of Obstetrics and Gynecology*, **155**, 166

Barcroft, J., Kennedy, J.A., and Mason, M.F. (1940). Oxygen in the blood of umbilical vessels of the sheep. *Journal of Physiology*, **97**, 347

Barry, M. and Bia, F. (1989). Pregnancy and travel. *Journal of the American Medical Association*, **261**, 728

Beall, C.M. (1983). Ages of menopause and menarche in a high-altitude Himalayan population. *Annals of Human Biology*, **10**, 365

Burton, G.J., Mayhew, T.M., and Robertson, L.A. (1989). Stereological re-examination of the effects of varying oxygen tensions on human placental villi maintained in organ culture for up to 12 h. *Placenta*, **10**, 263

Donayre, J. (1966). Population growth and fertility at high altitude. In *Life at High Altitudes*, Scientific Publication No. 140. Washington, DC; Pan American Health Organization, p. 74

Donayre, J. (1968). Endocrine studies at high altitude. IV. Seminal changes in men exposed to altitude. *Journal of Reproduction and Fertility*, **16**, 55

Eastman, N.J. (1930). Fetal blood studies. (1) The oxygen relationships of umbilical cord blood at birth. *Bulletin of the Johns Hopkins Hospital*, **47**, 221

Frisancho, A.R. (1970). Development responses to high altitude hypoxia. *American Journal of Physical Anthropology*, **32**, 401

Frisancho, A.R. (1978). Human growth and development among high-altitude populations. In *The Biology of High-Altitude Populations*, (P.T. Baker, Ed.). Cambridge; Cambridge University Press, p. 117

Gordon, A.S., Tornetta, F.J., d'Angelo, S.A., and Charipper, H.A. (1943). Effects of low atmospheric pressure on the activity of the thyroid, reproductive system, and anterior lobe of the pituitary in the rat. *Endocrinology*, **33**, 366

Greksa, L.P. (1990). Age of menarche in Bolivian girls of European and Aymara ancestry. *Annals of Human Biology*, **17**, 49

Guerra-Garcia, R. (1959). Hypofisis, adrenales y testiculo de cobayos a nivel del mar y en la altitud. B.S. thesis, Universidad Nacional Mayor de San Marcos, Facultad de Medicina

Haas, J.D., Frongillo, E.A., Stepick, C.D., Beard, J.L., and Hurtado, L.G. (1980). Altitude, ethnic and sex differences in birth weight and length in Bolivia. *Human Biology*, **52**, 459

Hellegers, A., Metcalfe, J., Huckabee, W.E., Prystowsky, H., Meschia, G., and Barron, D.H. (1961). Alveolar P_{CO_2} and P_{O_2} in pregnant and nonpregnant women at high altitude. *American Journal of Obstetrics and Gynecology*, **82**, 241

Huggett, A.St.G. (1927). Foetal blood-gas tensions and gas transfusion throughout the placenta of the goat. *Journal of Physiology*, **62**, 373

Hytten, F.E. and Thomson, A.M. (1965). Pregnancy, childbirth and lactation. In *The Physiology of Human Survival* (O.G. Edholm and A.L. Bacharach, Ed.). London; Academic Press, p. 327

Jackson, M.R., Joy, C.F., Mayhew, T.M., and Haas, J.D. (1985). Stereological studies on the true thickness of the villous membrane in human term placentae: a study of placentae from high-altitude pregnancies. *Placenta*, **6**, 249

Jackson, M.R., Mayhew, T.M., and Haas, J.D. (1987). The volumetric composition of human term placentae: altitudinal, ethnic and sex differences in Bolivia. *Journal of Anatomy*, **152**, 173

Jackson, M.R., Mayhew, T.M., and Haas, J.D. (1988). On the factors which contribute to thinning of the villous membrane in human placentae at high altitude. II. An increase in the degree of peripheralization of fetal capillaries. *Placenta*, **9**, 9

James, W.H. (1966). The effect of altitude on fertility in Andean countries. *Population Studies*, **20**, 97

Kaiser, I.H. and Cummings, J.B. (1957). Hydrogen ion and hemoglobin concentration, carbon dioxide and oxygen content of blood of the pregnant ewe and fetal lamb. *Journal of Applied Physiology*, **10**, 484

Kapoor, A.K. and Kapoor, S. (1986) The effects of high altitude on age at menarche and menopause. *International Journal of Biometeorology*, **30**, 21

Krüger, H. and Arias-Stella, J. (1970). The placenta and the newborn infant at high altitude. *American Journal of Obstetrics and Gynecology*, **106**, 586

Laurenson, I.F., Benton, M.A., Bishop, A.J., and Mascie-Taylor, C.G.N. (1985). Fertility at low and high altitude in Central Nepal. *Social Biology*, **32**, 65

Lichty, J.A., Ting, R.Y., Bruns, P.D., and Dyar, E. (1957). Studies of babies born at high altitude. I. Relation of altitude to birth weight. *Diseases of Children*, **93**, 666

Little, W.A. (1960). The significance of placental/fetal weight ratios. *American Journal of Obstetrics and Gynecology*, **79**, 134

MacLennan, A.H., Sharp, F., and Shaw-Dunn, J. (1972). The ultrastructure of human trophoblast in spontaneous and induced hypoxia using a system of organ culture. A comparison with ultrastructural changes in pre-eclampsia and placental insufficiency. *Journal of Obstetrics and Gynaecology of the British Commonwealth*, **79**, 113

MacLeod, J. (1965). Human seminal cytology following the administration of certain anti-spermatogenic compounds. In *Agents Affecting Fertility* (C.R. Austin and J.S. Perry, Ed.). Boston, Massachusetts; Little, Brown, p. 93.

Malcolm, L.A. (1970). Growth and development in the Bundi child of the New Guinea highlands. *Human Biology*, **42**, 293

Malik, S.L. and Hauspie, R.C. (1986). Age at menarche among high-altitude Bods of Ladakh (India). *Human Biology*, **58**, 541

Mayhew, T. (1986). Morphometric diffusing capacity for oxygen of the human term placenta at high altitude. In *Aspects of Hypoxia* (D. Heath, Ed.). Liverpool; Liverpool University Press, p. 187

Mayhew, T.M. (1991). Scaling placental oxygen diffusion to birthweight: studies on placentae from low- and high- altitude pregnancies. *Journal of Anatomy*, **175**, 187

Mayhew, T.M., Joy, C.E., and Haas, J.D. (1984). Structure–function correlation in the human placenta: the morphometric diffusing capacity for oxygen at full term. *Journal of Anatomy*, **139**, 691

Mayhew, T.M., Jackson, M.R., and Haas, J.D. (1986). Microscopical morphology of the human placenta and its effects on oxygen diffusion: a morphometric model. *Placenta*, 7, 121

McCullough, R.E., Reeves, J.T., and Liljegren, R.L. (1977). Fetal growth retardation and increased infant mortality at high altitude. *Archives of Environmental Health*, **32**, 36

Metcalfe, J., Meschia, G., Hellegers, A. Prystowsky, H., Huckabee, W., and Barron, D.H. (1962). Observations on the placental exchange of the respiratory gases in pregnant ewes at high altitude. *Quarterly Journal of Experimental Physiology*, **47**, 74

Monge-M, C. and Monge-C, C. (1966). High-altitude animal pathology. In *High Altitude Diseases: Mechanism and Management*. Springfield, Illinois; Charles C. Thomas, p. 67

Monge-M, C. and Mori-Chavez, P. (1942). Fisiologia de la reproduccion en la altura. *Anales de la Facultad de Medicina de Lima*, **25**, 34

Monge-M, C. and San Martin, M. (1942). Nota sobre la azoospermia de corneros recien llegados a la altura. *Anales de la Facultad de Medicina de Lima*, **25**, 58

Monge-M, C. and San Martin, M. (1944). Fisiologia de la reproduccion en al altiplano. *Ann III a Convención Agronómica*, Lima

Monge-M, C. and San Martin, M. (1945). Aclimatacion avina en los altiplanos andinos. Infertilidad reversible debida a la accion del viaje maritimo de Magallanes al Callae durante el varano. *Anales de la Facultad de Medicina de Lima*, **28**, 1

Moore, C.R. and Price, D. (1948). A study at high altitude of reproduction, growth, sexual maturity, and organ weights. *Journal of Experimental Zoology*, **108**, 171

Moore, L.G., Jahnigen, D., Rounds, S.S., Reeves, J.T., and Grover, R.F. (1982*a*). Maternal hyperventilation helps preserve arterial oxygenation during high-altitude pregnancy. *Journal of Applied Physiology*, **52**, 690

Moore, L.G., Rounds, S.S., Jahnigen, D., Grover, R.F., and Reeves, J.T. (1982*b*). Infant birth weight is related to maternal arterial oxygenation at high altitude. *Journal of Applied Physiology*, **52**, 695

Moore, L.G., Brodeur, P., Chumbe, O., D'Brot, J. Hofmeister, S., and Monge, C. (1986). Maternal hypoxic ventilatory response, ventilation, and infant birth weight at 4300 m. *Journal of Applied Physiology*, **60**, 1401

Mori-Chavez, P. (1936). Manifestacione pulmonares del conejo del llama transportado a la altura. *Anales de la Facultad de Medicina de Lima*, **19**, 137

Pawson, I.G. (1974). The growth and development of high altitude children with special emphasis on populations of Tibetan origin in Nepal. Ph.D. thesis, the Pennsylvania State University

Pawson, I.G. (1976). Growth and development in high altitude populations: a review of Ethiopian, Peruvian and Nepalese studies. *Proceedings of the Royal Society of London*, **194**, 83

Prystowsky, H. (1960). Proceedings of the conference. In *The Placenta and Fetal Membranes* (C.A. Villee, Ed.). Baltimore; Williams and Wilkins, p. 151

Shettles, L.B. (1947). Effects of low oxygen tension on fertility in adult male guinea pigs. *Federation Proceedings: Federation of American Societies for Experimental Biology*, **6**, 200

Tominaga, T. and Page, E.W. (1966). Accommodation of the human placenta to hypoxia. *American Journal of Obstetrics and Gynecology*, **94**, 679

Ulstein, M., Rana, G., Yangzom, K., Gurung, R., Karki, A. Gurung, G., and Pradhan, U. (1988). Some fetal and pregnancy parameters in Nepal. *Acta Obstetricia et Gynecologica Scandinavica*, **67**, 47

Unger, C., Weiser, J.K., McCullough, R.E., Keefer, S., and Moore, L.G. (1988). Altitude, low birth weight, and infant mortality in Colorado. *Journal of the American Medical Association*, **259**, 3427

Weitz, C.A., Pawson, I.G., Weiz, M.W., Lang, S.D.R., and Lang, A. (1978). Cultural factors affecting the demographic structures of a high altitude Nepalese population. *Social Biology*, **25**, 179

Yip, R. (1987). Altitude and birth weight. *Journal of Pediatrics*, **111**, 869

24

Cold

The other major hazard besides hypobaric hypoxia that confronts man at high altitude is cold. There is a central thermostatic mechanism in the hypothalamus to regulate body temperature. This receives sensory input from the skin, the reticular area of the mid-brain, and some large blood vessels like the internal carotid artery. However, man largely overcomes adverse environmental factors by evading them, and the native highlander in the Andes is able to live and work in mining areas permanently at altitudes around 4500 m through the protection of suitable clothing and accommodation (Fig. 24.1). In striking contrast to this is the impact of the extreme cold of high altitude on lowlanders who expose themselves in such occupations as mountaineering at great heights. Even air crew, commonly on military missions, may suddenly find themselves exposed to the severe cold. At high altitude the effects of extreme cold may be generalized, leading to hypothermia, or localized, leading to frostbite. We consider the pathophysiology, prevention, and treatment of both diseases in this chapter, noting that, as with the variants of acute mountain sickness, prevention is far preferable to attempted cure. Treatment is a great deal more complex than simply rewarming the affected subject.

ACUTE EXPOSURE TO COLD
The human body loses heat to its surroundings by several physical processes.

Convection
Heat is transferred directly from the body to its colder surroundings by the movement of air or water. Convective heat loss is of great importance in inducing hypothermia on mountainsides on account of the wind-chill factor described in Chapter 2. The combination of a high wind velocity and cold air will rapidly destroy the insulating layer of warm air around the body and induce hypothermia. Convective cooling is much greater in water than in air because the specific heat of water is far larger (Wilkerson 1986). Heat loss due to convection depends on the area of exposed skin and main-

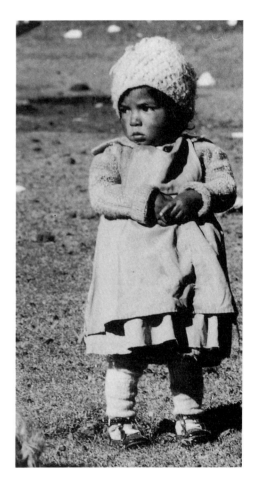

24.1 *A small Quechua girl from a settlement at 4500 m on the altiplano of Central Peru. She is well protected from the cold of the mountain environment.*

tenance of body temperature is dependent on the ratio of body mass to surface area.

Radiation
In this process, electromagnetic energy passes directly to the environment. Direct contact with air is

not necessary for this form of heat loss, which could take place in a vacuum. It is independent of air movement. As already seen in Chapter 2, the body also gains heat by this process through absorbing solar radiation, which is pronounced in the clear skies at high altitude and is exaggerated by reflection from snow. At sea level, up to two-thirds of the heat of metabolism is lost by radiation to temperate surroundings, but at high altitude the major cause of heat loss from the body is convection.

Conduction

In this process, heat loss is due to direct contact with cold surroundings. Air conducts heat poorly and still air, which does not cause convective heat loss, is an excellent insulator. Water has a conductivity 240 times greater than that of air, and contact with cold water, including wet clothing, will cause the body to lose much heat energy. Ice, stones on the mountainside, and metal implements will conduct heat away from the body very efficiently (Fig. 24.2). Alcohol is a good conductor and it remains liquid at temperatures well below the freezing temperature of water. Extremely cold alcohol, when imbibed, can almost instantly freeze the lips and tongue.

Evaporation

Evaporation of sweat leads to loss of heat in the transfer of energy required to change liquid to a vapour, the so-called latent heat of vaporization. This process is facilitated by the low humidity of cold air at high altitude (see Chapter 2). It is responsible for up to a third of heat loss from the body in temperate surroundings at sea level. The evaporative heat loss takes place from the skin as insensible water loss and sweating and from the air passages of the lungs. About 4 litres of water per day are required to humidify inhaled air, and its evaporation extracts some 2000 kcal (Wilkerson 1986). Evaporation of water from wet clothing causes great heat loss, particularly in a wind.

HYPOTHERMIA

Avoidance

The physical processes just described, which govern the loss of heat from the human body, are simple and well known and straightforward avoidance of them on the mountainside will avoid much hypothermia at high altitude. Failure to apply simple measures to avoid loss of body heat, on the other hand, may allow a slide into hypothermia, which may be very difficult to treat and even prove fatal. As

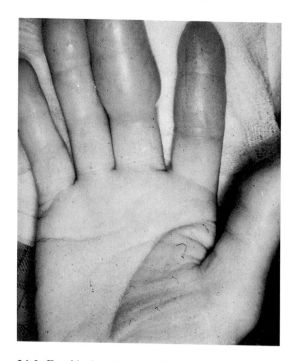

24.2 *Frostbite in a 36-year-old man caused by conductive heat loss to a metal jack he was using to change a tyre at high altitude. Metal conducts heat away from the body very efficiently.*

with the more severe forms of acute mountain sickness, it is much better to avoid profound hypothermia than to have to treat it.

Appropriate clothing will greatly reduce or eliminate increased convective or conductive heat losses, but it will have no effect on radiant or evaporative heat loss (Wilkerson 1986). Multiple layers of clothing will provide several zones of immobile warm air insulating the body, and outer layers may be shed to react to temperature changes in the environment. Loss of heat by convection is restricted by diminishing the area of skin exposed to the surrounding air, by avoidance of exposure to wind that destroys the still, insulating layer of warm air around the body, and by avoiding the 'bellows effect' of clothing loosely fitting around the neck that may force out the warm insulating air. Avoidance of direct contact of the body with snow will cut down heat loss due to conduction. So too will keeping dry, for water is a good conductor of heat and wet clothes lose their power for insulation. Furthermore, wet clothes require much heat to evaporate their water and this is drawn from the body. As noted in Chapter 2, humidity is low at high altitude, so that sweating is easy. The water can recondense on outer clothing and this again requires body heat for its evaporation. For such reasons it must be ensured that the protective clothing used does not induce excessive sweating on exercise.

Woollen fabrics contain innumerable small air pockets that provide excellent insulation even when the wool is wet. Down provides a similar level of insulation, but only when it is dry. Polyester fibres are less expensive and retain much of their insulation value when wet; they are heavier and much less compressible than down. Protection of the head is important; the unprotected scalp, especially in the bald-headed, exposes to the cold the warmest expanse of skin in the body richly supplied by blood. Balaclava woollen helmets cover the neck and most of the face and are desirable for severe conditions, particularly in strong winds. It is important to protect the lower extremities as well as the upper body from wind and water.

Shelters are as important as clothing on the mountainside. Snow shelters, ranging from igloos to a mere hole dug in the snow and covered by tarpaulin or tree trunks, are more effective than tents (Wilkerson 1986). They completely block the wind and eliminate severe convective cooling. Tent floors and lower walls must be waterproof to protect from conductive cooling. The upper portion of the tent must 'breathe' so that exhaled air can escape.

Hypothermia may be prevented not only by protection against cold but by heat generated by exercise. Heat production by the body can be increased significantly only by muscular exercise, be this shivering or voluntary muscular work, but it may also be generated to some extent by food. During physical activity most of the chemical energy from eating food is converted into heat. Body metabolism has to be increased to overcome the cold conditions. Usually the light meals taken during climbing do not provide the calories (energy) being expended, this shortfall being made up by an evening meal. For this reason light, concentrated foods of very high calorie value should be taken for any emergency.

Children and young people are especially vulnerable to hypothermia because they have less subcutaneous fat and are less insulated against the cold. In general, they are less willing to conserve energy, become easily fatigued, and are unable to keep up heat production.

Clinical features

The body may be considered to comprise a homeothermic core and a poikilothermic shell. The core consists of the deeper tissues of the body, including vital organs such as the heart and brain, whereas the shell is composed of the skin and superficial tissues. There is a great deal of argument as to the respective proportions of core and shell (Lloyd 1986). On the one hand it has been suggested that the shell is limited to 1.6 mm depth from the skin surface and comprises 10% of the body mass, the rest being core (Danzl 1983). Conversely, it has been calculated that in a man resting in an environmental temperature of 21°C, more than 50% of the body tissue will be at a temperature lower than that of the core (Burton and Edholm 1955). However, in spite of the lack of precision in the definition of core tissue, it is now generally accepted that for practical purposes a state of hypothermia in man is said to exist if the core temperature is below 35°C. This condition becomes lethal when the temperature of the vital organs falls below about 25°C. When the subject has a core temperature of between 35°C and 37°C he is said to be in a state of 'cold stress' (Lloyd 1986).

Table 24.1 gives specific temperatures, which form the only definitive way of documenting hypothermia, but few clinical thermometers available to the usual mountain party will register hypothermia of any degree since most record only down to 34°C. It is clear that the recognition of the stage of hypothermia reached depends on the assessment of symptoms and signs which may be subtle. The relation between different temperatures and clinical features is also shown in Table 24.1.

Mild hypothermia with a core temperature of 33°C or above may be subtle in onset. The subject on the mountainside complains of feeling cold and shows marked pallor due to peripheral vasoconstriction. Shivering is intense. The affected person loses interest in his activities and his mind is concentrated on only one thing, keeping warm. As he gets colder, he shows muscular incoordination. At first this presents as difficulty with precise hand movements, but later stumbling or clumsiness may appear. The deterioration in muscle function is also revealed in a progressive decrease in shivering which eventually disappears at about 32°C.

Once core temperature falls below this level, more serious clinical manifestations supervene. The patient becomes careless about protecting himself against cold. He may fail to wear gloves or blankets, or sleeping bags are not pulled up around the neck or head. A progressive impairment of cerebration takes place. The patient may appear to be uncooperative and this may be irritating and mis-

Table 24.1 Signs and symptons at different levels of hypothermia expressed as body core temperature. (After Harnett *et al*. 1983 and Lloyd 1986)

Body core temperature (°C)	Signs and symptoms
36	Increased metabolic rate in attempt to balance heat loss
35	Shivering at maximum; early cerebral dysfunction
34	Compatible with continued exercise; normal blood pressure still obtainable; still some shivering
32	Most shivering ceases; consciousness clouded
31	Blood pressure difficult to obtain
30–28	Progressive loss of consciousness; increased muscular rigidity; depressed respiration; slow pulse; cardiac arrhythmias develop; ventricular fibrillation easily provoked
27	Voluntary motion lost; papillary and deep tendon reflexes lost; subject appears dead
25	Ventricular fibrillation may appear spontaneuosly
24	Terminal pulmonary oedema

interpreted by companions who do not appreciate that this is a sign of deepening hypothermia. There is a failure to understand and respond to questions and directions. Thinking becomes slow. Decision-making is difficult and often erroneous. Memory for specific facts deteriorates. The patient has a strong desire to escape the cold by sleeping and he has lapses in his willingness to struggle for survival. Gradually, periods of unconsciousness become prolonged until the victim lapses into coma. Incoherent speech and loss of vision are late events, preceding coma or death by less than 1 hour (Bangs 1986).

When hypothermia becomes profound, the clinical picture may be very difficult to distinguish from death itself (Ward 1975; Lloyd 1986; Bangs 1986). There is extreme pallor and the skin may feel ice-cold and non-pliable. It may develop blue patches and the body may assume a corpse-like appearance. There may be evidence of frostbite. A chill may emanate from the body. The muscles and joints are still and simulate rigor mortis. No one should be pronounced dead from hypothermia until the body has been warmed to near normal temperature (Bangs 1986). The pulse becomes thready and may be difficult to palpate. It may be irregular due to atrial fibrillation.

The blood pressure is difficult to measure and may be low. Heart sounds may be unusually quiet and may become inaudible. These clinical effects on the heart are probably due to myocardial ischaemia. When haemoglobin is cooled, it releases oxygen less easily and when this effect is added to diminished coronary blood flow (Chapter 19) the supply of oxygen to the cardiac muscle is barely sufficient for its needs, even at rest. The myocardial ischaemia leads to the alterations in cardiac rhythm, with slowing of heart rate until the cardiac pacemaker fails. Eventually ventricular fibrillation may supervene to lead to cardiac arrest. The respiratory rate is slow and may become so shallow as to be practically imperceptible. Terminally the crepitations of incipient pulmonary oedema may become apparent. The patient's breath may have a fruity odour due to acetone bodies owing to incomplete fat metabolism (Bangs 1986).

MANAGEMENT OF HYPOTHERMIA

The treatment is different in the mild and severe forms of hypothermia. Treating a patient with the mild form as though he has the severe, causes unnecessary inconvenience, expense, and discomfort and may jeopardize other victims if resources are limited. On the other hand, treating profound hypothermia as though it were mild endangers the victim's life (Bangs 1986). Subjects with mild hypothermia, that is to say with a core temperature above 32°C, need only to be protected from further cooling and may be rewarmed by any convenient means. Placing the affected subject in a tent, sleeping bag, polythene bag, or something that is impermeable to heat will diminish heat loss and offer protection from the wind (Ward 1975). Wet clothing should be replaced by dry. Warm liquids may be given by mouth, even though they have little or no effect on core temperature. They engender a warm feeling by causing cutaneous vasodilatation, although this will lead to small further heat loss. Usually the subject can rewarm himself if further heat loss is stopped. External heat may be provided by anything, ranging from hot water bottles to the body warmth of a second person in a sleeping bag. Submersion in hot water or a hot shower is safe with mild hypothermia, but is dangerous if the condition is severe. On the mountainside, fit subjects may be 'walked out of trouble' by raising heat production by the body by exercise. Increased calorie intake by easily ingested foods such as glucose may also increase heat production. Alcohol should never be given.

The treatment of profound hypothermia when the core temperature sinks below 32°C is an entirely different matter, and the condition must be treated as a life-threatening emergency. The fundamental principle of care for patients with profound hypothermia consists of avoiding ventricular fibrillation while they slowly rewarm. The grossly hypothermic subject is very still for considerable periods of time and, when he is made to move, the muscles pump the cold, anaerobic blood back into the heart and the result of this is often fatal ventricular fibrillation. The cardiac arrhythmia may be induced by rough handling while lifting or transporting, by rapid external warming, by the insertion of needles, or the administration of drugs that stimulate the heart. Hence the victim of profound hypothermia must never be allowed to exert himself by walking or even be roughly moved when being lifted.

Ward *et al.* (1989) also stress that the treatment of profound hypothermia, with a body core temperature less than 32°C, requires treatment in the intensive care unit of a hospital. They believe it is vital to provide core temperature monitoring, an adequate airway, a central venous pressure line, monitoring of the ECG and blood gases, and restoration of fluid and electrolyte balance by warm fluids.

There is wide agreement that rewarming should not be attempted outside a hospital (Bangs 1986). During rapid rewarming the peripheral blood vessels dilate and the blood in the body core is shunted to the periphery, causing a severe fall in blood pressure and shock. The very cold, metabolically imbalanced blood in the limbs returns to the heart, causing a further drop in core temperature and perhaps fatal ventricular fibrillation. It is suggested that the safest procedure is to add external heat and initiate gentle transportation to a hospital.

The method of rewarming at the hospital differs greatly on the degree and type of hypothermia. Surface rewarming is advisable only for conscious patients suffering from mild acute accidental hypothermia (Ward *et al.* 1989). This peripheral rewarming may be carried out rapidly by placing the patient in a bath at 40°C for this is the fastest way of transferring heat, suppressing shivering and speeding the feeling of well-being (Ward *et al.* 1989). However, it should be used on only the mildest cases because of the dangers of dilating the peripheral circulation before body temperature has been fully restored. Slower rewarming by blankets and hot water bottles also carries the considerable risk of peripheral vasodilatation with return of cold blood to the heart and the risk of inducing irregularities of the heart's action including the dreaded ventricular fibrillation.

For such reasons central rewarming via the airways with warmed moist air or oxygen from a suitable apparatus via a mask or endotracheal tube is advocated. This method of treatment introduces heat slowly but directly into the lungs and then to the heart without the risks of prematurely dilating the peripheral circulation. Most of the heat is transmitted by the water used to humidify the air and is released when the water condenses in the respiratory passages. It should be noted that even warmed humidified gases administered through an endotracheal tube may induce ventricular fibrillation.

Intravenous therapy is commonly required, for most hypothermic subjects are dehydrated and have a reduced circulating blood volume. As the victim warms and the peripheral vessels dilate, the blood is lost to the core organs, impairing the circulation. Blood pressure rises, with rapid expansion of the blood volume, increasing blood flow to coronary arteries and increasing oxygen delivery to the heart muscle. This decreases the risk of rewarming shock and fatal ventricular fibrillation.

FROSTBITE

This is localized cold injury, characterized by freezing with ice crystal formation. It may affect any area of the body but most typically affects peripheral parts that do not include large heat-producing muscles and that are distant from the major sites of heat generation. Classically, frostbite affects the nose, ears, fingers, and toes but Ward *et al.* (1989) give a more comprehensive list of sites that may be involved together with brief comments on special risk factors for the particular area. Thus on the face they list not only the tip of the nose but its bridge due to spectacles. The ear-lobes, cheeks, lips, and tongue may be affected, the latter's involvement being due to drinking or sucking snow and ice. Ward and his colleagues (1989) make the interesting aside that double chins are especially vulnerable! The fingers and hands are prone to frostbite, especially if protective gloves and mittens are removed. Ward *et al.* (1989) point out that in the upper limb the head of radius, lower end of ulna, olecranon, and medial and lateral epicondyle of humerus may also be involved. During activity on the mountainside the feet are in contact with ice or snow and subject to great conductive heat loss. The toes are most commonly affected, but sometimes the rest of the foot is involved. In the lower limb frostbite may involve other areas such as the patella and head of fibula. The penis and testicles may become frostbitten due to difficulty in fastening zips and wetting due to overflow incontinence. The buttocks and perineum may be affected due to sitting on metallic seats.

Frostbite is frequently associated with generalized hypothermia. It is also predisposed to by obstruction of the blood supply to the extremities by constricting clothing such as boots laced too tightly (Fig. 24.3) and tight crampon straps. Contact with very cold metal can produce very rapid and severe freezing of tissues (see Fig. 24.2), while supercooled petrol, if spilled on to flesh, causes frostbite. The degree of cold and the time of exposure to it necessary to produce frostbite can vary considerably. In 812 cases of frostbite in the US army in Korea, four-fifths occurred on exposure to temperatures between $-7.5°C$ and $-18°C$ (Wilkerson 1986). In the majority of cases the duration of exposure was between 7 and 12 hours.

According to Wilkerson (1986) there are a number of factors that predispose to frostbite. Negroid subjects appear to be more susceptible than Caucasians, and it is conceivable that this reflects their ethnic origin from tropical countries where

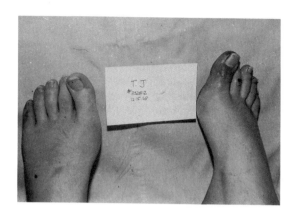

24.3 *Mild bilateral frostbite caused by the wearing of overtight ski boots for a day of skiing.*

evolutionary forces act to adjust to higher rather than lower temperatures. There is some evidence that smokers have a higher incidence than non-smokers, presumably due to the vasoconstrictive effects of nicotine.

Pathophysiology

Ice crystals form extracellularly in frostbite and raise the osmotic pressure in the interstitial tissue fluid. This leads to the withdrawal of fluid from the cells, which are damaged by the consequent dehydration, elevation of intracellular osmotic pressure, and associated biochemical imbalances (Ward 1975). Many of the cells, however, are not killed and survive for a long period, responding to rewarming of the tissues. The formation of ice crystals within cells themselves is a much more destructive process; fortunately it requires much faster freezing than occurs in frostbite. A second important factor in the pathophysiology is constriction of arteries, leading to a diminution in the blood flow to the peripheries (Ward 1975). There is also structural damage to the small arteries and veins, so that the endothelial cells are damaged allowing plasma to leak into the tissues to form blisters. This loss of fluid reduces the volume of blood in the peripheral vessels. The blood cells can no longer remain suspended in this lessened volume of slowly moving serum and they settle out as a sludge and predispose to local thrombosis. All these factors act together to diminish the blood supply to skin and subcutaneous tissues (Ward 1975; Wilkerson 1986).

Analysis of blister fluid reveals significant quantities of prostaglandin $F_{2\alpha}$ and thromboxane B_2, which promote clotting and which are derived from the damaged endothelial cells (Wilkerson 1986).

Obstruction of the circulation leads to changes in the tissue very similar to those produced by arteriosclerosis. One saving grace is that the tissues are kept in suspended animation by the cold, so that the deprivation of blood supply is not so catastrophic as it is when the tissues are rewarmed and become metabolically active. According to Ward (1975), arteriovenous shunts eventually come into operation, so that the supercooled blood remains in the affected area and is prevented from entering the general circulation. This increases the chance of survival, but at the expense of the frozen shell of tissue dying.

Non-specific changes occur in the tissues affected by areas of frostbite. They include swelling of nerve fibres, with axonal degeneration and coagulative necrosis of muscle fibres (Ward *et al.* 1989).

Clinical features

At first, frostbite causes pain in the involved tissue, but as the tissue freezes all sensation is lost and the pain goes. However, the symptoms are very variable. Some subjects never experience pain and a few never lose it (Wilkerson 1986). The loss of pain previously present must not be allowed to give the spurious impression that incipient frostbite is improving. Initially, frostbitten tissues are pale because of the intense vasoconstriction, but later they show a violaceous discolouration of the fingers and toes, and finally a purplish colour as a result of sludging of blood within the vessels (Fig. 24.4). This purplish change carries a poor prognosis, with the chance of loss of much tissue. Blisters filled with clear or bloody fluid develop within 1 or 2 days (Fig. 24.5). These blisters are especially common on the backs

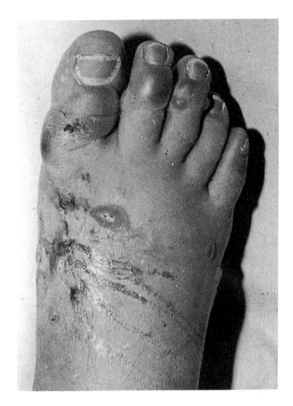

24.5 *Frostbite of foot with non-bloody blisters.*

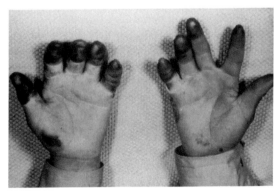

24.6 *Bilateral frostbite of hands, with blackening of the fingertips at 3 weeks.*

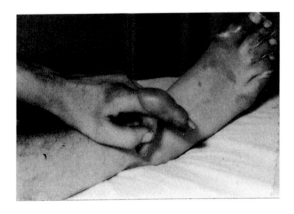

24.4 *Frostbite of hands and feet, with blistering and violaceous discoloration of the extremities.*

of the hands or the dorsa of the feet where the skin is lax (Ward *et al.* 1989). Finally, the initial violaceous discolouration of extremities may become black in the days and weeks following frostbite (Figs 24.6–24.8).

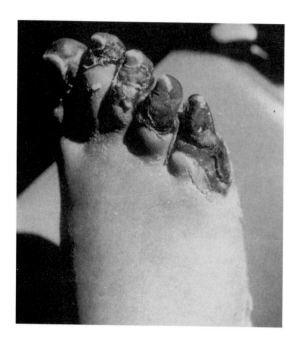

24.7 *Frostbite of foot, with blackening of the toes at 6 weeks. In this severe case the toes were eventually lost.*

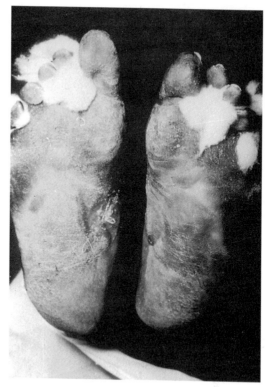

24.8 *Severe bilateral frostbite, with ultimate loss of forefeet.*

Finally, the frostbitten tissue turns black and hard and encases the finger or toe damaged by cold. It has been thought to resemble the shell of a tortoise and hence is sometimes termed a 'carapace'. This peels away in ensuing months to leave tender, pink underlying new epithelium. Frostbite may be superficial, when the skin and immediately adjacent subcutaneous tissues are affected, or deep, when such tissues as muscle, tendon, and bone are involved. Connective tissue, tendons, and bone are more resistant than skin to cold, so that the frostbitten tissues may be moved over still viable tendons.

A lesser degree of frostbite, termed 'frostnip', occurs when supercooling of the skin leads to blanching, numbness, and then tingling of the extremities. This process is reversible and can be cured by the simple expedient of exercise on the mountainside (Steele 1976). The affected part should be placed in the armpit or under clothing. It should not be rubbed (Ward *et al.* 1989). It commonly involves the ears and the tip of the nose.

Prevention

It is obvious that in general terms the preventive measures are those already presented above to avoid the onset of hypothermia. The most useful preventive measures are to limit the period exposed to the possibility of cold injury, to keep warm, maintain hydration, and keep the part dry and free from abrasion (Ward *et al.* 1989). Special care should be taken to protect the hands and feet. Removal of gloves and mittens in the extreme cold of high altitude can be a hazardous occupation. It is extremely important to dress for the temperature with which the limbs will be in contact (Ward 1975). Thus in deep powder snow it is possible for the feet to be in snow many degrees below freezing point, while at the same time the ambient temperature may be many degrees above freezing. Care should be taken not to obstruct the circulation to the feet in any way, such as overtight lacing of boots or crampon strips (Wilkerson 1986). The smoking of cigarettes is to be avoided, for the nicotine will induce peripheral vasoconstriction and aggravate the effects of the cold. Alcohol, while tending to dilate peripheral blood vessels and thus help to prevent frostbite, often lowers the critical faculties and induces forgetfulness about necessary safety precautions.

MANAGEMENT OF FROSTBITE

Although it is obvious that the basis for the treatment of frostbite is rewarming of the affected part, the matter is more complex than it might at first appear and several important problems have to be addressed. The rewarming of frostbitten hands and feet in front of the excessive, uncontrolled heat of campfires led to horrifying results in countless soldiers in the Napoleonic armies retreating from Moscow. The worst results undoubtedly follow thawing with excessive heat, especially dry heat at 60°C or above (Mills 1983; Flora 1985; Foray and Salon 1985). Such temperatures are produced by diesel exhausts, stoves and wood-fires. Another classical method of treating frostbite in the field is by rubbing the affected parts in ice and snow to effect a slower rewarming. This procedure does not melt the extracellular ice crystals or increase the blood supply to the injured area (Ward 1975). It carries the risk of breaking the surface of the damaged skin and blisters, thus allowing infection with the likelihood of increased loss of tissue (Mills 1983).

Attempts to treat frostbite at high camps on exposed mountainsides with inadequate facilities are ill-advised. Victims of frostbite can walk on frozen feet. If the subject is uninjured, he can make his own descent from the mountain, since walking on frostbitten feet does not appear to increase tissue loss (Ward 1975). People have walked on frozen feet for many hours (Mills and Rau 1983). The rewarming of frostbitten feet at high altitude on a mountain will result in thawed or partly thawed extremities on which the patient cannot walk. He will then have to be carried down under difficult circumstances. Thawing and refreezing leads to much greater tissue damage than walking on frozen feet. Repeated episodes of freezing lead to much greater risks of infection and to more extensive loss of tissue (Keatinge and Cannon 1960; Mills 1983). The most that should be attempted on the mountain are steps to combat the almost certainly associated hypothermia. The affected subject must be put into a sleeping bag and given hot liquids and food. Antibiotics should be given as a prophylaxis against infection. It is important to keep up morale. Mild analgesics such as aspirin may be used to alleviate the pain caused by rewarming.

Ward (1975) emphasizes the importance of treating frostbite at a hospital or in a well-equipped camp from which evacuation by air or some other means is easy. Here the preferred treatment is for rapid rewarming in a water bath, for which the temperature

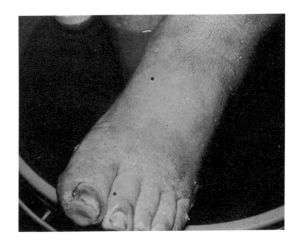

24.9 *Technique for rewarming frostbitten feet comprising container, water, and thermometer.*

can be precisely controlled at 37–41°C (Fig. 24.9). Rapid rewarming is associated with much less tissue damage due to a smaller area of circulatory arrest and the most adequate early function, especially in deep injury (Foray and Salon 1985; Mills 1983). Gradual spontaneous thawing appears to be satisfactory for superficial frostbite but not for deep injury (Mills 1983). Wilkerson (1986) also advocates that the water bath should be maintained at a temperature between 38°C and 42°C. Hotter water would further damage the tissues, and the water should not feel uncomfortable to an uninjured person's hand.

The frostbitten hand or foot obviously cools the water bath in which it is placed and the temperature of the bath must be maintained by adding warm water, and not by heating the container (Wilkerson 1986). The tissues must not be allowed to come into contact with the heated container, as the fragile tissues will be damaged still further. The injured hand or foot must be removed from the bath when hot water is being added and must not be returned to it until the water has been thoroughly mixed and the temperature checked. Warming takes 20–40 minutes and has to be continuous until the tissues are soft and pliable.

When rewarmed, frostbitten tissues that will survive lose their pallor and take on a flushed appearance. If there is no chance of tissue recovery, the part remains cyanotic and cold. Pain is commonly experienced during the rewarming and this may need analgesics, ranging from aspirin to morphine.

The current management in Alaska (Mills 1983) is to immerse the part or the whole person in a whirlpool bath (41°C) until the distal tip of the thawed part flushes. In Chamonix in the French Alps, the limb is placed in a 38–40°C bath for 30 minutes with the whirlpool effect being produced by bubbling oxygen through the water (Lloyd 1986). The whirlpool has the effect of removing necrotic and infected tissue without causing damage to healthy tissue. Thawing is not started until 15–20 minutes after the intravenous injection of a vasodilator. After thawing, the extremities are elevated and kept exposed on sterile sheets with cradles to avoid damage. Treatment is continued with whirlpool baths at 35°C twice daily for 20 minutes, with an antiseptic such as hexachlorophene.

Blisters should not be opened deliberately and, if any have ruptured spontaneously, they should be covered by dry, absorbent dressings (see Fig. 24.8). Blisters represent a potent source of infection. After thawing, the formation of oedema may result in a compartment pressure syndrome and fasciotomy is then essential to avoid extensive tissue necrosis (Mills 1983).

The blackened carapace acts as a protective covering for the regenerating tissue and will gradually separate itself without interference. Abscesses may occur in the damaged tissues and these may require drainage or removal of an overlying nail. Attempts to aid separation should be avoided, as it commonly leads to infection or excessive loss of tissue. Escharotomy should only be performed when the eschar is dry and causing splinting of the digits (Mills 1983). Debridement or amputation should be delayed till mummification and tissue demarcation are complete, which may take up to 90 days. This is a profound change in approach from former days when unnecessary amputations were carried out because of impatience at slow recovery. It has to be kept in mind that eschar may represent superficial rather than deep tissue damage. Commonly, the eventual outcome is much better than that originally envisaged. Premature surgery must be avoided at all costs, and when surgical intervention is considered eventually to be indicated it should be kept to a minimum.

Other supplementary methods have been tried in hospitals to improve the blood supply to the damaged periphery. There is some evidence that sympathectomy produces a reduction in pain, a decrease in oedema, and a tendency to less infection (Mills 1983; Flora 1985), but it does not significantly improve the amount of tissue preservation. Attempts have been made to achieve the same results pharmacologically by the use of the drug re-serpine, but the results have not been outstanding (Wilkerson 1986). Other measures include rehydration, especially with low-molecular-weight dextran (Mills 1983; Foray and Salon 1985), to try to reduce the sludging referred to above through haemodilution (Schmid-Schonbein and Neumann 1985).

Prognosis

The severity of frostbite injuries is notoriously difficult to judge accurately during the early stages (Wilkerson 1986). Frequently, even the extent of the injury cannot be determined accurately. A purple discoloration of the tissue, instead of pallor, is commonly a sign of severe damage. Predictive signs include a failure of the expected returning flush to the tissues, which indicates that circulation to these areas has not been resolved and that the tissue will probably be lost. Blisters filled with clear fluid that extend to the tips of the digits suggest that the underlying tissues will probably recover. On the other hand, blisters that are filled with bloody fluid, blisters that do not extend to the fingertips, or the failure of blisters to appear at all indicate that the tissues are probably damaged beyond recovery. In the ensuing weeks and months when the eschar is forming, and digits may become mummified, surgery may be needed for reconstruction or for amputation. Faced with a long period of recovery and perhaps severe permanent disability, the victims of frostbite may suffer sever emotional reactions. Continuing reassurance and psychological support are a significant part of their nursing care (Wilkerson 1986).

SHIVERING IN LOWLANDERS

Man's immediate response to cold on arriving at high altitude is to conserve heat by reducing the rate of blood flow to the skin (Fig. 24.10) with some erection of hairs that may make a minor contribution to insulation. Once the skin temperature falls below a thermoneutral zone of 25–35°C, cold-sensitive receptors in the skin, and probably in the viscera too, send stimuli via the spinal cord to the thermostatic centre in the hypothalamus (Ward 1975). This initiates stimulation of the motor centre for shivering (Fig. 24.10), which is a coordinated movement of voluntary skeletal muscle under involuntary nervous control that may increase heat production threefold. Shivering increases heat production by the body and is typical of the newcomer to high altitude adjusting to the cold.

The shivering response in lowlanders and highlanders was studied in Indians and Tibetans by

Sea-level man

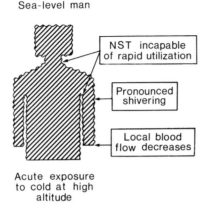

NST incapable
of rapid utilization

Pronounced
shivering

Local blood
flow decreases

Acute exposure
to cold at high
altitude

24.10 *Reactions of sea-level man to cold at high altitude. NST, Non-shivering thermogenesis.*

Native highlander

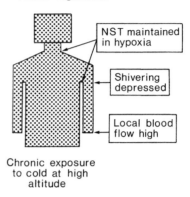

NST maintained
in hypoxia

Shivering
depressed

Local blood
flow high

Chronic exposure
to cold at high
altitude

24.11 *Reactions of the native highlander to cold at high altitude. NST, Non-shivering thermogenesis.*

Davis (1974) in Ladakh at an altitude of 3510 m. He studied five Indians from sea level, five Indian lowlanders who had become acclimatized to high altitude, and five Tibetan refugees native to elevations of 3960–4880 m. He measured skin and rectal temperature, oxygen consumption, and shivering rate in all 15 subjects who were exposed nude for 1 hour to an air temperature of 2°C. The 10 Indian lowlanders complained of severe pain in the extremities and half could not complete the hour; the shivering rate was significantly increased in all of them, although less in those acclimatized to mountain conditions. In contrast, the Tibetans had no difficulty in completing the test and they showed a much lower shivering rate. As seen below, this is an expression of their metabolic acclimatization to cold. The same phenomenon is seen in the aboriginal bushmen of Australia who may sleep virtually naked in the cold desert without shivering.

NON-SHIVERING THERMOGENESIS IN HIGHLANDERS

Native highlanders show a long-term acclimatization to cold, which is largely metabolic in nature and brought about by a process called 'non-shivering thermogenesis' (Fig. 24.11). This is the basis for the capacity of human infants and certain newborn and adult mammals to increase their heat production without shivering, when exposed to temperatures below thermoneutrality. In rats, cessation of shivering does not cause a fall in oxygen consumption due to this alternative form of heat production (Davis 1974). Rats acclimatized to cold whose muscles are paralysed by curare may actually increase their oxygen consumption in the cold.

The tissue primarily responsible for this increase in metabolic rate is 'brown fat' (Smith and Horowitz 1969). It is deposited in the abdomen, and in the cervical, interscapular, and axillary regions. The role of non-shivering thermogenesis in long-term acclimatization to cold in mountainous regions is modified by the fact that the process consumes oxygen, whereas the major adverse factor of life at high altitude is hypoxia. Indeed in some small mammals and their newborn under hypoxic conditions, the increase in oxygen consumption normally accompanying exposure to cold is suppressed. This decreased metabolic response is thought to be due to depression of non-shivering thermogenesis, presumably because there is insufficient oxygen in the ambient air to support it fully. Nevertheless, after acclimatization to hypoxia the deer mouse (*Peromyscus*) shows an increase in heat production to normal on exposure to cold (Roberts *et al.* 1969). This is accompanied by hyperplasia of brown fat.

In an attempt to assess thermal conditions in human infants naturally exposed to cold and hypoxia, Dufour *et al.* (1976) studied skin temperature on three infants in the high Andes. They chose the nape of the neck as an indirect measure of heat production by brown adipose tissue. The Quechua infants were aged respectively 8, 9, and 15 months and came from Nuñoa (4000 m). A disc thermistor probe was applied to six skin sites (forehead, nape at the level of the seventh cervical vertebra, chest over manubrium, right lateral thigh, and dorsal surfaces of the right hand and foot) every hour from 07.00 to 19.00 hours. They found that the nape temperatures were warmer than other skin sites, suggesting that in infant highlanders the brown adipose tissue associated with non-shivering thermogenesis is metabolically active despite the reduced oxygen availability at high altitude. Thus in naturally acclimatized infants at high altitude, non-shivering thermogenesis appears to be as important in thermoregulation as it is at sea level.

LOCAL REACTION TO COLD IN HIGHLANDERS

While most highlanders avoid generalized cold stress through appropriate clothing and accommodation (see Fig. 24.1), their extremities do not escape exposure to the cold inherent in life on high mountains. Thus, in Andean highlanders the rectal temperature is normal, but the surface temperature of the extremities is lower (Hanna 1970). Nevertheless, this lowered peripheral temperature is still higher than that of Caucasians exposed to the same environmental conditions. This is because the naturally acclimatized highlander maintains a high level of blood flow to the limbs (Hanna 1970; see Fig. 24.11). The same is true of Eskimos (Elsner *et al.* 1960). Thus it would appear that there are local vascular manifestations of acclimatization to cold as well as generalized mechanisms, which are metabolic in nature. The precise physiological processes that allow the microcirculation of the hand to be maintained under conditions that normally lead to vasconstriction are not fully understood.

Jones *et al.* (1976) studied the effects of these changes in peripheral blood flow in the daily lives of Andean Indians at Nuñoa (4000 m). They investigated thermal responses during acute exposure to cold while washing clothing in a river or creating a diversion of a stream. Men maintained equal temperatures in hands and feet during the exposure period, but the hands of women were slightly warmer than their feet. Women consistently maintained higher temperatures in the extremities than did men.

References

Bangs, C.C. (1986). Recognizing hypothermia- (p. 46) and Treating hypothermia (p. 54). In *Hypothermia, Frostbite and Other Cold Injuries* (J.A. Wilkerson, C.C. Bangs, and J.S. Hayward, Ed.). Seattle, Washington; The Mountaineers

Burton, A.C. and Edholm, O.G. (1955). *Man in a Cold Environment*. London; Edward Arnold

Danzl, D.F. (1983). Accidental hypothermia. In *Emergency Medicine. Concepts and Clinical Practice* (P. Rosen, F.J. Baker, G.R. Braen, R.H. Dailey, and R.C. Levy, Ed.), Vol. 2, Trauma. Boston; Mosby, p. 477

Davis, T.R.A. (1974). Effects of cold on animals and man. *Progress in Biometeorology*, **1** (1A), 215

Dufour, D.L., Little, M.A., and Brooke Thomas, R. (1976). Skin temperature at the nape in infants at high altitude. *American Journal of Physical Anthropology*, **44**, 91

Elsner, R.W., Nelms, J.D., and Irving, L. (1960). Circulation of heat to the hands of Arctic Indians. *Journal of Applied Physiology*, **15**, 662

Flora, G. (1985). Secondary treatment of frostbite. In *High Altitude Deterioration* (J. Rivolier, P. Cerretelli, J. Foray, and P. Segantini, Ed.). Basel; Karger, p. 159

Foray, J. and Salon, F. (1985). Casualties with cold injuries: primary treatment. In *High Altitude Deterioration* (J. Rivolier, P. Cerretelli, J. Foray, and P. Segantini, Ed.). Basel; Karger, p. 149

Hanna, J.M. (1970). A comparison of laboratory and field studies of cold responses. *American Journal of Physical Anthropology*, **32**, 227

Harnett, R.M., Pruitt, J.R., and Sias, F.R. (1983). A review of the literature concerning resuscitation from hypothermia. Part II. Selected rewarming protocols. *Aviation, Space, and Environmental Medicine*, **54**, 525

Jones, R.E., Little, M.A., Thomas, R.B., Hoff, C.J., and Dufour, D.L. (1976). Local cold exposure of Andean Indians during normal and simulated activities. *American Journal of Physical Anthropology*, **44**, 305

Keatinge, W.R. and Cannon, P. (1960). Freezing point of human skin. *Lancet*, **i**, 11

Lloyd, E.L. (1986). *Hypothermia and Cold Stress*. London: Croom Helm, p. 86

Mills, W.J. (1983). Frostbite. *Alaska Medicine*, **25**, 33

Mills, W.J. and Rau, D. (1983) University of Alaska. Anchorage-section of high altitude study and the Mt. McKinley project. *Alaska Medicine*, **25**, 21

Roberts, J.C., Hock, R.J., and Smith, R.E. (1969). Effects of altitude on brown fat and metabolism of the deer mouse, *Peromyscus*. *Federation Proceedings: Federation of American Societies for Experimental Biology*, **28**, 1065

Schmid-Schonbein, H. and Neumann, F.J. (1985). Pathophysiology of cutaneous frost injury:

disturbed microcirculation as a consequence of abnormal flow behaviour of the blood. Application of new concepts of blood rheology. In *High Altitude Deterioration* (J. Rivolier, P. Cerretelli, J. Foray, and P. Segantini, Ed.). Basel; Karger, p. 20

Smith, R.E. and Horowitz, B.A. (1969). Brown fat and thermogenesis. *Physiological Reviews*, **49**, 330

Steele, P. (1976). *Medical Care for Mountain Climbers*. London; William Heinemann

Ward, M. (1975). *Mountain Medicine. A Clinical Study of Cold and High Altitude*. London; Crosby, Lockwood, Staples

Ward, M.P., Milledge, J.S., and West, J.B. (1989). *High Altitude Medicine and Physiology*. London; Chapman and Hall Medical

Wilkerson, J.A. (1986). Avoiding hypothermia- (p. 12) and Frostbite (p. 84). In *Hypothermia, Frostbite and Other Cold Injuries* (J.A. Wilkerson, C.C. Bangs, and J.S. Hayward, Ed.). Seattle; The Mountaineers

25

Skin and nails

At high altitude the skin is exposed to increased levels of ultraviolet radiation with a shift of spectral intensity towards the shorter wavelengths (Chapter 2). This induces both acute and chronic effects, a notable exception being any tendency towards increased prevalence of skin cancer at high altitude. The hypoxia and hypocarbia of the mountain environment influence the cutaneous circulation. Finally, haemorrhages occur commonly in the nails of highlanders and we compare and contrast them with those found in lowlanders.

ACUTE EFFECTS OF ULTRAVIOLET RADIATION

The skin and the cornea both react to the increased intensity of ultraviolet radiation. The keratitis that may result is described in Chapter 27. The effects on the skin may be acute, in the case of the lowlander newly arrived in the mountains, or chronic as in the native highlander. The acute reaction takes the form of sunburn, which may produce a vivid erythema. The effects of ultraviolet radiation are enhanced not only by the increased intensity at high altitude but also by the change in its spectral quality, so that a higher proportion of it is composed of short wavelengths (Chapter 2). Ultraviolet radiation of short wavelength produces the severest degree of erythema, so that energy at 295 nm is about a hundred times more effective in producing erythema than that at 315 nm (Koller 1952). A further zone of maximal erythemic response is found with a wavelength of 380 nm. Hence the effects on the skin are due to amounts of radiation in narrow bands that are very small in comparison with the total ultraviolet. The erythema is not immediate and the time for it to appear is inversely proportional to the intensity of the radiation.

The erythema may proceed to vesiculation (Fig. 25.1) and crusting for the damaging radiation, of wavelength 280–310 nm with the maximum effect at 295 nm, has a destructive effect on proteins and nucleic acid causing injury to cells at the body surface. Even a short period of sufficient exposure to

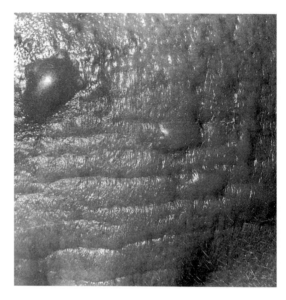

25.1 *Vesiculation of skin of scalp on acute exposure to ultraviolet radiation on the Jungfrau (3450 m). The intervening skin is severely oedematous and accentuates the furrows on the forehead above the left eyebrow (lower right-hand corner of figure).*

such radiation may lead to blistering, crusting, and desquamation of skin, which may be extensive on such areas as the unprotected scalp (Fig. 25.2) or chest (Fig. 25.3). The erythema usually takes 12–24 hours to become maximal, fades after 1–3 days, and is then replaced by pigmentation. Latent herpes simplex of the upper lip may be activated by the increased ultraviolet radiation at high altitude to lead to 'cold sores' (Chapter 26). Persons who have suffered from dendritic keratitis, an infection of the cornea with herpes simplex, at sea level should take care to protect their eyes by dark glasses at high altitude to prevent an activation of the virus by increased ultraviolet radiation.

After a single exposure to ultraviolet light, the skin of most Caucasians initially shows an increase in size

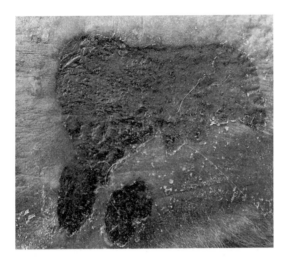

25.2 *Excoriation of skin of scalp after several hours of exposure to ultraviolet radiation at an altitude of 3450 m. There has been extensive loss of epidermis over the left eyebrow (lower right-hand corner of figure).*

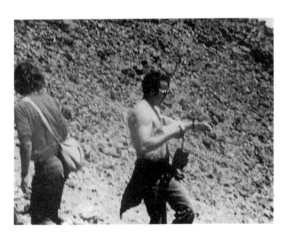

25.3 *Tourists walking near the summit of Mt Teide (3720 m), a volcano on the island of Tenerife off the coast of North Africa. Walking without a shirt in the increased intensity of ultraviolet radiation of shorter wavelength found at high altitude leads to rapid blistering, crusting, and desquamation of the skin, as shown here.*

and functional activity of existing melanocytes (Pathak *et al.* 1965). Repeated exposure leads to greater numbers of dopa-positive melanocytes as well as an enhancement of their size and activity (Quevedo *et al.* 1965). Repeated exposure of mice

to sun and vincristine reveals that the increased concentration of melanocytes is due to enhanced mitotic activity (Rosdahl 1978). These changes do not differ qualitatively from sunburn seen at sea level, but at high altitude they are usually more severe and there may be considerable oedema of the skin. Sunburn may be particularly severe in mountaineers and this is greatly enhanced by reflected radiation from the snow, the so-called albedo (Chapter 2). Snow reflects up to 90% of ultraviolet radiation compared to 9–17% reflected from ground covered by grass (Buettner 1969). Hence, on snow-covered ground at high altitude the combination of direct and reflected ultraviolet radiation leads to a much increased level compared to that found at sea level. The reflected ultraviolet radiation may lead to severe sunburn in areas not usually exposed such as the inside of nostrils and ears, and under the chin. Pigmentation of the skin is thought to be produced more by ultraviolet of longer wavelengths (Peemöller 1928). There is much individual variation in the susceptibility to the sunburn of high altitude, but in general fair-skinned persons are more sensitive than the dark-skinned.

PROLONGED EXPOSURE TO ULTRAVIOLET RADIATION

Prolonged exposure to solar radiation produces degenerative changes in the skin. Native highlanders, especially if they are peasants engaged in long hours in the fields exposed to fierce sunlight, develop pigmentation, thickening, and furrowing of the skin. This is prominent on the face and the back of the neck where the characteristic pattern leads to its being referred to as *cutis rhomboidalis nuchae*. Ageing of non-exposed skin manifests itself only as thinning with a decrease in the amount of subcutaneous fat; histologically there is a diminution in the number and diameter of the elastic fibres. However, on the face, hands, and any parts of the limbs exposed to solar radiation, degenerative changes occur. At first the elastic fibres become thicker, curled, and tangled. Later, in patients with clinically evident solar elastosis, staining with haematoxylin and eosin reveals in the upper dermis basophilic degeneration of the collagen separated from a somewhat atrophic epidermis by a narrow band of normal collagen (Fig. 25.4; Lever and Schaumburg-Lever 1983). In the areas of basophilic degeneration the bundles of eosinophilic collagen are replaced by amorphous basophilic granular material. The areas of degeneration stain like elastic tissue and are referred to as 'elastotic material'. This usually consists of aggregates of acid mucopolysaccharide. There is commonly an irregular distribution of melanin in the epidermis in some patients with solar degeneration.

HIGH-ALTITUDE DERMATOPATHY

Eguren (1972) believes that the histological changes induced in the exposed skin of the highlander are so characteristic that he terms them 'high-altitude dermatopathy'. He studied biopsy specimens from the lobe of the ear from 100 native inhabitants of Condoroma (4850 m) in southern Peru, most of them being young miners. He also examined biopsy specimens of skin from 50 citizens of Arequipa (2370 m) and, for comparison, from 50 natives of Camaná (20 m). Eguren found hyperkeratosis in the exposed skin of the native highlanders, with horny keratin plugs around hair follicles and sweat glands. There was some atrophy of the underlying Malpighian layer, especially where there was focally severe hyperkeratosis. Patchy focal dyskeratosis was present. Characteristically, there was loss of the interpapillary epithelial evaginations, so that the basal layer tended to even out horizontally. The skin of the native highlanders was hyperpigmented with hyperplasia of melanocytes and there was leakage of melanin both into the overlying cells of the Malpighian layer and into the underlying dermis. The phagocytosis of melanin granules in the dermis by a layer of enlarged, overloaded chromatophores in effect increased the thickness of the pigmented layer of the skin. The basal cells commonly showed hydropic degeneration with local thickening and disruption. Within the dermis Eguren (1972) found areas of basophilic elastotic degeneration like those we have described above. There was dilatation of blood vessels and lymphatics in the dermis with surrounding accumulations of lymphocytes.

It will be apparent that there is a close resemblance between Eguren's 'high-altitude dermatopathy' and the histological features associated with prolonged exposure to solar radiation which we describe above. It is in fact likely that the two conditions are identical and represent the reactions of skin to the increased intensity at high altitude of ultraviolet radiation and a shift of spectral intensity towards the shorter wavelengths. Electron microscopic studies by Everett *et al.* (1971) suggested that the lesions due to repeated exposure to ultraviolet radiation start in the epidermis. While they showed that early ultrastructural changes include loss of cellular cohesion, their findings also support the histological observations on the highlanders in the Andes in that they found increased formation of keratin, increased

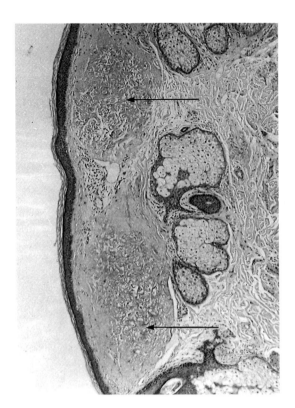

25.4 *Solar elastosis. In the upper dermis there are areas of basophilic degeneration of the collagen (arrows) separated from a somewhat atrophic epidermis by a narrow band of normal collagen. HE, × 70.*

thick interwoven bands but, when the degeneration becomes severe, it becomes granular.

Ultrastructurally the thick fibres of elastotic material comprise a fine granular matrix and, within it, homogeneous, electron-dense irregularly shaped inclusions. Collagen fibrils are diminished in number and show diminished electron density and cross-striation. Fibroblasts appear active with an extensive rough endoplasmic reticulum. In essence, solar elastosis appears to be due to altered function of fibroblasts, so that they are no longer capable of producing normal elastic fibres or collagen but produce instead the elastotic material (Lever and Schaumburg-Lever 1983); it should not be regarded as a degeneration-product of pre-existing elastic fibres. Nevertheless, the elastotic material has the same amino-acid composition as elastin and differs significantly from that of collagen, with a much lower content of hydroxyproline. The elastotic material is susceptible to digestion by elastase and contains a high proportion of size of melanosomes, and overloading of cells by melanin. Eguren (1972) thinks that the hyperpigmentation and leakage of melanin into the dermis, where it is taken up by melanophores, constitute a form of long-term dermal acclimatization to high altitude. The increased thickness and density of melanin form an increased barrier to ultraviolet radiation. An additional protection may be afforded by the increased layer of keratin.

SKIN TUMOURS

Localized areas of hyperkeratosis due to prolonged exposure to solar radiation may advance after several years to squamous carcinoma. Solar keratoses are usually seen as multiple lesions in sun-exposed areas of the skin in persons in or past middle life who have a fair complexion. They form erythematous areas, usually less than 1 cm in diameter, which are sometimes covered by adherent scales. Sometimes they are hyperkeratotic or pigmented. They are usually found on the face, the dorsa of the hands, and on the bald scalp. They are due to excessive exposure to sunlight and inadequate protection against it. Bowen's disease is an intraepidermal squamous-cell carcinoma that presents as an enlarging erythematous patch of sharp but irregular outline. It, too, develops in sun-damaged skin and is commonly found in association with areas of basophilic, elastotic degeneration in the dermis (Figs 25.5 and 25.6). It may develop into a squamous-cell carcinoma, although this malignant tumour may arise *de novo* in sun-damaged skin. Solar radiation will induce skin tumours at sea level if the intensity of the radiation and the exposure to it are high enough. In Australia, where there is a great amount of sunlight and a predominantly white population, skin tumours account for more than half of all diagnosed cancers (Mackie and Mackie 1963). Susceptibility to skin carcinoma is greater the smaller the amount of protective pigmentation in the skin.

Nevertheless, there are virtually no data on the prevalence of different types of skin tumour at high altitude. Such anecdotal evidence as there is suggests that skin tumours are not more prevalent than at low altitude. Krüger and Arias-Stella (1964) found that squamous carcinoma of the skin is not unduly common in highlanders. These Quechua Indians have a heavily pigmented skin as described above and the women have the added protection of the Andean custom of wearing wide-brimmed hats from youth, which shield the wearer from ultraviolet and other forms of solar radiation. Krüger and Arias-Stella (1964) carried out a study of the 20 ma-

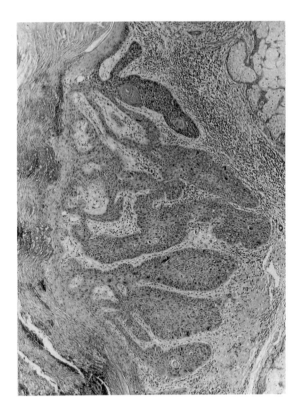

25.5 *Bowen's disease arising in skin affected by solar elastosis. The keratinous surface of the sun-damaged skin lies to the left. The columns of intraepidermal squamous cell carcinoma extend to the right in the dermis where there is a surrounding chronic inflammatory cell infiltrate. HE, × 60.*

lignant neoplasms that occurred in Cerro de Pasco (4330 m) during the years 1961 and 1962 when 152 biopsy and surgical specimens and 185 necropsies became available for study. Included were three malignant melanomas of the skin. One occurred on the upper lip of a woman of Yanahuanca (3540 m), the others on the toes in a man from Milpo (3990 m) and in a native of Yanahuanca. A basal-cell carcinoma was found on the right lower eyelid of an aged mestizo male from Ninacaca (4110 m). They did not find a single case of squamous-cell carcinoma. Jones (1975) is also sceptical that the increased level of ultraviolet radiation in the mountains represents a hazard that increases the risk of skin cancer. He notes that in Denver, Colorado (1600 m) the ultraviolet intensity at 295 nm is increased by 125%, whereas in the state as a whole the percentage of clear days (70%) is above the national average for

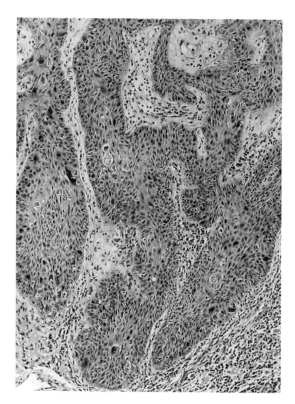

25.6 *Bowen's disease. Part of the lesion shown in Fig. 25.5 at higher magnification to show the histological features of the intraepidermal squamous-cell carcinoma. HE, × 117.*

the USA. However, in spite of these environmental factors, Colorado has one of the lowest skin cancer fatality rates in the USA.

NAIL HAEMORRHAGES

In lowlanders

Haemorrhages are common in the nails of healthy lowlanders and are due to repeated minor trauma. They have a characteristic distribution on the various fingers, and a characteristic form and position in the nails. Over half a century ago Horder (1920) associated their appearance with a diagnosis of subacute bacterial endocarditis. Some ascribed them to increased capillary fragility (Lewis 1942; White 1947), whereas others thought them to be embolic in origin (Bramwell and King 1942). Later, Wood (1956) had come to the conclusion that splinter haemorrhages were not diagnostic of bacterial endocarditis and this was confirmed in subsequent

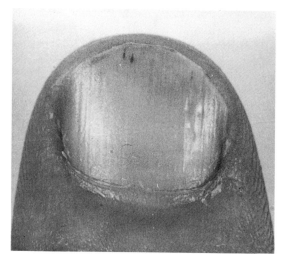

25.7 *Nail haemorrhages in a lowlander. They are linear in shape and occur at the line of separation of the nail-plate from the underlying nail-bed. This type of haemorrhage appears to be related to minor trauma.*

studies by Platts and Greaves (1958) and Gross and Tall (1963).

Platts and Greaves (1958) examined the finger-nails of 429 patients and normal subjects and 35 cadavers. They found nail haemorrhages in such a wide variety of diseases as to convince them that they were not diagnostic of subacute bacterial endocarditis or especially associated with any condition. Indeed they found nail haemorrhages in several of their healthy acquaintances. We have been able to confirm the common occurrence of such splinter haemorrhages both in ourselves and healthy colleagues. They are characteristically linear in shape and occur at the line of separation of the nail from the underlying nail-bed (Fig. 25.7; Heath and Williams 1978). They form in the deep part of the nail substance and pass distally with the nail, so that eventually they become available for histological examination in nail-parings. As they pass distally they become paler and move to a more superficial level in the nail-plate. As a consequence, nail haemorrhages in healthy lowlanders are largely confined to the crescent of nail-plate distal to the line of separation from the underlying nail-bed.

Nail-parings that contain splinter haemorrhages give the colour reactions of altered blood such as leuco-aniline blue peroxidase. We have studied the histological appearances of nail haemorrhages in methacrylate-embedded sections (Heath and

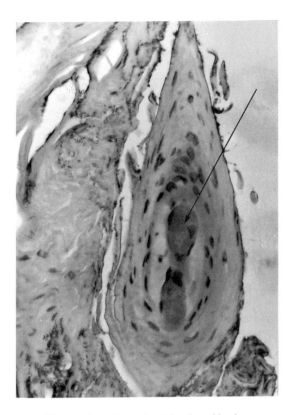

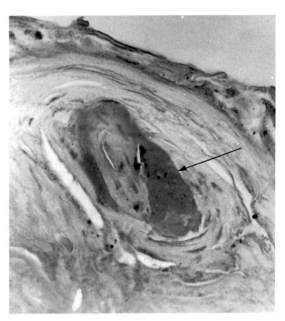

25.9 *An older, paler haemorrhage in the hard nail-plate (arrow) than that shown in Fig. 25.8. Methacrylate section, HE × 600.*

25.8 *Haemorrhage (arrow) arising from blood capillaries in the centre of whorl of squamous cells underlying soft nail-plate. HE, × 360.*

Williams 1978; Figs 25.8 and 25.9). They consist of a homogeneous mass of altered blood, embedded in a layer of squamous cells adherent to the undersurface of the cut nail. The haemorrhages seem to arise from capillaries in dermal papillae that could easily be damaged from trauma. In view of the characteristic line of origin of these haemorrhages at the separation of nail-plate from underlying nail-bed, we think it likely that they are traumatic in origin. This impression is strengthened by the fact that nail haemorrhages are commoner in the right hand in right-handed people and in the first three fingers, which are used more extensively than the fourth and fifth (Heath and Williams 1978). Platts and Greaves (1958) commented on the finding of haemorrhages in the nails of an emphysematous diabetic who was employed in making packing cases. Gross and Tall (1963) also believed the haemorrhages to be traumatic in origin. They examined 267 hospital in-patients for splinter haemorrhages and found them in 19.1% of subjects. They were found to occur more often in those patients whose occupations or activities exposed their hands to frequent trauma. They were also found more often in those patients who had recently been admitted to hospital, their incidence tending to decrease with increasing length of stay in hospital.

In climbers

Rennie (1974) reported that on an expedition to Dhaulagiri, Nepal (8170 m), the sixth highest mountain in the world, he developed numerous splinter haemorrhages in his fingernails. They appeared spontaneously during a restful evening at 5880 m. The following morning he had nearly 50 thin red longitudinal streaks under his finger- and thumbnails. They occurred near the distal part of the nail-bed. In the previous 5 weeks he had been engaged in manual work, transporting heavy loads from 760 to 5880 m. He had no purpura or ecchymoses. Eight fellow climbers had no splinter haemorrhages, three had one each, two showed two each, one had three, and one four. It would appear that climbing at high altitude with repeated minor trauma to the hands offers an acceptable explanation for the development of nail haemorrhages.

In native highlanders

Haemorrhages are as common in the nails of high-landers as they are in lowlanders, and, moreover, their distribution is the same, occurring as linear streaks at the line of separation of the nail-plate from the underlying nail-bed (Fig. 25.10(a)). We carried out a study of the prevalence and distribution of nail haemorrhages in subjects born and living at Lima (150 m), Cuzco (3400 m), and La Raya (4200 m). The incidence of nail haemorrhages at these three elevations was 34.9, 43.0, and 57.9%, respectively. In view of their position in the nail it seems very likely that such haemorrhages in healthy highlanders are traumatic in origin, just as they are in lowlanders (Heath *et al.* 1981).

In contrast, in subjects with Monge's disease the nail haemorrhages tend to have a different distribution, occurring throughout the nail, even to its base (Fig. 25.10(b)). We think it likely that they are related to hypoxaemia and a high haematocrit, leading to sludging of erythrocytes in small capillaries and associated bleeding. Haemorrhages of the same type and distribution occur in the nails of those patients with cyanotic congenital heart disease who have a high haematocrit.

KOILONYCHIA IN LADAKHIS

A high prevalence of koilonychia (Fig. 25.11) has been reported in Ladakhis living in the region of Leh (3800 m) by Anand and Harris (1988) and by Dolma *et al.* (1990), although these two groups of authors came to different conclusions as to its aetiology. Anand and Harris (1988) examined the fingers of men in the Indo-Tibetan Border Police, some being local Ladakhis born and bred at an altitude above 3600 m and others being lowlanders from other regions of India who had been transferred for duty to the high altitudes of the northern borders. They made observations on 29 Ladakhis and 28 lowlanders. Their ages (mean 34 years) and length of service (mean 14 years) were comparable and the average length of service at high altitude by the lowlanders was as long as 6.6 years. All 10 fingernails were inspected and the degree of koilonychia was graded into mild and severe.

Koilonychia was found to be more prevalent and severe in the Ladakhis. Because of the well-known association between iron-deficiency anaemia and koilonychia, measurements of haemoglobin were made on all the subjects studied. There was no substantial difference in the haemoglobin level between

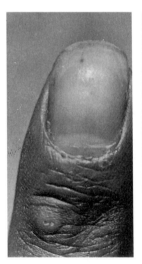
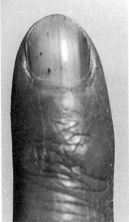

(a)   *(b)*

25.10 *(a) Fingertip of healthy male Quechua Indian, aged 23 years, showing a small haemorrhage in the nail. It is situated at the line of separation of the nail-bed from the underlying nail-plate, and this resembles the nail haemorrhages of healthy lowlanders shown in Fig. 25.7. Such bleeding into the fingernails of healthy highlanders is probably traumatic in origin.*
(b) Fingertip of a male Quechua Indian, aged 35 years, with Monge's disease. There are haemorrhages in the substance of the nail-plate, and they are scattered from the base to the edge of the nail. This distribution appears to be characteristic of extreme hypoxaemia and the resultant greatly elevated haematocrit.

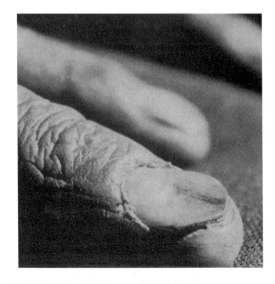

25.11 *Koilonychia in a male Ladakhi.*

the Ladakhis (15.9 ± 1.4 g/dl) and the lowlanders (15.5 ± 1.5 g/dl), the rather high levels clearly being related to the hypobaric hypoxia. The mean level of haemoglobin in the Ladakhis showing koilonychia was 15.8 g/dl and in those without was 16.0 g/dl. Thus the koilonychia did not appear to be related to anaemia. Neither did altitude seem to be a factor, for on average the lowlander had been living at high altitude for over 6 years which should have given them ample time to acclimatize to the same extent as the native population. Anand and Harris (1988) concluded that the tendency to koilonychia is a *racial* characteristic of the Ladakhi who forms part of a Tibetan population with a culture and facial appearance quite distinct from those of the rest of India.

In contrast, Dolma *et al.* (1990) found that the condition was much commoner in women. The prevalence of koilonychia was noted during a health survey of 364 subjects in the village of Chucot near Leh. The state of the nails was initially recorded in only 70 of them but 5 months later a more systematic examination of 226 of the same subjects was undertaken. Eight months later an attempt was made to contact the 38 subjects previously found to have koilonychia in order to investigate the underlying cause. Twenty-five were identified for interview and 23 of them were women. It emerged that, as well as being largely confined to women, the koilonychia was seasonal, being worse in summer; in winter the nails were normal or much improved.

Sociological studies revealed that most Ladakhi women repair walls or water channels in the spring when they expose their hands to cold, wet mud. Mud was also used with a coarse grass to clean cooking pots. In one case the koilonychia affected only the right hand, which was used for plastering wet mud between April and August. In September the fingers returned to normal after a few weeks. There was no association with iron deficiency anaemia. The mud in the region of Leh had a high silica content of 50% and was very alkaline (pH 8.1–8.6). The few cases of koilonychia in males occurred in migrant Bihari and Nepali workers who made mud-bricks. It is of interest that, without the benefit of medical investigations, the villagers of Chuchot called the condition 'chusent' or 'water nails'.

CUTANEOUS CIRCULATION AT HIGH ALTITUDE

Changes occur in the cutaneous circulation on initial exposure to high altitude and these seem to modify the flow and volume of blood in other organs. The circulation in the right hand, as representative of the cutaneous vascular bed, was studied in seven Europeans and 32 Bolivian highlanders at low altitude in Paris (50 m) and Santa-Cruz (400 m), respectively, and/or at high altitude in La Paz (3750 m) and Chorolque (5200 m) (Durand and Martineaud 1971). The study showed that in lowlanders cutaneous flow is reduced immediately on arrival at high altitude and then remains steady at a diminished level. There is a further significant reduction in cutaneous flow on further ascent. Durand and Martineaud (1971) interpret this reduction in cutaneous flow at high altitude as a result of arteriolar constriction, but we refer to evidence below that this may be the result of hypocapnia rather than hypoxia.

As well as changes in the resistance vessels of the skin there appear to be alterations in function of the capacitance vessels comprising capillaries and veins. Vascular pressure–volume curves obtained by plethysmography show a decrease in compliance at high altitude and this seems to reflect an increase in the tone of the capacitance vessels rather than a large volume of blood in them. Decrease in distensibility occurs immediately on arrival at high altitude, but even after 1 month is greater than in highlanders. The reduction in cutaneous blood flow and volume at high altitude is well established (Weil *et al.* 1969; Wood and Roy 1970).

The reduction in cutaneous blood flow is significant only when the skin temperature is above 33°C. Durand and Martineaud (1971) estimate that the fall in cutaneous flow redistributes less than 100 ml/min or some 2% of the total resting cardiac output. Hence the effect of high altitude on skin perfusion should not play any significant physiological role except on unusual exposure to heat. Increase in tone of the capacitance vessels is the more important physiological entity at high altitude. There is a pronounced overshoot of this venomotor response in highlanders returning from a lower altitude.

The increased tone in the capacitance vessels and the decrease in systemic venous compliance detected by Weil *et al.* (1969) is possibly of significance in the aetiology of high-altitude pulmonary oedema. Wood and Roy (1970) found that vascular compliance of the forearm was less in patients with high-altitude pulmonary oedema. Cruz *et al.* (1976) sought to determine whether the major cause of the sustained systemic venoconstriction at high altitude is hypoxia or hypocarbia. Five men were exposed to a simulated altitude of 4000–4400 m with supplemental carbon dioxide (3.8%) in a hypobaric chamber for 4 days. Similar alveolar oxygen tensions were obtained in four control subjects exposed to 3500–4100 m without carbon dioxide. A water-filled plethysmograph was used to determine forearm flow and venous compliance. Venous compliance at high altitude fell in both groups. Forearm flow and resistance were unaltered at altitude in the group with supplementation with carbon dioxide, while flow decreased and resistance increased in the hypocapnia group after 72 hours of exposure. It was concluded that hypoxia is responsible for decreasing venous compliance, whereas hypocapnia is responsible for increasing resistance and decreasing flow.

References

Anand, I.S. and Harris, P. (1988). Koilonychia in Ladakhis. *British Journal of Dermatology*, **119**, 267

Bramwell, C. and King, J.T. (1942). *Principles and Practice of Cardiology*. London; Oxford University Press, p. 386

Buettner, K.J.K. (1969). The effect of natural sunlight on human skin. In *The Biologic Effects of Ultraviolet Radiation with Special Emphasis on the Skin* (F. Urbach, Ed.). Oxford; Pergamon Press, p. 237

Cruz, J.C., Grover, R.F., Reeves, J.T., Maher, J.T., Cymerman, A., and Denniston, J.C. (1976). Sustained venoconstriction in man supplemented with CO_2 at high altitude. *Journal of Applied Physiology*, **40**, 96

Dolma, T., Norboo, T., Yayha, M., Hobson, R., and Ball, K. (1990). Seasonal koilonychia in Ladakh. *Contact Dermatitis*, **22**, 78

Durand, J. and Martineaud, J.P. (1971). Resistance and capacitance vessels of the skin in permanent and temporary residents at high altitude. In *High Altitude Physiology: Cardiac and Respiratory Aspects*, Ciba Foundation Symposium (R. Porter and J. Knight, Ed.). Edinburgh; Churchill Livingstone, p. 159

Eguren, V.L. (1972). Morfologia histologica de la piel expuesta en grandes altitudes. Dermatopatio de altura. Unpublished M.D. thesis. Universidad Nacional Mayor de San Marcos, Lima

Everett, M.A., Nordquist, J., and Olson, R. (1971). Ultrastructure of human epidermis following chronic sun exposure. *British Journal of Dermatology*, **84**, 248

Gross, N.J. and Tall, R. (1963). Clinical significance of splinter haemorrhages. *British Medical Journal*, **ii**, 1496

Heath, D. and Williams, D.R. (1978). Nail haemorrhages. *British Heart Journal*, **40**, 1300

Heath, D., Harris, P., Williams, D., and Krüger, H. (1981). Nail haemorrhages in native highlanders of the Peruvian Andes. *Thorax*, **36**, 764

Horder, T. (1920). Discussion on the clinical significance and course of subacute bacterial endocarditis. *British Medical Journal*, **ii**, 301

Jones, A. (1975). Ozone depletion and cancer. *New Scientist*, **68**, 14

Koller, L.R. (1952). *Ultraviolet Radiation*. London; Wiley

Krüger, H. and Arias-Stella, J. (1964). Malignant tumours in high altitude people. *Cancer*, **17**, 1340

Lever, W.F. and Schaumburg-Lever, G. (1983). Degenerative diseases. In *Histopathology of the Skin*, 6th edn. Philadelphia; J.B. Lippincott, p. 271

Lewis, T. (1942). *Diseases of the Heart*, 3rd edn. London; Macmillan, p. 89

Mackie, B.S. and Mackie, I.C. (1963). Cancer of the skin. In *Medical Biometeorology* (S.W. Tromp, Ed.). Amsterdam; Elsevier, p. 481

Pathak, M.A., Sinesi, S.J., and Szabo, G. (1965). The effect of a single dose of ultraviolet radiation on epidermal melanocytes. *Journal of Investigative Dermatology*, **45**, 520

Peemöller, F. (1928). Die physiologische Bedeutung des Pigments. *Strahlentherapie*, **28**, 168

Platts, M.M. and Greaves, M.S. (1958). Splinter haemorrhages. *British Medical Journal*, **ii**, 143

Quevedo, W.C., Szabo, G., Virks, J., and Sinesi, S.J. (1965). Melanocyte populations in UV-irradiated human skin. *Journal of Investigative Dermatology*, **45**, 295

Rennie, D. (1974). Splinter haemorrhages at high altitude. *Journal of the American Medical Association*, **228**, 974

Rosdahl, I.K. (1978). Melanocyte mitosis in UVB-irradiated mouse skin. *Acta Dermato-Venereologica (Stockholm)*, **58**, 217

Weil, J.V., Battock, D.J., Grover, R.F., and Chidsey, C.A. (1969). Venoconstriction in man upon ascent to high altitude; studies on potential mechanisms. *Federation Proceedings: Federation of*

American Societies for Experimental Biology, **28**, 1160

White, P.D. (1947). *Heart Disease*, 3rd edn. New York; Macmillan, p. 360

Wood, J.E. and Roy, S.B. (1970). The relationship of peripheral venomotor responses to high altitude pulmonary oedema in man. *American Journal of Medical Sciences*, **259**, 56

Wood, P.H. (1956). *Diseases of the Heart and Circulation*, 2nd edn. London; Eyre and Spottiswoode, p. 648

26

Infection and allergy

The question of infection at high altitude is complex. Many of the common infectious diseases found in native highlanders, such as tuberculosis, are more an expression of the poor socioeconomic conditions of the population than of the high-altitude environment in which it lives. In some instances, however, physical factors inherent in life in mountains seem to be directly related to the appearance of the inflammatory disease. An example is re-activation of herpes labialis in skiers by exposure to increased ultraviolet radiation. Sometimes the physical factors at high altitude are inimical to the growth of causative parasites or vectors predisposing to the disease. Thus, there is poor survival of oocysts of *Toxoplasma gondii* in the soil of high-altitude areas in Colorado, leading to a very low prevalence of congenital toxoplasmosis. The lower humidity of areas at altitude in East Africa is not conducive to proliferation of malarial mosquitoes so that the population is not afflicted with hyperendemic malaria and thus with Burkitt's lymphoma. On the more homely subject of mattresses in the Alps, the cold, dry conditions of even moderate altitude greatly reduce the population of house-dust mites and with it the prevalence of bronchial asthma. There are also infectious diseases classically associated with high altitude in the Andes, such as Oroya fever. In this chapter we shall consider all these differing manifestations of infectious disease and allergy at high altitude.

BRONCHIAL ASTHMA

It might be thought likely that asthmatic subjects who climb at high altitude are at increased risk from bronchospasm induced by exercise and cold, dry inspired air. The severity of the bronchospasm is directly related to the rate of respiratory heat loss and can be ameliorated or prevented by inhaling warm, humid air (Strauss *et al.* 1978). Boner *et al.* (1985*a*) found that an exercise challenge at moderate altitude produced a more intense stimulus than that experienced at sea level and thought this was related to the stress of low humidity added to the coldness of the

inspired air. On the other hand, Ward *et al.* (1989) report that asthmatics do well in general on high-altitude expeditions probably because any detrimental effects of inhaling cold air are more than outweighed by the beneficial consequences of the removal of the usual allergens of the subjects.

There is clinical evidence, supported by the results of lung function studies, to suggest that treatment for some months at asthma centres at moderate altitude below 2000 m is valuable in the management of refractory cases of bronchial asthma in children. Boner *et al.* (1985*a*) found that 23 children with bronchial asthma who had been resident at an altitude of 1756 m in the Dolomites reduced considerably their requirement for regular anti-asthma therapy, while steroids were discontinued altogether. Morrison-Smith (1981) reported on his experience of the treatment of 212 asthmatic children in Davos, Switzerland (1530 m) between 1954 and 1976 and of a further 37 children in Font-Romeu (1800 m) in the eastern Pyrenees. The length of stay in the mountains was from 6 months to 2 years. Some 80% of the children showed clinical improvement, becoming largely free of symptoms and able to take part in active exercise.

It is most unlikely that improvement is related in such children to altitude as such. It is more probable that children benefit from living in a stable, well-ordered environment where emotional factors and psychological problems are diminished or removed. Other important factors are the exclusion of air pollutants, especially tobacco smoke, and the common respiratory viral infections of life in urban society at sea level. Especially important is the absence from the mountain air of exogenous allergens. Clinicians working in these centres appear to be in little doubt that the elimination or curtailment of allergens accounts for much of the benefit of treatment in the mountains. Morrison-Smith (1981) thought that diminished exposure to pollen and house-dust was responsible for the improvement. Spieksma *et al.* (1971) thought that clinical improvement in asthmatic children was due to decreased exposure to house-dust mites in particular. Boner *et al.* (1985*b*) also thought the clinical improvement in 14 children with allergic bronchial asthma over an 8-month period of residence at Misurina (1756 m) in the Italian Alps was due to absence of such mites. Before considering house-dust mites at moderate altitude we should note that an improvement in lung function and a reduction in the use of medication are not confined to children treated at these mountain clinics. Speelberg *et al.* (1992) reported the benefit experienced by 34 adult patients with bronchial asthma and 116 subjects with chronic obstructive lung disease following a stay of 3 months at the Dutch Asthma Centre in Davos (1530 m).

HOUSE-DUST MITES AT ALTITUDE

It has been demonstrated many times that in the mountains there is a decrease in the number of mites that are known to be an important allergenic component of house-dust at sea level. Early reports by Dutch investigators working at Davos (1530 m) in the Swiss Alps had pointed out that house-dust mites decrease in number with increasing altitude (Voorhorst *et al.* 1969; Spieksma *et al.* 1971; Berrens *et al.* 1971). At about the same time, Rufli *et al.* (1969) failed to find *Dermatophagoides* in the house-dust of mountain treatment centres for bronchial asthma such as Celerina (1720 m) and Pontresina (1800 m).

A systematic study of this problem was made by Vervloet *et al.* (1982). They extracted, counted, and identified different species of mite during each season for 1 year on 218 mattress dust samples at sea level and at different altitudes in the Alps in the region of Briançon (1365 m) which is the highest city in Europe. Beds comprise the major site of mite infestation. They found that the percentage of dust samples containing mites and the number per-100 mg dust fell with increasing altitude. Thus at sea level 80% of 77 dust samples were positive, each 100 mg of dust containing 88 mites. At altitudes between 900 and 1100 m, only 40% of samples were positive and the number of mites was reduced to 7 per 100 mg. In the range of 1200–1350 m, 14% were positive with 4 mites per 100 mg dust. Between 1400 and 1600 m, 6% of the samples were positive with 2 mites per 100 mg. At higher altitudes, none of the samples contained mites.

This falling-off in the number of mites with increasing altitude does not seem to be related to their dislike of the elevation *per se*, but to its climatic associations. In particular, the fall in both temperature and relative humidity are detrimental to their prolif-

eration. Mites prefer an ambient temperature of about 25°C and cannot grow below 15°C. Even more critical for them is the relative humidity. They prefer a relative humidity of around 80% and, if this falls much below 70%, they succumb to desiccation. It is clear that the dry, cold atmosphere of mountains is not conducive to a happy life for mites.

The cold and low relative humidity of increasing altitude affects the proliferation of various species of house-dust mites to different extents. In general, *Dermatophagoides pteronyssinus* is less able to cope with the conditions of life at moderate altitude than is *Euroglyphus maynei*. At sea level, 65% of house-dust mites are *D. pteronyssinus*, 21% *D. farinae*, and 11% *E. maynei*. At moderate altitude the percentage of *D. farinae* remains roughly the same at 24%, but the percentage of *D. pteronyssinus* falls to 17% whereas the percentage of *E. maynei* rises to 51% (Vervloet *et al.* 1982). These changes presumably reflect the greater capacity of *E. maynei* to cope with the lower temperatures and relative humidity of high altitude. Such findings are consistent with the view that at moderate altitude there is a fall in the number of allergens provoking bronchial asthma. The fall-off in the number of house-dust mites is associated with less immunological reaction to them in the form of diminished levels of IgE, including immunoglobulin specific for mites. Vervloet *et al.* (1982) studied 42 asthmatic children, 36 boys and six girls, with positive skin tests to *D. pteronyssinus* first at sea level and then during a 9-month sojourn at Briançon (1365 m). At sea level the children had an initial mean total IgE level of 1047 u per ml; after 9 months at high altitude this level had fallen to 603 u per ml. The levels of IgE specific to *D. pteronyssinus* also fell.

POLLENS AND MOULD SPORES

Pollens represent another allergen in the atmosphere that is diminished at altitude. Environmental conditions and the flora vary from one mountain to another, so that generalizations concerning allergenic pollens in all high-altitude habitants cannot be drawn from individual reports based on a single area. Nevertheless, as an example we may consider the results of one such study. Buck and Levetin (1985) studied the subalpine environment at Gothic (2910 m) in the West Elk mountains in Colorado. They collected particles floating in the air on a Rotorod sampler whose impact surfaces were coated with silicone grease. Each day, 3283 litres of air were sampled and the rods were stained with Calberla's pollen stain, and examined microscopically for

Table 26.1 Pollen and allergenic mould spores found in the atmosphere at Gothic (2910 m) during June to August 1983 (after Buck and Levetin 1985)

Scientific name of plant	Common name	Per cent of sampling period during which pollen or mould was present
Pollens		
Poaceae	Grasses	100
Pinus	Pine	94.9
Picca; Abies	Spruce; Fir	78.0
Artemisia	Sagebrush	44.1
Amaranthaceae-Chenopodiaceae		100
Juniperus	Juniper	86.4
Plantago	Plantain	76.3
Betulaceae	Birch	52.5
Moulds		
Alternaria		47.5
Helminthosporium		100
Cladosporium		96.6

pollen and mould-spore identification and counting. They found 54 types of pollen, but only eight were regularly present in quantity (Table 26.1). It is clear from this study that allergenic pollens are still to be found in the mountain setting but that their level is low. Buck and Levetin (1985) found that pollen levels were generally low until late in the season, although some allergenic moulds were present in higher levels throughout the sampling period. They conclude that in general terms the mountain environment is a retreat for the sufferer from hay fever.

CYSTIC FIBROSIS

While bronchial asthma is improved by a period of treatment at moderate altitude, it has to be kept in mind that in patients with hypoxic lung disease holidays at altitude are potentially dangerous to the development of increased hypoxia associated with the lower inspired oxygen tension. Speechly-Dick *et al.* (1992) reported the cases of two young men in their early thirties with cystic fibrosis and poor lung function who went on skiing holidays at altitudes of 2000 and 2500 m, respectively. Neither sought medical advice before going on these holidays. The condition of both deteriorated sharply following their exposure

to high altitude, with the development of increased breathlessness, the production of more sputum, and the onset of fatigue. Response to subsequent therapy was slow. Speechly-Dick *et al.* (1992) point out that a sudden deterioration in relatively stable lung disease can be precipitated by strenuous physical exercise at high altitude. Patients who are active enough to contemplate such holidays should be made aware of the potential hazards and be carefully assessed including blood gases prior to departure.

BACTERIA IN MOUNTAIN AIR

The number of bacteria in ambient air decreases with altitude. They are relatively rare as low as 500 m, but can be found even at such extreme altitudes of 12 000 m as a result of upwinds (Rippel-Baldes 1952). A study on the Jungfraujoch (3450 m) showed that, despite the large number of tourists, very few bacteria were present in the air, the species represented being *Bacillus brevis*, *B. mesentericus*, *B. subtilis*, and diplococci (Keck and Buchmeiser 1964). The diminished barometric pressure does not appear to affect the growth of bacteria. Direct exposure to the increased solar radiation of the mountains severely inhibits the growth of some bacteria,

Staphylococcus aureus being particularly inhibited. This inhibitory effect of solar radiation is due to its ultraviolet components (Nusshag 1954). Mirrakhimov *et al.* (1979) found low staphylococcal antitoxins and antistreptolysin titres in native high-landers of the central Tyan-Shan (2800 m). Examination of nasal swabs in a high-altitude popu-lation in north Bhutan showed that there was only a 4% carrier rate of coagulase-positive staphylococci; normally the incidence is between 29 and 40% in Western communities. A high frequency of β haemolytic streptococci, highly sensitive to peni-cillin, was found in throat cultures, whereas in Western communities sensitivity to penicillin would be minimal (Selkon and Gould 1966).

The microbial flora of man appears to be uninfluenced by the high-altitude environment. The microbial flora of the skin, throat, and faeces of 16 subjects at 4300 m was studied by Weiser *et al.* (1969). In the throat were *Mycoplasma* species and harmless commensals and on the skin were *Staphylococcus*, *Candida*, *Aspergillus*, diphtheroids, and α and β haemolytic streptococci. Similar microorganisms are found at sea level. The average total organisms per g of faeces at 4300 m was 63.6 million as contrasted to 58 million at sea level. There are thus no qualitative or quantitative changes in microbial flora at high altitude.

TETANUS AT HIGH ALTITUDE

Ball *et al.* (1994) became aware that no deaths had been recorded from neonatal tetanus and only two from adult tetanus over the past 30 years in the Himalayan region of Ladakh. They thought this remarkable in an agricultural society where many people live in close contact with animal dung and trauma is common. Traditionally in this area dung is often applied to wounds and infants are placed in sacks of sheep dung as diapers. In many other moun-tainous regions such as Tibet, Nepal, Bhutan, and the Andes standards of hygiene are frequently equally low. Obstetric hygiene is minimal and dung may be used as a wound dressing. Tetanus is a readily recog-nized condition and so it is most unlikely that the diagnosis would be missed by Ladakhi doctors who had been trained in India where tetanus is common.

According to Ball *et al.* (1994) Dr Mohammed Deen of the Animal Husbandry Department in Ladakh believes that tetanus is also extremely rare in horses. Although they are susceptible to tetanus in the Vale of Kashmir and other parts of India, in Ladakh it is generally accepted in veterinary practice that horses do not require prophylactic immuniza-

tion even following large wounds. Tetanus in horses is also reported to be very rare in Peru and Bolivia. Ball *et al.* (1994) made extensive enquiries about the incidence of tetanus in other mountainous regions throughout the world and found it to be very low.

Ball *et al.* (1994) try to explain this extraordinary combination of frequent trauma, widespread expo-sure to dung, and rarity of tetanus at high altitude. They conclude that *Clostridium tetani* fails to sporu-late satisfactorily under the conditions of cold and low humidity at high altitude. High altitude alone in the absence of a low temperature such as is found in tropical regions of Kenya and Pakistan does not prevent the development of tetanus. Conversely cold alone at low altitude, such as in Scandinavia, does not prevent the appearance of the disease. It appears that a combination of cold and an additional factor inherent in the high-altitude environment is necess-ary to explain the rarity of tetanus in these moun-tainous areas. Hypobaric hypoxia is most unlikely to inhibit growth of an anaerobic organism at high alti-tude. Possibly the increased ultraviolet radiation of mountainous areas is responsible. Several unsuccess-ful attempts have been made to grow *Cl. tetani* from soil or dung in Ladakh (Ball *et al.* 1994).

The concept that at high altitudes tetanus spores occur in small numbers and are not in conditions conducive to sporulation is suppported by a report from Peru concerning anthrax, a disease caused by a spore-bearing aerobe (Manuel Moro 1967). Anthrax was not found above 2000 m in cattle, goats, and sheep. When cattle were brought down to the coastal areas, there were frequent outbreaks of anthrax if the animals were not vaccinated. There was lack of sporulation of *B. anthracis* when mouse-infected blood was poured into sterile soil.

Specimens of serum from some non-immunized Ladakhis contained tetanus antibodies. In a series of 19 men and 31 women between the ages of 15 and 69 years, the sera of eight men and two women contained levels of antibody between 0.04 and 0.36 iu/ml which were considered protective levels indicating exposure to antigen (Ball *et al.* 1994). These findings suggest that some Ladakhis may acquire natural immunity. Further studies need to be carried out to confirm, or refute, and explain the rarity of tetanus at high altitude.

LEUCOCYTES

Data available from the literature suggest that the native highlander, at any rate from the Andes, has normal total and differential white cell counts corre-sponding to those found in sea-level subjects. Figures obtained from 72 Quechua Indians at Morococha (4540 m) and from 140 mestizos of Lima on the coast by Hurtado (1964*a*) are shown in Table 26.2 . Under conditions of complete physical and mental relaxation, the leucocyte count lies between 5.0 and 7.0 $\times 10^9$/l (Wintrobe *et al.* 1974), so that the normal sea-level counts given by Hurtado are somewhat high. Nevertheless, the counts obtained at both altitudes were obtained by the same technique, so that his conclusion that there is no difference in leucocyte count at high altitude and sea level appears to be valid.

In contrast, it has been reported that in new-comers to high altitude there is for the first few days a leucocytosis accompanied by lymphopenia and eosinophilia (Verzar 1952). This is very likely to be brought about by the increased exercise indulged in by climbers, trekkers, and tourists on their arrival in the mountain environment. It has been known for a long time that a pronounced leucocytosis of segmented neutrophils occurs regularly with strenuous exercise. Counts as high as 22.0×10^9/l have been recorded for a runner after making a 100-yard (90 m) dash in 11 seconds and 35.0×10^9/l on completing a quarter-mile (400 m) run in less than 1 minute (Garrey and Bryan 1935). Leucocyte counts in excess of 20×10^9/l are regularly recorded for marathon runners covering 26 miles (42 km) in up to 3 hours and these values may take several hours to return to normal (Wintrobe *et al.* 1974). More recently, the same effectiveness of exercise in inducing a leucocytosis was reported by Schaefer *et al.* (1987) who studied the white cell count in 10 joggers at sea level. After running a distance of 2000 m the white cell count rose from 6.4 to 7.8×10^9/l and after a run of 10 000 m the count rose from 6.0 to 9.6×10^9/l.

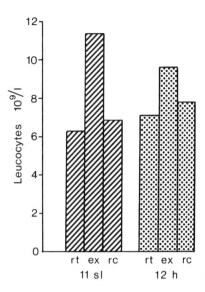

26.1 *Leucocyte counts at rest (rt), on exercise (ex), and on recovery(rc) in 11 non-athletes at sea level and in 12 highlanders native to 4520 m. (Based on data from Hurtado (1964b).)*

The exercise leucocytosis experienced by low-landers at sea level is greater than that shown in native highlanders at high altitude. Hurtado (1964*b*) studied this phenomenon in 12 athletes and 11 non-athletes at sea level and in 12 Quechuas at high altitude (Fig. 26.1). He found that the leucocytosis exhibited by highlanders on exercise to exhaustion (2.45×10^9/l) was only half of that shown at sea level by athletes (5.23×10^9/l) or non-athletes (5.09×10^9/l).

Table 26.2 Leucocyte and differential count at sea level and at high altitude. (After Hurtado 1964*a*).

	Sea level (Lima) (140 subjects)		4540 m (Morococha) (72 subjects)	
	Mean	SD	Mean	SD
Leucocytes ($\times 10^9$/l)	6.68	1.21	7.04	1.62
Neutrophils, stab. (%)	4.0	2.6	4.1	2.4
Neutrophils, segmented (%)	52.7	7.5	51.3	10.6
Neutrophils, total (%)	56.5	8.1	55.4	10.7
Eosinophils (%)	4.1	3.0	3.3	2.4
Basophils (%)	0.4		0.3	
Monocytes (%)	6.4	2.6	5.7	2.6
Lymphocytes (%)	32.4	10.4	35.8	10.4

The studies of Schaefer *et al.* (1987) demonstrate that this exercise leucocytosis is associated with the release of polymorphonuclear elastase. They measured plasma levels of this elastase in complex with α_1-proteinase inhibitor (E-α_1-PI). In 10 joggers there was an increase in the level of E-α_1-PI of 16% after running 2000 m and 186% after running 10 km. High plasma levels of elastase have been observed during bacterial infections. The implication is that the leucocytosis and associated release of polymorphonuclear elastase brought about by first exposure to high altitude, or by exercise at high altitude, are similar to those of an infectious or inflammatory challenge.

THE IMMUNE SYSTEM AT HIGH ALTITUDE

There are epidemiological data to suggest that hypobaric hypoxia may impair immune competence in man. In India a higher incidence of lobar pneumonia and amoebic hepatitis has been found among soldiers stationed at high altitude (Singh *et al.* 1977). Other infectious diseases, however, have been found to be either decreased or uninfluenced by exposure to high altitude (Singh *et al.* 1977). It is difficult to evaluate such epidemiological data so far as immune competence is concerned for, as we point out elsewhere in this chapter, other features of the high-altitude environment may directly reduce the viability of organisms or activate them. Thus the increased ultraviolet radiation in mountains may impair the growth of *Staphylococcus aureus* on the one hand or lead to reactivation of herpes virus on the other. Other direct effects on organisms may be effected through lower temperatures or the hypobaric hypoxia itself. We also note the effect of high altitude on reducing the population of mosquitoes, which are of importance in acting as vectors for various diseases. The same phenomenon has been reported by Clegg *et al.* (1970). Meehan (1987) has, nevertheless, presented data collected by various workers on the effects of exposure to high altitude on the immunization responses in animals to various immunogens (Table 26.3). It will be seen that there is a generally reported normal antibody response to bacteria.

The human immune system is a complex, highly regulated, and integrated network of circulating and fixed cells that are able to discriminate between self and non-self antigens (Meehan 1987). Circulating phagocytic cells in the form of granulocytes and macrophages and fixed tissue macrophages in the lymph nodes, spleen, alveoli, liver, and so on engulf and destroy invasive pathogens. An augmented phagocytic response is facilitated by circulating immunoglobulins, complement components, and C reactive protein. Specific immunity involves cellular co-operation between monocytes acting as antigen-presenting cells, B cells that produce immunoglobulins, and T cells that regulate by helper or suppressor capacity through the liberation of cytokines but that can also differentiate into cytotoxic effector cells (Meehan 1987).

Studies in human immunobiology are technically restricted. In general, only peripheral blood immunocompetent cells are available for study. Recent *in vitro* assays are sensitive enough to detect alterations in normal immune regulation following exposure to the hypoxia of high altitude. Thus, while most peripheral blood mononuclear cells circulate in a resting state, they must be transformed into immune effector cells to assess cellular immune responsiveness. This activation can be triggered *in vitro* by the addition of mitogenic lectins such as phytohaemagglutinin or pokeweed mitogen. Subsequent biochemical effects can be monitored sequentially including an increase in protein synthesis, the production of regulatory cytokines such as interleukins and interferons, DNA synthesis measured by thymidine incorporation, and cellular proliferation (Meehan 1987). Individual cells participating in activation events or immune effector function can be identified by isolation techniques or various immunoflourescence methods including flow cytometry.

In vitro T-cell function is commonly studied by measuring proliferation, the release of cytokines, or with cytotoxicity assays. Most investigators use mitogens to activate a large number of cells to facilitate the *in vitro* measurement and accuracy of responses. The mitogen-stimulated *in vitro* cellular responses are analogous to the *in vivo* antigen-stimulated responses. Such advances have allowed studies of the human immune response at high altitude. Operation Everest II in the United States provided, in particular, an opportunity to investigate scientifically the influence of progressive hypoxaemia on the human immune system. Seven healthy subjects in the age range of 21–31 years were studied during an exposure over 4 weeks in a hypobaric chamber simulating an ascent from sea level to 7620 m (Meehan *et al.* 1988). Multiple *in vivo* and *in vitro* variables of immune function, just referred to, were used to determine which aspect of the immune system is most sensitive to hypoxia.

Meehan (1987) reviewed the data on the immune response of man at high altitude reported before the

Table 26.3 Effects of exposure to high altitude on immunizaton responses in animals. (After Meehan 1987)

Immunogen	Animal	Altitude (m) × duration (days)	Reported results	Reference
BCG vaccine	Guinea-pigs	3200	Normal protection against tuberculosis	Mirrakhimov and Kitayev (1978)
TAB vaccine (tetanus toxoid, typhoid) and paratyphoid)	Mice	5500	Normal antibody response	Kaplanski *et al.* (1968)
Salmonella typhimurium	Mice	6100 × 21	Normal antibody response	Berry and Mitchell (1983)
Cytotransferrin	Rabbits	6100 × 21	Normal antibody response	Tengerdy and Kramer (1968)
Sheep red blood cells	Mice	6700 (16 h daily)	Decreased number of antibody forming cells. Day 3, normal to Day 7	Zhuravkin *et al.* (1978)
Sheep red blood cells	Mice	4310 × 30	Decreased number of antibody forming cells	Trapani (1969)
Sheep red blood cells	Rats	5000 × 90	Increased haemagglutinin titres	Meerson *et al.* (1980)
Sheep red blood cells	Rabbits	4880 × 35	Increased antibody responses	Singh *et al.* (1977)

results of the Operation Everest II project (Table 26.4). During this project Meehan *et al.* (1988) carried out simultaneous measurements of the multiple immune variables referred to above and found that the severe hypoxaemia of high altitude alters normal cellular immune regulation. Thus they found that mononuclear cell subset analysis by flow cytometry disclosed an increase in monocytes but not in B or T cells. However, these mononuclears were depressed in their ability to become activated *in vitro*. After 4 weeks of progressive hypoxaemia in the seven subjects in the Operation Everest II project there was a significant reduction in phytohaemagglutinin-stimulated thymidine uptake and protein synthesis by 33% and 50%, respectively (Meehan *et al.* 1988). There was much heterogeneity of *in vitro*

Table 26.4 Effects of exposure to high altitude on human immune responses reported before Operation Everest II project. (After Meehan 1987)

Altitude (m)	Reported results [*]	References
2300	Increased phagocytic index; increased influenza titres	Krupina *et al.* (1974)
3690	Increased IgM, IgA, and IgG levels after 2 years; increased Ab response to TAB vaccine	Chohan *et al.* (1975)
2100–4200	Increased phagocytic index; increased autoantibody production	Krupina *et al.* (1975)
6000	High titres of anticardiac Ab	Mirrakhimov and Kitayev (1978)
3200–3800	Decreased PHA-induced lymphocyte transformation after 5 days; normal by Day 25. Decreased complement and lysozyme after 5 days; normal by Day 25. Normal killing of Staphylococcus by PMN. Normal Ab responses to TAB vaccine. Normal plasma IgG, IgA, and IgM levels after 40 days	Mirrakhimov and Kitayev (1978)
3200	Decreased PHA-induced lymphocyte transformation after 5 days; normal by Day 25. Increased plasma IgM levels	Kitayev and Tokhtabayev (1981)

[*] Ab, Antibody; PHA, phytohaemagglutinin; PMN, polymorphonuclears.

cellular responses with regard to phytohaemagglutinin-stimulated interferon production and natural-killer cell cytotoxicity. The greater intersubject variations at 7620 m prevented statistical differences between altitude exposures being demonstrated. While T-cell function was impaired during hypoxaemia, B-cell function was not.

IMMUNOGLOBULIN LEVELS IN NEWCOMERS TO HIGH ALTITUDE

The concentration of circulating immunoglobulins and of antibodies to nuclear antigens was measured in plasma samples, in the subjects studied by Meehan *et al.* (1988) in the Operation Everest II project. There were significant increases in IgM and IgA but not IgG levels at 7620 m compared to values at sea level and 2290 m (Table 26.5). Mucosal immune function was assessed by quantifying total protein, IgA, and lysozyme levels in na-

sopharyngeal washings obtained weekly (Meehan *et al.* 1988). They found no significant effect of altitude exposure on either IgA or lysozyme levels in nasal washes. These results confirm the earlier findings of Mirrakhimov *et al.* (1979; see also Table 26.4) who studied the plasma levels of immunoglubins in 47 healthy subjects living in the foothills (760–980 m) before and after going to altitudes of between 3200 and 3800 m in the Tyan-Shan and Pamirs. These altitudes are considerably lower than those at which the studies of Meehan *et al.* (1988) were carried out but they too found significant increases of IgM and IgA but not IgG once the sixth day of acclimatization had passed. Until this stage all three classes of immunoglobulin were depressed.

Chohan *et al.* (1975) reported that blood levels of IgG were increased in Indian soldiers acutely exposed to the environment of the Himalaya. They suggested that the increased synthesis of IgG was as-

Table 26.5 Effects of exposure to simulated altitude on plasma immunoglobulin levels (after Meehan *et al.* 1988)

| Immunoglobulin | Plasma immunoglobulin levels (mg/dl) | | | |
	Normal range	Sea level	2290 m	7620 m
IgG	630–1349	1033 ± 58	996 ± 43	1011 ± 46
IgM	56–352	122 ± 17	120 ± 17	163 ± 22 *
IgA	70–312	154 ± 21	147 ± 22	181 ± 25 *

* Statistically different values from sea level and 2290 m.

sociated with increased resistance to viral infection and they note the decreased prevalence of such viral diseases as infectious hepatitis, chicken pox, and mumps in Indian soldiers stationed for long periods in the Himalaya, as noted in the paper by Singh *et al.* (1977). Until this observation of increased levels of IgG is confirmed by others, this suggestion of increased resistance to viral infection at high altitude must be treated with reserve.

Increased levels of IgA were also reported in newcomers to the Himalaya by Chohan *et al.* (1975) who thought them to have a protective role at mucous surfaces in those mountainous regions. It is known that this immunoglobulin is dominantly present in secretions such as colostrum, saliva, tears, nasal mucus, tracheobronchial secretions, and the lumen of the small intestine. As noted above, however, Meehan *et al.* (1988) did not detect alterations in mucosal immunity. They believed that their data supported the intepretation of results of a study at the South Pole that concluded that reduced IgA and lysozyme levels were caused by a combination of cold, isolation, and reduced humidity rather than by hypoxia as such (Muchmore *et al.* 1981).

IMMUNOGLOBULIN LEVELS IN NATIVE HIGHLANDERS

Memeo *et al.* (1982) studied the relation of the levels of the various classes of immunoglobulin in blood serum to age in Quechua Indians living at 4330 m in the Peruvian Andes. They investigated Indians of both sexes in the age range of 10–58 years and made the following observations (Fig. 26.2).

IgA. In the males there was a striking increase between the ages of 10 and 20 years. Maximal values were maintained until the age of 30 years, after which there was a slow decrease. In contrast to

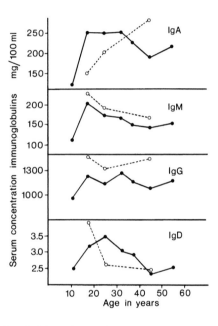

26.2 *Level of four classes of immunoglobulin at different ages in Quechua Indians in the Peruvian Andes. Solid lines, males; broken lines, females. (After Memeo* et al. *(1982).)*

this, in the female there was a constant increase of the serum levels of IgA from the ages of 20 to 45 years. IgA levels in 45-year-old female Indians were one-third higher than in males of the same age, and similar to values observed in males between 20 and 30 years.

IgM. Serum levels of this class of immunoglobulin also increased in the same group of 5–15 years. Thereafter there was a progressive decline. The values for females were consistently but slightly higher than those found in males.

IgG. In this class of immunoglobulin there were no significant changes with advancing age, with the exception of the increment observed in male Indians from 10 to 20 years of age. As with IgM, the values found in females exceeded those in males.

IgD. In this class there were considerable differences between serum levels with age and sex.

These studies show that in native highlanders certain classes of immunoglobulins show a consistent decline with advancing age, thus supporting the concept that at high altitude, as at sea level, the efficiency of the immune system is substantially diminished with old age. The decreased levels of IgA, IgM, and IgD in male highlanders with increasing age are in agreement with those found in sea-level residents (Buckley and Dorsey 1970). It is not possible to evaluate the age-dependence of IgG concentrations, since there are conflicting data on the levels of immunoglobulin of this class in residents at sea level. In conclusion it would seem that immunoglobulin patterns in male and female highlanders undergo the same manifestations with age as those seen at sea level. However, the absolute values may be different.

In high-altitude pulmonary oedema, IgM and IgA immunoglobulins are said to be raised further. According to Singh and Chohan (1972), IgG and IgM may get absorbed on to the surface of platelets, altering their mobility and increasing aggregation. IgG may promote the release of platelet factor 3 and ADP, the implications of which are referred to in Chapter 9.

SPECIFIC B-CELL RESPONSES IN HYPOBARIC HYPOXIA

The fact that serum immunoglobulin levels are not depressed significantly on exposure to hypobaric hypoxia (Table 26.3) suggests that high altitude does not impair B-cell function as noted by Meehan *et al.* (1988). However, evaluation of total serum immunoglobulins does not provide reliable information on specific immune responses elicited by a given antigen. Antigen-induced activation of specific B lympocytes follows different routes depending on whether or not T-cell co-operation is required. Biselli *et al.* (1991) examined the effects of the hypobaric hypoxia of high altitude on the immune response to a T-independent immune antigen in

man. As the model, vaccination with polysaccharides A and C of *Neisseria meningitidis* was chosen. Eighteen males (18–40 years) were given a single subcutaneous injection 5 days after arrival on Mt. Poumori (4930 m). Control subjects were vaccinated at sea level. Biselli and his colleagues (1991) found that B lymphocytes retain their full competence to generate a normal antibody response at high altitude. Serum immunoglobulin levels did not change after 4 weeks' exposure to hypobaric hypoxia. The study of Biselli *et al.* (1991) indicates that the suggested susceptibility to bacterial infections at high altitude is not related to any impairment of the specific antibody response to antigens on the part of B lymphocytes.

IMMUNE SUPPRESSION AT HIGH ALTITUDE

All these studies on man and animals suggest that hypoxia probably blunts cell-mediated immune responses, whereas B-cell function remains intact (Meehan 1987). It is well established that human T cells are more sensitive to the immunosuppressive effects of glucocorticoids than are B cells. At the same time it is well known that on initial ascent to high altitude there is increased secretion of steroids from the adrenal cortex (Chapter 22). The mechanism of such cortisol-mediated immune suppression has been extensively investigated and involves the inhibition of cytokines by activation of the cytoplasmic glucocorticoid receptor (Munck *et al.* 1984). The excessive output of ACTH and beta endorphins may also be involved.

BURKITT'S LYMPHOMA AND ALTITUDE

Some diseases are rare at moderate altitude because the mountain environment is not favourable for associated organisms that are involved in the development of that disease. One such condition is Burkitt's lymphoma. This oncogenic process is initiated by infection with the Epstein–Barr virus early in life. However, a heavy and prolonged burden of malaria at a later stage is necessary to trigger the development of the tumour (Morrow *et al.* 1976). Even moderate altitude is unattractive to malarial mosquitoes and hence it comes about that the level of altitude has a considerable influence on the distribution of Burkitt's lymphoma in East Africa. The lymphoma is prevalent in the tropical lowlands of Africa, but is rare at altitudes higher than 1500 m. Geser *et al.* (1980) carried out serological surveys in Uganda and Tanzania to see whether the variation in prevalence of the lymphoma from high to low areas is paralleled by a variation in the extent of infection with the Epstein–Barr (EB) virus. Sera were collected from samples of the general child population living in the tropical lowlands at altitudes between 600 and 1200 m in the West Nile District of Uganda, and living at moderate altitude (1200–1750 m) in North Mara, Tanzania. The sera from these surveys were tested for anti-EB virus antibodies to viral capsid antigens and to early antigens. The prevalence and strength of positive virus titres of both types were very similar in the lowlands and on the high plateaux. Clearly there is no direct relation between the prevalence of Burkitt's lymphoma and the extent of infection by the EB virus. In contrast, hyperendemic malaria is closely associated geographically with a high incidence of Burkitt's lymphoma. In the tropical lowlands of the West Nile District the prevalence of parasitaemia in children under 10 years of age is about 60–70% (Geser *et al.* 1980). On the other hand, in North Mara, Tanzania on the plateau at 1750 m the prevalence of parasitaemia varies from 5 to 25%. It would appear that malaria is an essential factor in the aetiology of Burkitt's lymphoma and that the absence of malarial transmission above an altitude of 1500 m accounts for the absence of the tumour there (Dalldorf *et al.* 1964; Burkitt 1969). Thus altitude exerts an indirect but important effect on the prevalence of the lymphoma in different areas of East Africa.

There is reason to believe that this freedom from malaria at moderate altitude is being lost. The whole of Zambia lies in the range of 900–1200 m and up to 1969 there was practically no malaria in the principal urban centres and copper-belt towns, but since then there has been a deterioration of urban antimalarial control measures and towns are now as vulnerable as at the turn of the century. In the past, areas over 1200 m in Zimbabwe were considered largely malaria-free, but it is probable that the situation has now changed (Bruce-Chwatt 1985).

TOXOPLASMOSIS

Some parasitic diseases are rare at high altitude because the mountain environment has a deleterious effect on the life cycle of the parasite. As an example, we may quote the case of congenital toxoplasmosis, which is rarely diagnosed in Colorado. To test whether this apparent rarity is the result of underreporting or a true state of affairs Hershey and McGregor (1987) tested the sera of 120 consecutive pregnant women for antibodies to *Toxoplasma gondii*. Only four of their patients had a

positive Sabin–Feldman dye test and none of them had acute infection as evidenced by IgM antibodies. This prevalence of 3% is very low, being one-tenth of the rate found in a large, broad-based population of pregnant women in the United States (Sever 1982). The four affected women showed no differences in exposure to the well known causes of toxoplasmosis such as exposure to domestic cats, the eating of uncooked meat, and so on. The low prevalence of toxoplasmosis in Colorado seems to be more closely related to the features of the mountain environment such as cold, low humidity, and, perhaps, increased ultraviolet radiation. In particular, low humidity is thought to shorten the survival of oocysts in the soil. This is reminiscent of the deleterious effects of low humidity on house-dust mites in the Alps as described earlier in the chapter.

CHAGAS' DISEASE

In Bolivia half the population lives at altitudes above 3000 m and moves up and down from the Andes to the lowlands, where Chagas' disease is endemic. This condition is due to infestation with *Trypanosoma cruzi* and commonly leads to serious heart disease. Ribante *et al.* (1986) sought to ascertain if asymptomatic subjects with Chagas' disease as proven by positive serology had normal cardiovascular responses and normal work capacity at high altitude. They studied two groups of 21 male Quechua Indians living permanently at Chivisivi (2850 m) in the Sapahaqui valley; one group was serologically positive for *T. cruzi*, whereas the other was negative. The two groups were similar with regard to age, stature, nutritional status, blood parameters, and heart and lung function. In absolute values, rises in systemic arterial pressure after half an hour's exercise, and maximal oxygen uptake, were identical in the two groups. They found no differences in the cardiovascular responses of the two groups at high altitude. This demonstration is of social and economic impact because it suggests there is no basis to support any political move to eliminate workers with positive serology from working at high altitude.

RECURRENT HERPES LABIALIS IN SKIERS

There is one viral disease that appears to be reactivated by physical factors in the high-altitude environment. Little certain is known about the factors that reactivate the herpes simplex virus (Fig. 26.3) but there is much anecdotal evidence to suggest that exposure to sunlight and specifically to ultraviolet radiation may be involved. We pointed out in

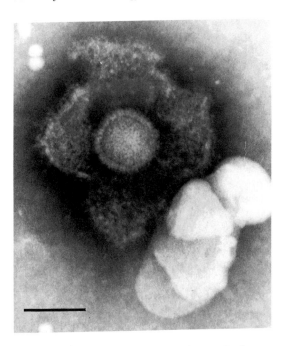

26.3 *Direct negative stain electronmicrograph of a vesicle fluid from herpes labialis. A typical herpes virion with a lipid envelope and eicosahedral nucleocapsid is visible. Scale bar, 100 nm.*

Chapter 2 that one of the characteristic features of the mountain environment is increased ultraviolet radiation. Mills *et al.* (1987) attempted to assess the risk of reactivation of herpes simplex virus in skiers. They studied 51 subjects engaged in skiing for 1 week at altitudes between 2290 and 3610 m who were known herpes simplex subjects and who had suffered from herpes labialis on previous ascent to high altitude. They found that reactivation of herpes labialis occurred in 12% of those studied. The recurrences developed in the usual location and were neither unusually severe nor mild. The median interval between first exposure to the sun and the development of skin lesions was 3.5 days. In two of the six affected skiers reactivation was delayed to as much as 6 days after the beginning of exposure to the sun when the subjects had left the mountain. In the four subjects who showed reactivation during the period of study at high altitude, herpes simplex type I was isolated. As to the mechanism of reactivation of the virus at high altitude, it is possible that the ultraviolet radiation stimulates nerve fibres originating in the trigeminal ganglion so that virions are transported to the epidermis where herpetic lesions

develop. Mills *et al.* (1987) found no correlation between the degree of skin pigmentation and the risk of reactivation.

A sunscreen ointment with a sun protection factor of 15 failed to influenced the reactivation rate as compared with a placebo. Possibly cold or other stress of exposure to high altitude may also be involved in the reactivation of herpes labialis and such factors would not be protected against by a sunscreen. Some of the subjects studied volunteered that an occlusive zinc oxide ointment was the most effective measure to prevent reactivation. Such an ointment would probably offer better protection against wind and cold than a sunscreen.

DANIEL CARRION'S EXPERIMENT

There is one bacterial infection classically associated with the Andes that afflicts the native highlanders of Peru, Colombia, Chile, and Ecuador. It is of considerable historical interest and is linked for all time with the name of Daniel Alcides Carrion (Fig. 26.4). As a boy he made frequent trips through the Peruvian mountains with his uncle, Manuel Ungaro, going to school in Lima from his home in Cerro de Pasco (4330 m) and travelling by way of La Oroya. During these journeys he saw how many of the Quechua Indians had wart-like nodules on their skin and mucous membranes. It was well known that the disease was restricted to the steep Peruvian valleys as it had been for centuries (Sutton 1971). Indeed, modern research has revealed a case of this disease in a mummy of the Tiahuanoco culture of southern Peru, the subject having apparently been sacrificed and some of his organs used in rituals (Allison *et al.* 1974).

An interesting account has been given by Schultz (1968) of the circumstances traditionally believed to surround the experiment of Daniel Carrion that shed light on the disease that has now become to be associated with his name. When Daniel became a medical student, he became vaguely aware that the cutaneous eruption of this mountain disease was preceded by fever, anaemia, and joint pains and he became obsessed with the need for early diagnosis of the warts so that treatment could be effective. It seemed to him that the most direct way of determining the early signs and symptoms of Peruvian warts was to inject fragments of them into himself and study the effects. On the morning of 27 August 1885, he carried out this procedure in the Nuestra Señora de las Mercedes ward of the Dos de Mayo Hospital in Lima (Schultz 1968). We are very familiar with this hospital with its central tropical garden

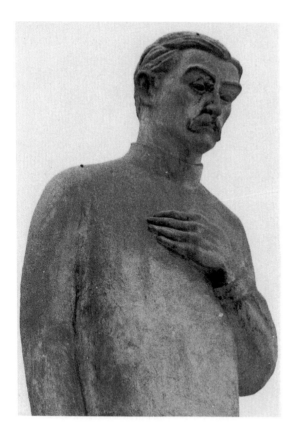

26.4 *Daniel Alcides Carrion (1857–1885), from a memorial outside the Dos de Mayo Hospital in Lima, Peru.*

with religious statues from which radiate the wards. In bed number 5 was a 14-year-old boy, Carmen Paredes, with a wart on his right eyebrow. The medical student tried to inoculate himself with material from this wart, but he was not dextrous enough to complete the task on his own. Accordingly a young medical graduate, Dr Chavez, completed the task. Daniel was delighted with the success of his minor operation and began to keep a diary of any symptoms that might appear.

On 17 September he began to feel unwell and had pain in his left ankle. Two days later he became ill with fever, chattering of the teeth, abdominal cramp, and pains in all the bones and joints of the body. His urine became dark and scanty and he became jaundiced. By 26 September he was too weak to record his symptoms any longer, so his fellow medical students took over the task so that the project for his thesis should not be disturbed. At this stage Daniel felt ill but had the satisfaction, as he thought, that he

was at last discovering the symptoms that precede the eruption of Peruvian warts. Soon, however, he became dangerously ill. A systolic murmur became audible over the base of the heart and could be felt over the carotid arteries. The pulse became rapid, he developed abdominal pain and diarrhoea, and vomited frequently.

The onset of these serious symptoms led him to recall the events of his boyhood. He remembered that, when the workers had striven to drive a railway through the Andes at La Oroya in 1871, many of them had died from fever and anaemia. The fatal condition was unknown to the medical profession and so, in deference to the route, was designated 'Oroya fever'. It began to dawn on Daniel that as a consequence of his inoculation he was developing not the symptoms of the invasive stage of the verruga, but the dreaded Oroya fever. By 3 October he was still in his lodgings and was visited by a Dr Flores who found that his total red cell count had fallen to just over $1.0 \times 10^{12}/l$. He was sent to hospital for a blood transfusion and became delirious. On 5 October, 39 days after inoculation and after 18 days of illness, he became comatose. Looking at one of his friends he muttered 'Enrique, c'est fini' and died at 23.30 hours. He was just 28 years of age.

Daniel Carrion thus demonstrated that verruga peruana and Oroya fever are but phases of one and the same disease. A historic medical advance had been made, but Lima was appalled. The experiment was described by a prominent Peruvian physician as a 'horrible act by a naive young man that disgraces the profession'. The necropsy was a scene of terrible confusion, for the body had already begun to decompose. Professor Villar made an eloquent plea in defence of martyrs and initial charges against Dr Chavez were dropped. The remains of the dead medical student were carried on the shoulders of his classmates, past his university to the cemetery.

The small pleomorphic microorganism that causes this severe, usually fatal, febrile anaemia, known as Oroya fever, was first seen by Barton in or on red cells (Barton 1909). Early in the disease the organism presents in a bacillary form and hence it has come to be designated *Bartonella bacilliformis*. Members of the 1937 Harvard Expedition to Peru were able to confirm hat this organism is the cause of both Oroya fever and verruga peruana. Pinkerton and Weinman (1937*a*) were able to grow *B. bacilliformis* in leptospira medium from blood or tissues from patients with Oroya fever or from the cutaneous lesions of verruga peruana, and found it behaved as a facultative intracellular parasite when cultivated *in vitro* with growing or surviving guinea-pig mesenchymal cells. The different forms of Carrion's disease as seen in man were reproduced in rhesus monkeys by Weinman and Pinkerton (1937*a*).

VARIOUS FORMS OF CARRION'S DISEASE

Carrion's disease occurs along the Andean range in Colombia, Ecuador, Peru, and Chile. Clinically, it presents incubative, invasive, pre-eruptive, and eruptive stages (Ricketts 1949). The incubation period varies from 3 to 14 weeks. After that time the causative organism, *B. bacilliformis*, parasitizes the red blood cells (Fig. 26.5), leading to a rapidly progressive febrile anaemia. The anaemia is macrocytic and frequently hypochromic. There is no spherocytosis, and the saline fragility of the erythrocytes is normal (Ricketts 1949). Nearly every erythrocyte is involved, so that the red cell count is commonly below $1.0 \times 10^{12}/l$. The anaemia does not respond to liver extract.

The pathological lesions in fatal cases of Oroya fever are those of a severe infectious haemolytic anaemia. The skin and conjunctiva may be icteric.

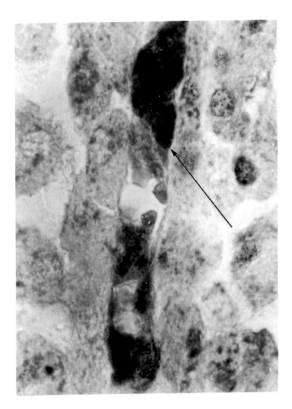

26.6 *Clusters of* Bartonella bacilliformis *(arrow) within endothelial cells lining small capillaries in the adrenal cortex. Wolbach's modification of Giemsa's stain after Regaud fixation,* × *1200.*

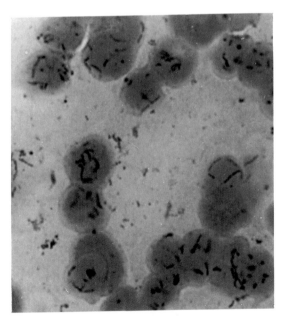

26.5 Bartonella bacilliformis *within the red cells of a patient with Oroya fever. Both bacilliform and coccal forms are seen. Adjacent rods give a criss-cross appearance in places. Blood film; Giemsa's stain,* × *1500.*

There is red hyperplasia of the bone marrow. The liver shows fatty infiltration. The reticulo-endothlial cells of the body, in lymph nodes, spleen, bone marrow, and hepatic Küpffer cells are crowded with *B. bacilliformis*, which form spherical clusters in the cytoplasm (Pinkerton and Weinman 1937*b*). They are also to be found in the adrenal (Fig. 26.6), pancreas, thyroid, testicle, and kidney and there may be degeneration of renal tubules. More than 90% of the cells contain organisms. The laboratory diagnosis is readily made in the anaemic stage by finding the organism in the red cells in Giemsa-stained blood smears.

Bartonella bacilliformis is polymorphous in human blood. Usually it is found in red cells as minute Gram-negative rods, 0.3–2.5 μm in length and 0.25–0.50 μm in width (Weinman 1944; see Fig. 26.5). However, coccal forms of 0.75 μm in diameter, also occur, especially when the organism is about to disappear from the blood. At such times they may also show hourglass and pear-shaped forms. The extremities of *B. bacilliformis* appear thicker and darker in colour when stained reddish-violet by Giemsa methods. Up to 90% of erythrocytes may be infected and several organisms may be found in one red cell. Often the organisms are distributed in rows of three or more, suggesting prior segmentation. Frequently adjacent rods are at an angle giving a V, Y, or criss-cross appearance (Weinman 1944). This organism is actively motile, possessing flagella that are always unipolar and that vary in number from one to four and in length from 3 to 10 μm. No spores or capsules are seen. Cultures are obtained in semi-solid leptospira medium (Noguchi and Battistini 1926) and on solid blood media but not in ordinary broth or agar. The optimum temperature is 25–28°C. The organisms can survive in blood or cultures for many weeks, months, or even years after recovery. During the acute phase of the disease the organisms disappear in a few days from the erythrocytes and they change from the bacilliform to the coccoid form. This tendency to degenerate from sharply stained bacillary rods to clusters of less discrete, coccoid, granular or amorphous forms was also seen in *Bartonella* grown in mesenchymal cells of the guinea-pig (Pinkerton and Wienman 1937*a*).

The *pre-eruptive stage* is characterized by pains in joints, muscle, and bones. Inflammatory reactions in various organs, such as parotitis and phlebitis, occur most often in this stage. The bacterial infection may also involve the central or peripheral nervous system and the meninges (Ricketts 1949). Encephalitis may occur.

Finally the *eruptive stage* occurs several weeks after recovery from the severe febrile anaemia. Cherry-red nodules, referred to as verruga, appear in the skin. They are 2–20 mm in diameter and are located chiefly on the extremities and face, but may be situated anywhere on the skin. Such lesions constitute the 'verruga peruana' that was investigated by Carrion. The nodules are soft and deep-red in colour when sectioned. Histologically they resemble a capillary haemangioma, with blood vessels of small calibre, proliferating endothelial cells, and organisms (Fig. 26.7). *Bartonella bacilliformis* is usually found in large numbers when Giemsa's stain is used. Large inclusions may be found in the endothelial cells and may represent clusters of degenerating organisms (Pinkerton and Weinman 1937*b*). Patients in the eruptive phase have little in the way of systemic symptoms. Verruga peruana usually confers immunity for a lifetime, although sometimes it is only transitory.

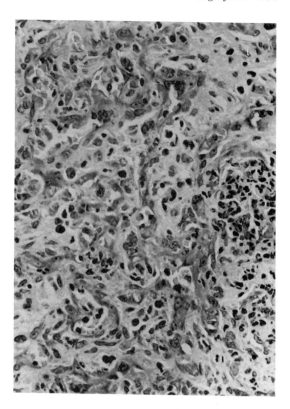

26.7 *Section of a verruga peruana showing it to consist of small blood capillaries and proliferating endothelial cells, thus resembling a capillary haemangioma. To the right is seen an infiltrate of acute inflammatory cells. Wolbach's modification of Giemsa's stain after Regaud fixation, × 375.*

Persons may carry *B. bacilliformis* without any signs or symptoms of Carrion's disease. Weinman and Pinkerton (1937*b*) showed that, while some carriers residing in Callahuanca remembered having had verruga peruana some months before, others gave no such history. Most carriers endure living conditions that make them only too accessible to haematophagous arthropods. Hence they constitute an important reservoir of *B. bacilliformis*. The insect vectors for Carrion's disease are two species of sandfly, *Phlebotomus verrucarum* and *P. noguchii* (Hertig 1937). It is likely that transmission of the disease by *Phlebotomus* is nocturnal. The sandflies leave caves for houses after twilight. Intermediate mammalian hosts have not been discovered. Other representatives of *Bartonella* at high altitude are *B. muris* in rats, *B. canis* in dogs, and *B. tyzzori* in guinea-pigs.

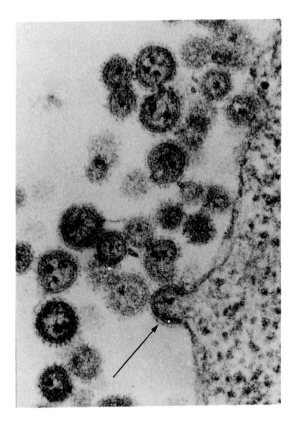

26.8 *Machupo virus budding (arrow) from marginal membrane of a 33H cell and accumulating extracellularly. x 114 000.*

The ultrastructure of the verrugas was studied by Recavarren and Lumbreras (1972). They found that, while most of the histiocytes between the endothelium-lined capillaries had clear cytoplasm, some contained numerous lamellar structures that they thought might represent destroyed organisms. Intact organisms within the cells were not seen, but in places cytoplasmic extensions of clear cells around *B. baccilliformis* were seen and were interpreted as suggestive of phagocytosis.

BOLIVIAN HAEMORRHAGIC FEVER

The highlands of Bolivia constitute one of the widely separated areas of the world afflicted by 'haemorrhagic fevers'. Although this group of diseases is regarded as infectious and caused by a virus, direct spread from person to person is not a predominant feature (Wilson and Miles 1975). Bolivian haemorrhagic fever is a representative of this class of condition that occurred in the Andes but is no longer seen.

The disease was first recognized in the Department of Beni, Bolivia in 1959. Four years later a laboratory was established in San Joaquin to study the aetiology, epidemiology, and ecology of the disease that was epidemic in that town and proving to have a mortality rate of over 20%. It is caused by the Machupo virus (Fig. 26.8 and 26.9), which has been isolated from human cases during the acute fever (Johnson *et al.* 1965) and from the wild rodent *Calomys callosus*, which suffers from a chronic infection excreting virus in the saliva and urine (Johnson *et al.* 1966). No arthropod vector has been found. It is closely related to Junin virus and other members of the Tacaribe complex of viruses (Fig. 26.10). These viruses have now been assembled into a taxonomic group called arenoviruses (Rowe *et al.* 1970), which also includes Lassa fever and lymphocytic choriomeningitis (Murphy *et al.* 1969, 1970). The name 'arenoviruses' (from *arenosus*, Latin: sandy) was proposed to reflect the characteristic fine granules seen in the virion in ultrathin sections. These RNA viruses share a group-specific antigen. The virus particles are round, oval, or irregular in shape and range in diameter from 50 to 300 nm, usually between 110 and 130 nm. The particles consist of a dense, well-defined unit-membrane envelope with closely spaced projections

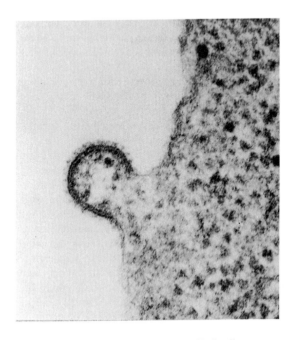

26.9 *Machupo virus budding from a Raji cell. × 140 000.*

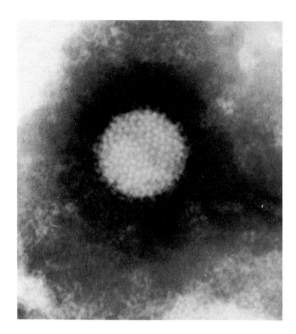

26.10 *Tacaribe virus particle in negative contrast from ultracentifuged Vero cell culture supernatant; rather closely spaced surface projections cover its surface.* × 330 000.

and an unstructured interior containing a variable number of electron-dense granules. These granules form the most striking, unique feature of these viruses; they are 20–30 nm in diameter and closely resemble host ribosomes. Virus particles are formed by budding, chiefly from plasma membranes. The pathology of human haemorrhagic fever caused by Machupo virus is generalized lymphadenopathy with haemorrhagic necrosis and haemorrhages and moderate congestion in many organs (Andrewes and Pereira 1972).

HAEMORRHAGIC EXANTHEM OF BOLIVIA

There has been one report of an epidemic of a haemorrhagic exanthematous disease that occurred in highland Bolivian recruit soldiers during May 1967 (Noble *et al.* 1974). After lifelong residence at high altitude the men had been transferred to a tropical area. This disease was initially considered to be an outbreak of an atypical Bolivian haemorrhagic fever, described above, or even of haemorrhagic smallpox. However, exhaustive clinical and epidemiological studies did not reveal any evidence of man-to-man transmission and serological studies failed to substantiate a viral or other infections aetiology.

Noble *et al.* (1974) came to the conclusion that the syndrome was similar to reported cases of haemorrhagic vesicular lesions following bites from small blackflies (*Simuliidae*, locally called 'marigui'). They point out that species of blackflies are present on the altiplano, but these bite small mammals not man. Hence the soldiers, native to high altitude, never had the opportunity to develop immunity to the allergens of these tropical insects. The hypersensitivity angiitis may be enhanced by the concurrent vascular fragility and hyperaemia that characterizes the highlander and of which we have noted examples throughout this book. In addition to headache and malaise, many of those affected showed haemorrhagic manifestations such as bleeding gums, haematuria, or gastrointestinal haemorrhage.

References

Allison, M.J., Pezzia, A., Gerszten, E., and Mendoza, D. (1974). A case of Carrion's disease associated with human sacrifice from the Huari Culture of Southern Peru. *American Journal of Physical Anthropology*, **41**, 295

Andrewes, C. and Pereira, H.G. (1972). Arenavirus. In. *Viruses of Vertebrates*, 3rd edn. London; Baillière Tindall, p.171

Ball, K., Norboo, T., Gupta, U., and Shafi, S. (1994). Is tetanus rare at high altitudes? *Tropical Doctor*, **24**, 78

Barton, A.L. (1909). Descripción de elementas endo-globulares hallados en los enfermos de fiebre verrucosa (Articulo preliminar). *Cronica Medica (Lima)*, **26**, 7

Berrens, L., Young, E., and Zuidema, P. (1971). A comparative chemical and clinical investigation of house-dust extracts from alpine and lowland regions. *Acta Allergologica*, **26**, 200

Berry, I.L. and Mitchell, R.B. (1983). Influence of simulated altitude on resistance–susceptibility to S. typhimurium infection in mice. *Texas Reports on Biology and Medicine*, **11**, 379

Biselli, R., Le Moli, S., Matricardi, P.M., Farrace, S., Faltorossi, A., Nisini, R., and D'Amelio, R. (1991). The effects of hypobaric hypoxia on specific B cell responses following immunization in mice and humans. *Aviation, Space, and Environmental Medicine*, **62**, 870

Boner, A., Niero, E., Antolini, I., and Warner, J.O. (1985a). Biphasic (early and late) asthmatic responses to exercise in children with severe asthma, resident at high altitude. *European Journal of Pediatrics*, **144**, 164

Boner, A.L., Niero, E., Antolini, I., Valletta, E.A., and Gaburro, D. (1985*b*). Pulmonary function and bronchial hyperreactivity in asthmatic children with house dust mite allergy during prolonged stay in the Italian Alps (Misurina, 1756 m). *Annals of Allergy*, **54**, 42

Bruce-Chwatt, L.J. (1985). Malaria at high altitudes in Africa. *British Medical Journal*, **291**, 280

Buck, P. and Levetin, E. (1985). Airborne pollen and mold spores in a subalpine environment. *Annals of Allergy*, **55**, 794

Buckley, C.E. and Dorsey, F.C. (1970). The effect of ageing on human serum immunoglobulin concentrations. *Journal of Immunology*, **105**, 964

Burkitt, D.P. (1969). Etiology of Burkitt's lymphoma — an alternative hypothesis to a vectored virus. *Journal of the National Cancer Institute*, **42**, 19

Chohan, I.S., Singh, I., Balakrishnan, K., and Talwar, G.P. (1975). Immune response in human subjects at high altitude. *International Journal of Biometeorology*, **19**, 137

Clegg, E.J., Harrison, G.A., and Baker, P.T. (1970). The importance of high altitude on human populations. *Human Biology*, **42**, 486

Dalldorf, G., Linsell, C.A., Barnhart, F.E., and Martyn, R. (1964). An epidemiological approach to the lymphomas of African children and Burkitt's sarcoma of the jaws. *Perspectives in Biology and Medicine*, **4**, 435

Garrey, W.E. and Bryan, W.R. (1935). Variations in white cell blood cell counts. *Physiology Reviews*, **15**, 597

Geser, A., Brubaker, G., and Olwit, G.W. (1980). The frequency of Epstein–Barr virus infection and Burkitt's lymphoma at high and low altitudes in East Africa. *Revue d'Epidemiologie et Santé Publique*, **28**, 307

Hershey, D.W. and McGregor, J.A. (1987). Low prevalence of Toxoplasma infection in a Rocky Mountain prenatal population. *Obstetrics and Gynecology*, **70**, 900

Hertig, M. (1937). Carrion's disease V. Studies on *Phlebotomus* as the possible vector. *Proceedings of the Society for Experimental Biology and Medicine*, **37**, 598

Hurtado, A. (1964*a*). Animals in high altitudes: resident man. In *Handbook of Physiology*, Section 4:

Adaptation to the Environment (D.B. Dill, Ed.). Washington DC; American Physiological Society, p.843

Hurtado, A. (1964*b*). Some physiologic and clinical aspects of life at high altitudes. In *Aging of the Lung* (L. Cander and J.H. Moyer, Ed.). New York; Grune and Stratton, p.257

Johnson, K.M., Wiebenga, N.H., Mackenzie, R.B., Kuns, M.L., Tauraso, N.M., Shelokov, A., Webb, P.A., Justines, G., and Beye, H.K. (1965). Virus isolations from human cases of haemorrhagic fever in Bolivia. *Proceedings of the Society for Experimental Biology and Medicine*, **118**, 113

Johnson, K.M., Kuns, M.L., Mackenzie, R.B., Webb, P.A., and Yunker, C.E. (1966). Isolation of Machupo virus from wild rodent *Calomys callosus*. *American Journal of Tropical Medicine and Hygiene*, **15**, 103

Kaplanski, A.S., Durnova, G.N., and Roschchina, N.A. (1968). Problemy Kosmicheskov Biologii. In *Problems in Space Biology*, Vol. 8. Moscow; 12d-vo Nauta, p.129

Keck, G. and Buchmeiser, R. (964). Existence and growth of bacteria at high altitude. In *The Physiological Effects of High Altitude* (W.H. Weihe, Ed.). Oxford; Pergamon Press, p.153

Kitayev, M.I. and Tokhtabayev, A.G. (1981). T and B lymphocytes as related to adaptation to high altitudes. *Kosmicheskaia Biologiia i Aviakosmicheskaia Meditsina*, **15**, 87

Krupina, T.N., Korotaev, M.M. Pukhova, IaI., *et al.* (1974). Characteristics of the human immunologic state during hypoxic hypoxia. *Kosmicheskaia Biologiia i Aviakosmicheskaia Meditsina*, **8**, 56

Krupina, T.N., Korotaev, M.M., and Pukhova, IaI. (1975). Comparative evaluation of studies of different levels of hypoxia on the human immunological status. *Kosmicheskaia Biologiia i Aviakosmicheskaia Meditsina*, **11**, 38

Manuel Moro, S. (1967). Influence of altitude in the incidence of anthrax in Peru. *Federation Proceedings*, **26**, 1593

Meehan, R.T. (1987). Immune suppression at high altitude. *Annals of Emergency Medicine*, **16**, 974

Meehan, R., Duncan, U., Neale, L., Taylor, G., Muchmore, H., Scott, N., Ramsey, K., Smith, E., Rock, P., Goldblum, R., and Houston, C. (1988). Operation Everest II: Alterations in the immune system at high altitudes. *Journal of Clinical Immunology*, **8**, 1988

Meerson, F.Z., Evseev, V.A., Davydove, T.V., *et al.* (1980). Effect of adaptation to high altitude hypoxia on non specific resistance, haemaglutinin production and the development of adjuvant arthritis in rats. *Byulleten Eksperimental Noi Biologii i Meditsiny*, **89**, 12

Memeo, S.A., Piantanelli, L., Mazzufferi, G., Guerra, L., Nikolitz, M., and Fabris, N. (1982). Age related patterns of immunoglobulin serum levels in the Quechua Indians of Andean Mountains. *International Journal of Biometeorology*, **26**, 49

Mills, J., Hauer, L., Gottlieb, A., Dromgoole, S., and Spruance, S. (1987). Recurrent herpes labialis in skiers. Clinical observations and effect of sunscreen. *American Journal of Sports Medicine*, **15**, 76

Mirrakhimov, M.M. and Kitayev, M.I. (1978). Basic trends of immunologic studies of high altitude adaptation. *Zdravookhranenie Kirgizii*, **6**, 3

Mirrakhimov, M.M., Tulebekov, B.T., Kitaev, M.I., Amanturova, K.A., and Saburov, K.A. (1979). Immunophysiological aspects of human adaptation to life at high altitudes. *Human Physiology*, **5**, 203

Morrison-Smith, J. (1981). The use of high altitude treatment for childhood asthma. *The Practitioner*, **225**, 1663

Morrow, R.H., Gutesohn, N., and Smith, P.G. (1976). Epstein–Barr virus malaria interaction models for Burkitt's lymphoma: implication for preventing trials. *Cancer Research*, **36**, 667

Muchmore, H.T., Parkinson, A.J., and Scott, E.N. (1981). Nasopharyngeal secretory immune and nonimmune substances in personnel at South Pole, 1978 winter-over period. *Antarctic Journal of the United States*, **16**, 181

Munck, A., Guyre, P.M., and Holbrook, N.I. (1984). Physiological functions of glucocorticoids in stress and their reaction to pharmacologic actions. *Endocrine Reviews*, **5**, 25

Murphy, F.A., Webb, P.A., Johnson, K.M., and Whitfield, S.G. (1969). Morphological comparison of Machupo with lymphocytic choriomeningitis virus. Basis for a new taxonomic group. *Journal of Virology*, **4**, 535

Murphy, F.A., Webb, P.A., Johnson, K.M., Whitfield, S.G., and Chappel, W.A. (1970). Arenovirus in Vero Cells: ultrastructural studies. *Journal of Virology*, **6**, 507

Noble, J., Valverde, L., Eguia, O.E., Serrate, O., and Antezana, E. (1974). Hemorrhagic exanthem of Bolivia. Studies of an unusual hemorrhagic disease in high altitude dwellers at sea level. *American Journal of Epidemiology*, **99**, 123

Noguchi, H. and Battistini, T.S. (1926). Etiology of Oroya fever I. Cultivation of *Bartonella bacilliformis*. *Journal of Experimental Medicine*, **43**, 851

Nusshag, W. (1954). *Hygiene der Haustiere*. Leipzig; Verlag S., Hirzel, p.86

Pinkerton, H. and Weinman, D. (1937a). Carrion's disease I. Behaviour of the etiological agent without cells growing or surviving *in vitro*. *Proceedings of the Society for Experimental Biology and Medicine*, **37**, 587

Pinkerton, H. and Weinman, D. (1937b). Carrion's Disease. II. Comparative morphology of the etiological agent in Oroya fever and *Verruga peruana*. *Proceedings of the Society for Experimental Biology and Medicine*, **37**, 591

Recavarren, S. and Lumbreras, H. (1972). Pathogenesis of verruga of Carrion's disease. *American Journal of Pathology*, **66**, 461

Ribante, E., Lemesre, J.L., Rodriguez, C., Carrasco, R., Breniere, F., Antezana, G., Raynaud, J., and Carlier, Y. (1986). Bioenergetic and cardiovascular responses to exercise in residents at 2,850 m with asymptomatic Chagas' disease. *Tropical and Geographical Medicine*, **38**, 150

Ricketts, W.E. (1949). Clinical manifestations of Carrion's disease. *Archives of Internal Medicine*, **84**, 751

Rippel-Baldes, A. (1952). *Grundriss der Mikrobiologie*. Berlin; Springer Verlag, p.281

Rowe, W.P., Murphy, F.A., Bergold, G.H., Casals, J., Hotchin, J., Johnson, K.M., Lehmann-Grube, F., Mims, C.A., Traub, E., and Webb, P.A. (1970). Arenoviruses: proposed name for a newly defined virus group. *Journal of Virology*, **5**, 651

Rufli, M., Rufli, T., and Schuppli, R. (1969). Étude comparative experimentale et clinique de l'allergie aux mite. *Medecine et Hygiene*, **887**, 1139

Schaefer, R.M., Kokot, K., Heidland, A., and Plass, R. (1987). Jogger's leukocytes. *New England Journal of Medicine*, **316**, 223

Schultz, M.G. (1968). Daniel Carrion's experiment. *New England Journal of Medicine*, **278**, 1323

Selkon, J. and Gould, J.C. (1966). In *Report on IBP Expedition to North Bhutan* (F.S. Jackson, R.W.D. Turner, and M.P. Ward. Ed.). London; Royal Society, p.88

Sever, J.L. (1982). Infections in pregnancy. Highlights from the collaborative perinatal project. *Teratology*, **25**, 227

Singh, I. and Chohan, I.S. (1972. Abnormalities of blood coagulation of high altitude. *International Journal of Biometeorology*, **16**, 283

Singh, I., Chohan, I.S., Lal, M., Khanna, P.K., Srivastava, M.C., Nanda, R.B., Lamba, J.S., and Malhotra, M.S. (1977). Effects of high altitude stay on the incidence of common diseases in man. *International Journal of Biometeorology*, **21**, 193

Speechly-Dick, M.E., Rimmer, S.J., and Hodson, M.E. (1992). Exacerbations of cystic fibrosis after holidays at high altitude — a cautionary tale. *Respiratory Medicine*, **86**, 55

Speelberg, B., Folgering, H.T., Sterk, D.J., and van-Herwaarden, C.L. (1992). Lung function of adult patients with bronchial asthma or chronic obstructive lung disease prior to and following a 3-month-stay in the Dutch Asthma Center in Davos. *Nederlands Tijdschrift voor Geneeskunde (Amsterdam)*, **136**, 469

Spieksma, F.T.M., Zuidema, P., and Leupen, M.J. (1971). High altitude and house dust mites. *British Medical Journal*, **1**, 82

Strauss, R.H., McFadden, E.R., Ingram, R.H., Peal, E.C., and Jaeger, J.J. (1978). Influence of heat and humidity on the airway obstruction induced by exercise in asthma. *Journal of Clinical Investigation*, **61**, 433

Sutton, J. (1971). Daniel Carrion and Oroya fever. *Medical Journal of Australia*, **2**, 589

Tengerdy, R.P. and Kramer, T. (1968). Immune response of rabbits during short term exposure to high altitude. *Nature*, **217**, 367

Trapani, I.L. (1969). Environment, infection and immunoglobulin synthesis. *Federation Proceedings*, **28**, 1104

Vervloet, D., Penaud, A., Razzouk, H., Senft, M., Arnaud, A., Boutin, C., and Charpin, J. (1982). Altitude and house dust mites. *Journal of Allergy and Clinical Immunology*, **69**, 290

Verzar, F. (1952). Die Zahl der Lymphocyten und eosinophilen. Leukocyten in 1800 und 3450 m Hohe. *Schweizerische Medizinische Wochenschrift*, **82**, 324

Voorhorst, R., Spieksma, F.T., Varekamp, H., Leupen, M.J., and Luklema, A.W. (1969). Recent progress in the house dust mite problem. *Acta Allergologica*, **24**, 115

Ward, M.P., Milledge, J.S., and West, J.B. (1989). Reaction to Cold. In *High Altitude Medicine and Physiology*. London; Chapman and Hall Medical, p.350

Weinman, D. (1944). Infectious anaemia due to Bartonella and related red cell parasites. *Transactions of the American Philosophical Society*, **33**, 243

Weinman, D. and Pinkerton, H. (1937*a*). Carrion's Disease. III. Experimental production in animals. *Proceedings of the Society for Experimental Biology and Medicine*, **37**, 594

Weinman, D. and Pinkerton, H. (1937*b*). Carrion's Disease. IV. Natural sources of Bartonella in the endemic zone. *Proceedings of the Society for Experimental Biology and Medicine*, **37**, 596

Weiser, O.L., Peoples, N.J., Tull, A.H., and Morse, W.C. (1969). Effect of altitude on the microbiota of man. *Federation Proceedings: Federation of American Societies for Experimental Biology*, **28**, 1107

Wilson G.S. and Miles, A. (1975). Virus diseases. Group characterized by general infection. In *Topley and Wilson's Principles of Bacteriology, Virology and Immunology*, 6th edn. London; Edward Arnold

Wintrobe, M.M., Lee, G.R., Boggs, D.R., Bithell, T.C., Athens, J.W., and Foerster, J. (1974). *Clinical Haematology*, 7th edn. Philadelphia; Lea and Febiger

Zhuravkin, I.N., Lozovoi, V.P., and Kozlov, V.A. (1978). Antibody-forming capacity of mouse spleen cells after hypoxic hypoxia and injection of erythropoietin. *Byulleten Eksperimental Noi Biologii i Meditsiny*, **85**, 565

27

High-altitude retinopathy and special senses

The retinal circulation is of interest in high-altitude studies because it presents for direct ophthalmoscopic examination a sample of systemic arteries and veins under the stimulus of chronic hypoxia.

RETINAL CIRCULATION ON EXPOSURE TO HYPOXIA

Pronounced changes occur in the retinal circulation in most subjects on acute exposure to high altitude. After only 2 hours at 5330 m retinal arteries and veins increase in diameter by about a fifth (Fig. 27.1; Frayser *et al.* 1971). Under these conditions retinal blood flow increases by some 90% (Fig. 27.2), the retinal circulation time decreases (Fig. 27.3), and

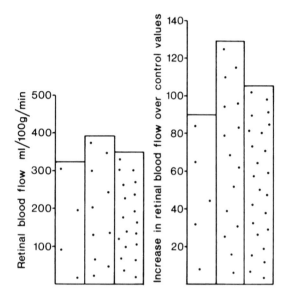

27.2 *Retinal blood flow expressed in ml/100 g per min and as a percentage increase over control values in the same subjects as in Fig. 27.1. The identification of the columns is as in that figure.*

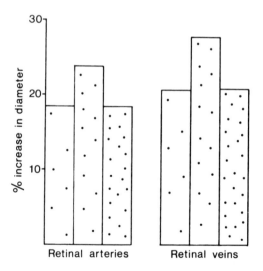

27.1 *Percentage increase in diameter in the retinal arteries and veins in nine males between 20 and 40 years of age (mean age 25.9 years) after 2 hours at 5330 m (very lightly stippled columns), and after 5 days at the same altitude (lightly stippled columns) and in nine males between 21 and 40 years of age (mean age 27.3 years) who had been at 5330 m for 5–7 weeks (medium stippled columns). (Data in this figure and in Figs 27.2–27.4 are from Frayser* et al. *(1971).)*

the retinal vascular blood volume increases (Fig. 27.4). These trends increase over the following 5 days at this altitude and then revert to the levels found initially on exposure to high altitude (Frayser *et al.* 1971). Duguet *et al.* (1947) had reported earlier that dilatation of the retinal vessels became apparent at 1830 m and maximal at 5490 m. In contradistinction to the later studies of Frayser *et al.* (1971) they found no further increase in vessel size after 15 minutes at this altitude.

Hypocapnia without hypoxia significantly reduces retinal blood flow (Hickam and Frayser 1966). Thus, at an elevation of 5330 m, restoration of the systemic arterial oxygen saturation from 70% to 95% at the prevailing arterial carbon dioxide tension of 24 mmHg will decrease retinal flow by about half to approximately sea-level values (Frayser *et al.* 1974). There is a significant decrease in retinal flow

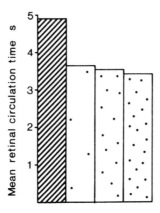

27.3 *Mean retinal circulation time in seconds in the same subjects as in Fig. 27.1. The identification of the columns is as in that figure, with the addition that the hatched column shows values obtained on nine subjects at 790 m.*

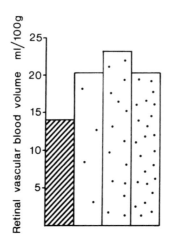

27.4 *Retinal vascular blood volume (ml/100 g) in the same subjects as in Fig. 27.1. The identification of the columns is as in Fig. 27.3.*

after 9 days at high altitude as compared with 5 days, suggesting that the tone of retinal vessels may become reset at the prevailing tension of carbon dioxide and that hypoxia becomes the predominant controlling factor in regulating retinal flow at high altitude. There is an analogy here to the resetting of the medullary respiratory receptor to lower partial pressures of carbon dioxide, as described in Chapter 4. Meehan *et al.* (1986) investigated and disproved the hypothesis that vasodilator prostaglandins are involved in the pathogenesis of hypoxia-induced

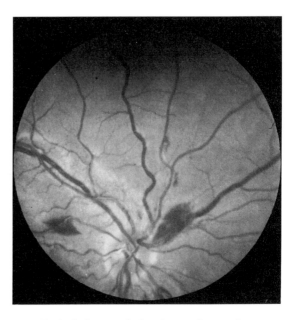

27.5 *Retinal photograph showing two haemorrhages which occurred in a climber ascending above 5000 m.*

retinal vasodilatation by using the cyclooxygenase inhibitor, naproxen, to see if it prevents the retinal engorgement. This non-steroidal anti-inflammatory drug proved to have no effect.

RETINAL HAEMORRHAGES

Retinal haemorrhages (Fig. 27.5) may occur on ascending to above 4000 m. The first report of their occurrence appears to have been made in July 1968 when they were found in two persons working at 5330 m on Mt Logan in the Yukon territory. One of them developed papilloedema and became semicomatose. The following year the Arctic Institute undertook a pilot study of the retinal circulation at high altitude. Twenty-five subjects were studied in groups exposed to different conditions of ascent (Frayser *et al.* 1970). Eight mountaineers climbed to the laboratory at 5330 m and stopped there for 7 weeks. Seven scientists and 10 volunteers were flown directly to the area and remained for 2–10 days. Some of them were given acetazolamide before ascent or frusemide for 1–3 days after arrival. None of the subjects going to high altitude had retinal disease. Three of the eight mountaineers who ascended slowly developed retinal haemorrhage, as did six of 17 subjects who ascended rapidly. Hence there was no correlation between the occurrence of retinal haemorrhages and the speed of ascent.

Similarly, there was no relation to the severity of headache or other symptoms of acute mountain sickness. Neither acetazolamide nor frusemide prevented the retinal haemorrhages. All but one of the affected subjects were unaware of the presence of bleeding. However, in the ninth subject the haemorrhage occurred at the macula and resulted in a scotoma. This man developed the haemorrhage while he was sitting quietly after having been at altitude for 9.5 days. On examination he had papilloedema with prominently tortuous retinal arteries and veins.

High as the incidence of retinal haemorrhage (36%) was in this group, changes in the blood vessels of the retina of the type described above were even higher. Indeed pronounced hyperaemia around the optic disc, tortuosity, and increased diameter of veins and arteries appeared in all subjects within a few days of arrival at high altitude and persisted throughout the whole length of the stay. Frayser *et al.* (1970) injected fluorescein and were unable to detect leakage from the vessels. There was a substantial increase in retinal blood flow, with a fall in retinal mean circulation time from 4.9 seconds at 610 m to 3.4 seconds at 5330 m. Hence the retinal vessels were maximally dilated in the presence of increased retinal blood flow. However, fluorescein leakage was noted after exercise in eight of 20 climbers tested and was associated with exercise-induced retinal haemorrhages (McFadden *et al.* 1981).

Schumacher and Petajan (1975) studied 39 subjects who spent up to 24 days above 4330 m on Mt McKinley. No fewer than 14 of the group developed retinal haemorrhage, which was commoner in those with high-altitude headache. There was an association with rapid ascent above 4200 m. 'Quick dashes' to the summit of Mt McKinley from 3000 m gave rise to retinal haemorrhage in six of nine climbers. Such bleeding is unlikely to occur at rest below 5300 m.

Retinal haemorrhage is now recognized as a well-documented complication of ascent to high altitude (Rennie and Morrissey 1975; Wiedman 1975; Shults and Swan 1975). They occur in about one-third to one-half of all persons exposed to altitudes above 5000 m (McFadden *et al.* 1981). Rennie and Morrissey (1975) described retinal changes that occurred in the members of the American Expedition to Dhaulagiri, Nepal (8170 m), the sixth highest mountain in the world. They studied 15 subjects, retinal photographs being taken at sea level and at 5880 m, after each climber had descended from his highest point. Five Nepali Sherpas were also studied. Vascular engorgement with tortuosity was observed, with an increase of 24% in retinal arterial diameter and an increase of 23% in diameter of retinal veins. Retinal haemorrhages were seen in one-third of the American climbers, but in none of the Sherpas. Shults and Swan (1975) reported their occurrence in four of six surviving members of a climbing expedition on Aconcagua (6920 m) in Argentina, the highest mountain in the Western Hemisphere. Two were left with permanently disturbed vision with paracentral scotomas. Clarke and Duff (1976) reported the development of retinal haemorrhages in four of six Britons of the successful 1975 British Everest Expedition who were newcomers to altitudes over 6000 m, in two of 14 Britons who had previously visited these altitudes, and in two of the 75 Sherpas with the expedition. Thirty-nine healthy subjects were examined before and after a stay on Mt Logan (5360 m) in the Canadian Yukon by ophthalmoscopy and by retinal photography by McFadden *et al.* (1981). Eleven were acclimatized mountaineers, 16 newly-arrived climbers, and 12 were persons flown up from 3280 m. Twenty-three were men and 11 were women. No fewer than 22 of these subjects (56%) developed retinal haemorrhages. Even more remarkable observations were made on an expedition to Peak Communism (7495 m) during which 15 of the 16 members were afflicted by retinal haemorrhages (Nakashima 1983). In contrast to this only small asymptomatic retinal haemorrhages were found in five eyes of four of the 14 members of the 1989 American Everest Expedition after 6 weeks of exposure to altitudes between 5300 and 8200 m (Butler *et al.* 1992). It is of interest that this low incidence of retinal haemorrhages was associated with a carefully controlled rate of ascent. Nevertheless, an additional eye of one of the affected climbers had a central retinal vein occlusion with vitreous haemorrhages. High-altitude retinopathy does not seem to have been reported in studies with decompression chambers and this is probably because the simulated altitude in these investigations is usually limited in duration and magnitude (McFadden *et al.* 1981).

Form

Retinal haemorrhages are usually located throughout the fundus without involving the macula. They may be diffuse, punctate, confluent, or flame-shaped (see Fig. 27.5). Clarke and Duff (1976) described several flame-haemorrhages near the left optic disc of a 28-year-old Briton on the successful ascent of the south-west face of Everest in 1975. Duff himself developed them near the right optic disc, together with gross retinal venous tortuosity. Retinal haemorrhages at high altitude may extend into the vitreous (Wiedman 1975). Those involving the macula are infrequent and may be solitary or occur in conjunction with diffuse haemorrhage into the posterior pole of the fundus.

Relation to intraocular pressure

It has been suggested that hypoxic vasodilatation makes retinal vessels more vulnerable to sudden rises in intraocular pressure and the site of haemorrhage (Rennie and Morrisey 1975). However, the relationship remains controversial. Clarke and Duff (1976) measured the intraocular pressure of climbers ascending Mt Everest with a Perkins tonometer. Readings had to be confined to the early part of the expedition because the investigation was unpopular with the climbers. Readings were normal, however, up to an elevation of 6000 m. On the other hand, Butler *et al.* (1992) found a statistically significant association between the development of retinal haemorrhages at high altitude and a higher intraocular pressure at sea level.

Cause

Only rarely are retinal haemorrhages developing in subjects ascending to high altitude a warning sign of impending cerebral oedema. Here they become associated with bilateral papilloedema and herald the onset of cerebral mountain sickness (Chapter 14). Under these circumstances a sudden increase of cerebral pressure leads to effusion of cerebrospinal fluid into the optic nerve-sheath causing it to swell and compress the central retinal vein. Compression of the retinochoroidal anastomosis produces retinal venous hypertension and haemorrhage (Muller and Deck 1974; *British Medical Journal* 1975).

Far more commonly, high-altitude retinal haemorrhages are benign and they appear to be related to the increased blood flow through the dilated retinal vessels described earlier in the chapter. Many authorities believe that this vascular congestion is exaggerated by the extreme physical exertion and concomitant Valsalva manoeuvre required in mountain climbers (Shults and Swan 1975). McFadden *et al.* (1981) found that after maximal exertion on a cycle ergometer at 5360 m fresh retinal haemorrhages were found in seven of 34 subjects. Even the persistent, non-productive cough characteristic of high altitude has been held to be a factor in the causation of this bleeding (Butler *et al.* 1992).

In the early report on high-altitude retinal haemorrhages by Frayser *et al.* (1970) it was concluded that there was no relation between their development and the speed of ascent. A recent study by Butler *et al.* (1992) has suggested otherwise. They found a low incidence of retinal haemorrhages in members of the American Everest Expedition in 1989. The bleeds were few in number and small, although the altitudes concerned were extreme and the climbers included many who had no recent exposure to conditions of high altitude and who had suffered prolonged exposure to altitude before examination of the eyes. In spite of all these factors the incidence of retinal haemorrhage was low and Butler *et al.* (1992) thought that this was due to the carefully controlled gradual ascent used in trekking to base camp. Arterial oxygen saturation at 5300 m was not found to have a significant correlation with high-altitude retinal haemorrhage (Butler *et al.* 1992).

Another factor that has been suggested as involved in the causation of these haemorrhages is occasional-to-frequent medication by non-steroidal anti-inflammatory drugs (Butler *et al.* 1992). Retinal haemorrhages may be produced in monkeys and rabbits by exposing them to simulated high altitude (Sakaguchi *et al.* 1988).

Course

The majority of the high-altitude retinal haemorrhages absorb spontaneously without loss of visual acuity. Descent is the immediate treatment. Both Everest climbers with flame-haemorrhages reported by Clarke and Duff (1976) had normal fundi at 1500 m after leaving the mountain. The use of frusemide or acetazolamide for prevention or therapy is inconclusive (Wiedman 1975). Subjects in whom retinal haemorrhages have once occurred should be advised against returning above 3050 m, so as to avoid recurrences.

The clinical effects and prognosis are not always so encouraging. As noted earlier in the chapter, scotomata may develop if the retinal haemorrhages occur in the region of the macula (Frayser *et al.* 1970). One of the climbers in the 1989 American Everest Expedition developed central retinal vein occlusion with vitreous haemorrhage which reduced visual acuity to counting fingers (Butler *et al.* 1992).

'COTTON-WOOL SPOTS'

Hackett and Rennie (1982) reported 'cotton-wool' spots in the retina of a Japanese high-altitude climber who spent 17 days at altitudes between 5200 and 6600 m. This young man of 29 years complained of 'blind spots' and 'foggy vision' that affected central vision. By the time he had descended to 4250 m, he had regained normal visual acuity and visual fields were unimpaired. Funduscopic examination revealed retinal haemorrhages and cotton-wool spots. One year later he was reported to be in good health.

Such so-called 'soft exudates' form ill-defined small white areas resembling cotton wool in the inner retina. On histological examination the cotton-wool spot in most ophthalmological conditions represent microinfarction of the nerve-fibre and ganglion-cell layers of the retina. The damaged segment becomes oedematous and contains the bulbous tips of disrupted axons called cytoid bodies (Hume Adams and Graham 1985). This change occurs as the result of focal occlusive disease in the retinal blood vessels. Cotton-wool spots are characteristic of hypertensive and diabetic retinopathies. In the case of systemic hypertension the focal retinal ischaemia is thought to be caused by angiospastic arteriolar disease. Hence it is possible that the cotton-wool spots occurring rarely in the retina of high-altitude climbers may be the result of temporary spasm of the retinal arterioles, perhaps as a consequence of hypocapnia. McLeod *et al.* (1977) believed that the cotton-wool spots of ischaemic necrosis were the result of a combination of hypoxia and hypoperfusion. Since hypoxia alone does not cause hypoperfusion, another mechanism must be involved, possibly microembolization from platelet aggregates that are known to develop during hypoxia or hypobaria. Such platelet aggregates may cause the pale centre occasionally seen in high-altitude retinal haemorrhages (McFadden *et al.* 1981). Extensive 'cotton-wool spots' were reported as developing in association with numerous retinal haemorrhages in an acclimatized and asymptomatic female mountaineer by McFadden *et al.* (1981).

SNOW BLINDNESS

This condition is brought about by exposure of the corneal epithelium to ultraviolet radiation, which at high altitude is both increased in amount and shows a change in spectral intensity to the more damaging short wavelengths (Chapter 2). At the same time the effects are enhanced at high altitude under snow conditions by the extreme reflection of ultraviolet rays by the snow surface, the so-called albedo (Chapter 2). Initially, there is damage to the corneal epithelium and this solar keratitis may proceed to actual blistering of the cornea. This damage leads to severe symptoms a few hours after exposure to the intense ultraviolet radiation. Commonly there is severe photophobia and blepharospasm. Because of the intense pain the affected subject can hardly bear to open his eyes to the light and so is, in effect, blind — hence the term 'snow blindness'. There is intense congestion of the conjunctiva. Areas of ulceration of the cornea will stain with fluorescein.

The condition may be prevented by wearing goggles or dark glasses with side protectors. The latter are recommended because even light entering from the side can be strong enough to damage the corneal epithelium (Brandt and Malla 1982). In an emergency, horizontal slits can be cut into a piece of cardboard that can be tied around the head with string. The pain and spasm may be treated by anaesthetic drops (Steele 1976). Brandt and Malla (1982) recommended application of ointment and a patch for 24 hours after which the cornea is generally healed without complication.

SUBCONJUNCTIVAL HAEMORRHAGE

This condition is common enough at sea level in middle-aged people, especially if they are hypertensive. It has been reported as occurring with the onset of acute mountain sickness (Brandt and Malla 1982), but it is harmless and requires no treatment as it is resorbed spontaneously within 1 or 2 weeks.

VISUAL ACUITY

It has been known for many years that visual acuity is impaired at high altitude (McFarland and Evans 1939). Sensitivity to light and ability to make out objects is already somewhat impaired at elevations as low as 1220–1520 m and at 4880 m it may be only half of what it is at sea level (McFarland 1972). When the intensity of illumination is high, there is little or no impairment of vision until an altitude of some 5490 m is exceeded, but, when it is low, diminished visual acuity becomes apparent at elevations as low at 2440 m (McFarland and Halperin 1940). Denison (1986) believes this failure to see faint objects in subdued light is highly characteristic of acute exposure to the hypoxia of altitudes as moderate as 1200–2400 m.

Deterioration in night vision appears to be a pure response to hypoxia (Denison 1986). Halperin *et al.* (1959) found that the inhalation of 100% oxygen reversed within a few minutes the diminution in visual acuity induced by exposure for 3–4 hours to a simulated altitude of between 2130 and 5030 m. During the Battle of Britain, night blindness became a problem in fighter pilots. It was almost complete at an altitude of 3660 m, but found to be totally reversible, not by large amounts of vitamin A but by oxygen inhalation (Robinson 1973). It is clear that the retinal rods, which are responsible for night vision, are very sensitive to hypoxia.

Kobrick *et al.* (1984) studied eight subjects who were exposed to a simulated altitude of 4600 m for 48 hours. They were periodically measured for near and far visual acuity, stereopsis, binocular depth perception, dark adaptation, and response time to peripheral visual signals. Performance on all visual tasks showed similar decrements, which occurred rapidly and reached their maximum extent within approximately 1 hour of exposure. Thereafter there was a gradual recovery over the remaining interval. The impairment noted appeared to be due to the effects of hypoxia acting directly on the visual system.

COLOUR VISION

Colour vision is affected by exposure to the hypobaric hypoxia of high altitude and the alterations observed have interesting clinical and endocrinological associations. Richalet *et al.* (1989) studied eight healthy male lowlanders between the ages of 25 and 40 years with normal colour vision. Colour vision tests were performed every 2 hours from 08.00 to 20.00 hours at Créteil (60 m) and at the Observatoire Vallot on Mont Blanc (4350 m) over a period of 79 hours. Colour vision was tested with two portable anomaloscopes, both exploring the green/red axis. One was derived from the Chromotest (Essilor) apparatus and the other from the OSCAR tester (Objective Screening of Colour Anomalies and Reductions). The principle of the first apparatus was to produce a mixed colour with a bicolour light-emitting diode (green 565 nm, red 635 nm) in order to balance a reference, fixed yellow of 583 nm. Alterations in colour vision are indicated by changes in the green/red luminance, an increased value of the green–red ratio corresponding to a relative decrease in sensitivity to green compared to sensitivity to red. At the same time these workers attempted to quantify the severity of acute mountain sickness by awarding points to the extent of a list of symptoms. At the same time plasma cortisol and adrenocorticotrophic hormone (ACTH) concentrations were measured at various times during the day.

The results of this study showed a decrease in sensitivity to green compared to red in the environment of hypobaric hypoxia at high altitude. This confirms the findings of other workers (Kobrick *et al.* 1984). Alterations in colour vision were particularly clear in the morning, and values tended to return to nor-

moxic levels during the course of the day. Other studies have reported modifications of colour sensitivity to be greater for blue (Menu and Santucci 1985).

Significant diurnal variations were noted with both anomaloscopes. A significant decrease in the green/red luminance ratio was found according to the hour of the day. As we note in Chapter 22, one of the components of disturbed endocrinology at high altitude is the increase of cortisol levels on ascent. The diurnal rhythm in plasma cortisol concentrations is well known and Richalet *et al.* (1989) found that this diurnal rhythm was maintained at high altitude. They found that the peak concentration generally observed around 05.00 in normoxia is maintained in hypobaric hypoxia. They suggest that exposure to altitude hypoxia induces an increase in plasma cortisol that can transiently alter diurnal rhythm on the day of exposure but that this rhythm is restored after the first night at high altitude.

Diurnal variations in acute mountain sickness (AMS) were also found and they were parallel to those of plasma cortisol and modifications of colour vision. Instant AMS scores were found to be correlated significantly to corresponding plasma cortisol levels. Parallel variations in colour vision, plasma cortisol levels, and severity of acute mountain sickness suggested to Richalet *et al.* (1989) that the use of anomaloscopes may quantify in a simple and objective way the intensity of symptoms of acute mountain sickness. In this respect luminance threshold shifts at selected wavelengths (red, green, and blue) might be worth exploring. No causal relationship between the parallel variations in colour vision, acute mountain sickness, and plasma cortisol could be established but cerebral oedema may be involved.

AUDITORY SENSITIVITY

In contrast to the decrement in visual acuity at high altitude, auditory sensitivity appears to be resistant to hypoxia. Curry and Boys (1956) found no difference between initial threshold values at sea level for both air- and bone-conducted hearing and those found after an exposure to a simulated altitude of 4570 m for 30 min. On the other hand, Klein *et al.* (1961) found that exposure to hypobaric hypoxia led to a diminution in auditory sensitivity at the lower frequencies and a slight improvement at 4096 Hz. A subsequent study by Klein (1961) under similar hypoxic conditions confirmed a significant loss of bone-conducted thresholds at frequencies lower than 1024 Hz, but enhancement at 4096 Hz.

Singh *et al.* (1976) studied 54 healthy Indian troops between the ages of 17 and 30 years at low altitude (210 m) and at an elevation of 3500 m after passive transport there by air. A pure-tone audiogram showed loss of both low and high tone on arrival at high altitude. This was reversible and returned to normal after a stay of 4 days at high altitude. The threshold of hearing under the conditions of the test carried out by these authors was consistently better in native highlanders than in lowlanders, but this was possibly attributable to the absence of background noise in the mountains.

VESTIBULAR FUNCTION

Studies by Singh *et al.* (1976) on soldiers in the Himalaya suggest that there is a reversible alteration in vestibular function on exposure to high altitude. More than half of 53 soldiers from sea level showed signs of vestibular upset, in the form of swaying, soon after arrival at 3500 m. After a period of 6 months of acclimatization all signs of disturbance had gone in 26 of these men. There was never evidence of swaying at any time in 36 highlanders native to the same region. About one-third of these soldiers freshly arrived in the mountains also developed spontaneous nystagmus at the same time as the swaying. These Indian investigators point out that abnormalities of the cerebral blood flow run parallel with abnormal findings on audiological and vestibular testing, both returning to normal after 4–5 days' sojourn at high altitude. This suggests to them that disturbances of inner ear function are the result of the altered haemodynamics induced by acute exposure to high altitude.

THE MIDDLE EAR AND RAPID ASCENT TO HIGH ALTITUDE

The middle ear is an air-containing cavity surrounded on all sides by bone (Fig. 27.6). It is lined by mucous membrane and contains the three auditory ossicles. If this cavity were completely closed, a sudden change in barometric pressure such as occurs on rapid ascent to high altitude would lead to a different pressure on the outside of the tympanic membrane from that on the inside. This dangerous situation is, however, avoided because there is a communication between the middle ear and pharynx (Fig. 27.6). This is the pharyngotympanic (Eustachian) tube, which opens at the posterior extremity of the inferior turbinate bone, but which is not permanently open. It is shut by a valve that is relaxed during the act of swallowing and, while it is open, it permits the pressure in the middle ear to

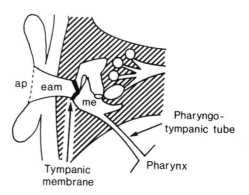

27.6 *Connections of the pharyngotympanic tube, which allows equalization of the pressure in the middle ear (me) with the atmospheric pressure (ap) in the external auditory meatus (eam).*

become the same as that of the ambient air. Variation in pressure on either side of the ear drum is thus prevented. Nevertheless, an uncomfortable feeling of pressure in the ears associated with temporary deafness is not uncommonly associated with rapid ascent to altitude as occurs at take-off in aircraft or in cable-cars travelling to the summits of volcanoes or Swiss peaks. Avoidance of this unpleasant sensation is achieved by repeated swallowing, and many airlines offer their passengers sweets to chew to equalize pressure on either side of the tympanic membrane. A cold in the head will prevent proper equalization of pressure due to blockage of the Eustachian tube by exudate or by pressure from without by inflammatory exudate or swollen lymphoid tissue. Such upper respiratory infections may lead to a persistence of aural symptoms for several days after descent from high altitude.

GUSTATORY SENSITIVITY

The four basic tastes of salt, sour, bitter, and sweet appear to become less sensitive on ascent to moderate altitude. Increasing molar concentrations of sodium chloride, citric acid, caffeine, and sucrose, representative of the four tastes, were presented to six women and their threshold value for each taste determined at sea level and various levels of simulated moderate altitude by Maga and Lorenz (1972). The composite taste response was most sensitive at sea level and there was a significant fall in this sensitivity even on ascending to an altitude as modest as 1520 m. No further decrement resulted on moving up to 3050 m. Grandjean (1955) had previously found that the thresholds of gustatory sensitivity to glucose, salt, tartaric acid, and quinine were diminished during exposure to a natural high altitude of 3450 m on the Jungfraujoch. The taste thresholds returned rapidly to normal on return to sea level. At higher altitudes it does not seem to be possible to detect further changes in gustatory sensitivity. Thus, Finkelstein and Pippett (1958) found that exposure to a simulated altitude of 7620 m for 2 hours with or without administration of 100% oxygen had no effect on taste perception.

References

Brandt, F. and Malla, O.K. (1982). Eye problems at high altitudes. In *High Altitude Physiology and Medicine* (W. Brendel and R.A. Zink, Ed.). New York; Springer Verlag, p.212

British Medical Journal (1975). High altitude retinal haemorrhage. *British Medical Journal*, **iii**, 663

Butler, F.K., Harris, D.J., and Reynolds, R.D. (1992). Altitude retinopathy on Mount Everest, 1989. *Ophthalmology*, **99**, 739

Clarke, C. and Duff, J. (1976). Mountain sickness, retinal haemorrhages, and acclimatization on Mount Everest in 1975. *British Medical Journal*, **ii**, 495

Curry, E.T. and Boys, F. (1956). Effects of oxygen on hearing sensitivity of simulated altitudes. *Eye, Ear, Nose and Throat Monthly*, **35**, 239

Denison, D. (1986). Where and how hypoxia works. In *Aspects of Hypoxia* (D. Heath, Ed.). Liverpool; Liverpool University Press, p. 241

Duguet, J., Dupont, P. and Baillant, J.P. (1947). The effects of anoxia on retinal vessels and retinal arterial pressure. *Journal of Aviation Medicine*, **18**, 516

Finkelstein, B. and Pippett, R.G. (1958). Effect of altitude upon primary taste perception. *Journal of Aviation Medicine*, **29**, 386

Frayser, R., Houston, C.S., Bryan, A.C., Rennie, I.D., and Gray, G. (1970). Retinal haemorrhage at high altitude. *New England Journal of Medicine*, **282**, 1183

Frayser, R. Houston, C.S., Gray, G.W., Bryan, A.C., and Rennie, I.D. (1971). The response of the retinal circulation to altitude. *Archives of Internal Medicine*, **127**, 708

Frayser, R., Gray, G.W., and Houston, C.S. (1974). Control of the retinal circulation at altitude. *Journal of Applied Physiology*, **37**, 302

Grandjean, E. (1955). The effect of altitude on various nervous functions. *Proceedings of the Royal Society*, **B 143**, 12

Hackett, P.H. and Rennie, D. (1982). Cotton-wool spots: a new addition to high altitude retinopathy. In *High Altitude Physiology and Medicine* (W. Brendel and R.A. Zink, Ed.). New York; Springer Verlag, p. 215

Halperin, M.H., McFarland, R.A., Niven, J.I., and Roughton, F.J.W. (1959). The time course of the effects of carbon monoxide on visual thresholds. *Journal of Physiology*, **146**, 583

Hickam, J.B. and Frayser, R. (1966). Studies of the retinal circulation in man. *Circulation*, **33**, 302

Hume Adams, J. and Graham, D.I. (1985). Nervous system and voluntary muscle. In *Muir's Textbook of Pathology*, 12th edn (J.R. Anderson, Ed). London; Edward Arnold, Ch. 21, p. 81

Klein, S.J. (1961). Effects of reduced oxygen intake on bone conducted hearing thresholds in a noisy environment. *Perceptual and Motor Skills*, **13**, 43

Klein, S.J., Mendelson, E.S., and Gallagher, T.J. (1961). The effects of reduced oxygen intake on auditory threshold shifts in a quiet environment. *Journal of Comparative and Physiological Psychology*, **54**, 401

Kobrick, J.L., Zwick, H., Witt, C.E., and Devine, J.A. (1984). Effects of extended hypoxia on night vision. *Aviation, Space, and Environmental Medicine*, **55**, 191

Maga, J.A. and Lorenz, K. (1972). Effects of altitude on taste thresholds. *Perceptual and Motor Skills*, **34**, 667

McFadden, D.M., Houston, C.S., Sutton, J.R., Powles, A.C.P., Gray, G.W., and Roberts, R.S. (1981). High-altitude retinopathy, *Journal of the American Medical Association*, **245**, 581

McFarland, R.A. (1972). Psychophysiological implications of life at altitude and including the role of oxygen in the process of aging. In *Physiological Adaptations. Desert and Mountain* (M.K. Yousef, S.M. Horvath, and R.W. Bullard, Ed.). New York; Academic Press, p. 157

McFarland, R.A. and Evans, J.N. (1939). Alterations in dark adaptation under reduced oxygen tensions. *American Journal of Physiology*, **127**, 37

McFarland, R.A. and Halperin, M.H. (1940). The relation between foveal visual acuity and illumination under reduced oxygen tension. *Journal of General Physiology*, **23**, 613

McLeod, D., Marshall, J., Kohner, E.M., and Bird, A.C. (1977). The role of axoplasmic transport in the pathogenesis of retinal cotton-wool spots. *British Journal of Ophthalmology*, **61**, 177

Meehan, R.T., Cymerman, A. Rock, P., Fulco, S.C., Hoffman, J., Abernathy, C., Needleman, S., and Maher, J.T. (1986). The effect of naproxen on acute mountain sickness and vascular responses to hypoxia. *American Journal of Medical Sciences*, **292**, 15

Menu, J.P. and Santucci, G. (1985). Contribution of contrast sensitivity to aerospace ergonomics. *Aviation, Space, and Environmental Medicine*, **56**, 497

Muller, P.J. and Deck., J.H.N. (1974). Intraocular and optic nerve sheath haemorrhage in cases of sudden intracranial hypertension. *Journal of Neurosurgery*, **41**, 160

Nakashima, M. (1983). High altitude medical research in Japan. *Japanese Journal of Mountain Medicine*, **3**, 23

Rennie, D. and Morrissey, J. (1975). Retinal changes in Himalayan climbers. *Archives of Ophthalmology*, **93**, 395

Richalet, J-P., Rutgers, V., Bouchet, P., Rymer, J-C., Kéromès, A., Duval-Arnould, G., and Rathat, C. (1989). Diurnal variations of acute mountain sickness, colour vision, and plasma cortisol and ACTH at high altitude. *Aviation, Space, and Environmental Medicine*, **60**, 105

Robinson, D.H. (1973). *The Dangerous Sky. A History of Aviation Medicine.* Henley-on-Thames, England; G.T. Foulis and Co

Sakaguchi, E., Osada, H., and Yurugi, R. (1988). Retinal hemorrhages under simulated altitude conditions in monkeys and rabbits. In *High-Altitude Medical Science* (G. Ueda, S. Kusama, and N.F. Voelkel, Ed.). Matsumoto, Japan; Shinshu University, p. 289

Schumacher, G.A. and Petajan, J.H. (1975). High altitude stress and retinal haemorrhage. *Archives of Environmental Health*, **30**, 217

Shults, W.T. and Swan, K.C. (1975). High altitude retinopathy in mountain climbers. *Archives of Ophthalmology*, **93**, 404

Singh, D. Kochhar, R.C., and Kacker, S.K. (1976). Effects of high altitude on inner ear functions. *Journal of Laryngology and Otology*, **90**, 1113

Steele, P. (1976). *Medical Care for Mountain Climbers.* London; William Heinemann

Wiedman, M. (1975). High altitude retinal haemorrhage. *Archives of Ophthalmology*, **93**, 401

28

Sleep

When lowlanders ascend to significant high altitude, they show disturbances of their sleep pattern and an onset of nocturnal periodic breathing associated with periods of apnoea. Native highlanders, on the other hand, do not appear to exhibit a similar sleep fragmentation. To understand these disturbances it is necessary first to consider the nature and types of sleep.

TYPES OF SLEEP

There are two varieties of sleep. The first, called 'orthodox sleep', is characterized by falls in peripheral vascular tone, systemic blood pressure, respiratory rate, and basal metabolic rate (by 5–25%). The heart beat is regular, the throat muscles tense, and the eyes quiescent. This variety of sleep is dreamless and restful. Orthodox sleep is considered to be composed of four stages. Stage I is a light, drowsy phase, the transition from wakefulness to sleep. Stage II is the first real stage of sleep. In the early stages of orthodox sleep the typical alpha rhythm (8–13 Hz) of wakefulness becomes more obvious and 'sleep spindles' (14–16 Hz) and 'K complexes' appear in the electroencephalogram (EEG) (Shapiro and Flanigan 1993). Stages III and IV are known collectively as 'slow-wave sleep' because in this deep sleep the EEG is characterized by delta waves of high voltage occurring at a rate of 1–2 per second. These big, slow delta waves appear to originate in the cerebral cortex in the face of reduced stimulation from the reticular activating system.

As people fall asleep they progress through the four stages of orthodox sleep and then, at low altitude, some 80 to 90 minutes after falling to sleep begin to show a second type of sleep that is characterized by rapid horizontal eye movements and that is, therefore, termed 'REM sleep'. There is a cycle of orthodox and REM sleep throughout the night. Bouts of REM sleep last 5–20 minutes and appear every hour and a half or so (Ward *et al.* 1989). As the night progresses the episodes of orthodox sleep become shorter and those of REM sleep longer. At low altitude most slow-wave sleep occurs during the first third of the night, and most REM sleep during the last third (Shapiro and Flanigan 1993). The EEG is much more like that of wakefulness with low-voltage waves but in spite of this it is more difficult to rouse the subject from sleep. In this deep 'paradoxical sleep' the throat muscles are relaxed and the heart rate and respiration become irregular (Oswald 1974). The brain remains active and dreaming is common. While muscle tone throughout the body is depressed there may be occasional muscle-twitching and limb-jerking (Ward *et al.* 1989).

It is generally accepted that energy that is expended during the day must be balanced by a recuperative period during sleep. Metabolic rate is reduced by 5–25% at night during sleep. Oxygen consumption, heart rate, and body temperature decline during the first few hours of sleep and particularly during slow-wave sleep (Shapiro and Flanigan 1993). Infants have the most slow-wave sleep and the amount declines with age. High energy expenditure during the day and sleep deprivation, perhaps producing a delayed drop in metabolic rate, are both associated with increased duration of sleep and increased deep-wave orthodox sleep. Thus the primary function of sleep appears to be to preserve energy.

In addition to the preservation of energy it is believed that sleep may be concerned with total body or neurological restoration. It is commonly believed that more orthodox sleep, particularly of the slow-wave type, is required when there has been weight loss or starvation as in hyperthyroidism. Low metabolic rates during sleep allow the net concentration of protein to increase as a result of both an increase in synthesis and a reduction in degradation. Growth hormone is released mainly at night, also in association with slow-wave sleep (Shapiro and Flanigan 1993).

It has been suggested that it is particularly the brain that recuperates during sleep. It has been postulated that REM sleep in particular is thought to allow protein synthesis in the brain. It predominates in infancy when the brain is growing, falls off in old age or in mentally retarded children, and may be important in the synthesis of durable memory proteins (Oswald 1974). Others believe that it is the cycling of orthodox and REM sleep that is fundamental to the restoration accomplished during sleep (Shapiro and Flanigan 1993). Each sleep cycle results in partial restoration of the brain, and after a number of cycles recuperation is complete, which reduces the need for further slow-wave sleep. This theory explains to some extent why the duration of periods of slow-wave sleep reduces over the course of a night's sleep (Shapiro and Flanigan 1993).

SLEEP IN EXPERIMENTAL RATS EXPOSED TO SIMULATED HIGH ALTITUDE

The effects of high altitude on sleep pattern and quality have been investigated experimentally in rats by Pappenheimer (1977). He studied how hypobaric hypoxia, simulating an altitude of 5500 m, altered the duration and depth of sleep in rats in which cortical electrodes had been chronically implanted. He found that during the daytime the proportion of time spent in slow-wave sleep fell from 45% when the rats were breathing air to 27% when they were exposed to 10% oxygen. The normal pattern of episodes of 5–15 minutes of slow-wave sleep was changed by hypoxia to a series of brief, incompletely developed episodes lasting 2–3 minutes. These effects on sleep were not altered by inhalation of carbon dioxide and appear to be due to hypoxia *per se*. With the fall in slow-wave sleep there was an increase in respiratory rate. Behaviourally, the hypoxic rats appeared to be restless and frequently turned around to curl up again as if to seek a more comfortable position (Pappenheimer 1977). REM sleep accounts for about 15% of the total daytime sleep of rats (Weiss and Roldan 1964). It is easily recognized in rats by twitching of their ears and vibrissae. REM sleep was found to be largely absent during prolonged hypoxia (Pappenheimer 1977).

SLEEP PATTERNS IN NEWCOMERS TO HIGH ALTITUDE

Newcomers to high altitude show disturbances of their sleep pattern reminiscent of those seen in rats. They wake more frequently during the night than at sea level (Reite *et al.* 1975; Weil *et al.* 1978). It is difficult to exclude the possibility that some of these awakenings are the result of periodic breathing, described below, that leads to apnoea, perhaps by the exertions of hyperventilation. There is deterioration

of the quality of sleep at high altitude. Light sleep (stages I and II of orthodox sleep referred to above) is increased but deep sleep (stages III and IV of orthodox sleep and REM sleep) is decreased. There is a deterioration in the quality of orthodox sleep at high altitude and Pappenheimer (1984) found that the amplitude of the cortical delta waves is much reduced at simulated high altitude.

In our personal experience in the Andes, rapid ascent to high altitude commonly induces feelings of tiredness and sleepiness to an extent that are quite disproportionate to the degree of physical activity undertaken. However, sleep is not the answer to this sense of tiredness but instead brings its own problems. In addition to the frequent arousals from light sleep, itself of poor quality, and the decrease in REM sleep, at high altitude there is the additional complicating factor of nocturnal period breathing described below. These disturbances lead to restless nights and the affected subject wakes up feeling unrefreshed and the persistent tiredness seeks relief from more sleep of this disturbed nature. A vicious circle is thus brought about and disturbances of sleep may persist for many days or even weeks at high altitude.

From a practical standpoint it has to be appreciated that disturbances of sleep experienced by lowlanders at high altitude are influenced by factors other than hypobaric hypoxia. Williams (1959) kept records on the sleeping habits of four subjects during 2 months of their normal life and during an expedition to the Karakorams where the elevations reached ranged form 3050 to 6100 m, the greater part of the time being spent at over 4570 m. He found that the new sleep patterns that emerged reflected the exigencies of mountaineering as much as the effects of high altitude. There was a tendency for the diurnal sleep–wakefulness pattern to coincide with the light–darkness cycle. All four subjects tended to sleep longer, with the hours of sleep moving forward to stretch from the early hours of the evening to very early the following morning, this being dictated by the sudden evening drop in temperature and the necessity for early morning starts.

NOCTURNAL PERIODIC BREATHING

One of the most characteristic features of sleep at high altitude is the development of periodic breathing with apnoea. It is a very common occurrence in newcomers to the mountains and has been reported at altitudes as low as 2440 m (Waggener *et al.* 1984). The phenomenon was studied by two groups during the American Medical Research Expedition to Mt Everest in 1981. Periodic breathing in lowlanders takes the form of three or four large breaths in quick succession, followed by cessation of breathing for about 10 seconds. The first respiratory movement after the apnoea is usually an inspiration and the volume and frequency of the succeeding breaths go through a crescendo, as seen in Cheyne–Stokes breathing. The sleep apnoea observed by Lahiri *et al.* (1983) was of central type, as both abdominal and rib-cage movements stopped, suggesting that the apnoeic periods are of central nervous origin rather than caused by airway obstruction.

West *et al.* (1986) described the patterns of nocturnal periodic breathing in nine Caucasian members of the expedition during several week' residence at an altitude of 6300 m with excursions to 8050 m, elevations that come within our definition of 'extreme altitude' (Chapter 32). The proportion of sleeping time occupied by periodic breathing increases with increasing altitude. Thus it rises from 24% at 2440 m to 40% at 4270 m (Waggener *et al.* 1984) and to 72.5% at 6300 m (West *et al.* 1986). In parallel with this, there is a fall in the duration of the respiratory cycles. Thus at sea level the cycle length is about 30 seconds (Douglas and Haldane 1909), but it falls to 24 seconds at 2440 m and to 20 seconds at 4270 m (Waggener *et al.* 1984). At extreme altitudes of 6300 m the cycle duration varies from 18 to 24 seconds, with a mean of 20 seconds, the duration of the apnoeic periods ranging from 6.2 to 9.2 seconds (mean 7.9 seconds) (West *et al.* 1986). There was no evidence in these climbers at extreme altitude that the percentage of time during which periodic breathing was observed was reduced by an increase in duration of acclimatization. With regard to the type of sleep involved it has been shown that periodic breathing is uncommon during REM sleep (Berssenbrugge *et al.* 1983), a type of sleep that as we note above, is uncommon at high altitude.

Pronounced fluctuations in systemic arterial oxygen saturation occur during nocturnal periodic breathing, ranging from 73 to 63% at an altitude of 6300 m (West *et al.* 1986). The most severe arterial hypoxaemia over the course of 24 hours probably occurs during sleep as a consequence of the periodic breathing. There is a phase difference between the apnoeic portion of the periodic cycle and the minimal value of arterial oxygen saturation as measured at the ear. The lowest arterial saturation is found just after the point of maximal ventilation and the highest saturation is observed at the end of the apnoeic period just before breathing starts to in-

crease again. The period of reduction in breathing is associated with a gradual decline in heart rate, while maximum heart rate occurs shortly after the peak of the hyperpnoea (West *et al.* 1986). Abnormalities of cardiac rhythm are seen infrequently during nocturnal periodic breathing. Ventricular extrasystoles may occur during apnoea.

BASIS FOR OSCILLATORY RESPIRATION

The basis for the oscillatory nature of these disturbances in respiration during sleep was considered by West *et al.* (1986) with reference to an analysis of the problem by Khoo *et al.* (1982). According to this model, two factors are necessary for self-sustained oscillatory behaviour in a control system. One is a 'disturbance', such as a change in alveolar ventilation caused by a sigh or alteration of body position. The second is a 'corrective action' tending to suppress the disturbance, such as an increase in alveolar ventilation caused by the sigh, which would lower arterial carbon dioxide tension and thus tend to reduce ventilation by diminished stimulation of central and peripheral chemoreceptors. For sustained oscillatory behaviour the corrective action must be of a magnitude exceeding that of the disturbance and must be presented $180°$ out of phase with the disturbance, so that what would otherwise inhibit the change in ventilation now augments it. The main corrective action is increased activity of the chemoreceptors in the face of hypoxia. The findings of West *et al.* (1986) in climbers at an extreme altitude are consistent with a very unstable system of respiratory control and suggest that periodic breathing is most likely to occur and present in the most pronounced manner in subjects with the greatest ventilatory response to hypoxia. This hypothesis had been put to the test by a companion study carried out by Lahiri *et al.* (1983) on lowlanders and Sherpas at 5400 m on Mt Everest.

PERIODIC BREATHING IN LOWLANDERS AND SHERPAS

Lahiri *et al.* (1983) studied respiration during sleep at night over a period of 6–8 hours in two groups of men at 5400 m. One group was composed of six high-altitude Shepas (20–44 years of age), all born and continuously residing above 3500 m, and one low-altitude Sherpa (30 years of age) who had spent most of his life at or below 1220 m. The other group comprised seven lowlanders of Caucasian extraction, 25–48 years of age, who had spent at least 32 days at or above 5400 m before the study.

It emerged that nocturnal periodic breathing was highly characteristic of the lowlanders who showed a high respiratory sensitivity to hypoxia, but it also occurred in the low-altitude Sherpa who showed a high ventilatory sensitivity to hypoxia. In contrast, it was not manifested in high-altitude Sherpas who had an attenuated ventilatory sensitivity (Chapter 4) or in the one lowlander who had a low ventilatory sensitivity to hypoxia. In other words there was a close relation between the strength of the peripheral chemoreflex respiratory response and instability of breathing during sleep. Inhalation of oxygen stabilized the breathing pattern of the lowlanders, so that it came to resemble that of Sherpas breathing air. It did this by diminishing the stimulation of the peripheral arterial chemoreceptors; the resulting decrease in ventilation raised the partial pressure of carbon dioxide in the alveolar spaces, which provided an enhanced central respiratory stimulus to eliminate the period of apnoea. Direct inhalation of carbon dioxide also eliminated the apnoea by ameliorating the respiratory alkalosis and stimulating the medullary respiratory centres, but it did not stop the periodicity of the breathing, suggesting that this is independent of central stimulation by carbon dioxide and hydrogen ions.

Returning to the model referred to above, it is clear that a low arterial oxygen tension is critical in the development and maintenance of periodic breathing with apnoea. There is an initial disturbance brought about by stimulation of the carotid bodies. The large breaths bring about an abrupt alveolar hyperoxia and hypocarbia. This corrective action, diminishing the level of stimulation of central and peripheral chemoreceptors, is likely to be enhanced to a magnitude exceeding the initial disturbance by the rate sensitivity of the carotid bodies. It is well known that the chemosensors of the carotid body are sensitive to the rate of change of blood gases, particularly to levels of partial pressure of carbon dioxide in the blood, so that there is an undershoot in response to a diminishing stimulus of carbon dioxide (Black *et al.* 1971). These responses of the carotid body are augmented by hypoxia (Lahiri *et al.* 1982), so the chemoreceptor activity may disappear during a fall in the stimulus by blood carbon dioxide even when there is a considerable hypoxic stimulus (Black *et al.* 1971).

We have already seen above that there is a phase difference between the apnoeic portion of the periodic cycle of breathing and the minimal value of arterial oxygen saturated as measured at the ear. Hence the conditions are fulfilled for an unstable system of respiratory control. There is thus a natural mechanism for the oscillations of the carotid chemosensory input with the oscillation of alveolar and arterial gases (Lahiri *et al.* 1983). The reduced level of peripheral arterial chemoreceptor activity brought about by these mechanisms induces a period of apnoea. This decreases tissue and arterial oxygen tension, which then induce a rapid rise in the arterial chemosensory input stimulating breathing.

PERIODIC BREATHING AND ACCLIMATIZATION

Since well-established nocturnal periodic breathing brings about severe hypoxaemia during the hours of sleep at high altitude, it might be thought that it would be associated with a poor tolerance of extreme altitude. Because, as we have seen, nocturnal periodic breathing is characteristic of persons with a vigorous ventilatory response to hypoxia and is associated with periods of severe arterial hypoxaemia, it would seem logical to deduce that their unstable respiratory control would make them least likely to acclimatize well to high altitude. Direct investigation of this point demonstrates that precisely the opposite is the case. Schoene *et al.* (1984), in a companion study on the subjects studied by West *et al.* (1986), found that climbers who were able to attain and spend nights at altitudes in excess of 8000 m showed a stronger hypoxic ventilatory response and a better arterial blood oxygenation than those who were forced to keep to lower altitudes.

In the face of this controversy Masuyama *et al.* (1986) studied the control of ventilation in 10 climbers ascending to 8500 m in the Nepal–Japan Kangchenjunga Expedition in the spring of 1984. They also found that five climbers who reached an altitude higher than 8000 m exhibited a significantly higher hypoxic ventilatory response than five who did not. In a later paper Masuyama *et al.* (1989) studied the relationship between periodic breathing during sleep at high altitude and ventilatory chemosensitivity in nine Japanese climbers who participated in the expedition to the Kunhun Mountains (7170 m) in China in 1986. They found there was a significant correlation between periodic breathing during sleep and ventilatory response to hypoxia. All the climbers showed severe desaturation during sleep but climbers with a high hypoxic ventilatory response can maintain their arterial oxygenation during sleep, due to hyperventilation induced by periodic breathing. The success at high altitude of those climbers with a strong ventilatory response to hypobaric hypoxia and a propensity to develop nocturnal periodic breathing has to be contrasted with the successful long-term acclimatization to high altitude of Sherpas with an attenuated ventilatory response and little tendency to show periodic breathing. This seeming paradox is referred to briefly in Chapter 4, and the relative advantages and disadvantages of a brisk ventilatory response to hypoxia for the high-altitude climber are considered further in Chapter 32.

SLEEP AT EXTREME SIMULATED ALTITUDE

It is important to gain a better understanding of the severity of sleep disturbances and oxygen desaturation at extreme altitudes. As part of Operation Everest II five healthy male volunteers aged 27.2 ± 1.5 years were subjected during 6 weeks to a progressive hypobaric hypoxia in a decompression chamber to a barometric pressure of 282 mmHg simulating an altitude of 7620 m (Anholm *et al.* 1992). In general, the data collected showed that quality of sleep worsens progressively as arterial oxygen saturation decreases. Changes in various factors in sleep are shown in Table 28.1. It goes without saying that studies of sleep in a decompression chamber in a laboratory may not reflect the effects of natural high altitude on a cold and windy mountainside but this is more than counterbalanced by the collection of a large volume of scientific data to replace the anecdotal evidence of climbers. Other factors that adversely affect sleep studies in decompression chambers are movements from normal beds

or bunks under control conditions to mattresses on the floor, the effects of the noise of equipment and ventilation system, the wearing of face masks, and so on. The studies of Anholm *et al.* (1992) showed that the number of awakenings and the decrease in REM sleep were nearly as much at 4572 m as they were at 7620 m. Similarly, sleep efficiency did not deteriorate above 4572 m.

At 7260 m the longest period of undisrupted sleep was less than 10 minutes. Such severe sleep fragmentation can have an important effect the following day on psychomotor performance and feelings of sleepiness and lack of freshness on awakening. Anholm *et al.* (1992) speculate that breathing supplemental oxygen for as little as 2 or 3 hours of sleep high on a mountain might be beneficial in preventing frequent arousals and would significantly improve performance the next day.

At extreme altitude arterial oxygen saturation was similar in all sleep stages suggesting that the effects of sleep state on ventilatory control during sleep at high altitude are overridden by the chemoreceptor input. Sleep is no exception to the general principle that wide individual differences exist in tolerance to altitude. Some of the subjects involved in the Operation Everest II project had to be removed prematurely from the decompression chamber at 5500 and 7620 m because of transient hypoxic episodes.

SLEEP OF NATIVE ANDEAN HIGHLANDERS

Such studies as we have just referred to confirm that the structure of sleep in lowlanders exposed to

Table 28.1 Arterial oxygen saturation and sleep at extreme simulated altitude (after Anholm *et al.* 1992)

Factor	Barometric pressure 760 mmHg (sea level)	Barometric pressure 282 mmHg (simulated altitude 7620 m)
Nighttime awakenings	14.8	37.2
Total sleep time (min)	337 ± 30	167 ± 44
Rapid eye movement (REM) sleep (% of sleep time)	17.9 ± 6.0	4.0 ± 3.3
Sleep continuity (brief arousals per hour of sleep)	22 ± 6	161 ± 66
Arterial O_2 saturation (Sa_{O2}) (whole night) (%)	96.6 ± 1.5	52 ± 2
Apnoea index (no. of events per hour of sleep)	0.7 ± 1.2	75.2 ± 37.8

Table 28.2 Duration in minutes of sleep stages in native highlanders (after Coote *et al.* 1992)

| Sleep stage | Duration of sleep stages (min) | | | | | |
| | All ages (*n* = 8) | | Under 40 years (18–31 years) (*n* = 5) | | Over 40 years (40–69 years) (*n* = 3) | |
	Mean	SD	Mean	SD	Mean	SD
Awake	38.2	30.7	13.0	3.4	63.4	57.3
Orthodox sleep						
I	42.8	22.9	24.0	8.3	61.7	19.3
II	203.4	41.5	201.7	48.3	205.2	36.8
III	27.8	23.5	46.0	17.6	9.7	8.1
IV	14.3	22.6	28.6	22.7	0.0	0.0
REM sleep	96.2	27.8	94.0	34.5	98.3	17.6
Total sleep time	382.8	57.9	399.1	67.9	366.6	43.1

natural or simulated high altitude is grossly disturbed. In contrast, until very recently there were no data on sleep in long-term residents. This hiatus has been filled by Coote *et al.* (1992) who carried out an electroencephalographic study of sleep in eight native highlanders of Cerro de Pasco (4330 m). To allow for adjustment to sleeping with electrodes only data from the third night were used in the analysis.

It was found that the native highlanders took a long time to get to sleep and woke early so that total sleep time was less that 400 minutes (Table 28.2). Their sleep was disturbed by periods of awake activity. The duration of stage I was greatly increased in those over the age of 40 years but the duration stage II sleep was similar in both young and old subjects. There were significant amounts of slow-wave sleep (stages III and IV) in young highlanders but this was much reduced in subjects over the age of 40 years (Table 28.2). The amount and percentage (25%) of REM sleep were large and did not differ between the two age groups. The onset of REM sleep occurred early in the night (mean 36.1 minutes) and this was particularly evident in the older subjects (Coote *et al.* 1992).

It emerged from this study that the sleep patterns of native highlanders closely resemble those normal lowland populations sleeping at sea level. It is different absolutely from the sleep of lowlanders ascending to similar altitudes (Nicholson *et al.* 1988) and from that of rats chronically exposed to hypoxia (Pappenheimer 1977, 1984). The earlier onset of REM sleep seemed to be characteristic of highlanders over the age of 40 years. Coote *et al.* (1992) make the interesting observation that a very early onset of REM sleep often indicates a depressive illness (Kupfer and Foster 1972).

References

Anholm, J.D., Powles, A.C.P., Downey, R., Houston, C.S., Sutton, J.R., Bonnet, M.H., and Cymerman, C. (1992). Operation Everest II: Arterial oxygen saturation and sleep at extreme simulated altitude. *American Review of Respiratory Disease*, **145**, 817

Berssenbrugge, A.J., Dempsey, C., Iber, C., Skatrud, J., and Wilson, P. (1983). Mechanisms of hypoxia-induced periodic breathing during sleep in humans. *Journal of Physiology, London*, **343**, 507

Black, A.M.S., McCloskey, D.I., and Torrance, R.W. (1971). The responses of carotid body chemoreceptors in the cat to sudden changes in hypercapnia and hypoxic stimuli. *Respiration Physiology*, **13**, 36

Coote, J.H., Stone, B.H., and Tsang, G. (1992). Sleep of Andean high altitude natives. *European Journal of Applied Physiology*, **64**, 178

Douglas, C.G. and Haldane, J. S. (1909). The causes of periodic or Cheyne–Stokes breathing. *Journal of Physiology, London*, **38**, 401

Khoo, M.C.K., Kronauer, R.E., Strohl, K.P., and Slutsky, A.S. (1982). Factors inducing periodic breathing in humans: a general model. *Journal of Applied Physiology*, **53**, 644

Kupfer D.J. and Foster, F.G. (1972). Interval between onset of sleep and rapid eye movement sleep as an indicator of depression. *Lancet*, **ii**, 684

Lahiri, S., Mulligan, E., and Mokashi, A. (1982). Adaptive responses of carotid body chemoreceptor to CO_2. *Brain Research*, **234**, 137

Lahiri, S., Maret, K., and Sherpa, M.G. (1983). Dependence of high altitude sleep apnea on ventilatory sensitivity to hypoxia. *Respiration Physiology*, **52**, 281

Masuyama, S., Kimura, H., Sugita, T., Kuriyama, T., Tatsumi, K., Kumitomo, F., Okita, S., Tojima, H., Yuguchi, Y., Watanabe, S., and Honda, Y. (1986). Control of ventilation in extreme-altitude climbers. *Journal of Applied Physiology*, **61**, 500

Masuyama, S., Kohchiyama, S., Shinozaki, T., Okita, S., Kunitomo, F., Tojima, H., Kimura, H., Kuriyama, T., and Honda, Y. (1989). Periodic breathing at high altitude and ventilatory responses to O_2 and CO_2. *Japanese Journal of Physiology*, **39**, 523

Nicholson, A.N., Smith, P.A., Stone, B.M., and Bradwell, A.R. (1988). Altitude insomnia: studies during an expedition to the Himalayas. *Sleep*, **11**, 554

Oswald, I. (1974). *Sleep*, 3rd edn. Harmondsworth; Penguin Books

Pappenheimer, J.R. (1977). Sleep and respiration of rats during hypoxia. *Journal of Physiology, London*, **266**, 191

Pappenheimer, J.R. (1984). Hypoxic insomnia: effects of carbon monoxide and acclimatization. *Journal of Applied Physiology*, **57**, 1696

Reite, M., Jackson, D., Cahoon, R.L., and Weil, J.V. (1975). Sleep physiology at high altitude. *Electroencephalography and Clinical Neurophysiology*, **38**, 463

Schoene, R.B., Lahiri, S., Hackett, P.H., Peters, R.M., Milledge, J.S., Pizzo, C.J., Sarnquist, F.H., Boyer, S.J., Graber, D.J., Maret, K.H., and West, J.B. (1984). Relationship of hypoxic ventilatory response to exercise performance on Mount Everest. *Journal of Applied Physiology*, **56**, 1478

Shapiro, C.M. and Flanigan, M.J. (1993). Function of sleep. *British Medical Journal*, **306**, 383

Waggener, T.B., Brasil, P.J., Kronauer, R.E., Gabel, R.A., and Inbar, G.F. (1984). Strength and cycle time of high-altitude ventilatory patterns in unacclimatized humans. *Journal of Applied Physiology*, **56**, 576

Ward, M.P., Milledge, J.S., and West, J.B. (1989). *High Altitude Medicine and Physiology* . London; Chapman and Hall Medical, p. 267

Weil, J.V., Kryger, M.H., and Scoggin, C.H. (1978). Sleep and breathing at high altitude. In *Sleep Apnea Syndromes* (C. Guilleminault and W. Dement, Ed.). New York; Liss, p. 119

Weiss, T. and Roldan, E. (1964). Comparative studies of sleep cycles in rodents. *Experientia*, **20**, 280

West, J.B., Peters, R.M., Aksnes, G., Maret, K.H., Milledge, J.S., and Schoene, R.B. (1986). Nocturnal periodic breathing at altitudes of 6,300 and 8,050 m. *Journal of Applied Physiology*, **61**, 280

Williams, E.S. (1959). Sleep and wakefulness at high altitudes. *British Medical Journal*, **i**, 197

29

Cerebral function

The brain is very susceptible to the effects of hypobaric hypoxia, and cerebral function is commonly disturbed in the mountain environment. This manifests itself in a variety of ways. Hypoxia affects accurate and rapid decision-making and this may assume significance in military operations at high altitude. It may also affect scientific work such as the maintenance and operation of the infrared telescope by astronomers on the summit of the volcano Mauna Kea (4200 m) (Chapter 30). The demonstration of man's ability to climb Mt Everest without the protection of supplementary oxygen has encouraged others to follow the same path and risk the same effects on the brain. It has now become apparent that there are persistent defects of function of the central nervous system upon return to sea level after periods of severe hypoxia at high altitude. Irrational decisions made by climbers in the dangerous environment of extreme altitude may lead to disasters. Exposure to great heights may lead to exotic manifestations of hypoxia such as hallucinations. Excluding the factor of hypoxia, the mountain environment *per se* affects higher cerebral function. The psychological reactions of lowlanders and native highlanders to mountains are quite distinct. To the high-altitude climber the mountains are goals for conquest. To the highlander they commonly have a religious significance and frequently spawn mountain myths.

DECISION-MAKING AND TESTS OF MENTAL REACTION AT HIGH ALTITUDE

A considerable literature exists on assessing mental reaction at high altitude by somewhat artificial tests, but it was criticized by Tune (1964) who found it less convincing and developed than other areas of physiological research in this environment. Even with these reservations, the results of such tests suggest that decision-making tends to be impaired at altitude. Most of the early studies were connected with 'choice-reaction time' and they showed that, when subjects were required to discriminate between five different coloured lights, their reaction times

were a positive function of altitude up to 6100 m (McFarland and Dill 1938).

In recent years the tests have become ever more complex. Thus, Cahoon (1972) studied the reactions of eight volunteer soldiers after short-lived exposure to a simulated altitude of 4570 m for 3, 20, 24, and 45 hours. They were asked to perform four tasks. One was a simple psychomotor task of sorting 96 blank cards into two bins alternately. One was a complex psychomotor task of sorting 96 blank cards into 16 bins sequentially. A simple cognitive task involved sorting the 96 cards into two bins according to whether the central figure was red or green. Finally, a complex cognitive task involved sorting 96 cards into 16 bins according to colour, shape, and size of central figure and presence or absence of a black dot. The results showed that cognitive tasks showed a greater decrement at 4570 m in speed and accuracy than psychomotor tasks. Complex decision-making tasks were more affected than simple tasks. Speed was sacrificed to maintain accuracy.

This impairment of mental performance and decision-making during prolonged stay at high altitude was studied by Sharma *et al.* (1975). They investigated the sequential changes in eye–hand co-ordination in terms of speed and accuracy that occurred over a period of 2 years at an altitude of 4000 m in the Western Himalaya. The subjects were 25 healthy soldiers between 21 and 30 years of age who were natives of the plains of southern India. They were required to move a stylus along a groove of 0.5 cm, cut to form a multicornered star. Errors were sounded automatically. The time to trace the design was recorded by stopwatch. The test was applied after 1, 10, 13, 18, and 24 months' residence at high altitude. Psychomotor efficiency was found to be adversely affected both in terms of speed and accuracy during the early stages of residence at high altitude. After living in the mountains for 10 months there was a gradual return towards the original level of psychomotor efficiency. The interpretation of the initial impairment of mental performance as an effect of high altitude and its subsequent recovery as an expression of acclimatization is open to question. The early fall-off in mental agility in lowlanders exposed to high altitude could equally well be attributed to the considerable psychological stress they might experience with, for example, the onset of symptoms of acute mountain sickness, rather than to a direct effect of hypoxia on higher cerebral function involved in decision-making. The improvement in performance after a few months at high altitude could similarly be explained by the growing familiarity of the subjects with the tests rather than by any process of acclimatization.

Effects of motivation

Further studies of Cahoon (1973) are enlightening in that they demonstrate that motivation and training can effectively compensate for the stress imposed by a high-altitude atmosphere on the successful performance of tasks of short duration. He sought to determine the effects of high altitude on the performance of a simulated radiocommunication task. The subjects studied had to monitor and respond to tapes of simulated radio traffic at four different altitudes, namely, sea level, 3960 m, 4570 m, and 5180 m. Two groups were tested in this manner. The first consisted of nine volunteers. Above an altitude of 3960 m they detected significantly fewer messages, the percentage falling from nearly 80% at 3960 m to only 40% at 5180 m. Furthermore, reaction time increased from 1.3 seconds at 3960 m to 1.8 seconds at 5180 m. Apparently the environmental conditions had led to a deterioration in performance. The second group consisted of highly motivated trained soldiers. Four had received radio training and four had not. The difference in the responses of this group was significant. It performed better in all forms of monitoring. At 3960 m the trained soldiers achieved a 95% detection rate of messages and it still exceeded 90% at 5180 m. Their reaction time actually fell from 1.0 second at 3960 m to 0.9 seconds at 5180 m. There was a striking difference in attitude as well as in performance. The results were not significantly different in those trained and not trained in radiocommunications indicating that motivation is a more important factor than training in maintaining performance at high altitude. Such findings do not exclude the possibility that, in extended operation where motivation may drop, say, through lack of sleep, the stress of high altitude may affect performance in soldiers so that it falls towards that achieved by the volunteers referred to above.

The effects of exercise and high altitude (3700–4300 m) on marksmanship accuracy and sighting time were quantified in 16 experienced marksmen by Tharion *et al.* (1992). The subjects studied fired a disabled rifle equipped with a laser-based system from a free-standing position. The 2.3-cm circular target was at a distance of 5 m. Acute altitude exposure reduced marksmanship accuracy and increased sighting time. However, after residence at high altitude, accuracy and sighting time at rest returned to sea-level values. Exercise and acute altitude exposure had similar but independent detrimental effects on marksmanship.

It is apparent from these somewhat artificial tests that there are decrements in psychomotor and cognitive skills at high altitude. These are moderate and appear to improve with time, either as a result of acclimatization or familiarity with the tests. Motivation appears to overcome the fall-off in performance. It is necessary to relate the results of these artificial tests to what actually occurs in routine skills being applied in real programmes of work at high altitude. The opportunity to do this arose from a study of astronomers working on the summit of the volcano Mauna Kea in Hawaii.

EFFECTS ON SCIENTIFIC WORK AT HIGH ALTITUDE

Astronomers working on the United Kingdom infrared telescope at 4200 m on the summit of the volcano Mauna Kea in Hawaii have to operate complex scientific equipment routinely over a period of months and years (Chapter 30). When we visited the site, we were told by several members of staff that they had experienced difficulties in using or repairing equipment. Forster (1986) reports that he carried out on them tests of numerate memory (Wechsler digit span forwards and digit span backwards (DSB)), and motor speed and recoding of information (digit symbol substitution (DSS)). In shiftworkers he found deterioration of the DSB tests on the first day at 4200 m, whereas there was no decrement in the performance of the DSS or digit span forwards. After 5 days on the mountain, even the DSB tests scores were similar to the scores obtained at sea level. Numerate memory (for DSB) and psychomotor ability (for DSS) were impaired in commuters on Mauna Kea. The conclusion from this investigation is that impairment of ability to handle complex scientific equipment at high altitude in the region of 4200 m is but moderate and short-lived. Hence it comes about that the greatest concentration of telescope power in the world is sited at high altitude in Hawaii and functions very effectively.

CEREBRAL FUNCTION AT MODERATE ALTITUDE

The effects of hypobaric hypoxia on cerebral function depend on the level of altitude involved. Denison *et al.* (1966) found that, at a simulated altitude of only 2440 m, subjects were slower to learn complex mental tasks than at sea level. Even at the considerably lower altitude of only 1525 m, eight subjects were slower to learn complex tasks than a matched group breathing an enriched oxygen mixture. The tests involved recognizing the posture of man-like figures having different orientations and presented in random sequence on a screen. Thus, even at the cabin altitudes of commercial aircraft, sensitive psychometric tests can pick up minor degrees of impairment.

CEREBRAL FUNCTION AT HIGH ALTITUDE

McFarland (1937*a,b*, 1938*a,b*) had much earlier carried out a series of experiments at higher altitudes during the International High Altitude Expedition to Chile in 1935. He studied the psychophysiological effects of sudden ascents to 5000 m in unpressurized aircraft and compared the results with ascents by train and car to villages at high as 4700 m in Chile. The most important factor was the rate of ascent, rapid increase to altitude by plane being the most damaging. Simple and complex psychological functions were significantly impaired at high altitudes including arithmetical tests and writing ability. There were errors in memory and perseverance, and reductions in auditory threshold and the understanding of words.

Studies of sensory and motor responses during acclimatization were studied at altitudes up to 6100 m. There were significant reductions in hearing, vision, and eye–hand co-ordination. Impairment was not significant below 5330 m. Mental and psychosomatic tests were carried out at the same altitudes. Mental flexibility and immediate memory were significantly impaired. There was increased distractability and lethargy, which tended to reduce the ability to concentrate. However, complex mental work could be carried out if the subjects increased their concentration, a feature that we have already considered above (Cahoon 1973).

Sensory and circulatory responses were measured on sulfur-miners residing permanently at Aucanquilcha (5330 m). They were compared with a group of workers at sea level similar in age and race. It was found that the high-altitude miners were slower in simple and choice reaction times. They were less acute in auditory sensitivity than workers at sea level.

CEREBRAL FUNCTION AT EXTREME ALTITUDE

Disturbances of cerebral function at extreme altitude are more pronounced and may be long-lasting. Townes *et al.* (1984) reported studies of cerebral function on 21 members of the 1981 American Medical Research Expedition to Mt Everest. They carried out neuropsychological tests immediately before and after the expedition but also included follow-up tests. They found that performance improved between the pre- and post-expedition periods on tests of complex problem-solving, including spatial problem-solving and abstract reasoning, and this improvement was thought to be due simply to practice. This study demonstrated that disturbances of cerebral function at extreme altitude may be transient or long-lasting. Verbal learning and memory declined significantly after the time on the mountain. There were expressive language difficulties such as errors in reading, writing, and spelling. These mild impairments in learning, memory, and verbal expression were still present 3 days after descent to Kathmandu (1500 m) and they took up to 1 year to return to pre-expedition levels. The observed decrements in verbal memory were regarded as being due to effects on the hippocampus or temporal areas of the brain. The speed of finger-tapping decreased significantly over the course of the expedition. This bilateral reduction in motor speed was characterized by rapid muscle fatigue. This effect was probably primarily on cerebellar or motor cortex function and, significantly, persisted for 1 year after completion of the study. The findings are supported by previous studies (Sharma *et al.* 1975; Sharma and Malhotra 1976) that revealed that lowlanders living for 10 months at high altitude initially experienced impairment of both motor co-ordination and speed. The incoordination resolved within 1 year, but the loss of speed persisted for 2 years. In contrast, Clark *et al.* (1983) found no evidence of permanent cerebral dysfunction due to altitude exposure. They studied 22 mountaineers prior to, and 16–221 days after, Himalayan climbs above 5300 m with an extensive battery of psychological and neuropsychological tests.

Altitudes exceeding 5500 m represent the limit for acceptable performance for mental tests requiring decision-making (McFarland 1972). At such elevations hypoxia exerts an increasingly severe effect on higher cerebral functions. Shipton had aphasia at

7010 m after returning from his attempt to reach the summit of Mt Everest with Smythe (Shipton 1943): 'I suddenly found that I was suffering from aphasia and could not articulate words properly. For example, if I wished to say "Give me a cup of tea", I would say something entirely different — maybe tramcar, cat, feet. I was perfectly clear headed: I could even visualise the words I wanted to say but my tongue just refused to perform the required movements.' Attention fluctuates more easily and mental block is common. Calculations are unreliable, judgement becomes faulty, and emotional responses are unpredictable. Above 6700 m there is an onset of significant mental impairment with serious lapses of judgement. At such great altitudes one has left the realms of the physiology of acclimatization for those of heroic endurance and deliberate exposure to extreme conditions.

A significant new finding arose from the Operation Everest II project and was referred to by Ward *et al.* (1989) from at that time unpublished observations by Townes and his colleagues. During this project eight normal subjects spent 40 days in a low-pressure chamber and were gradually decompressed, ultimately being exposed to the simulated altitude of the summit of Mt Everest. Impairments in motor speed, memory, and verbal expressive abilities were found after the simulated ascent just as with the 1981 Everest expedition. The new observation was a significant negative correlation between hypoxic ventilatory response and neuropsychological function measured after the completion of the project. This was opposite to what was anticipated. According to Ward *et al.* (1989), Townes and his associates believed that subjects with the highest hypoxic ventilatory response would reduce their arterial carbon dioxide tension to the greatest extent, thereby developing the most pronounced cerebral vasoconstriction. This would cause the most severe cerebral hypoxia even though their arterial oxygen tension would actually be higher than in the subjects with the smaller ventilatory response to hypoxia. This correlation between hypoxic ventilatory response and residual impairment of CNS function leads to an interesting paradox (Ward *et al.* 1989). A brisk hypoxic ventilatory response is necessary for a climber to reach extreme altitudes and yet he is likely to suffer the most severe cerebral dysfunction.

HALLUCINATIONS

Hallucinations may occur in climbers at extreme altitude. One of the most characteristic phenomena is that of the *phantom companion*. Smythe (1934)

gave a graphic account of this curious sensation and we quote here his account of his experience during the attempted ascent to Everest in 1933. It has become a classic description.

> All the time that I was climbing alone I had a strong feeling that I was accompanied by a second person. This feeling was so strong that it completely eliminated all loneliness I might otherwise have felt. It even seemed that I was tied to my 'companion' by a rope, and that if I slipped 'he' would hold me. I remember constantly glancing back over my shoulder, and once, when, after reaching my highest point, I stopped to try to eat some mint cake, I carefully divided it and turned round with one half in my hand. It was almost a shock to find no one to whom to give it. It seemed to me that this 'presence' was a strong, helpful and friendly one, and it was not until Camp VI was sighted that the link connecting me, as it seemed at the time to the beyond, was snapped and, although Shipton and the camp were but a few yards away, I felt suddenly alone.

Two members of the British Everest team of 1975 dug a snow-hole on the mountain and spent the night at 8800 m without oxygen. Both reported the curious sensation that they had been accompanied by a third person (Clarke 1976).

Smythe (1934) also reported that during the same ascent at an altitude of 8290 m:

> I was still some 200 feet above Camp VI and a considerable distance horizontally from it when, chancing to glance in the direction of the north ridge, I saw two curious-looking objects floating in the sky. They strongly resembled kite-balloons in shape, but one possessed what appeared to be squat under-developed wings, and the other protuberance suggestive of a beak. They hovered motionless but seemed slowly to pulsate, a pulsation incidentally much slower than my own heartbeats, which is of interest supposing that it was an optical illusion. The two objects were very dark in colour and were silhouetted sharply against the sky, or possibly a background of a cloud. So interested was I that I stopped to observe them. My brain appeared to be working normally, and I deliberately put myself through a series of tests. First of all I glanced away. The objects did not follow my vision, but they were still there when I looked back again. Then I looked away again, and this time identified by name a number of peaks, valleys and glaciers by

way of a mental test. But when I looked back again, the objects still confronted me.

One is aware that large mountain birds such as lammergeyers frequent the extreme altitudes of the Himalaya, but it seems most likely that these bird-like creatures observed by Smythe (1934) were hallucinations.

The dramatic and disastrous effects that the hallucinations induced by hypoxia may have are illustrated by a description of an ill-fated climb of Aconcagua (6920 m) in Argentina, the highest mountain in the Western hemisphere (Shults and Swan 1975). Eight climbers between 25 and 52 years of age, one a woman, climbed the mountain too rapidly after ascending as much as 610 m in a single day. At 5370 m one developed pulmonary oedema and another cerebral oedema; the doctor accompanying the party remained with them. The remaining five continued the climb, but one soon became grossly disorientated. The last four camped at 6400 m and what transpired above this altitude was open to doubt for only two of the climbers survived and their recall of events was fragmentary. When the two survivors arrived back at base camp, they reported having seen on the summit highway equipment, dead mules, skiers, and trees. They recalled the presence of voices of an Argentinian mountain patrol that was in fact never there. Such bizarre effects of deprivation of oxygen on the brain have commended themselves to the popular press. One such press report included an interview with Alfredo Magnani, a guide on Aconcagua, who referred to the cerebral symptoms in the following terms: 'It is like dreaming on your feet. I saw a horse dancing once, many years ago' (Lindley 1975).

HIGH-ALTITUDE CLIMBING WITHOUT OXYGEN

With the conquest of all the major peaks in the world and of the most dangerous ascents on them, fewer and fewer goals have been left to be attained. One, however, that has emerged is the challenge of reaching Whymper's 'loftiest summits of the earth' (see Chapter 1) without the use of oxygen. Habeler (1979) describes the mental effects induced by the hypoxia of extreme altitude without the protection of supplementary oxygen. He and Messner climbed the main summit of Mt Everest (8850 m) without the use of a supply of oxygen on 8 May 1978. At the summit they found that their attentiveness and concentration declined dramatically. The capacity for clear logical thinking was lost. Slowly they become

overwhelmed by a dangerous sense of euphoria: 'I felt somehow light and relaxed, and believed that nothing could happen to me. Undoubtedly, many of the men who have disappeared for ever in the summit region of Everest had also fallen victim to this *treacherous euphoria*.' After this fleeting sense of triumph, Habeler felt exhausted and suddenly afraid of death or severe damage to the brain. This led him to descend as rapidly as possible by sliding down the mountain. After his heroic climb, Habeler suffered nightmares and lapses of memory that persisted to the time of writing his book. Cavaletti *et al.* (1987) reported brain damage after high-altitude climbs without oxygen. They studied seven climbers, five male, who ascended, without supplementary oxygen, Mount Satopanth (7075 m). Tests at base camp (5200 m) were carried out after 2 days of complete rest, to rule out the possibility of low performance of memory due to physical exhaustion. In all cases memory performance decreased either at base camp or, to a lesser degree, at sea level 75 days after the climb. West (1986) suggests that high-altitude climbing without the use of oxygen should be grouped together with professional boxing as a sport leaving its participants open to brain damage.

INTERACTION OF DRUGS AND HYPOXIA

Ravenhill (1913) was of the opinion that alcohol increased the severity of the symptoms of acute mountain sickness. Nettles and Olson (1965) studied the effects of alcohol upon the time of useful consciousness of a subject when he is suddenly subjected to hypoxia, conditions that might obtain in sudden decompression in a civilian aircraft. They studied 10 normal subjects at a simulated altitude of 7620 m. After their oxygen masks were removed, they performed various tasks requiring mental and physical co-ordination until definite hypoxic symptoms were manifested. Later the same subjects were submitted to identical conditions after the administration of 0.5 ml of 100% alcohol per lb (0.5 kg) of body weight. With blood alcohol levels of between only 22 and 49 mg/100 ml there was a reduction of 38% in the time of useful consciousness under these hypoxic conditions. The interrelation of the effects of alcohol and altitude on man during rest and work has also been studied by Mazess *et al.* (1968).

Marijuana impairs the performance of complex behavioural tasks in animals and man (US Department of Health, Education and Welfare, 1974). Lewis *et al.* (1976) have studied the effects of marijuana on two female adolescent baboons to see if the impairment produced by the drug is potentiated by the hypoxia of simulated high altitude. The animals were trained to perform a delayed matching-to-sample task on red, white, and green lamps. Both baboons were subjected to various combinations of oral doses of marijuana, ranging from 0.25 to 2.0 mg/kg body weight and exposure to simulated altitudes of 390–3660 m, before performing the matching tests. The study showed that, while accuracy of matching performance was unaffected by the combination of hypoxia and marijuana, the level of the work output was greatly reduced due to deterioration in the speed of response.

ELECTROENCEPHALOGRAM AT HIGH ALTITUDE

Ryn (1971) found electroencephalographic abnormalities in 11 of 30 climbers who had been at altitudes exceeding 5500 m. The main abnormality was a decreased frequency of alpha waves and a diminution of their amplitude. Zhongyuan *et al.* (1983) also studied electroencephalographic changes occurring above 5000 m in members of a Chinese expedition to Mt Everest. They also found a reduced amplitude of the alpha rhythm but an increase in its frequency.

PSYCHOLOGICAL REACTION OF THE LOWLANDER TO MOUNTAINS

The mountain environment may exert powerful psychological influences on the human mind. These differ greatly in the lowlander and the native highlander. Over the centuries the response of the lowlander has changed from fear of mountains into seeing them as objects for challenge and conquest. To the native highlander they are commonly subjects of awe and reverence, and a rich source of myths.

A love of mountains and a desire to scale them is not innate in the lowlander. During the Middle Ages Europeans feared that the Alps were infested with dragons that dropped stones as they flew between the peaks. These 'dragon-stones' were thought to have the power to effect miraculous cures in such diseases as dysentery and cholera. One of them is exhibited in the Museum of Natural History in Basle (Fig. 29.1). Jacob Scheuchzer of Zurich made nine journeys to the Alps from 1702 and concluded that the large number of caves suitable for habitation by dragons was proof of their existence (Sanuki and Yamada 1974). The villagers at the foot of the Matterhorn were convinced that the summit of the mountain was inhabited by 'djinns and efreets'. In the Italian valley of Breuil, mothers frightened their children with threats that 'the wild man of Becca'

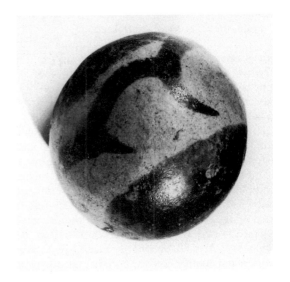

29.1 *Dragon stone exhibited at the Natural History Museum in Basle.*

(that is the Matterhorn) would carry them away (Sanuki and Yamada 1974). Even today grotesque carvings of faces from the rough bark of trees abound in the alpine valleys (Fig. 29.2). While produced nowadays for the tourist, they almost certainly have their origins in a belief in mountain monsters by the people of the alpine valleys of bygone days. This terror of mountains persisted for centuries and exceptional indeed were such events as the ascent of Mont Aiguille (2100 m) by de Beaupré in the South of France in July 1492, a few weeks before Columbus set sail for the New World.

A change in attitude began in the eighteenth century under the influence of people like Albrecht von Haller, a noted Swiss physiologist who was one of the first to identify the carotid bodies, whose role in acclimatization to high altitude is discussed in Chapter 7. The era of climbing began in August 1786 with the ascent of Mont Blanc (4810 m) by Balmat and Paccard for the prize offered by de Saussure. Once the taste for this activity had been whetted, there was a slow but inexorable movement to climb ever higher peaks, where the climber had to contend not only with the dangers of the mountain but also with those of high altitude.

The peaks were no longer conceived as objects of fear but as challenges to be overcome. The very language of mountaineering became military in nature, suggesting that the mountain peak was an adversary to be vanquished. The talk has become that of the

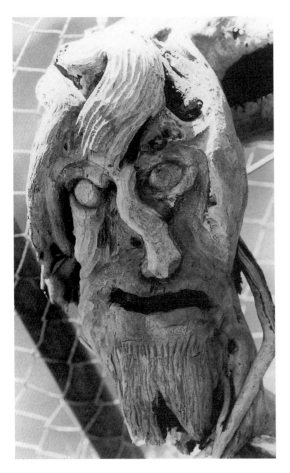

29.2 *One of the grotesque carvings of tree bark and roots that are to be found in the valleys of Valais in Switzerland. The carving shown was seen in Zermatt at the foot of the Matterhorn, the summit of which was thought to be the site of a ruined city populated by demons.*

expedition, assault, conquest, or defeat. The camps on the ascent are, like army corps, identified with Roman numerals from I to VIII (Nicolson 1975).

Mood states on ascent to high altitude

Anecdotal evidence and personal experience suggest that ascent to altitudes between 2500 and 5500 m is often associated with changes of mood. Shukitt and Banderet (1988) attempted to assess these by applying the Clyde Mood Scale to 19 men and 16 women between the ages of 18 and 28 years who ascended to 1600 and 4300 m. This scale consists of 48 adjectives rated on a four-point scale that can be clustered into six principal mood factors, which are sleepiness,

dizziness, clear thinking, aggressiveness, friendliness, and unhappiness. Mood changes were found to be related to both the level and duration of altitude. The only change noted at 1600 m was an increase in sleepiness. The newcomer to high altitude commonly feels tired and sleepy to an extent that is quite disproportionate to the degree of physical activity to be undertaken. At 4300 m there was an elevation of spirit that, as we have seen earlier in this chapter, may escalate into treacherous euphoria at extreme altitudes. Sleepiness and dizziness worsened at the higher altitude. The affected subjects became less friendly but aggressiveness remained the same. Their capacity for clear thinking diminished. Sleepiness was greatest at 1–4 hours after ascent at both 1600 and 4300 m. All the mood changes at the higher altitude were greatest on the first day of exposure, 18–24 hours after ascent. The time course of mood changes was similar to that of the symptomatology of acute mountain sickness. All mood changes recovered to baseline values 42–52 hours after ascent.

The personality and motivation of alpinists

Ryn (1988) gives an account of research carried out into the psychology of a group of 80 Polish alpinists who had been on expeditions to the Andes, Himalaya, and Karakorams during the quarter of a century from 1960. The group comprised 70 men and ten women aged 20–49 years, the average age being 35 years. All were members of the Polish Alpine Club and had practised mountain climbing for 6–25 years, average 15 years. Their personality was assessed by the Cattell Personality Questionnaire. They were classified as schizothemic being withdrawn and detached. They tended to be aggressive, self-centred, and highly competitive. They were unconventional, being independent of thought and ready to break accepted social norms of conduct. Other characteristics were emotional lability, stubbornness, a strong need to dominate, and a desire for recognition by society at large. They felt the need for new exciting experiences.

As regards the motivation for high-altitude climbing, Ryn (1988) found the strongest motive to be the need to experience strong emotional states and looking for inner strengths and possibilities. Elsewhere in this book we note that man largely overcomes his environmental difficulties by avoiding them. Not so the high-altitude climber, who exposes himself to physical injury and to extreme conditions of cold and hypoxia that will not support life indefinitely and that may prove fatal.

Clark (1976) does not subscribe to the view that climbing offers the means for fulfilment of deep psychological goals. He finds worrying 'the overtones of high seriousness which today are sometimes tacked onto a simple sport'. He believes that 'the tendency to see in the sport dark depths that would have intrigued most of the pioneers and set many of them into roars of laughter is probably a passing fad'. We find it difficult to accept this view and believe, on the contrary, that powerful psychological forces motivate the high-altitude climber. The prolonged assault on Nanga Parbat (8125 m) by German mountaineers illustrates the terrifying determination, regardless of cost, that can be brought to the ascent and conquest of mountains when personal and national pride is felt to be at stake. After the first unsuccessful attempt on the summit in 1932 by a party led by Merkl, a second under the same leader was organized for 1934. During this climb Drexel died from high-altitude pulmonary oedema and Merkl and the Welzenbachs and seven porters were lost soon after in the blizzard-ridden expedition. In 1937 seven climbers and nine porters from a party led by Dr Karl Wien were buried under a vast avalanche. Sixteen years later the German climbers returned and on 3 July 1953 Hermann Buhl reached the summit on his own. The ever-present risk of injury or death appears to be readily accepted and may in fact be one of the fascinations of alpine and high-altitude climbing: 'It is true that great ridges sometimes demand their sacrifice, but the mountaineer would hardly forgo his worship though he knew himself to be the destined victim' (Mummery 1894). The year after he wrote that Mummery died while trying to scale the summit of Nanga Parbat.

PSYCHOLOGICAL REACTION OF THE SHERPA TO MOUNTAINS

This almost mystical approach to the great mountain ranges is more developed in peoples living in and around the Himalaya which is central to the religious faith of the Hindus. Shiva is believed to sit on the celestial heights of the mountain peaks in a state of perpetual meditation, generating the spiritual force that sustains the cosmos (Nicolson 1975). To the Tibetans the high places are the sacred ground of a multitude of gods and devils. In 1955 a British climbing team planned to ascend Kangchenjunga (8600 m), but this expedition was immediately recognized as a threat to the divinity of the Mountain God of Wealth and the governments of India, Nepal, and Sikkim refused to allow the climb. They feared the god of Kangchenjunga might be provoked

to exact retribution. A compromise was reached when the climbers agreed to halt a few metres beneath the summit in order for the Sherpas to bury offerings. While the Sherpa accepts the daily hazards and difficulties of his mountain home, the isolated and desolate country in which he lives is a fertile breeding ground for strange myths that appear to meet deep psychological needs. It has led him to create mountain monsters.

The Yeti

For countless generations the Sherpas have recounted stories of a Yeti, a wild, hairy humanoid creature of the Himalaya. The first mention of this mythical creature in Western literature appears to be that of Hodgson (1832). He reported that his native hunters were frightened by a *rakshas* (Sanskrit: demon) with long dark hair and no tail. It is of interest to note that Hodgson considered this intruder to be an orang-utan. In 1921 Howard-Bury was shown tracks like those of a human foot and they were ascribed by his porters as those of 'the wild man of the snows', the *Metoh-Kangmi*, later translated as the Abominable Snowman. In 1961 a special licence was issued by the government of Nepal to authorize the hunting of Yetis at 400 pounds sterling per animal. Yeti-seeking expeditions in the Himalaya were undertaken in 1954 and 1957. These had been promoted by the finding of a giant footprint, 13 in × 8 in (33 cm × 20 cm), at 5490 m on the Menlung glacier by Shipton and Ward in 1951 during an Everest reconnaissance expedition. Photographs of this and a line of footprints at the edge of the glacier have never been explained and they stimulated great public interest in the Yeti myth.

Napier (1976) presents a fascinating account of the beliefs of the native highlanders of the Himalaya as to the nature and behaviour of the Yeti, based on 18 separate Sherpa reports gathered from the literature. It is thought to live in caves high in the mountains between 4370 and 6100 m, although some are considered to live in the impenetrable thickets of the mountain forests at some 3050 m. It is said to be nocturnal and carnivorous. It eats the small Himalayan mouse-hare, the pika, but it has been reported as devouring yaks. On occasion, it has been reported as raiding villages and carrying off human beings. It has a vile pungent smell and mews, yelps, whistles, and roars. Yetis are traditionally considered to have tremendous physical strength and can uproot trees and lift and hurl boulders over vast distances. The breasts of the females are so large that they have to throw them over their shoulders when running or when bending down. They are impeded, when running down slopes, by their long head-hair, which falls over their eyes and thus blinds them. Yetis are reported as being inordinately fond of alcohol. So far as social behaviour is concerned, they are solitary.

Belief in the Yeti seems to have a deep psychological significance for the Sherpas and provides at the same time an opportunity for sensationalism and publicity for visitors to these isolated area. It is likely that the creation of a mountain monster creates a common danger and thus binds the group together. It may act as a traditional bugbear, used to frighten children by Sherpa parents (Napier 1976). The Yeti may represent a form of cultural grooming, providing a feeling of togetherness and comfort in the face of a common external enemy, namely the adverse mountain environment. There appears to be no reasonable doubt that the Yeti is an idea rather than an animal. There is no hard evidence of its existence such as a skull, or a captive animal, or a photograph of it of unquestionable probity (Napier 1976). The scalps and hair that have been presented as evidence have not been authenticated by the institution investigating them.

Two forms of soft evidence abound in quantity. There are numerous sightings of the Yeti in the Himalaya, but individuals, especially newcomers, at high altitude are susceptible to the mental disturbances and even hallucinations referred to. As with the Loch Ness monster, one cannot exclude always the desire for sensationalism and publicity in those who claim to have seen the phenomenon. There have been many instances of footprints. Many mammals frequent high altitudes for shorter or longer periods and their footprints may be misinterpreted. Pilgrims and lamas undertake dedicated plodding through this region of Tibet, Bhutan, and Sikkim. Certainly the excessive size of the feet is highly characteristic of the Yeti. A step of 1.5–2 feet (46–61 cm) would be acceptable for a man walking in snow, and a foot length of 10–12 in (25–30 cm) is within the normal human range, but the crux comes in trying to explain away a foot width of 8 in (20 cm). The broadness of the foot is what makes the photograph of Shipton and Ward, taken in 1951, so difficult to explain away. However, it has to kept in mind that, when footprints melt and then resolidify, with the rising and setting of the sun, they enlarge. Figs 29.3–29.6 provide examples of how big footprints in snow at high altitude can be explained simply without invoking the existence of the Yeti. We are indebted for these photographs to a col-

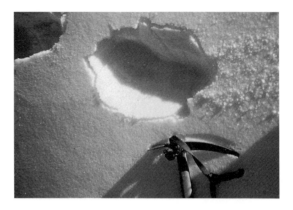

29.3 *This illustration and Figs 29.4–29.6 provide examples of how big footprints in snow at high altitude can be explained simply without involving the existence of the Yeti. Here a print has been made by a climbing boot and the surrounding snow has fallen in to produce a much larger footprint. Melting and subsequent freezing perpetuate the large print. These photographs of footprints were taken by Kevin Marsh at Camp I (4880 m) on Cherichor peak (6750 m) in the Karakorams, on 28 September 1976.*

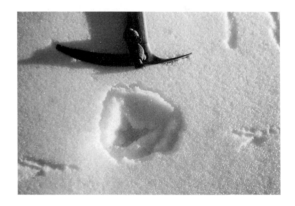

29.4 *Various species of bird frequent high altitudes and some of them may be responsible for the mysterious appearance of big footprints at the tops of mountains. To the left and right of the picture are typical bird-tracks in firm snow. In the centre area the snow was soft and the bird has sunk into it, replacing a footprint with a body-print. When freshly made, the footmarks can still be seen in the floor of the body-print, but with melting and subsequent freezing a print of a 'Bigfoot' would be produced.*

league Kevin Marsh who took them while he was climbing in the Karakorams. So characteristic of the mountain monster is the large footprint, that Napier

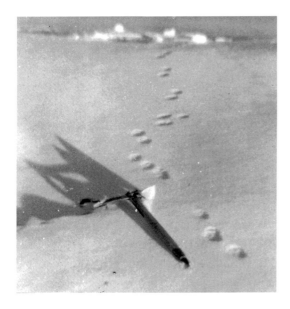

(a)

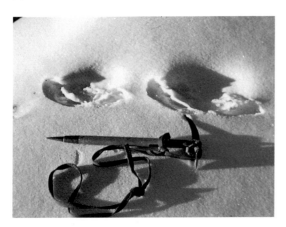

(b)

29.5 (a) *Footprints of a small quadruped in snow;*
(b) *when this small animal runs across soft snow, the footprints (left) become converted with body-prints (centre and right). Some species of small animals live at high altitude. The ice-axe is 21 in (53 cm) in length.*

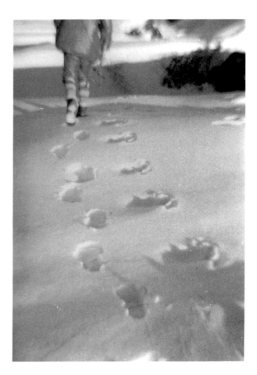

29.6 *Typical footprints produced by the bipedal gait of man (left) and the single line of large body-prints produced by an unknown animal in the snow at high altitude (right). The single nature of the 'Bigfoot' prints makes it clear that they have been produced as body prints of a small animal leaping through the snow.*

(1976) refers to both the Yeti and its North American counterpart by the group-name 'Bigfoot'.

There have been attempts to substantiate the *idea* of the Yeti as an *animal*. Some still maintain that the Yeti is real and represents a relict form of *Gigantopithecus*. Others believe the animal exists as a form derived from this. It is believed that a species of orang-utan (Fig. 29.7) roamed southern China

and Tibet for the last quarter of a million years and may have acted as the physical expression of the Yeti legend of such psychological need and importance to the indigenous peoples of the area. Belief in the Yeti exists even to the present day. Loudon reports that in April 1978 the government of Sikkim sent four expeditions to the heights of Kishong La following reports that the Yeti had killed several yaks in the area, hurling them for a distance of 200 yards (180 m) (Loudon 1978). Ara Singh, a forest guard, stated that he saw a Yeti face-to-face in 1978. It was a 'man-like animal with brown hair on the body. It had a red face and red lips'.

There have also been reports of a 'wild man' in the mountains of central China. Only soft evidence to support the existence of such a creature has been forthcoming, taking, once again, the form of footprints and hairs. Once again, the hair is of an orange-brown colour reminiscent of the orang-utan. In May 1976 a sighting was reported of a wild man somewhat taller than a man with a protuberant belly

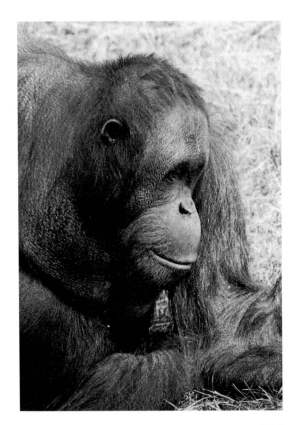

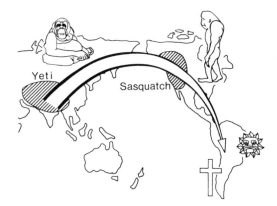

29.8 *With the emigration of mongoloid peoples from Asia across the Bering Strait into the North American continent went the legend of 'Bigfoot'. The concept of the Yeti based on the orang-utan appears to have been translated into the idea of the Sasquatch, itself a humanoid creature based on a North American animal, the bear, rather than the Asiatic orang-utan unknown to the population. In the Andes the Sun God of the Incas and the Cross of Roman Catholicism left no place for an Andean mountain deity.*

29.7 *Face of an orang-utan (*Pongo pygmaeus*). With its humanoid qualities it is easy to see why this species has been regarded by some authorities as forming the basis of the Yeti legend in the Himalaya.*

and covered in red-brown hair. This prompted the Chinese Government to instigate a year-long hunt to determine whether or not this creature existed. This unidentified primate was once again regarded by the Chinese as a relict form of *Gigantopithecus*.

The Sasquatch

It is now generally accepted that mongoloid people emigrated into North America across the Bering Strait, and the legend of 'Bigfoot' seems to have travelled with them to give rise to the legend of the Sasquatch, an Amerindian word meaning 'the wild man of the woods' (Fig. 29.8). On its introduction into North America the concept had to be transferred to a different kind of animal. There are no orang-utans in the New World, so the physical features of the Sasquatch had to be those of an animal native and common in the north-west of this continent, namely the bear. Thus the reddish shaggy fur

changes to black, brown, or grey, the partly quadrupedal gait of the Yeti has become wholly bipedal, and the cone-shaped head is lost.

Napier (1976) presents an interesting profile of the Sasquatch based on reports of 72 incidents from British Columbia, Alberta, Washington, Oregon, and northern California. Its reported estimated stature has ranged between 6 and 11 ft (1.8 and 3.4 m). Its footprints range in length from 12 to 22 in (30–56 cm) — the commonest quoted range being 14–18 in (36–46 cm), and the width being most frequently reported as 7 in (18 cm). The Sasquatch is seen most often during June and July (the holiday season) and October and November (the hunting season). Males are more commonly observed than females. A Sasquatch was captured on cinefilm by Roger Patterson in 1967 in the Bluff Creek Valley of northern California. The validity of this controversial film record is examined at length by Napier (1976). The acquisition of frankly human attributes does not help the credibility of the Sasquatch as an animal species.

Los Muquis

In the Andean mines of Cerro de Pasco, Huancavelica, and the district of Junin live 'Los Muquis', the spirits of the mines, appearing as dwarfs with long white beards (Bravo 1967). They wear ponchos trimmed with bright colours and have a liking for red and green hats. Los Muquis are nocturnal and noisy. They like to dance, sing, whistle, and blow horns. Like the Yeti, however, they are not altogether pleasant, for while they may save some mine-workers from death they allow others to perish (Bravo 1967). The Quechuas who work in these high-altitude mines treat Los Muquis with respect and depend for protection from their possibly malign influence on a combination of coca, *pisco* (Peruvian brandy), and prayer.

References

Bravo, C.A.E. (1967) In *The Man of Junin Looking at His Country and Folklore*, Vol. 2. Lima. Peru; P.L. Villanueva, p. 593

Cahoon, R.L. (1972). Simple decision-making at high altitude. *Ergonomics*, **15**, 157

Cahoon, R.L. (1973). Monitoring army radio-communications networks at high altitude. *Perceptual and Motor Skills*, **37**, 471

Cavaletti G., Moroni, R., Garavaglia, P., and Tredici, G. (1987). Brain damage after high-altitude climbs without oxygen. *Lancet*, **i**, 101

Clark, C.F., Heaton, R.K., and Wiens, A.N. (1983). Neuropsychological functioning after prolonged high altitude exposure in mountaineering. *Aviation, Space, and Environmental Medicine*, **54**, 202

Clark, R.W. (1976). In *Men, Myths and Mountains*. London; Weidenfield and Nicolson

Clarke, C. (1976). On surviving a bivouac at high altitude. *British Medical Journal*, **i**, 92

Denison, D.M., Ledwith, F., and Poulton, E.C. (1966). Complex reaction times at simulated cabin altitudes of 5000 feet and 8000 feet. *Aerospace Medicine*, **57**, 1010

Forster, P. (1986). Telescopes in high places. In *Aspects of Hypoxia* (D. Heath, Ed.). Liverpool; Liverpool University Press, p. 217

Habeler, P. (1979). *Everest Impossible Victory*. London; Arlington Books, pp. 179–80

Hodgson, B.H. (1832). On the Mammalia of Nepal. *Journal of the Asiatic Society of Bengal*, **1**, 335

Lewis, M.K., Ferrado, D.P., Mertens, H.W., and Steen, J.A. (1976). Interaction between marihuana and altitude on a complex behavioural task in baboons. *Aviation, Space, and Environmental Medicine*, **47**, 121

Lindley, R. (1975). Secrets of killer mountain. *Sunday Times*, 22 June

Loudon, B. (1978). Yak-hurling Yeti hunted in Sikkim. *Daily Telegraph*, 13 April, p. 4

Mazess, R.B., Picón-Reátegui, E., Thomas, R.D., and Little, M.A. (1968). Effects of alcohol and altitude on man during rest and work. *Aerospace Medicine*, **39**, 403

McFarland, R.A. (1937a). Psycho-physiological studies at high altitude in the Andes. I. The effects of rapid ascent by aeroplane and train. *Comparative Psychology*, **23**, 191

McFarland, R.A. (1973b). Psycho-physiological studies at high altitude in the Andes. II. Sensory and motor responses during acclimatization. *Comparative Psychology*, **23**, 227

McFarland, R.A. (1938a) Psycho-physiological studies at high altitude in the Andes. III Mental and psycho-somatic responses during gradual adaptation. *Comparative Psychology*, **24**, 147

McFarland, R.A. (1938b). Psycho-physiological studies at high altitude in the Andes. IV. Sensory and circulatory responses of the Andean residents at 17 500 feet. *Comparative Psychology*, **24**, 189

McFarland, R.A. (1972). Psychological implications of life at high altitude and including the role of oxygen in the process of aging. In *Physiological Adaptations, Desert and Mountain* (M.K. Yousef, S.M. Horvath, and R.W. Bullard, Eds). New York; Academic Press, p. 157

McFarland, R.A. and Dill, D.B. (1938). A comparative study of reduced oxygen pressure on man during acclimatization. *Journal of Aviation Medicine*, **9**, 18

Mummery, A.F. (1894). Quoted by Samuki and Yamada (1974)

Napier, J. (1976). *Bigfoot. The Yeti and Sasquatch in Myth and Reality*, Abacus edition. London; Cox and Wyman

Nettles, J.L. and Olson, R.N. (1965). Effects of alcohol on hypoxia. *Journal of the American Medical Association*, **195**, 1193

Nicolson, N. (1975). *The Himalayas. The World's Wild Places*. Amsterdam; Time-Life Books

Ravenhill, T.H. (1913). Some experience of mountain sickness in the Andes. *Journal of Tropical Medicine and Hygiene*, **16**, 313

Ryn, Z. (1971). Psychopathology in alpinism. *Acta Medica Polonica*, **12**, 453

Ryn, Z. (1988). Psychopathology in mountaineering — mental disturbances under high-altitude stress. *International Journal of Sports Medicine*, **9**, 163

Sanuki, M. and Yamada, K. (1974). Climbing to fame. In *The Alps*. Tokyo; Kodansha International, pp. 15 and 29

Sharma, V.M. and Malhotra, M.S. (1976). Ethnic variations in psychological performance under altitude stress. *Aviation, Space, and Environmental Medicine*, **47**, 248

Sharma, V.M., Malhotra, M.S., and Baskaran, A.S. (1975). Variations in psychomotor efficiency during prolonged stay at high altitude. *Ergonomics*, **18**, 511

Shipton, E. (1943). *Upon That Mountain*. London; Hodder and Stoughton, p. 129

Shukitt, B.L. and Banderet, L.E. (1988). Mood states at 1600 and 4300 meters terrestrial altitude. *Aviation, Space, and Environmental Medicine*, **59**, 530

Shults, W.T. and Swan, K.C. (1975). High altitude retinopathy in mountain climbers. *Archives of Ophthalmology*, **93**, 404

Smythe, F.S. (1934). The second assault. In *Everest 1993*. London; Hodder and Stoughton, p. 164

Tharion, W.J., Hoyt, R.W., Marlowe, B.E., and Cymerman, A. (1992). Effects of high altitude and exercise on marksmanship. *Aviation, Space, and Environmental Medicine*, **63**, 114

Townes, B.D., Hornbein, T.F., Schoene, R.B., Sarnquist, F.H., and Grant, I. (1984). Human cerebral function at extreme altitude. In *High Altitude and Man* (J.B. West and S. Lahiri, Eds). Bethesda, Maryland; American Physiological Society, p. 31

Tune, F.S. (1964). Psychological effects of hypoxia. Review of certain literature from the period 1950 to 1963. *Perceptual and Motor Skills*, **19**, 551

US Department of Health Education and Welfare (1974). *Marihuana and health*, DHEW Report No. 74–50. Washington, DC; US Government Printing Office

Ward, M.P., Milledge, J.S., and West, J.B. (1989). *High Altitude Medicine and Physiology*. London; Chapman and Hall Medical

West, J.B. (1986). Do climbs to extreme altitude cause brain damage? *Lancet*, **ii**, 387

Zhongyuan, S., Deming, Z., Changming, L., and Miaoshen, Q. (1983). Changes of electroencephalogram under acute hypoxia and relationship between tolerant ability to hypoxia and adaptation ability to high altitudes. *Scientia Sinica*, **26**, 58

30

Astronomers at high altitude

This chapter is about the astronomers and supporting staff who man the United Kingdom infrared telescope on the summit of the volcano Mauna Kea (4200 m) on Hawaii. When this telescope was planned and commissioned it set the British Science Research Council and the Royal Observatory at Edinburgh some unique physiological and medical problems. Lowlanders were to be repeatedly exposed to high altitude only to withdraw to moderate or low altitude before acclimatization was achieved. A code of practice had to be drawn up to cover working arrangements for the astronomers, and investigations were carried out to determine whether or not intermittent subjection to hypobaric hypoxia can allow sea-level man to achieve acclimatization. It was also paramount to assess the dangers of the astronomers developing acute mountain sickness and pulmonary and cerebral oedema.

TELESCOPES ON MAUNA KEA

An important advance in modern astronomy has been the development of infrared telescopes, which have to operate at high altitude to avoid absorption by water vapour of the infrared radiation streaming in from space. An ideal environment for such a telescope is the dry, clear atmosphere of the summit of a volcano, high above its cloud inversion layer, in a subtropical area. Thus it comes about that one of the great concentrations of telescope power in the world has taken place on the summit of the volcano Mauna Kea, at an altitude of 4200 m, on the 'big island' of Hawaii, situated at the volcanically active southern extremity of the Hawaiian archipelago (Fig. 30.1). Six telescopes, making observations at optical and infrared wavelengths, are situated on the site. One of these is the 3.8 m United Kingdom Infrared Telescope (UKIRT) that was commissioned by the (then) Science Research Council and is operated by astronomers from the Royal Observatory at Edinburgh (Fig. 30.2). In 1980 we were approached to undertake an investigation into the health and safety of the staff manning the telescope. Dr Peter Forster was appointed to carry out

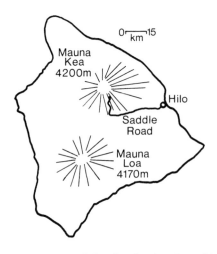

30.1 *Island of Hawaii showing the situations of its two volcanoes, and demonstrating the accessibility of the summit of Mauna Kea by the Saddle Road from the port of Hilo. The newcomer from sea level can reach an altitude of 4200 m in 1.5 hours.*

studies on the astronomers and these occupied 2 years. His findings were reported at length by the Observatory (Forster 1983) and later at a symposium on 'Aspects of Hypoxia' at the University of Liverpool (Forster 1986).

At the summit of the volcano barometric pressure is 468 mmHg and the ambient partial pressure of oxygen is 60% of that at sea level. The partial pressure of oxygen in inspired air is 95 mmHg, compared with 150 mmHg at sea level, and in alveolar air is 57 mmHg, compared with 105 mmHg at sea level. Workers on the high-altitude telescopes live in the small coastal town of Hilo and are able to reach the summit at 4200 m by car within 90 minutes. They do this repeatedly.

Forster investigated two groups of workers — shiftworkers and commuters. The British telescope was operated on a shift system that involved work for 40 days at Hilo, followed by duties on the volcano for a further 40 days (Fig. 30.3). The moun-

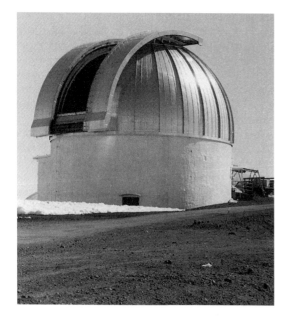

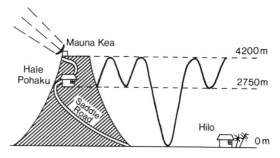

30.3 *Movements of astronomers and supporting staff working on the infrared telescope situated on the summit of Mauna Kea (4200 m). They oscillate between working at the summit, sleeping in the acclimatization lodge at Hale Pohaku (2750 m), and spending time in between tours of duty on the mountain at Hilo on the coast.*

30.2 *United Kingdom Infrared Telescope (UKIRT) at the summit (4200 m) of the Hawaiian volcano, Mauna Kea.*

tain duties comprised four shifts on Mauna Kea, each lasting 5 days, with an initial night for acclimatization at a sleeping lodge at Hale Pohaku at an altitude of 2750 m (Fig. 30.3). Shifts on the mountain were interspersed by periods of rest for 5 days at sea level. The 3.0 m NASA telescope was operated by staff who commuted daily from Hilo to the summit. They left the coast at 08.00 hours and arrived at Hale Pohaku 1 hour later by car. After half an hour at the lodge they travelled by car on a winding dirt-track road to the summit (Fig. 30.4), arriving there at 10.00 hours. At 16.00 hours they left the telescope site to arrive back in Hilo 90 minutes later.

ACUTE MOUNTAIN SICKNESS

Eighty per cent of the shiftworkers developed symptoms of acute mountain sickness on the first day at the summit. The commonest complaints were breathlessness (50%) and headache (41%). Other common symptoms were insomnia, lethargy, poor concentration, poor memory, and unsteadiness of gait (Forster 1986). Headache was the most disabling symptom and caused several shiftworkers to descend from the summit. After 5 days only 40% had symptoms. A fifth of the shiftworkers had no symptoms at any time. In contrast to this, only 40% of the commuters had symptoms on the first day.

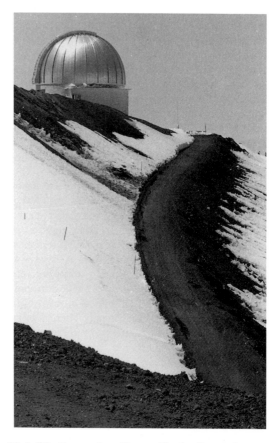

30.4 *Winding road on Mauna Kea leading to the infrared telescope at its summit.*

The rapid ascent in cars gave rise to minimal discomfort, but after a lag period of 5 hours at high altitude they too began to experience breathlessness, headache, poor concentration, and lethargy. None of the shiftworkers or commuters developed nail-haemorrhages (see Chapter 25). Half of them showed engorgement of retinal veins (see Chapter 27) that disappeared rapidly on descent to sea level. None of them developed papilloedema.

At first sight the commuters seem to have acclimatized better than the shiftworkers, but this impression is spurious. The reason for their early freedom from symptoms is that they entered and left the hypoxic environment during the lag period of 6–9 hours that precedes the onset of acute mountain sickness (see Chapter 12). During a visit to the telescope site we were impressed by the paucity of symptoms compared with what we had experienced during the stay at an identical altitude of 4200 m in La Raya, Peru. The difference was the fleeting nature of the exposure to high altitude in Hawaii and the ease and speed of retreat from the hypoxic environment. This comparative freedom from symptoms is bought at the expense of failing to develop full acclimatization, which ultimately would allow a better overall work performance. Forster (1986) found that after 5 days on Mauna Kea the somewhat acclimatized shiftworkers experienced fewer symptoms, performed better at psychometric tests, and recorded a higher arterial oxygen tension than did the commuters.

ARTERIAL BLOOD GASES

Analysis of arterial blood samples was carried out on 27 shiftworkers on the first and last days of a total of 40 shifts. During this period, arterial oxygen tension rose from a mean level in the group of 42 mmHg to one of 44.2 mmHg, a rise of statistical significance. Arterial carbon dioxide tension was reduced at exposure to high altitude compared with sea-level values and was lower on the fifth day, indicating a more sustained respiratory effort. Hydrogen ion concentration was also reduced. There was no association between individual symptoms and the level of arterial oxygen tension. In the commuters (28 subjects, 35 ascents) mean arterial blood-gas tensions for the group were 39.7 mmHg for oxygen and 27.7 mmHg for carbon dioxide.

There was a pronounced individual susceptibility to the symptoms of acute mountain sickness and individuals responded reproducibly on every ascent to high altitude. Forster (1983) measured arterial blood oxygen tensions in 12 subjects during two

successive shifts on the mountain. On the first day of the two ascents to the summit the level ranged from 33 to 57 mmHg, with a group mean of 41.3 mmHg. It was found that the value recorded in any individual on the first day of the first shift correlated with that found on the first day of the second shift. The subject with the highest arterial oxygen tension on the first shift (49 mmHg) recorded the highest on the second (57 mmHg). The worker with the lowest value on the first shift (33.0 mmHg) registered a value of 38.2 mmHg on the second. The values for individual shiftworkers were similar on the fifth day of the two shifts. Mean arterial carbon dioxide tension was higher on the first shift than on the second but once again there was a significant correlation between the measurements of this on the two ascents in individuals.

Six other shiftworkers were added to make a group of 18 subjects in which the severity of acute mountain sickness was assessed on the two successive shifts. It was found that five of the subjects were asymptomatic on both shifts, while the remainder developed symptoms. There was a significant correlation between the order of the 18 men ranked according to severity of symptoms of altitude sickness on the first day of the two shifts. These results make it clear that there is a reproducible degree of hypoxia and hyperventilation on each exposure to high altitude in individual subjects. There is also a reproducible individual susceptibility to the symptoms of acute mountain sickness. The reasons for this are not known. It has been suggested that it may be related to the individual sensitivity of hypoxic drive (Lakshminarayan and Pierson 1975). In this respect it is of interest to note that Flenley (1986) reported that he had found a sevenfold variability in the sensitivity of the hypoxic drive, which he believed to be mediated by the carotid chemoreceptors, in apparently healthy human subjects. If this is the case, clearly some lowlanders ascend into the mountains far better equipped to cope with the hypobaric hypoxia than some of their fellows. Others have suggested that the inherent characteristic which determines susceptibility to altitude sickness is related to the magnitude of the ventilatory response to carbon dioxide under conditions of hypocapnic hypoxia (Miller *et al.* 1983).

SYSTEMIC BLOOD PRESSURE AND HEART RHYTHM

Among the shiftworkers systemic blood pressure was elevated at 4200 m compared with sea level (Forster 1983). The diastolic pressure was increased by about 10% of the pre-ascent level and remained elevated throughout the stay on the volcano. Systolic pressure was increased from the second day onwards. On descent the systemic blood pressure fell to pre-ascent levels. No difference was found in the height of systemic blood pressure between subjects with or without acute mountain sickness and, in particular, there was no relation to the presence of headache. Systemic blood pressure did not rise in the commuters and, in fact, both diastolic and systolic pressure fell marginally at the summit. The resting pulse rates rose after about 5 hours at 4200 m and reached a peak on the first day on the mountain, with an average increase of 10 beats/min greater than the count at sea level. The systemic circulation at high altitude is considered in Chapter 18.

One 45-year-old engineer working on Mauna Kea had multifocal ventricular extrasystoles occurring in a bigeminal pattern following a standard exercise test (see Fig. 19.3). He experienced no discomfort other than awareness of the irregular pulse. A 37-year-old technician showed unifocal ventricular extrasystoles in a bigeminal pattern following exercise at 4200 m. When both men underwent submaximal exercise tests on a bicycle-ergometer, there were no electrocardiographic abnormalities other than occasional extrasystoles in the older man. Both continued to work on Mauna Kea without ill effects.

Changes occurred in the electrocardiographs of the astronomers. At sea level the mean QRS axis was 58.1°, but there was a progressive right-axis shift at high altitude, so that on the first day at 4200 m it rotated to 63.9° and by the fifth day to 65°. There was no significant alteration in the P- or T-wave axes. At sea level, inversion of the T wave in lead VI was found in a quarter of the subjects, but within hours arrival at the summit this was seen in half the workers. The electrocardiogram at high altitude is considered in Chapter 19.

RESPIRATORY RATE AND MINUTE VOLUME
There was a slight but statistically significant increase in respiratory rate from 16.5 breaths/min (SD 3.4) at sea level to 18.2 breaths/min (SD 3.2) on arrival at 4200 m and 18.7 breaths/min (SD 3.7) after 5 days on the mountain. On return to sea level the respiratory rate returned to the pre-ascent value. Four subjects exhibited periodic breathing at high altitude, but only two of them were aware of their disordered respiratory rhythm. Minute volumes did

not increase to any extent. At sea level the minute volume was 10.7 litres (SD 3.4) and at the summit it remained at 10.6 litres (SD 3.0) on the first day but rose slightly to 12.5 litres (SD 3.5) on the fifth day.

Reports that a pronounced reduction in peak expiratory flow rate occurred in acute mountain sickness (Singh *et al.* 1969; Stockley and Green 1979) led Forster (1983) to employ a Mini Wright Peak Flow Meter in an attempt to predict the development of altitude sickness. However, his observations suggested that the observed fall in peak expiratory flow rate at high altitude was a consequence of the effect of reduced air density on the performance of the peak flow meter and not a reflection of disordered pulmonary physiology. Experiments with the meter demonstrated that peak flow readings were universally proportional to the density of the ambient air when tested at sea level, 3000 m, and 4200 m (Forster and Parker 1983). It was concluded that the peak flow meter has no value in predicting the development of acute mountain sickness.

BLOOD
Following exposure for 5 days to hypobaric hypoxia, significant increases were seen in red blood cell count, haemoglobin concentration, packed cell volume, and platelet count. Within 20 days of the return to sea level all had returned to pre-ascent values (see Chapter 5).

SEVERE ACUTE MOUNTAIN SICKNESS
Only three cases occurred during the period of study over 2 years. One was a presumed case of high-altitude pulmonary oedema in a 29-year-old computer engineer with suggestive symptoms, but with no confirmatory clinical or radiological findings. After treatment with oxygen and descent to sea level, he recovered rapidly and continued to work thereafter without incident on the mountain. A 30-year-old engineer developed cerebral oedema that resolved rapidly on treatment with oxygen and descent to sea level. A 30-year-old computer engineer experienced severe acute mountain sickness at the start of every shift on the mountain. These symptoms were not prevented by acclimatization or medication. The latter two subjects discontinued their duties on the volcano.

GROUPS AT SPECIAL RISK
Some groups of people are at special risk so far as working on the telescopes is concerned. Forster (1994) considers that modest increases in cardiac output at 4200 m will have little deleterious effect

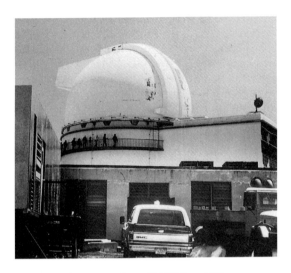

30.5 *Ambulances on site at UKIRT at 4200 m on Mauna Kea, providing the facility for rapid descent to sea level in the event of a sudden medical emergency.*

on asymptomatic subjects with ischaemic heart disease and they can work on such projects safely. On the other hand patients with angina or exertional dyspnoea at sea level may well suffer a worsening of symptoms shortly after arrival at high altitude. Those patients whose level of activity is severely curtailed by symptoms related to ischaemia at sea level are likely to suffer a marked deterioration at high altitude and must be cautioned against ascent. For such people who do visit the telescopes at 4200 m, facilities for rapid retreat down the mountain are mandatory (Fig. 30.5). A single cardiac death has occurred at the telescopes on Mauna Kea in the last decade while the population at risk has numbered about 60 personnel each working day (Forster 1994). The fatal event involved a 37-year-old astronomer, a cigarette smoker, who suffered a myocardial infarction at the summit. Post-mortem examination revealed severe coronary artery disease.

We have already pointed out in Chapter 26 that lowlanders rendered hypoxic by chronic lung disease will experience a further reduction in alveolar oxygen tension at high altitude. In that chapter we also pointed out that, while bronchonspasm in asthmatics can be provoked by the inhalation of cold, dry air, this is in the main outweighed by the absence of exogenous allergens such as house-dust-mites and pollutants such as tobacco smoke. In the Mauna Kea study a 32-year-old asthmatic was unaffected by work at 4200 m (Forster 1994). The risks attached to

sickle-cell disease at high altitude were dealt with in Chapter 8. Potential workers for projects at high altitude should be screened for the sickle-cell trait before they are employed to work at high altitude.

CODE OF PRACTICE FOR WORK ON MAUNA KEA

The studies of Forster (1983) have shed light on the problems of sea-level man whose work involves intermittent exposure to high altitude at an easily accessible site. They show first that commuters can enter and leave such areas without developing severe symptoms of acute mountain sickness or being exposed to serious danger, provided they do not remain at high altitude for longer than the 'lag' period of 6–9 hours referred to in Chapter 12. However, employing this 'snatch and grab' technique of working does not allow the development of even the limited degree of acclimatization achieved on the shift system, which is not comparable to that acquired by permanent residence at high altitude. There is little danger of serious medical emergencies arising, provided facilities are available for a rapid, efficient retreat from high altitude. Just as one can get into trouble by too rapid an ascent to high altitude, so one can get out of it by an equally rapid descent. The main tenets of the code of practice at UKIRT are that no astronomer is allowed to work alone at the telescope and vehicles must be available at all times at the summit to allow rapid descent to sea level (Fig. 30.5). It is, nevertheless, thought necessary to maintain generous supplies of oxygen (60 000 litres) in the telescope dome for use in the event of a medical emergency such as a telescope-user developing pulmonary or cerebral oedema when descent is made impossible by snowstorms on the volcano blocking the dirt-track road. The repeated exposure of the astronomers to high altitude for short periods of time does not allow them to develop a degree of acclimatization sufficient to allow them to treat such possible periods of isolation at such high places with impunity.

Forster (1986) concludes that the experience on Mauna Kea demonstrates that high altitude can be a safe working environment provided that certain precautions are taken. Education of the staff is essential and telescope operators are taught to recognize the signs of altitude sickness. A 'red alert' notice is shown to all visitors to UKIRT and is displayed in the telescope dome. This comprises summaries of the cerebral and respiratory symptoms of acute mountain sickness. The action to be taken centres on the administration of oxygen at 6 l/min, rapid descent to sea level, and the prompt seeking of medical attention. It is stressed, as we do in different contexts in other places in this book, that it is better to be safe than sorry and to descend from the telescope if in doubt. As Forster (1986) points out, it is a testimony to the good sense of the UKIRT staff that supplemental oxygen was needed on but a single occasion during the preceding 5 years of operation of the telescope.

INTERMITTENT EXPOSURE TO HYPOBARIC HYPOXIA IN FLIGHT PERSONNEL

The investigation of the effects of intermittent exposure to the hypoxia of high altitude on the astronomers of Mauna Kea had in fact been preceded by a study of pilots and other flight personnel working in non-pressurized aircraft by Hurtado and co-workers as early as 1947. They studied a group of American pilots and Peruvian cabin crew working for a commercial airline in South America whose unpressurized aircraft commonly flew at altitudes between 3600 and 6000 m to cross the Andes. Three routes were followed. A typical one was of 9 hours' duration and involved flying between altitudes of 4500 and 6000 m for 5–6 hours. On this route there were stopovers of 15–20 minutes at airports between 3900 and 4500 m and, not infrequently, overnight stops were necessary at these altitudes. Fifty healthy pilots and co-pilots were studied. Their ages ranged from 22 to 52 years, with a mean of 30 years; all had resided on the coast at Lima for between 1 and 10 years. The period of exposure to intermittent hypobaric hypoxia was considerable, for no less than one-fifth of the pilots had logged up flying time of over 5000 h, while a few had flying time of over 10 000 h. The pilots and co-pilots inhaled oxygen by means of a tube carried in the mouth, with a continuous inflow of gas at altitudes of 3600 m and higher. The cabin staff did not have access to oxygen.

The degree of acclimatization to high altitude being achieved on intermittent exposure to hypobaric hypoxia was assessed by Hurtado *et al.* (1947) on the basis of six criteria. These were changes in the total lung capacity and its subdivisions, in haematological parameters, in acid–base balance, in the position of the oxygen–haemoglobin dissociation curve, in the transverse diameter of the heart measured radiographically, and finally in the subjective experience of the flight personnel. Only two physiological variants were detected that could be related to intermittent exposure to a low-pressure environ-

ment. One was a slight elevation of haemoglobin concentration in some of the staff, although there was considerable variation in this. Thus, while the haematocrit was more than 50% in three subjects, it was less than 42% in three others. In contrast to the constant polycythaemia found in native highlanders in Peru, there was only a very moderate polycythaemia in the flight personnel.

The position of the oxygen–haemoglobin dissociation curve was determined in eight healthy Peruvian cabin staff between the ages of 21 and 28 years who did not have access to oxygen. Some of them had a total flying time of over 1 year. At a pH of 7.4 the P_{50} (see Chapter 5) of these personnel was 25.16, in comparison with values of 25.99 in healthy highlanders at 4470 m and of 24.55 for non-flight personnel at sea level. Hurtado and co-workers interpret these findings as indicating a slight decrease in the affinity of haemoglobin for oxygen in the cabin staff, as found in native highlanders.

There was an increase in the residual lung volume in some of the pilots. As seen in Chapter 4 this is defined as the volume of air remaining in the lung and respiratory dead space after a forced expiration. Its mean absolute and relative values, 1.80 ± 0.13 litres and $28.1 \pm 1.10\%$, were higher than obtained in healthy subjects at sea level. In 15 of the 48 subjects studied the absolute residual air volume was higher than 2.00 litres and in 11 men the relative volume exceeded 30%. In newcomers to, and residents at, high altitude there is a frequent increase in the residual lung volume, but the degree is greater than in flight personnel. No changes were found in heart size or acid–base balance of the blood. Hurtado *et al.* (1947) came to the conclusion that intermittent exposure to high altitude, such as that experienced by air crew, does not give rise to constant physiological variations that can be interpreted as evidence of acclimatization.

MENTAL FATIGUE

Nevertheless, these authors found that in these pilots intermittent exposure to a high-altitude environment gave rise not infrequently to symptoms of chronic mental fatigue accompanied at times by a state of what they term 'mental irritability'. For this reason they concluded that it was desirable at that time to place air crew employed on very high routes in unpressurized aircraft under close medical observation. It is intriguing to note that, 40 years on, Forster (1986) found some deterioration of the results of psychometric tests on the astronomers on Mauna

Kea. Tests of numerate memory (Wechsler digit span forwards and digit span backwards) and motor speed and recoding of information (digit symbol substitution) were performed by telescope staff. In the shiftworkers, no decrement in the performance of the digit symbol substitution or digit span forwards was found at high altitude. Performance of the digit span backwards test, however, did deteriorate on the first day at 4200 m but, after 5 days on the volcano, the scores for this test were similar to those attained at sea level. These results suggest that on immediate ascent to operate high-technology equipment there may be some slight blurring of higher cerebral functions. It is also clear, however, that adequate motivation and familiarity with the techniques to be followed can overcome such problems.

References

Flenley, D. (1986). Long-term oxygen therapy and the pulmonary circulation. In *Aspects of Hypoxia* (D. Heath, Ed.). Liverpool; Liverpool University Press, p. 48

Forster, P.J.G. (1983). Work at high altitude: a clinical and physiological study at the United Kingdom Infrared Telescope, Mauna Kea, Hawaii. Occasional Reports, Edinburgh Royal Observatory

Forster, P.J.G. (1986). Telescopes in high places. In *Aspects of Hypoxia* (D. Heath, Ed.). Liverpool; Liverpool University Press, p. 217

Forster, P.J.G. (1994). Working at high altitudes. In *Hunter's Diseases of Occupations*, 8th edn (P.A.B. Raffle, P.H. Adams, P.J. Baxter, and W.R. Lee, Eds). London; Edward Arnold, p. 363.

Forster, P.J.G. and Parker, R.W. (1983). Peak expiratory flow at high altitude. *Lancet*, **ii**, 100

Hurtado, A., Aste-Salazar, H., Merino, C., Velasquez, T., Monge-C, C., and Reynafarje, C. (1947). Physiological characteristics of flight personnel. *Journal of Aviation Medicine*, **18**, 406

Lakshminarayan, S. and Pierson, D.J. (1975). Recurrent high altitude pulmonary edema with blunted chemosensitivity. *American Review of Respiratory Disease*, **111**, 869

Miller, M.R., Pincock, A.C, and Wright, A.D. (1983). Predicting susceptibility to acute mountain sickness. *Lancet*, **ii**, 164

Singh, I., Khanna, P.K., Srivastava, M.C., Lal, M., Roy, S.B., and Subramanyam, C.S.V (1969). Acute mountain sickness. *New England Journal of Medicine*, **280**, 175

Stockley, R.A. and Green, I.D. (1979). Cardiopulmonary function before, during and after a twenty-one day Himalayan trek. *Postgraduate Medical Journal*, **55**, 496

31

Athletic performance at moderate altitude

Throughout this book we have given an account of the numerous physiological and frequently associated structural changes that occur in many tissues on the ascent of the lowlander to high altitude. At the onset we defined 'high altitude' as one exceeding 3000 m but, as we point out, the physiological consequences of exposure to hypobaric hypoxia start to develop at considerably lower elevations. The effects of moderate altitude assume importance when international sports meetings are held at such elevations. Even the relatively slight degree of hypobaric hypoxia may affect deleteriously the performance of the athletes. This has led to controversy over the wisdom of holding major sports meetings at altitude, for the performance of competitors depends not only on their innate ability but also on their idiosyncratic capacity to cope with the environment. Some believe that the effects may be alleviated by previous acclimatization including altitude training. This in itself has proved controversial for the efficacy of altitude training has been much debated.

THE 19TH OLYMPIAD

In October 1963 the International Olympic Committee chose Mexico City (2380 m) as the venue for the 19th Olympiad. Although many of the effects of high altitude on the human body were known at the time, it was not clear whether or not this moderate elevation would be deleterious to athletes coming from sea level. Some considered that as a little as 48 hours would be sufficient for adequate acclimatization. On the other hand, in June 1965 the British Olympic Association, on the advice of its medical committee, decided to send a research team to Mexico to study the time necessary to acclimatize and the type of training schedules the athletes would require. Its report concluded that in events requiring endurance, such as track events exceeding 1500 m, 4 weeks would be the minimal acceptable time for acclimatization. It also concluded that athletes other than those in such endurance events would benefit from acclimatization and that there was no evidence of any risk of permanent injury.

Predictions for athletic performance prior to the 19th Olympiad were based on comparisons drawn from the results of the 1955 Pan American Games, also held at Mexico City, with the results of previous and subsequent Pan American competitions held at sea level (Faulkner 1967; Jokl and Jokl 1968). This comparison had shown a small gain in running events between 100 and 400 m, because of a decrease in wind resistance, and a slowing of times for more long-distance and endurance events. This slowing amounted to 6–7% in the 5000 and 10 000 m events and rose to 17–22% in the marathon (42 000 m). In some instances it was possible to compare the performance of individuals both at sea level and at moderate altitude. Although the apparent effect of such altitude varied, there was an immediate loss of performance of 6–8%. When high-altitude natives competed at sea level, the gain in performance was 2–4%.

The results from Mexico City in 1968 were in fact better than those predicted (Craig 1969; Faulkner 1971). Twenty-nine per cent of competitors broke world records and the average winning margin was only 0.9% below the world record. This compares with the margin of 2.9% below the world record in previous Olympiads held at sea level (Shephard 1973). To assist the interpretation of the results and to separate short- and long-term events, Craig (1969) expressed the results as a percentage of the world record plotted against their duration. When a linear regression was applied to both track and swimming events, it showed that, although world records were exceeded in short events, there was a steady decline in events lasting longer than a minute. This fall ranged from 3% at 4 minutes to 8% at 1 hour.

Information on the effects of hypoxia at altitudes of less than 3000 m is somewhat sparse, for most of the studies on the cardiopulmonary effects of hypoxia are based on much higher altitudes, as seen earlier in this book. Consequently, it is important to differentiate between the studies carried out on high mountains and those concerned with the more subtle problems of altitudes below 3000 m. In

Mexico City the effects of moderate altitude were normally slight and may be confused with the symptoms of anxiety before the contest. Sime *et al.* (1974) carried out a study at Arequipa (2370 m) in southern Peru, the altitude of which is similar to Mexico City. They studied eight male amateur soccer players between the ages of 16 and 21 years. These men were subjected to right heart catheterization and studies by bicycle-ergometer at moderate and submaximal exercise (300 and 600 kg m/min per m² BSA, respectively), initially at sea level and subsequently at Arequipa 4–6 hours after arrival and, in some instances, after a 5-day sojourn at this altitude.

VENTILATION AND OXYGEN UPTAKE

We may now consider the effects of moderate altitude on some specific physiological factors concerned in exercise as determined principally by the studies of Sime *et al.* (1974) and by the earlier investigations of Pugh (1967). Specifically, we may consider the effects on ventilation and oxygen uptake, heart rate and cardiac output, and pulmonary and systemic blood pressures.

Athletic exercise at high altitude is associated with increased ventilation, a fall in arterial oxygen saturation, and a decrease in oxygen uptake. Sime *et al.* (1974) found that minute ventilation did not change at 2370 m at rest, but it increased by some 12% on submaximal exercise, compared with sea level. Following ascent, systemic arterial oxygen saturation fell 4% at rest and 4–7% on exertion. Oxygen uptake decreased 10% at rest and 7% during exercise. This confirmed the earlier results of Pugh (1967) in a series of investigations carried out prior to the Olympics in Mexico. The major difference between the two groups was that, while Sime's group was composed of amateur soccer players, Pugh's group consisted of six international middle-distance runners. Although they were still technically amateurs, it is reasonable to assume that their intensity and level of training was much higher than in the case of the soccer players. Pugh (1967) also used a bicycle-ergometer and the work load was adjusted so that the subjects could just undertake 5 minutes' work at sea level. The data for maximum oxygen uptake was obtained from 1-minute gas samples obtained at the third to fourth and fourth to fifth minute, and usually these samples agreed to within 50 ml, indicating a steady intake of oxygen.

The initial tests undertaken at Mexico City were on the second day of exposure to the altitude. They showed a mean reduction of 14.6% of oxygen intake for all individuals, compared with the mean values at sea level. This reduced with exposure to altitude, until by the fourth test undertaken on the 27th day of exposure the reduction was 9.6%. Although all six athletes were of international standing, the individual variation was considerable. Three improved progressively, one showed little improvement, and in two cases the results were so varied that little use could be made of them. This wide range was reflected in the ventilatory response. At sea level the minute volume varied from 122 to 196 l/min, with a mean of 148 l/min. In Mexico City, ventilation increased by between 3 and 22 l/min to a mean value of 160 l/min.

Maximum oxygen uptake in sea-level subjects falls on their ascent to high altitude and this applies even at the moderate altitude of Mexico City (2380 m). The decrease in oxygen uptake occurs in spite of a slight increase in pulmonary ventilation. It is clear, therefore, that the limiting factor in oxygen consumption is not ventilation. It is more likely to be a combination of the lowering of arterial oxygen saturation and the depression of cardiac output referred to below that interfere with the diffusion of oxygen at tissue level (Sime *et al.* 1974). The fall in resting arterial oxygen saturation down the oxyhaemoglobin dissociation curve with increasing altitude takes place up to an elevation of about 6000 m. Above this at extreme altitudes there is a slight rise in arterial oxygen saturation due to the profound alkalosis that occurs causing a leftward shift of the curve (Wood *et al.* 1988). As work rate increases there is a further sharp drop in arterial oxygen saturation. While some believe that impaired cardiac function at high altitude contributes to the decline in maximal oxygen uptake (Reeves *et al.* 1987), others suggest that reduced cardiac output is the result rather than the cause of the reduced oxygen uptake (Houston 1988).

To take the extreme example, at the summit of Mt Everest (8848 m) exercise performance should be nil as maximal oxygen uptake is predicted to be only slightly above the oxygen level required for basal metabolism (Pugh *et al.* 1964). For prolonged running at sea level, oxygen consumption must be below the anaerobic threshold, that is 70–80% of maximal oxygen uptake for most subjects (Costhill 1970). Running at 7.5 mph requires an oxygen consumption of about 40 ml O_2/kg/minute so that a maximal oxygen uptake of 50 ml O_2/kg/minute is necessary (Wood *et al.* 1988). It becomes impossible to provide such a supply of oxygen in the mountain environment so that one of the striking consequences of going to high altitude is reduced exercise tolerance and we refer to this important aspect below.

HEART RATE AND CARDIAC OUTPUT

The heart rate at an altitude like that of Mexico City does not increase significantly in its response to exercise from that at sea level. Sime *et al.* (1974) found that the heart rate did not change either at rest or during moderate exercise, but decreased significantly on submaximal exercise both immediately after ascent and after some days' sojourn at high altitude. Pugh (1967) also found no significant differences in heart rate. The mean values for individuals at sea level after exercise varied from 159 to 185 beats/min, with a mean of 168 beats/min, and at 2270 m after comparable exercise the individual mean range was 147–184 beats/min, with a mean of 166 beats/min.

Sime *et al.* (1974) found that the cardiac index was reduced by 10% at rest at 2370 m on the first day, but fell by 20% at rest and by 15% on exercise by the fifth day. Since heart rate at moderately high altitude does not differ significantly in its responses from that at sea level, it seems that a diminution in stroke volume is far more likely to account for the diminution in cardiac output. This could arise from a defective contractile myocardial force resulting from a lower coronary arterial tension or flow. However, Sime *et al.* (1974) were unable to find any correlation between the degree of lowering of cardiac output or stroke volume and the altitude or degree of work performed. An alternative view is that there may be a lowering of venous return from a diminished circulating blood volume due to redistribution of blood flow occurring early on exposure to altitude.

BLOOD PRESSURES

In Sime's group the pulmonary arterial mean pressure increased by 18% at rest and 30% on submaximal exercise above sea-level values. On ascent to 2370 m there was an increase of total pulmonary resistance of 29% and this rose to 42% after a 5-day sojourn at high altitude. Pugh (1967) did not subject his athletes to this type of investigation, but measured the systemic blood pressure by auscultation. He obtained values of 200–230 mmHg in submaximal exercise at sea level and at altitude. During the period of maximal exercise the systolic pressure was measured by means of a cuff and transducer and showed pressures of up to 300 mmHg.

Newcomers to high altitude are exposed to a degree of hypoxaemia that is different to that found in the long-term residents at the same altitude due to the lower systemic arterial oxygen saturation. Since the extent of hypoxaemia is greater in newcomers to the mountains, it might be anticipated that they would experience higher levels of pulmonary arterial pressure secondary to exaggerated hypoxic pulmonary vasoconstriction. According to Sime *et al.* (1974), the reverse is true. It seems likely that the higher degree of pulmonary hypertension in long-standing high-altitude residents both at rest and during exercise is related to the muscularization of pulmonary arterioles which is described in Chapter 10.

DIMINISHED WORK CAPACITY OF LOWLANDERS AT HIGH ALTITUDE

At 2370 m the soccer players studied by Sime *et al.* (1974) were exhausted on completing a work intensity of 600 kg m/min per m^2 BSA, indicating that submaximal exercise at sea level becomes nearly maximal at high altitudes. Pugh (1967) found that the oxygen debt mechanism was unchanged at Mexico City and that in his opinion a reduction in performance in endurance events arises from a reduction in oxygen uptake. The reduction in work performance must clearly be related to the reduction in oxygen intake, but the diminution in cardiac output and arterial oxygen saturation with an increase in pulmonary arterial pressure must play an important role in the overall mechanism. The decreased exercise capacity of sea-level subjects at high altitude has also been reported by Grover and Reeves (1966) at a medium altitude of 3100 m and Pugh *et al.* (1964) at an extreme altitude of 5790 m. Certainly all the results of the physiological studies of Pugh (1967) and Sime *et al.* (1974) indicate that moderately high altitude has a deleterious effect on work capacity and suggest that at the altitude of Mexico City submaximal exercise entails a handicap for sea-level athletes.

In short-duration athletic events the speed at which oxygen debt increases is the main physiological determinant of performance, the event having finished before the athlete reaches the maximum tolerable debt (Shephard 1973). In events of a longer duration, 50% of the energy expenditure can come from the build-up of a large oxygen debt.

HIGH EXERCISE TOLERANCE IN NATIVE HIGHLANDERS

Hurtado (1964) found that, in sharp contrast to the diminished work-capacity of lowlanders at high altitude, the native highlander showed a high exercise tolerance (see Chapter 36). He found that the Quechua Indian had a very high level of tolerance to maximal exercise on a treadmill. Indeed at a meeting of a Pan American Health Organization Advisory

Committee on Medical Research he stated: 'We observed that no matter how long a man from sea level stays at high altitude, his efficiency and his tolerance for maximal work were a great deal lower' (Hurtado 1966). In his opinion this high work capacity was perhaps the best index of successful natural acclimatization in these native highlanders of the Andes. He studied 11 non-athletes at 150 m and 12 native highlanders at 4540 m. They were asked to run on a treadmill until exhausted. The highlanders tolerated the exercise twice as long and showed a greater degree of hyperventilation. They showed smaller increases in their pulse rate and systemic systolic blood pressure. It seems likely that the increased exercise tolerance of native highlanders is due in part to acclimatization, as envisaged by Hurtado, and habitual exercise in childhood as described above. In Chapter 32 we describe the intriguing situation that maximal exercise in acclimatized subjects at high altitude brings about only very low levels of blood lactate. The oxygen debt is prominently reduced in the native highlander.

In travelling through the Andes one cannot fail to be impressed by examples of the high exercise tolerance of native highlanders. Every spare piece of ground around mining communities like Cerro de Pasco (4330 m) is converted into a football pitch and the local youth engage in vigorous matches (Fig. 31.1). The authors have sometimes been breathless while merely standing still to watch local schoolboys playing a hard game of soccer on the school playground (Fig. 31.2).

ATHLETES AND ACUTE MOUNTAIN SICKNESS

Acute mountain sickness can be of considerable importance to an international athlete, for its many manifestations (see Chapter 12) may severely handicap him in any competition. He is particularly vulnerable, as he must adhere to his training programme of vigorous exercise despite feelings of headache, sickness, dizziness, or any of the other symptoms he may encounter. Fortunately, as the symptoms tend to resolve themselves within 48 hours, conservative treatment with a temporary lightening of training is generally sufficient.

ATHLETIC PERFORMANCE IN PERSONS NATIVE TO MODERATE ALTITUDE

During the course of the 19th Olympiad in Mexico City it became apparent that this moderate altitude had a particularly significant effect on athletic performance in long-distance events. Athletes who were

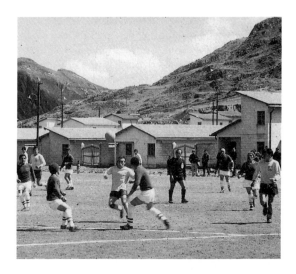

31.1 *A football match between teams of Quechua inhabitants of Cerro de Pasco (4330 m) in the Peruvian Andes.*

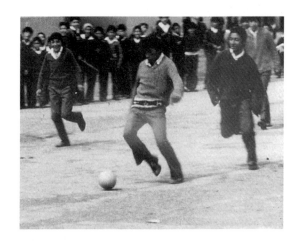

31.2 *Schoolboys play a hard game of soccer on their school playground at Cerro de Pasco.*

capable of world record performances at sea level were adversely affected. In the final of the 10 000 m race Ron Clarke, who was the world record holder in this event, finished sixth and in a state of collapse, although he was not reported as suffering from any other illness (Fig. 31.3). The pace had been unremarkable and yet Clarke could not accelerate when necessary. In contrast, athletes originating from high-altitude areas performed well in long-distance events. Thus in the 10 000-m race

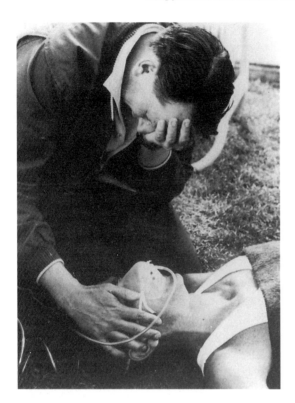

31.3 *Dr Corrigan, the Medical Officer to the Australian Olympic Team in 1968, weeps as he administers oxygen to Ron Clarke who collapsed as he crossed the finishing line of the men's 10 000 m event at the 1968 Olympic Games held in Mexico City (2380 m). (Popperfoto).*

referred to above, the first five places were achieved by athletes either native to high altitude or domiciled there for a prolonged period. First was Naftali Temu of Kenya, second Mamo Wolde of Ethiopia, third Mohamed Gammoudi of Tunisia, fourth Juan Martinez of Mexico, and fifth Nikolay Sviridov of the Soviet Union of that period, who was thought to have been domiciled at Alma-Ata (1000 m) or Leninakhan (1500 m).

The origin of the winner seemed to confirm the long-standing impression that Kenyans have outstanding ability in middle- and long-distance events. The British Broadcasting Corporation Television Service was so intrigued by this that it sent a unit to East Africa to investigate the matter. Its findings were incorporated into a television programme, *Kenya Runner* (BBC 1975). It was found that the successful middle-distance runners originated from

two areas of the plateau near Lake Victoria at an altitude of 1500–2000 m. The tribes concerned were the Kalenjin and the Kipsigis (sometimes called Kisii). The natives of these tribes have a physical advantage in that their femora are longer than those of Caucasians. However, what is probably more important is that from early childhood they run long distances to school at this moderate altitude. Boys from the local population who are interested in athletics find their way into the army or the prision service, during which they are encouraged to undertake training at an altitude of some 1500 m. As already noted in Chapter 4, the development of these Kenyan children during daily exercise in the mildly hypoxic conditions of life on the plateau may well influence the magnitude of vital capacity achieved.

LUNG FUNCTION AND HABITUAL ACTIVITY IN CHILDHOOD IN THE HIGHLANDERS OF NEW GUINEA

The concept that exercise in children at moderate altitude improves lung function and thereby the potential for improving athletic performance for distance events is supported by the investigations of Cotes *et al.* (1973). They carried out lung function tests on coastal dwellers and highlanders in New Guinea. The sea-level people were studied at Kaul Village on Kar Kar Island, approximately 10 miles off the mainland of New Guinea. The highlanders, who were 17–30 years of age, came from Lufa, situated at an altitude of 2000 m, and the studies were carried out in a laboratory situated at 1700 m in Goroka. Cotes *et al.* (1973) studied the lung volume and ventilatory capacity of their young adult male and female subjects, but in addition they carried out an investigation of the transfer factor which estimates the diffusing capacity of the lung. The results were carefully standardized for age, height, and, in the case of the transfer factor, the haemoglobin concentration.

They found that lung function in the coastal dwellers in New Guinea resembled that of people of Indian and West African descent. Thus the inspiratory capacity (Fig. 31.4) and the expiratory reserve volume (Fig. 31.4) were smaller than for comparable Europeans (Fig. 31.5). However, the highlander of this area of New Guinea was found to have a larger total lung capacity (Fig. 31.4), similar to that of Europeans and mainly due to a larger inspiratory capacity (Fig. 31.5). The transfer factor, measuring diffusing capacity, was greater in the highlander than in either the native sea-level resident or in Europeans (Fig. 31.6).

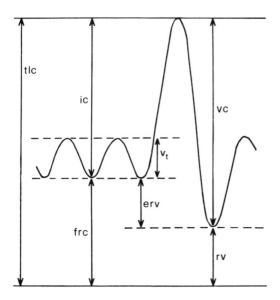

31.4 *Definitions of the various functional lung compartments referred to in the text. tlc, total lung capacity; frc, functional residual capacity; ic, respiratory capacity; erv, expiratory reserve volume; V_t tidal volume; vc, vital capacity; rv, residual volume.*

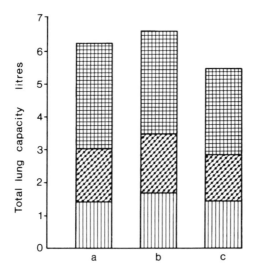

31.5 *Total lung capacity and its subdivisions for young men (height 1.7 m) in: (a) Europeans; (b) highlanders in New Guinea; and (c) coastal people in New Guinea. Area occupied by vertical line, residual volume; dot-dash area, expiratory reserve volume; squares, inspiratory capacity. (Based on data from Cotes* et al. *(1973).)*

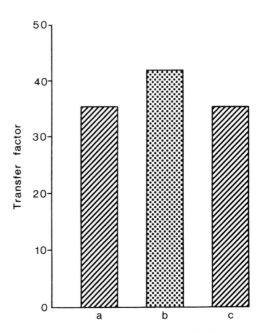

31.6 *Transfer factor for young men (height 1.7 m) in: (a) Europeans; (b) highlanders in New Guinea; and (c) coastal people in New Guinea (Based on data from Cotes* et al. *(1973).)*

It has been known for many years that both the ventilatory and diffusing capacities of highlanders are increased compared with those of sea-level dwellers (Cotes and Ward 1966; De Graff *et al.* 1970; see Chapter 4, this volume). In the case of the natives of New Guinea, however, the increased total lung capacity occurred in highlanders living at the moderate altitude of only 2000 m and the greater lung size noted by Woolcock *et al.* (1972) was in subjects living at a mere 1200 m. This raises the interesting possibility that the unusual lung function of the highlanders of New Guinea depends on another factor in addition to that of moderate altitude. This seems to be the high level of physical activity characteristic of the highlanders of the area (Durnin *et al.* 1972) and it probably exerts its greatest effect on lung size during infancy, childhood, and adolescence when these organs are developing (Cotes *et al.* 1973). In this respect the physiological responses to exercise in childhood resemble those of the athlete in Western countries (Sinnett and Solomon 1968; Cotes *et al.* 1972). Hence from New Guinea we have evidence that a population with a lung size comparable with that of African Negroes, Malayans, Chinese, and Indians may increase this to a volume more appropriate to Europeans because of habitual exercise undertaken at moderate altitude during childhood. The improvement in lung function is shown in both sexes. Should these highland populations of underdeveloped countries assume in the future a Western style of living, the advantage of increased lung volume and oxygen transfer may well be lost (Cotes *et al.* 1973). The significantly increased pulmonary diffusing capacity of these highlanders may be due to attenuation and increase in area of the alveolar capillary membrane, consequent upon the increase in total lung capacity. Such physiological investigations add weight to the view that highland populations of this type would be placed in an unusually advantageous position with regard to long-distance events in international athletics meetings held at moderate altitude.

ALTITUDE TRAINING

It has long been believed by many athletes that there is some advantage to be gained for their performance from a period of training at high altitude. The anecdotal nature of much of the evidence for this belief is exemplified by opening remarks made by Bannister (1974) at a meeting over which he was presiding. He said:

> I remember some early results from a group of American world record holders, including Jim Ryun, who went to altitude for 14 days. After coming down Jim Ryun set up a world record for the mile of 3 min. 51.3 sec., a record in which I have a little personal interest. Five out of six of the other athletes also achieved best performances. They then went to altitude for another 14 days and after coming down Ryun lowered the 1500 metre world record. After a third spell at altitude, five out of six athletes again produced best performances. That was the moment at which it seemed to me that there was something rather special going on.

This joint meeting to discuss 'altitude training' was held between the British Association of Sport and Medicine and the British Olympic Association at the Royal Society of Medicine in London in November 1973. The proceedings were subsequently published in Volume 8 of the *British Journal of Sports Medicine* in April 1974. By the time of the concluding panel discussion it had become clear from the papers that had been read that many of the participants were confused as to whether altitude training bestowed any benefits at all and, even if it did, whether such training was ethically desirable. Many expressed the view that training athletes together in a training-camp atmosphere might in itself be expected to bring advantages excluding altogether the factor of altitude.

The same uncertainty exists 20 years later and Levine *et al.* (1992) have given an excellent, perceptive review of altitude training to highlight where the problems exist. They believe that it is difficult to evaluate the reports on altitude-training on four main accounts. These are the small numbers of subjects employed in the studies, the lack of a clearly defined training programme at altitude, the use of subjects of widely differing degrees of fitness, and inadequate controls undergoing the same testing and training programme at sea level. Thus Balke *et al.* (1965) studied five untrained men before and after 10 days of training at 2800 m. Maximal oxygen uptake increased in all subjects after altitude training. This is an example of a study where the use of untrained subjects without controls is an important limitation. A simple training effect related to increased physical activity at altitude as well as the training and testing procedures can easily explain their observations (Levine *et al.* 1992). The same comments can be made on the studies of Klausen *et al.* (1966). Hansen *et al.* (1967) studied 16 untrained subjects before and after a stay of 2 weeks at 4300 m. Eight of them undertook a course of calisthenics while the remaining eight had 'reduced activity'. A third group of eight subjects lived at sea level and presumably carried through the same programme of calisthenic exercises. In this study it was found that there was no greater increase in maximal oxygen uptake in the altitude activity group compared to the sea-level group.

There was a plethora of studies before, during, and after the Olympic Games in Mexico City in 1968. According to Levine *et al.* (1992) several conclusions drawn from the results of these studies apparently rested on firm ground by 1970 but some of them were soon to be challenged. Their analysis suggested to them that soon after the 19th Olympiad there was a consensus on the following points.

1. Maximal work capacity decreases roughly 1% for each 100 m above 1500 m but returns slightly toward sea-level values during an extended stay at high altitude.
2. Long residence at high altitude does not enhance endurance performance at sea level.
3. In endurance competition at medium altitudes, athletes who have spent a lifetime at moderate or high altitude appear to have a physiological

advantage over those from, and raised at, low altitude.

4. In the case of brief, intense athletic exertion neither prior acclimatization nor altitude training makes an appreciable difference.

5. There is no agreement as to whether intermittent exposure to altitude has an adverse or beneficial effect in training for competitive sports or for slow-paced climbing.

6. There are great differences in speed and work capacity between individuals. Further differences are thought to arise from the type of work or exercise involved, the level of training, and the length of time spent at altitude. Many of these factors are unpredictable and explain the contradictory results found in different studies.

Levine *et al.* (1992) point out that many of the features of acclimatization are very similar to those induced by endurance training. These include improvement in substrate utilization by increasing mobilization of free fatty acids and increasing dependence on blood glucose, thus sparing muscle glycogen. This is manifested by decreased accumulation of metabolites such as lactate or ammonia. Such similarities have led many athletes to seek training at altitude but the evidence supporting this practice remains controversial (Jackson and Sharkey 1988).

Levine *et al.* (1992) give an account of recent altitude-training studies and readers are referred to their review for details of these investigations. We may, however, quote here in full their conclusions as to the value of altitude training representing as they do the present consensus of opinion on the subject. Levine *et al.* (1992) say:

Both altitude acclimatization and hypoxic exercise appear to play important roles in improving oxygen-carrying capacity of the blood and altering the training stimulus at the skeletal muscle level. It is reasonable to conclude that for performance at altitude, acclimatization and training at altitude carry important benefits. The situation for performance at sea level is probably divergent, depending on the level of fitness and training, the training altitude and the specifics of the training program. For untrained individuals, there is probably minimal benefit in maximal aerobic power training at altitude compared to equivalent training at sea level. Endurance and work-capacity, however, are likely to be most improved at the training altitude. For elite athletes, training at altitudes above 3000 m limits absolute training

intensity and precludes any favourable impact of altitude acclimatization. Training at lower altitudes, if sufficiently intense, may carry added advantages; this remains to be proved. The most efficient technique may well be to live at altitude and train at sea level, although logistical difficulties may limit the utility of this approach in practice.

A crucial question is how long any improvement achieved are maintained on return to sea level. Recent investigations suggest that training at altitude enhances oxygen transport and activity to the tissues beyond levels anticipated from passive acclimatization.

EFFECTS OF HIGH-ALTITUDE TRAINING ON OXYGEN TRANSPORT AND RELEASE

'High-altitude training' is in fact usually carried out at moderate altitude. The effects of ascent to an elevation of 2300 m and training there on the transport and delivery of oxygen to the tissues have been studied by Mairbäurl and Schobersberger (1986) and by Mairbäurl *et al.* (1986). They studied 12 men, of mean age 21 years, over a period of study of 13 days at moderate altitude. Half of the subjects rested as controls and half, 'the training subjects', worked a bicycle-ergometer, training at 75% of their maximal exercise performance capacity for 45 min daily. Incremental bicycle-ergometer tests were performed before ascent, within 48 hours of arrival at 2300 m, at the end of the stay at altitude, and after the descent. The beginning work load was 50 W and this was increased by 50 W every 2 minutes until subjective exhaustion. Measurements were made of the maximal work capacity (W/kg) and of the heart rates at each work load.

Studies of oxygen transport and delivery included measurements of haemoglobin concentrations, haematocrit, red cell and reticulocyte counts, and maximal oxygen uptake. Measurements were also made of levels of 2,3-DPG and the value of P_{50} and of metabolic substrates such as the concentration of lactate in venous blood in exhaustion. It was found that in both groups haemoglobin concentration fell slightly during the stay at moderate altitude, but reticulocytes increased significantly within 2 days of ascent. The reticulocyte count continued to increase at altitude, and this was more pronounced in training subjects. On descent, reticulocyte counts decreased but were still above pre-altitude values. Levels of 2,3-DPG increased after the ascent. In controls the level was 0.7 μmol/g Hb at the start of the stay at high altitude and decreased slightly below pre-altitude values. In the training subjects the level reached 1.9 μmol/g Hb and then decreased after descent, but even so the values remained significantly above pre-altitude levels. Within 1 day of ascent, P_{50} increased from 25.8 to 28.4 mmHg in both groups and this level was maintained at altitude, becoming higher by the thirteenth day in the training subjects. After descent the P_{50} values decreased, but still remained about 1 mmHg higher than pre-altitude values. One factor that might increase the production of the intraerythrocytic phosphates is stimulation of glycolysis by such endocrinological factors as increased catecholamine or corticosteroid production (see Chapter 22). Another is a stimulation of erythropoiesis, since young red cells have a higher metabolic activity and produce more 2,3-DPG. Respiratory alkalosis is not a factor involved in view of the moderate altitude. These data seem to indicate that exercise and training at moderate altitude act as a separate stimulus for decreasing the affinity of haemoglobin for oxygen, thus adding to the effect of hypobaric hypoxia *per se*.

Ascent to altitude resulted in a decreased maximal work performance capacity for some 10% but both groups recovered during the stay. In training subjects, maximal exercise performance was increased after descent. After descent the maximal work capacity was unchanged in controls, but was elevated significantly by about 8% in training subjects as compared with pre-altitude values. The maximal heart rate in exhaustion was significantly lower at moderate altitude. This effect was greater in training subjects than in controls and there was a further decrease in heart rate of some 15–20 beats/min during the exercise tests at the end of the stay at altitude. This association of falling heart rate with recovery of maximal work performance suggests that the initial decreased work capacity at altitude is not due to the decreased cardiac output.

The concentration of lactate in venous blood collected in exhaustion was significantly lower during the stay at moderate levels compared with pre- or post-altitude values. This effect was greater in training subjects. We refer in the following chapter to lowered blood lactate levels on exercise at high altitude in native highlanders. This implies that, due to the greater release of oxygen from haemoglobin referred to above, there is more oxygen available for metabolic needs during exercise at high altitude. Anaerobic energy production is not required to the same extent.

In summary, the studies of Mairbäurl and co-workers seem to indicate that training and exercise in themselves augment the enhanced transport and release of oxygen to the tissues, as described in Chapter 5. The increased levels of 2,3-DPG and the resultant shift to the right of the oxygen–haemoglobin dissociation curve associated with exercise augment the passive acclimatization at high altitude and improve tissue oxygenation. This increased oxygenation diminished anaerobic energy production and blood lactate levels. Exercise performance at high altitude remains at comparable strength to that seen at lower elevations with a decreased cardiac output. Mairbäurl and Schobersberger (1986) express the view that, since some of the advantageous effects induced by training at moderate altitude are maintained for 'a certain period of time even after descent', a higher exercise performance capacity in healthy subjects might result for a time after the return to sea level. The all-important question, however, is what is meant by 'a certain period of time after descent', for this will determine whether or not altitude training has any value for athletes with regard to their subsequent performances at sea level.

Whether there are any longer-term advantages from altitude training appears to be dubious. As soon as the athlete descends to sea level or lower altitudes there is a decrease in the production of reticulocytes. Erythropoietin becomes undetectable and there is a progressive decrease in the activity of the bone marrow. There is an increase in red-cell destruction and the phenomenon of 'overshoot' may lead even to the development of anaemia in subjects descending to sea level (see Chapter 33). The consequence of this is that the haematological gains of several years may disappear in a matter of weeks. In addition, the disruption of the training programme and the less vigorous training while at altitude may cause lessening of the subject's overall fitness. For these reasons athletic training at high altitude cannot be recommended as a panacea for improving physical fitness.

Undoubtedly the performance of athletes who are native highlanders suggests that there is some advantage from growing up as a child at high altitude, as described earlier in this chapter, but the advantages of short periods at altitude training camps are much more open to dispute. It seems to us that little improvement in lung function can be expected if the adult fully developed lung is exposed to the hypoxia of high altitude for a period of a few short weeks. Improvement in lung function of the type that could enhance performance in middle- or long-distance running at sports meetings must depend on the exposure for many years of the developing lung of the child and adolescent accustomed to the hypoxia and habitual activity of the native highlanders at moderate altitude. The advantages derived by the children of native highlanders from their high-altitude habitat cannot hope to be achieved in a temporary visit by an adult European. Adams *et al.* (1975) also share this view. They found from study of 12 trained athletes that hard endurance training at an altitude of 2300 m had no advantage over equivalently severe training at sea level either on the maximum oxygen uptake or on the performance time for a 2-mile (3000 m) race in already well-conditioned middle-distance runners.

References

Adams, W.C., Bernauer, E.M., Dill, D.B., and Bomar, J.B. Jr (1975). Effects of equivalent sea level and altitude training on VO$_2$ max and running performance. *Journal of Applied Physiology*, **39**, 262

Balke, B., Nagle, F.J., and Daniels, J.T. (1965). Altitude and maximum performance in work and sports activity. *Journal of the American Medical Association*, **194**, 176

Bannister, R. (1974). Chairman's opening remarks and panel discussion. *British Journal of Sports Medicine*, **8**, 3 and 56

BBC (1975). Television Programme: *Kenya Runner*, 14 December

Costhill, D.L. (1970). Metabolic responses during distance running. *Journal of Applied Physiology*, **28**, 251

Cotes, J.E. and Ward, M.P. (1966). Ventilatory capacity in normal Bhutanese. *Journal of Physiology*, **186**, 88P–89P

Cotes, J.E., Davies, C.T.M., Patrick, J.M., Reed, J.W., and Saunders, M.J. (1972). Cardio-respiratory response to submaximal exercise, comparison of young adults in New Guinea and U.K. *Ergonomics*, **15**, 484

Cotes, J.E., Saunders, M.J., Adam, J.E.R., Anderson, H.R., and Hall, A.M. (1973). Lung function in coastal and highland New Guineans — comparison with Europeans. *Thorax*, **28**, 320

Craig, A.B. (1969). Olympics 1968: a post mortem. *Medicine and Science in Sports*, **1**, 177

DeGraff, A.C., Grover, R.F., Johnson, R.L., Hammond, J.W., and Miller, J.M. (1970). Diffusing capacity of the lung in Caucasians native to 3,100 m. *Journal of Applied Physiology*, **29**, 71

Durnin, J.V.G.A., Ferro-Luzzi, A., and Norgan, N.G. (1972). An investigation of a nutritional enigma – studies on coastal and highland populations in New Guinea. *Human Biology in Oceania*, **1**, 318

Faulkner, J.A. (1967). Training for maximum performance at altitude. In *The Effects of Altitude and Athletic Performance* (R. Goddard, ed.). Chicago; Athletic Institute, p. 88

Faulkner, J.A. (1971). Maximum exercise at medium altitude. In *Frontier of Fitness* (R.J. Shephard, ed.). Springfield, Illinois; Charles C. Thomas, p. 360

Grover, R.F. and Reeves, J.T. (1966). Exercise performance of athletes at sea level and 3,100 m altitude. *Medicina Thoracalis*, **23**, 129

Hansen, J.E., Vogel, J.A., Stelter, G.P., and Consolazio, C.F. (1967). Oxygen in man during exhaustive work at sea level and high altitude. *Journal of Applied Physiology*, **26**, 511

Houston, C.S. (1988). Acclimatization to hypoxia. Operation Everest I and II. *Annals of Sports Medicine*, **4**, 171

Hurtado, A. (1964). In *Aging of the Lung* (L. Cander and J.H. Moyer, eds). New York; Grune and Stratton, p. 270

Hurtado, A. (1966). In *Life at High Altitudes*, Scientific Publication No. 140. Washington; Pan American Health Organization, p. 68

Jackson, C.G. and Sharkey, B.J. (1988). Altitude, training and human performance. *Sports Medicine*, **6**, 279

Jokl, E. and Jokl, P. (ed.) (1968). The effect of altitude on athlethic performance. In *Exercise and Altitude*. Baltimore; University Park Press, p. 28

Klausen, K., Robinson, S., Michael, E.D., and Myhre, L.G. (1966). Effect of high altitude on maximal working capacity. *Journal of Applied Physiology*, **21**, 1191

Levine, B.D., Roach, R.C., and Houston, C.S. (1992). Work and training at altitude. In *Hypoxia and Mountain Medicine*, Proceedings of the 7th International Hypoxia Symposium, Lake Louise, Canada, 1991. (J.R. Sutton, G. Coates, and C.S. Houston, Ed.). Oxford; Pergamon Press, p. 192

Mairbäurl, H. and Schobersberger, W. (1986). Red cell O$_2$ transport at altitude and altitude training. *Advances in Experimental Medicine and Biology*, **191**, 495

Mairbäurl, H., Schobersberger, W., Humpeler, E., Hasibeler, W., Fischer, W., and Raas, E. (1986). Beneficial effects of exercising at moderate altitude on red cells oxygen transport and on exercise performance. *Pflügers Archiv*, **406**, 594

Pugh, L.G.C.E. (1967). Athletes at altitude. *Journal of Physiology*, **192**, 619

Pugh, L.G.C.E., Gill, M.B., Lahiri, S., Milledge, J.S., Ward, M.P., and West, J.B. (1964). Muscular exercise at great altitudes. *Journal of Applied Physiology*, **19**, 431

Reeves, J.T., Groves, B.M., Sutton, J.R., Wagner, P.D., Cymerman, A., Malconian, M.K., Rock, P.B., Young, P.M., and Houston, C.S. (1987). Operation Everest II: Preservation of cardiac function at extreme altitude. *Journal of Applied Physiology*, **63**, 531

Shephard, R.J. (1973). The athlete at high altitude. *Canadian Medical Association Journal*, **109**, 207

Sime, F., Peñaloza, D., Ruiz, L., Gonzales, N., Covarrubias, E., and Postigo, R. (1974). Hypoxaemia, pulmonary hypertension and low cardiac output in newcomers to low altitude. *Journal of Applied Physiology*, **36**, 561

Sinnett, P.F. and Solomon, A. (1968). Physical fitness in a New Guinea highland population. *Papua New Guinea Medical Journal*, **2**, 56

Wood, S.C., Appenzeller, O., and Riedel, C.E. (1988). Physiology of running at high altitudes. *Annals of Sports Medicine*, **4**, 270

Woolcock, A.J., Colman, M.H., and Blackburn, C.R.B. (1972). Factors affecting normal values for ventilatory lung function. *American Review of Respiratory Disease*, **106**, 692

32

Exposure to extreme altitudes

The various aspects of acclimatization described in the earlier chapters enable man to carry on a comparatively normal social and economic life at high altitude. Thus Cerro de Pasco, the centre of the Peruvian mining industry, is situated at 4330 m (Fig. 32.1). Even at a slightly higher elevation, however, daily community life is less easy and the authors can vouch for the appreciably less comfortable feel of working at Morococha (4540 m). There is a critical altitude above which successful, permanent acclimatization cannot take place and this limit appears to be somewhere around an elevation of 5500 m. From his experience in the Himalaya, Pugh (1962) is of the opinion that 5790 m is too high for what he calls 'complete adjustment'. An arbitrary definition of the beginning of 'high altitude' is one exceeding 3000 m on the grounds that it is at this elevation that unequivocal symptoms associated with the ascent appear (Chapter 2). In the same way,

'extreme altitude' is here defined as one exceeding 5800 m because above this elevation permanent successful acclimatization cannot be achieved and maintained.

HIGHEST INHABITANTS IN THE WORLD

The behaviour of the workers at the Aucanquilcha sulfur mine in the Andes of northern Chile is of interest in determining the highest altitude at which men are prepared to live and work permanently. Native miners live in the area at an altitude of 5330 m and prefer to climb 500 m every day to their work, refusing to occupy a camp built for them at the higher elevation on account of difficulty in sleeping. The altitude of the mine was given as 5800 m when members of the International High Altitude Expedition visited it in 1935, but during a visit there West (1986a) recorded the barometric pressure as 373 mmHg and established its true altitude as 5950 m. During his visit West was astonished to find four caretakers living at the mine in a galvanized iron hut. One of them had been living there for 2 years, but like his three companions he descended each Sunday to the relative lowland conditions of 4200 m to play football! West (1986a) estimates that in these men the partial pressure of oxygen was 68 mmHg in their inspired air and 42 mmHg in their alveolar spaces. The mean haematocrit in three of them was 61%. These caretakers appear to be the highest inhabitants in the world, but few can tolerate living at such altitudes for this period of time.

HIGH-ALTITUDE PHYSIOLOGY AT THE LIMITS OF HUMAN ENDURANCE

This book is concerned with the physiology and pathology of the numerous native highlanders and the considerable numbers of lowlanders who reside permanently or for long periods at high altitude. Since the critical elevation above which successful, permanent acclimatization cannot be achieved is 5800 m we regard this as the entrance to 'extreme altitude'. This term has also been used by others to describe the considerably greater heights reached by

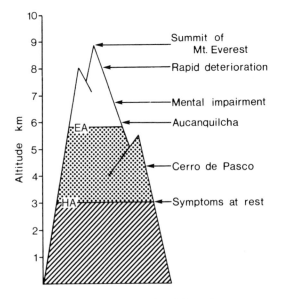

32.1 *Definition of high altitude (HA) and extreme altitude (EA) on the criteria considered in the text.*

small groups of climbers and physiologists at the limit of human endurance on peaks exceeding 8000 m. Studies on human physiology in such heroic circumstances reveal the extremes that the body can reach for very short periods of time in the face of environmental conditions incapable of supporting life. Most of the data in this specialized area have been obtained from three large investigations. Two were at natural high altitude. These were the Himalayan Scientific and Mountaineering Expedition of 1960–61 (Pugh 1962) and the American Medical Research Expedition to Everest in 1981. A third investigation was carried out at simulated high altitude in Operation Everest II in 1985 (Houston *et al.* 1987). In this, eight subjects were gradually decompressed to a barometric pressure of 240 mmHg over a period of 40 days in a low-pressure chamber.

In mountainous areas approaching the equator the barometric pressure is higher than that estimated from the Standard Atmosphere (Chapter 2). Thus, the barometric pressure at the summit of Mt Everest was estimated by this method to be 236 mmHg. However, direct measurement on the summit found it in fact to be 253 mmHg (West *et al.* 1983). This explains the capacity for climbing the mountain without supplementary oxygen; in winter months the barometric pressure falls (Chapter 2) and oxygen is required. At such great heights the very low barometric pressure leads to a greatly diminished partial pressure of oxygen in the alveolar spaces. This is improved by the dramatic hyperventilation which occurs at these great heights. West (1988) notes that at the summit of Mt Everest Pizzo had to gasp for breath every three or four words. This profound augmentation of breathing also diminishes alveolar carbon dioxide pressure, which is inversely proportional to alveolar ventilation and thus a good measure of its level. Subjects who can generate this remarkable ventilation can tolerate extreme altitude better than those with a more modest response. There is an approximately linear fall in alveolar carbon dioxide pressure so that at the summit of Mt Everest it falls to a remarkably low level of 7.5 mmHg with an alveolar ventilation five or six times greater than at sea level (West 1988; Table 32.1). The ventilation did not reach this level in the subjects of Operation Everest II probably because the period of acclimatization was shorter. Once an altitude of 7000 m is exceeded alveolar oxygen pressure settles out at a value of about 35 mmHg maintained by extreme hyperventilation (West 1988; Table 32.1).

At the same time that alveolar oxygen pressure is kept at this level arterial oxygen tension is considerably lower. This is because there is difficulty in transfer of oxygen from the alveolar spaces across the alveolar-capillary wall at high altitude. Arterial

Table 32.1 Data at rest from six subjects subjected to a simulated altitude of 8840 m (Operation Everest II) and from one subject at the summit of Mt Everest (after Houston 1988 and West 1988)

| Factor | Simulated altitude in Operation Everest II | | Summit of Mt Everest (8840 m) |
	Sea level	8840 m*	
Atmospheric pressure (mmHg)	760	240	253
Ventilation (1/min BTPS)			
At rest	11	42	
Maximal work	124	184	
$P_{A_{O_2}}$ (mmHg)	104	30	35
Pa_{O_2} (mmHg)	99	30	28
$P_{A_{CO_2}}$ (mmHg)	38	12	7.5
Pa_{CO_2} (mmHg)	34	11	7.5
Arterial pH	7.43	7.56	7.76
Pulmonary arterial pressure (mmHg)	15	33	
$P\bar{v}_{O_2}$ (mmHg)	35	22	

* Fortieth day of experiment.

oxygen tension on the summit of Mt Everest was found to be 28 mmHg (West 1988; Table 32.1). When oxygen loading is so low on the oxygen-dissociation curve, the rate of rise of oxygen tension in the pulmonary capillary is extremely slow and end-capillary oxygen tension does not reach the alveolar value.

There is a striking degree of respiratory alkalosis. Two climbers at the summit were able to take blood samples from each other and the calculated arterial pH exceeded 7.7 (Table 32.1). This alkalosis has important implications, for the oxygen affinity of haemoglobin is greatly increased and thus the loading of oxygen by the pulmonary capillaries is enhanced. The benefits of the increased oxygen-loading in the lung outweigh the disadvantages of the decreased unloading in the tissues. It is of interest to note that HbF in the fetus has a P_{50} of only 19 mmHg at pH 7.4. In the climber at the summit of Mt Everest, due to the severe respiratory alkalosis that increased the oxygen affinity of haemoglobin, P_{50} was also 19 mmHg (West 1988).

Subjects at these extreme altitudes show a chronic depletion of blood volume despite an adequate intake of fluid and subjects at 6300 m were found to have a significantly higher serum osmolality than in control values at sea level. In spite of this their vasopressin concentration remained unchanged (West 1988). A likely factor in producing this chronic dehydration is the large insensible loss of fluid as a result of hyperventilation. It would seem that the kidney gives a higher priority to maintaining fluid balance than to correcting acid–base balance. To correct respiratory alkalosis the excretion of bicarbonate ions must be increased, or their absorption decreased; this entails the loss of a cation, which inevitably aggravates the hyperosmolality. This may explain the slow metabolic compensation of the respiratory alkalosis at very high altitudes in the presence of volume depletion (West 1988).

HIGH-ALTITUDE DETERIORATION IN CLIMBERS

Man can survive at elevations considerably greater than 5800 m for short periods. High-altitude climbers are exposed to such extreme conditions for a comparatively short time after a preparatory period of acclimatization walking up through the foothills. During scientific expeditions the stay at extreme altitudes may be prolonged beyond what is customary for mountaineering trips. Early signs of deterioration become apparent at 5800 m (Ward 1975), which, it will be recalled, is the same altitude at which

Chilean miners refuse to live permanently. Above this elevation there is a progressive worsening in their mental and physical condition which has been termed 'high-altitude deterioration'. During the Makalu expedition of 1960–61, a stay of 90–100 days at this altitude led to early deterioration despite the fact that the party enjoyed good living conditions with adequate food and fluid intake and protection from the environment.

At first there is an exaggeration of signs and symptoms that may initially be encountered at much lower elevations. Thus, the anorexia that afflicts most people ascending mountains becomes more severe. The higher the altitude and the longer the stay there, the greater is the hypophagia with resulting loss of weight. The physiological basis for the loss of weight was discussed in Chapter 21. The appetite for sweet foods is said to increase and Ward (1975) comments that some climbers may develop a craving for certain food such as tinned salmon or pineapple cubes. Headache, nausea, and vomiting may become pronounced if the ascent to extreme altitudes has been made too rapidly to avoid acute mountain sickness. At this altitude there is no fall in the capacity for work and Sherpas may carry heavy loads all day without undue signs of fatigue. However, already at this elevation there are the early signs of impairment of mental capacity, which may be detected by psychometric tests of the type described in Chapter 29.

Above 5800 m heavy loads can still be carried and extreme exertion is possible, but such muscular activity is commonly followed by great exhaustion. The working day tends to be shortened to 6 hours. Anorexia and loss of weight may become acute. From 6000 to 6700 m there is a wide variation in performance and feeling of well-being from day to day. Muscular fatigue becomes very pronounced and beneficial results in allaying this by the ingestion of easily assimilated carbohydrate such as sugar become apparent according to Ward (1975).

Between altitudes of 6700 and 7900 m evidence of significant mental impairment appears. Although routine tasks can still be carried out without too much trouble, any activity requiring initiative takes much longer. At the same time, weakness and fatigue become striking and cases of total exhaustion are not uncommon. Weight loss, nausea, and dyspnoea become even more exaggerated. Finally, at altitudes between 7900 and 8850 m one passes from any semblance of physiological acclimatization to high altitude to a state of rapid deterioration in which mental aberrations occur and survival itself becomes the central issue. Mental depression is common. The ability to perform routine mechanical tasks in an orderly way takes much longer. Insight into one's behaviour is lost and climbers may embark on foolhardy procedures oblivious of the risks involved. Hallucinations may occur (Chapter 29).

At these great heights the combination of severe hypoxia and extreme cold may lead to loss of consciousness. Oxygen inhalation increases endurance and enables climbers to take an interest in their surroundings. Men have, however, scaled Mt Everest (8850 m) without oxygen as described above. The reasons for this ability are described in Chapter 2.

VENTILATORY RESPONSE TO HYPOXIA IN HIGH-ALTITUDE CLIMBERS

The brisk ventilatory response that occurs in the lowlander ascending to high altitude is a component of acquired acclimatization (see Chapter 4). In contrast, one of the characteristics of the native highlander showing successful natural acclimatization is a blunted response to hypoxia. These conflicting responses to altitude raise the interesting problem as to what are the relative advantages and disadvantages of a brisk ventilatory response to hypoxia for the high-altitude climber. Milledge (1987) argues that two criteria should be employed to assess the value of any change in the ventilatory response to hypoxia. The first is the ability to acclimatize rapidly, including freedom from acute mountain sickness. The second is the ability to perform well at extreme altitudes.

It is apparent that a brisk ventilatory response protects against acute mountain sickness. Hackett *et al.* (1982) studied at Pheriche (4250 m) 42 subjects on a trek to the Everest Base Camp, inferring changes in the ventilatory response to hypoxia by changes in arterial carbon dioxide tension. They found that those who lost more than 2% of their body weight had the lowest carbon dioxide tension, the highest oxygen saturation, and very little acute mountain sickness. In contrast, those who gained more than 2% of their body weight due to water retention had a lower oxygen saturation and pronounced acute mountain sickness. In Chapter 12, reference is made to studies that have demonstrated that prophylactic acetazolamide brings about the same changes in blood gases as those achieved by a brisk ventilatory response to hypoxia with the same ameliorating effect on acute mountain sickness.

There has also been recent evidence to suggest that an intense ventilatory response to extreme high altitude is important to achieving a high performance while mountain climbing. Schoene *et al.* (1984) found that climbers who were able to attain and spend nights at altitudes in excess of 8000 m showed a stronger ventilatory response to hypoxia and a better arterial blood oxygenation than those who were forced to keep to lower altitudes. Indeed a higher ventilatory response at sea level has been suggested as an indicator of a climber's capability at high altitude. Masuyama *et al.* (1986) studied the hypoxic ventilatory responses of 10 climbers in the Nepal–Japan Kangchenjunga Expedition (8500 m) in the spring of 1984. They found that five climbers who reached an altitude higher than 8000 m exhibited a significantly higher ventilatory response to hypoxia than five climbers who did not. Successful climbers achieving altitudes over 8000 m are very few in number. An increase of 2–3 mmHg in alveolar oxygen tension at this height results in an increase in oxygen uptake of more than 100 ml. Hence climbers with a high ventilatory response to hypoxia can accomplish such elevation of alveolar oxygen tension by intense hyperventilation, and enhance performance at very high altitude.

On the other hand it has been known for many years that native highlanders both in the Andes (Severinghaus *et al.* 1966) and in the Himalaya (Milledge and Lahiri 1967) have a blunted ventilatory response (see Chapter 7). Severinghaus and co-workers believed that this blunting of ventilatory response was a loss of acclimatization, since in chronic mountain sickness (Chapter 15) the diminution in response was even greater. Milledge (1987) points out the difficulty of accepting that Sherpas are anything but well adjusted to their mountain environment. They can usually carry more and climb faster while at the same time ventilating less and being less dyspnoeic than lowlanders climbing with them. It has also been shown that endurance runners have a lower ventilatory response to hypoxia in contrast to high-altitude climbers (Schoene 1982). Milledge (1987) argues that for native highlanders and endurance runners a reduced ventilatory response to hypoxia is appropriate and beneficial. This blunting does not have a racial or genetic basis, for it occurs in Whites born at high altitude, requiring 10–30 years to develop (Weill *et al.* 1971).

There appears to be some blunting of response even in ascending to stop at high altitude (Weill *et al.* 1971). Milledge *et al.* (1983) reported that four highly experienced mountaineers who formed the climbing team on an expedition to Mt Kongur had a less brisk ventilatory response to hypoxia than four members of the scientific party who were 'moun-taineers of more modest achievement'. It was seen in Chapter 28 that a brisk ventilatory response is necessary to produce periodic breathing, but this results in profound hypoxia during the periods of apnoea. Thus a mountaineer with a brisk ventilatory response and periodic breathing could in the final analysis be worse off than a native highlander who has a lower response and avoids periodic breathing.

Milledge (1987) concludes that different ven-tilatory responses are optimal for different con-ditions. He thinks a brisk response is an advantage for a lowlander ascending to high altitude for the first time. He would be likely to have less severe acute mountain sickness, to be more dyspnoeic on exertion, and to be at greater risk of developing peri-odic breathing at a lower altitude. A blunted ventila-tory response to hypoxia he thinks is advantageous to the native highlander who may have adjusted to a chronically lower arterial oxygen tension by the changes in the tissues which are described in Chapter 6. This leaves the question as to the level of ventilatory response that is more beneficial to the high-altitude climber. It is possible that a vigorous hypoxic ventilatory response is desirable at extreme altitudes, say over 8000 m, to improve arterial oxygen tension in a situation where the inspired oxygen is so critically low. Even so, as Milledge (1987) points out, Sherpas have climbed Mt Everest. In this respect, Hackett *et al.* (1980) found no significant difference in hypoxic ventilatory re-sponse between 25 Sherpas and 25 White trekkers. They also reported that the mean resting ventilation in the Sherpas at low (1377 m) and high (4243 m) altitudes was higher than in Westerners.

EXERCISE AT EXTREME ALTITUDE

The vigorous exercise necessitated in the climbing of very high mountains cannot be sustained above the altitude at which the maximum uptake of oxygen by the body is less than that required by the contracting muscles. The quantity of oxygen consumed by the tissues of the body at rest each minute is in the range of 220–260 ml (Harris and Heath 1977). This is easily supplied, taking the ventilatory responses to hypoxia into account. Even at extreme altitude the bodily requirements of oxygen can be met at rest. Thus, Ward (1975) notes that on the first ascent of Mt Everest (8850 m) Sir Edmund Hillary removed his oxygen mask at the summit for about 10 minutes before symptoms occurred.

However, the oxygen requirements of the tissues may increase tenfold on exercise, so that some

2.2–2.6 l/min is required. Difficulties now arise because oxygen requirements for a given level of ex-ercise remain the same at high altitude at they are at sea level. At the same time, however, the maximum oxygen uptake of the body per minute falls with in-creasing altitude. At sea level this maximum uptake is 3.5–4.0 l/min but at 5800 m, corresponding to our definition of 'extreme altitude', this capacity for uptake of oxygen falls to 2.0–2.5 l/min (Pugh *et al.* 1964). This uptake is only just sufficient to provide the quantity of oxygen necessary for severe exercise referred to above. Ward (1975) gives the somewhat lower value of 1.7 l/min as the necessary oxygen intake of a man weighing 70 kg during normal climbing activity. This means that, as man ascends into extreme altitude, breathing and exercise become progressively more difficult. Ward (1975) reckons that up to about 6100 m the acclimatized climber from sea level can proceed at a normal pace appro-priate for Alpine climbing (Fig. 32.2). By the time, however, that man reaches an altitude of 7460 m his maximum oxygen uptake is only in the range of 1.3–1.5 l/min (Pugh *et al.* 1964). This will no longer sustain necessary muscular activity.

In Fig. 32.2 are shown the levels of ventilation with increasing altitude that accompany a work rate of 900 kg m/min, which may be taken as appropriate for normal Alpine climbing (Milledge 1975). It is clear from this diagram that, at a certain critical

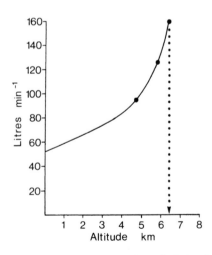

32.2 *Ventilation at a work rate of 900 kg/min which is approximately the preferred work rate of Alpine climbing. At an altitude of about 6100 m it becomes very difficult to climb continuously without oxygen. (Data from Milledge (1975).)*

range of altitude, ventilation becomes inadequate to sustain continuous muscular exercise, so that climbing becomes progressively intermittent with the oxygen debt being repaid during periods of rest. The critical altitude at which this takes place is given as 6100 m by Ward (1975) and 5790 m by Milledge (1975). Breathlessness at rest is noted at 5180 m (Milledge 1975) and eventually at extreme altitudes exceeding 8000 m several breaths may have to be taken for each step. Climbing with oxygen becomes worthwhile at 7010 m. Below this altitude oxygen reduces ventilation and makes the climber feel more comfortable, but the extra weight burden makes it hardly worthwhile. As we note elsewhere, individuals have scaled Mt Everest without oxygen. This is possible because the barometric pressure at its summit is marginally greater than had been stated before (Chapter 2); this minor modification, however, is of critical physiological importance in elevating the partial pressure of oxygen in the alveolar spaces.

Lactic acid production

Exhaustive muscular activity at sea level is accompanied by high levels in blood lactate as the muscles exceed their capacity for aerobic work and revert to aerobic glycolysis. At high altitude the amount of oxygen consumption for a given level of work remains the same and independent of P_{O_2}. Acute exposure to the hypoxia of high altitude does not diminish the formation of lactic acid during severe exercise so that blood lactate levels are increased. On the other hand, the intriguing fact has been known for many years (Edwards 1936) that maximal exercise in acclimatized subjects at high altitude brings about very low levels of blood lactate. The greater the altitude the smaller the increase in blood lactate. The early report of Edwards (1936) was confirmed by Hurtado (1971) who reported that after significant exercise was taken by native highlanders of the Andes living at 4540 m the accumulation of blood lactate was lower than in sea-level subjects after comparable work (Fig. 32.3). Its rate of disappearance was also faster. After maximal exercise at altitudes exceeding 7500 m during the American Everest Expedition of 1981 there was no more increase in the lactate level in the blood in spite of extreme oxygen deprivation (West 1986*b*).

It is commonly believed that this anomalous finding of low blood lactate levels after exercise in the acclimatized at high altitude is related to the depletion of plasma bicarbonate that characterizes acclimatization to the hypobaric hypoxia (Chapter

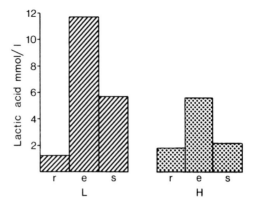

32.3 *Lactic acid levels in 11 lowlanders (L) and 12 highlanders (H) at 4540 m at rest (r), on exercise (e), and on recovery (s). Exercise was specified as running to exhaustion on a treadmill at a speed of 135.3 m/min and gradient of 18.9%. (After Hurtado (1964).)*

4). This depletion reduces buffering and results in large increases in H^+ concentration for a given release of lactate. The consequent local fall in pH may inhibit such enzymes as phosphofructokinase in the glycolytic pathway (West 1986*b*). This effectively slows up glycolysis and thus lactate production. Cerretelli (1980) has shown that the changes in blood H^+ concentration as a result of increase in blood lactate are higher in acclimatized than in unacclimatized subjects.

Other factors thought to be involved in the production of low lactate levels were considered by Binns *et al.* (1987) to be a diminution of muscle glycogen, a greater use of free fatty acids, and a reduction in muscle blood flow. These authors studied blood lactate levels in 18 normal subjects who walked to 4850 m over 11 days. Exercise studies designed to maintain heart rate at 85% of maximum for 15 minutes were carried out after they had been at high altitude for 2–4 days. They found that the blood lactate response to exercise at high altitude was reduced in all subjects. The concentration at the end of exercise at high altitude was 2.7 ± 1.0 mmol/m compared with 5.9 ± 2.6 mmol/l at sea level. Blood lactate concentrations at the end of exercise correlated with both pH and arterial oxygen tension in the pre-exercise period. Binns *et al.* (1987) thought the changes in pH were most important in reducing lactate concentrations. This is consistent with the striking reduction in blood lactate found in normal subjects exercising while acidotic on ammonium chloride (Fletcher *et al.*

1985). Half of the subjects studied were given prophylactic acetazolamide but this group, although having higher hydrogen ion concentrations than the placebo group, did not show lower lactate responses.

Effects of acetazolamide on exercise at extreme altitude

Hackett *et al.* (1985) studies the effect of acetazolamide on exercise performance at extreme altitude. They studied four climbers at an altitude of 6300 m. After an initial progressive exercise test to exhaustion on a bicycle-ergometer, they were re-studied after taking acetazolamide, 250 mg every 8 hours for three doses. They found that even at this extreme altitude the drug causes partial inhibition of carbonic anhydrase, producing metabolic acidosis of a degree produced at lower altitude, despite a pre-existing respiratory alkalosis. The mechanism of action of the drug has already been described in Chapter 12.

Hackett *et al.* (1985) found that during exercise the drug caused increased ventilation, an increased heart rate, and a slight increase in oxygen consumption at a given work level. The diuretic effect led to an increase in haemoglobin and haematocrit, probably due to a decreased plasma volume. This study is of unusual interest in that it illustrates what happens in climbers who acclimatize at altitudes of 4000–6000 m and then climb to extreme altitudes exceeding 7000 m. It reveals that even at these great elevations benefits in the form of prevention of acute mountain sickness, faster acclimatization, improved ventilation at rest, and better sleep are to be gained from the administration of acetazolamide. However, Hackett *et al.* (1985) found that the drug failed to improve work performance and suggested that it may even impair exercise performance at extreme altitude. They think that there are a number of theoretical reasons for this, such as decreased plasma volume, and the metabolic acidosis reducing the ability to buffer organic acids such as pyruvate and lactate. Dyspnoea on exercise may become excessive and inhibit exercise performance. The conclusions of Hackett *et al.* (1985) are in disagreement with those of Bradwell *et al.* (1986), referred to in Chapter 21, who found that acetazolamide is beneficial to acclimatized climbers at extreme altitude in slowing loss of muscle mass and body weight and thus helping to maintain exercise performance.

AVIATION AND SYMPTOMS RELATED TO HIGH ALTITUDE

Modern commercial aircraft are pressurized to simulate an altitude of 1520–1830 m in order to avoid the effects of hypobaric hypoxia, and an emergency oxygen supply is available should pressurization fail. In former years unpressurized aircraft flew Andean routes and reference is made in Chapter 30 to studies carried out on the crew by Hurtado *et al.* (1947). Even today it is possible to fly in unpressurized aircraft in this region; under such circumstances the crew and passengers will develop signs and symptoms of hypoxia if certain critical altitudes are exceeded. The oxygen saturation of arterial blood will fall below the acceptable level of 85% at 3660 m when the aviator is breathing air and at 12 190 m when he is breathing 100% oxygen (Robinson 1973). With increasing altitude, water vapour and carbon dioxide occupy more of the volume of the lungs until at 15 240 m they are filled entirely with these gases and even 100% oxygen at this altitude cannot sustain life (Robinson 1973). Table 32.2 outlines the symptoms experienced by aviators with progressive increase in altitude.

ACUTE EXPOSURE TO EXTREME ALTITUDE

Early balloonists ascended rapidly to great heights without appreciating the risks to which they were exposing themselves. Robinson (1973) gives an account of such an ascent by Glaisher from Wolverhampton on 17 July 1862. The balloon was inflated by an unusually light gas mixture specially prepared at the Stafford Road Gasworks and it shot up to 7990 m. Glaisher experienced palpitation, cyanosis, and a feeling of seasickness. Undeterred, on 5 September of the same year he ascended to 12 180 m and lost the power of his limbs and then became unconscious, but he survived. On 4 November 1927, Gray ascended from Scott Field, Illinois, and rose to 12 940 m. Later that afternoon his balloon returned to earth with its occupant dead.

Such episodes have not been lost entirely in the era of modern aircraft for, although the pilot is able to climb to great altitudes in safety, occasionally he has to bale out. Robinson (1973) pointed out that with an open parachute a man would die during the 10 minutes or so that it would take to descend from 10 670 m to 6100 m. It was apparent that with a free fall and closed parachute the drop could be made in 1 minute. However, early studies showed that even during a short period of free fall a test subject became cyanotic and began to lose consciousness after only 30 seconds, forgetting to open the valve of an emergency oxygen cylinder. After a further 5 seconds he became unconscious and

Table 32.2 Symptoms of hypoxia recorded in aviators with increasing altitude (after Robinson 1973)

Range of altitudes (m) at which symptoms occur, when breathing		Symptoms
Air	**100% O$_2$**	
0–3050	10 360–11 890	Impaired night vision (see Chapter 27)
3050–4570	11 890–12 960	Hyperventilation: tachycardia, increased cardiac output
4570–6100	12 960–13 660	Fatigue, lassitude, headache, sleepiness, euphoria resembling alcoholic intoxication; impaired vision; faulty judgement; poor memory; delayed reaction time; impaired muscle co-ordination; fine muscle movements impossible
6100–7000	13 660–13 870	Loss of consciousness, failure of respiratory centre; convulsions; death

moved convulsively. Subsequently one subject survived a parachute jump from an altitude of 12 192 m using an open parachute but having a supply of oxygen from a small cylinder carried in the leg pocket of his flying suit. From these two examples it will be appreciated that very short exposure to extreme altitude can be lethal.

The symptoms of acute exposure to the hypoxia of high altitude, as would be experienced by passengers when an aircraft suddenly loses cabin pressure or by experimental subjects in a decompression chamber, have been summarized by Milledge (1975). Sudden exposure to an altitude as low as 1220 m gives rise to a purplish tinge to the vision and night vision is measurably affected (see Chapter 29). Precipitate exposure to elevations of 1830 m and above causes slight breathlessness on exertion and such dyspnoea is more pronounced the higher the altitude. Sudden exposure to 4880 m brings about tingling of the lips and fingers, feelings of unreality, and dizziness. The higher functions of the brain are affected, with disturbances of association, memory, and fine movement. Difficulty is experienced in recognizing the orientation of stylized figures presented to subjects in a decompression chamber (Purves and Ponte 1977) and writing becomes slurred. Once the initial exposure is to an altitude of 6100 m or above, loss of consciousness takes place with increasing speed so

that only 2 minutes of useful consciousness can be expected after immediate exposure to 8840 m (Fig. 32.4).

In one remarkable case a young man of 18 years became a stowaway in the confined space of the unpressurized landing gear cell of a DC-8 which flew for 9 hours at an altitude of 8840 m from Havana to

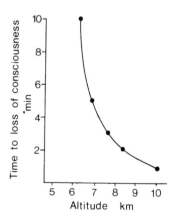

32.4 *Time in minutes for which consciousness is maintained on sudden exposure to altitudes exceeding 6100 m. (After Milledge (1975).)*

Madrid (Pajares and Merayo 1970). During a period of 8 hours the temperature fell to −6°C. On arrival he was unconscious and hypothermic and showed pronounced peripheral cyanosis. He was deaf. An ECG showed slurring of the QRS complexes, elevation of the ST segments, and flattening or inversion of the T waves. The electrocardiographic changes were thought to be the result of a combination of hypoxia and hypothermia. The electroencephalogram was normal. This extraordinary case shows that exceptionally the human body is capable of surviving acute exposure to a combination of extremes of hypoxia and hypothermia.

References

Binns, N., Wright, A.D., Singh, B.M. Coote, J.H., and Bradwell, A.R. (1987). Blood lactate changes during exercise at high altitude. *Postgraduate Medical Journal*, **63**, 177

Bradwell, A.R., Dykes, P.W., Coote, J.P., Forster, P.J.E., Miles, J.J., Chester, I., and Richardson, N.V. (1986). Effect of acetazolamide on exercise performance and muscle mass at high altitude. *Lancet*, **i**, 1001

Cerretelli, P. (1980). Gas exchange at high altitude. In *Pulmonary Gas Exchange* Vol. 2, (J.B. West, Ed.). New York Academic Press

Edwards, H.T. (1936). Lactic acid at rest and work at high altitude. *American Journal of Physiology*, **116**, 367

Fletcher, R.F., Wright, A.D., Jones, G.T., and Bradwell, A.R. (1985). The clinical assessment of acute mountain sickness. *Quarterly Journal of Medicine*, **54**, 91

Hackett, P.H., Reeves, J.T., Reeves, C.D., Grover, R.F., and Rennie, D. (1980). Control of breathing in Sherpas at low and high altitudes. *Journal of Applied Physiology*, **49**, 374

Hackett, P.H., Rennie, D., Hofmeister, S.E., Grover, R.F., Grover, E.B., and Reeves, J.I. (1982). Fluid retention and relative hypoventilation in acute mountain sickness. *Respiration*, **43**, 321

Hackett, P.H., Schoene, R.B., Winslow, R.M., Peters, R.M., and West, J.B. (1985). Acetazolamide and exercise in sojourners to 6,300 meters: a preliminary study. *Medicine and Science in Sports and Exercise*, **17**, 593

Harris, P. and Heath, D. (1977). The relation between ventilation and perfusion. In *The Human Pulmonary Circulation. Its Form and Function in Health and Disease*, 2nd edn. Edinburgh; Churchill Livingstone, p. 567

Houston, C.S. (1988). Acclimatization to hypoxia: Operations Everest I and II. *Annals of Sports Medicine*, **4**, 171

Houston, C.S., Sutton, J.R., Cymerman, A., and Reeves, J.T. (1987). Operation Everest II. Man at extreme altitude. *Journal of Applied Physiology*, **63**, 877

Hurtado, A. (1964). Some physiologic and clinical aspects of life at high altitudes. In *Aging of the Lung* (L. Cander and J.H. Mayer, ed.). New York, Grune and Stratton, p. 257

Hurtado, A. (1971). The influence at high altitude on physiology. In *High Altitude Physiology: Cardiac and Respiratory Aspects* (R. Porter and J. Knight, Ed). Edinburgh; Churchill Livingstone, p. 3

Hurtado, A., Aste-Salazar, H., Merino, C., Velasquez, T., Monge-C, C., and Reynafarje, C. (1947). Physiological characteristics of flight personnel. *Journal of Aviation Medicine*, **18**, 406

Masuyama, S., Kimura, H., Sugita, T., Kuriyama, T., Tassumi, K., Kumitomo, F., Okita, S., Tojima, H., Yuguchi, Y., Watanabe, S., and Honda, Y. (1986). Control of ventilation in extreme-altitude climbers. *Journal of Applied Physiology*, **61**, 500

Milledge, J.S. (1975). Physiological effects of hypoxia. In *Mountain Medicine and Physiology* (C. Clarke, M. Ward, and E. Williams, ed. London Alpine Club, p. 73

Milledge, J.S. (1987). The ventilatory response to hypoxia: how much is good for a mountaineer? *Postgraduate Medical Journal*, **63**, 169

Milledge, J.S. and Lahiri, S. (1967). Respiratory control in lowlanders and Sherpa highlanders. *Respiration Physiology*, **2**, 310

Milledge, J.S., Ward, M.P., Williams, E.S., and Clarke, C.R. (1983). Cardiorespiratory response to exercise in men repeatedly exposed to extreme altitude. *Journal of Applied Physiology*, **55**, 1379

Pajares, J. and Merayo, F. (1970). Unique clinical case both of hypoxia and hypothermia studied in an 18 year old aerial stowaway on a flight from Havana to Madrid. *Aerospace Medicine*, **41**, 1416

Pugh, L.G.C.E. (1962). Physiological and medical aspects of the Himalayan Scientific and Mountaineering Expedition 1960–61. *British Medical Journal*, **i**, 621

Pugh, L.G.C.E., Gill, M.B., Lahiri, S., Milledge, J.S., Ward, M.P., and West, J.B. (1964). Muscular exercise at great altitudes. *Journal of Applied Physiology*, **19**, 431

Purves, M. and Ponte, J. (1977). Film: *Hypoxia and the Role of Peripheral Chemoreceptors*. Directed by D. Ponting; distributed by John Wiley & Sons, London

Robinson, D.H. (1973). *The Dangerous Sky. A History of Aviation Medicine*. Henley-on-Thames, England; G.T. Foulis

Schoene, R.B. (1982). Control of ventilation in climbers to extreme altitude. *Journal of Applied Physiology*, **53**, 806

Schoene, R.B., Lahiri, S., Hackett, P.H., Peters, R.M. Jr, Milledge, J.S., Pizzo, C.J., Sarnquist, F.H., Boyer, S.J., Graber, D.J., Maret, K.H., and West, J.B. (1984). Relationship of hypoxic ventilatory response to exercise performance on Mount Everest, 1984. *Journal of Applied Physiology*, **56**, 1478

Severinghaus, J.W., Bainton, C.R., and Carcelen, A. (1966). Respiratory insensitivity to hypoxia in chronically hypoxic man. *Respiration Physiology*, **1**, 308

Ward, M. (1975). *Mountain Medicine. A Clinical Study of Cold and High Altitude*. London; Crosby Lockwood Staples

Weill, J.V., Byrne-Quinn, E., Sodal, I.E., Filey, G.F., and Grover, R.F. (1971). Acquired attenuation of chemoreceptor function in chronically hypoxic man at high altitude. *Journal of Clinical Investigation*, **50**, 186

West, J.B. (1986a). Highest inhabitants in the world. *Nature (London)*, **324**, 517

West, J.B. (1986b). Lactate during exercise at extreme altitude. *Federation Proceedings*, **45**, 2953

West, J.B. (1988). Physiology at the summit of Mount Everest. *Annals of Sports Medicine*, **4**, 224

West, J.B., Lahiri, S., Maret, K.H., Peters, R.M., and Pizzo, C.J., (1983). Barometric pressures at extreme altitudes on Mt. Everest; physiological significance. *Journal of Applied Physiology*, **54**, 1188

33

Descent to sea level

The many adjustments of the human body to hypobaric hypoxia and other adverse factors of the environment are initially of a physiological functional nature. As the period of residence at high altitude lengthens, many become associated with structural changes at histological or ultrastructural level. On descent to low altitude many of these functional changes would be expected to be reversed rapidly to sea-level values. The associated microanatomical alterations, however, commonly slow up the regression. What is more, in some instances the principle of overshoot seems to apply so that not only do the physiological changes revert to sea-level values but many continue to fall until they are below the normal range.

The most complete study of the effects of long-term descent to sea level has been made by Sime *et al.* (1971). They studied 11 healthy native highlanders of Cerro de Pasco (4330 m) aged 18–23 years. These young men were taken to Morococha (4540 m) where the investigations listed in Table 33.1 were carried out. They were then taken to Lima (150 m) and the investigations were repeated after they had been living at sea level for 2 years. Where appropriate, the investigations were carried out at rest and after exercise.

ANAEMIA
After 2 years of continuous residence at sea level healthy native highlanders show a fall in haemoglobin level and haematocrit (Table 33.1). It will be recalled from Chapter 15 that similar drops occur in patients with Monge's disease on descent to sea level. Peñaloza *et al.* (1971) studied the haematological changes that occured in three patients with the condition after 3, 11 and 60 days' sojourn at low altitude. After residence at sea level for 2 months the haematocrit and haemoglobin levels fell substantially. In one patient the haematocrit fell from 86 to 50% and the haemoglobin level from 23.2 to 17.0 g/dl.

As we note in Chapter 18 increased red-cell mass at high altitude is associated with a hypervolaemia

(Hurtado *et al.* 1945; Merino 1950). With the fall in haematocrit on descent to sea level there is a proportionate increase in plasma volume. After some 4 months at sea level the total blood volume falls since red-cell mass drops to subnormal values leading to anaemia. This gradually improves over the following months. This overshoot in fall in haemoglobin levels in native highlanders after 2 years' residence at sea level commonly occurs so that they actually become anaemic after this period.

These changes in plasma volume associated with fall in haemoglobin level may have some importance in predisposing the highlander at sea level to the onset of pulmonary oedema on his return to the mountains (see Chapter 13).

VENTILATION
After residence at sea level for 2 years the characteristic hyperventilation of those previously permanently domiciled at high altitude (Chapter 4) disappears. This change in ventilation at sea level becomes more apparent on exercise (Table 33.1). Differences in oxygen uptake in individuals at high altitude and sea level are not significant (Table 33.1) and increments from rest to exercise are very similar for the same work load in the two environments. The arterial oxygen saturation rises significantly at sea level.

The diminished hypoxic ventilatory response of the enlarged carotid bodies at high altitude (Chapter 7) does not improve on descent to sea level. We know of no evidence to support the view that the enlarged carotid bodies of the highlander return to a normal size after a period of residence at low altitude. Such enlarged glomera with histological and ultrastructural changes of the type described in Chapter 7 cannot be compared with the carotid bodies of such laboratory animals as rats in decompression chambers. In rats the enlargement is due entirely to vascular engorgement after a brief exposure to simulated high altitude. As might be anticipated, on withdrawal of the hypoxic stimulus the carotid bodies lose their engorgement and rapidly

Table 33.1 Changes in haematological and cardiopulmonary parameters in high-altitude natives after residence at sea level for 2 years (after Sime et al. 1971)

	Morococha (4540 m)		Lima (150 m)	
	At rest	On exercise*	At rest	On exercise*
Haemoglobin (g/dl)	18.5 ± 0.55		13.5 ± 0.24	
Haematocrit (%)	55.4 ± 1.6		41.9 ± 0.8	
Mean oxygen uptake (ml/min per m² BSA)	158 ± 4.7	802 ± 28.8	161 ± 3.7	866 ± 24.0
Ventilation (l/min per m² BSA)	5.24 ± 0.36	24.74 ± 1.07	4.80 ± 0.25	19.88 ± 0.75
Arterial oxygen saturation (%)	78.48 ± 1.25	69.20 ± 1.28	97.31 ± 0.68	94.33 ± 0.57
Heart rate (beats/min)	77 ± 3.9	144 ± 6.9	59 ± 2.1	114 ± 3.8
Cardiac index (l/min per m² BSA)	3.83 ± 0.21	7.57 ± 0.29	4.32 ± 0.20	8.79 ± 0.32
Stroke index (ml/beat per m² BSA)	50.2 ± 2.7	54 ± 3.7	74.2 ± 3.6	
Pulmonary arterial pressure (mmHg)	24 ± 1.6		12 ± 0.6	25 ± 1.1
Pulmonary resistance (dyn/s per cm⁻⁵)	334 ± 27.4		145 ± 10.7	

* Exercise, 300 kg m/min per m² BSA.

return to a normal size. These conditions and the microanatomical changes in the carotid bodies are totally dissimilar to those found in native highlanders.

BRADYCARDIA

The heart rate falls on descent from high altitude and, after 2 years' residence at the coast, highlanders may show bradycardia. The slowing of the heart occurs very shortly after arrival at low altitudes. Thus, Hartley *et al.* (1967) describe a slight fall in heart rate in residents of Leadville, Colorado (3100 m) after only 10 days' residence at sea level. The same rapid slowing of heart rate has been detected during electrocardiographic studies on children and adults taken down to sea level from the Andes. An acute reduction in heart rate at high altitude following the administration of oxygen has been reported by Hultgren *et al.* (1965).

CARDIAC OUTPUT

The decrease in heart rate just referred to is associated with an increased stroke volume and an increase in cardiac output (Table 33.1). Thus the normal or slightly diminished cardiac output of the Andean native that is referred to in Chapter 18, described by several authors including Peñaloza *et al.* (1963) and Sime *et al.* (1963), and confirmed by Sime *et al.* (1971) is increased on descent to sea level.

REVERSAL OF PULMONARY HYPERTENSION

A good example of the complex nature of the reversibility of the changes induced by long-term residence at high altitude, especially in native highlanders, is provided by the pulmonary circulation. As we have seen in Chapter 10, native highlanders have pulmonary hypertension from infancy associated with the chronic alveolar hypoxia brought about by the diminished barometric pressure. The elevation of pulmonary arterial pressure is moderate in early childhood but is maintained into adult life to a limited extent. The pulmonary hypertension becomes associated with remodelling of the lung vasculature with muscularization of the pulmonary arterioles, the development of a layer of longitudinal muscle in the intima of pulmonary arteries and arterioles, and the formation of inner muscular tubes (Heath and Williams 1991). Thus, the pulmonary hypertension of native highlanders has a basis in two different factors. One is functional and due to hypoxic vasoconstriction of the muscularized periph-

eral portions of the pulmonary arterial tree. The other is structural and due to the components of the pulmonary vascular remodelling referred to above. These functional and structural elements behave differently on descent to sea level.

Inhalation of oxygen will produce only a partial alleviation of raised pulmonary arterial pressure in long-standing residents at high altitude, as was noted by Grover *et al.* (1966) during an investigation at Leadville, Colorado (3100 m). The ineffectiveness of the increased partial pressure of oxygen in the ambient air of low altitudes in immediately reversing the pulmonary hypertension in former residents at high altitude was reported by Hartley *et al.* (1967) who did not find a significant drop in pulmonary arterial pressure after 10 days' residence at low altitude following domicile at 3100 m. In one of their cases Grover *et al.* (1966) noted a fall of pulmonary arterial pressure of only 17 mmHg after 11 months' residence at sea level following descent from 3100 m. Peñaloza and Sime (1971) reported that in three cases of chronic mountain sickness the fall in pulmonary arterial pressure was related to the time spent at sea level after descent from high altitude and had not returned to normal even after 60 days. Such data support the concept that *partial* reversal of hypoxic pulmonary hypertension by relief of vasoconstriction in the lung by oxygen is rapid. An additional factor that may be involved, especially in chronic mountain sickness, is a progressive fall in polycythaemia.

In sharp contrast to this, total reversal of pulmonary hypertension may take up to 2 years to achieve while regression of the pulmonary vascular remodelling described in Chapter 10 takes place. In this respect there is an interesting parallel with the lack of regression of the identical form of pulmonary vascular remodelling that occurs in pulmonary emphysema, even after long-term oxygen therapy. We carried out a pathophysiological study of 10 cases of hypoxic cor pulmonale half of whom had been treated by long-term oxygen therapy for between 2 and 8 years (Wilkinson *et al.* 1988). In spite of this therapy all five showed musculoelastic thickening of the intima, while four showed muscularization of the pulmonary arterioles or precapillaries. Muscular tubes were found in pulmonary arterioles in two of the five. It is apparent that long-term oxygen therapy had had no effect in reversing the pulmonary vascular changes in these patients. It seems that the pulmonary vascular remodelling of the native highlander likewise takes a long time to regress if it ever does.

We regard the various functional features of acclimatization to high altitudes as normal physiological responses to abnormal environmental stimuli. On descent to sea level these stimuli are removed. There seems to be no convincing evidence that descent to the sea-level environment carries a risk for the highlander. The only hazard appears to be that the increase in plasma volume in the highlander that occurs on his moving to sea level may predispose to the development of high-altitude pulmonary oedema when he returns to the mountains.

References

Grover, R.F., Vogel, J.H.K., Voight, G.C., and Blount, S.G. Jr (1966). Reversal of high altitude pulmonary hypertension. *American Journal of Cardiology*, **18**, 928

Hartley, L.H., Alexander, J.K., Modelski, M., and Grover, R.F. (1967). Subnormal cardiac output at rest and during exercise in residents at 3100 m altitude. *Journal of Applied Physiology*, **23**, 839

Heath, D. and Williams, D. (1991). Pulmonary vascular remodelling in a high-altitude Aymara Indian. *International Journal of Biometeorology*, **35**, 203

Hultgren, H.N., Kelly, J., and Miller, H. (1965). Effect of oxygen upon pulmonary circulation in acclimatized man at high altitude. *Journal of Applied Physiology*, **20**, 239

Hurtado, A., Merino, C., and Delgado, E. (1945). Influence of anoxemia on the hemopoietic activity. *Archives of Internal Medicine*, **75**, 284

Merino, C.F. (1950). Studies on blood formation and destruction in the polycythaemia of high altitude. *Blood*, **5**, 1

Peñaloza, D. and Sime, F. (1971). Chronic cor pulmonale due to loss of altitude acclimatization (chronic mountain sickness). *American Journal of Medicine*, **50**, 728

Peñaloza, D., Sime, F., Banchero, N., Gamboa, R., Cruz, J., and Marticorena, E. (1963). Pulmonary hypertension in healthy men born and living at high altitudes. *American Journal of Cardiology*, **11**, 150

Peñaloza, D., Sime, F., and Ruiz, L. (1971). Cor pulmonale in chronic mountain sickness: present concept of Monge's disease. In *High Altitude Physiology: Cardiac and Respiratory Aspects*, Ciba Foundation Symposium (R. Porter and J. Knight, Ed.). Edinburgh; Churchill Livingstone

Sime, F., Banchero, N., Peñaloza, D., Gamboa, R., Cruz, J., and Marticorena, E. (1963). Pulmonary hypertension in children born and living at high altitudes. *American Journal of Cardiology*, **11**, 143

Sime, F., Peñaloza, D., and Ruiz, L. (1971). Bradycardia, increased cardiac output, and reversal of pulmonary hypertension in altitude natives living at sea level. *British Heart Journal*, **33**, 647

Wilkinson, M., Langhorne, C.A., Heath, D., Barer, G.R., and Howard, P. (1988). A pathophysiological study in 10 cases of hypoxic cor pulmonale. *Quarterly Journal of Medicine*, **NS66**, 65

34

Cancer in the Andes

The incidence of various types of cancer at high altitude could theoretically be influenced by physical factors characteristic of the elevation *per se* such as hypobaric hypoxia and enhanced ultraviolet radiation. Another factor is the genetic make-up of the particular group of highlanders being studied such as Aymaras versus Ladakhis, for example. However, probably the most important factor is the life-style of the community being studied. In other words the physical features of high altitude *per se* are probably less important that the socio-economic influences of the environment. It is difficult to acquire data on the incidence of various forms of cancer at high altitude, for native highlanders tend to live in isolated communities in remote areas where facilities for accurate clinical and laboratory diagnosis are sparse. One notable exception to this general rule is La Paz, Bolivia, the highest capital city in the world. Built in a narrow valley at the edge of the Andean altiplano it slopes down from its international airport at 4120 m to 3200 m, the central plaza being at 3600 m. This city offers a population of over 650 000 inhabitants with a network of hospitals and an acceptable level of diagnostic capabilities. It also offers a population in which are included different ethnic groups, which include Whites, Aymara Indians, and mestizos. Hence in this city we have a unique opportunity to gain insight into the prevalence of various tumours in a large community at high altitude. However, the frequency of different types of cancer in La Paz relates only to this particular area and this is why this chapter is entitled 'Cancer in the Andes', rather than 'Cancer at high altitude'.

In La Paz the local factors in addition to the anticipated hypobaric hypoxia of high altitude are an exceptionally dry climate, high levels of background radiation, intensive ultraviolet radiation, cold that demands the use of heavy clothing, and ingestion of dietary items characteristic of the area. Against this background of unusual opportunity a study of the morbidity from cancer in La Paz was carried out by Rios-Dalenz *et al.* in 1981 using a cancer registry in the city which started collecting data in January 1978. Average annual age-specific incidence rates for 1978–79 for all forms of tumour were calculated using data from the last national census as denominator. For international comparisons, age-adjusted incidence rates were calculated and compared with those published in the third volume of *Cancer Incidence in Five Continents* (Waterhouse *et al.* 1976). In this highland city the population over 65 years of age makes less use of diagnostic facilities and for international comparisons it is necessary to make use of 'truncated rates' for subjects in the age range of 35–64 years. In overall terms it is clear that by international comparison the city of La Paz has a low average annual rate of cancer incidence (Table 34.1). Illness from all forms of cancer in the city is much greater in females than in males. Superimposed on these general terms it is possible to study the incidence of specific types of tumour, which reveals fascinating and often surprising insights into cancer in this one city. No doubt, when other communities at high altitude are studied with the same degree of attention, other trends peculiar to those areas will emerge.

ORAL CAVITY AND PHARYNX

Coca-chewing is a common custom of the high-altitude Indians of Bolivia. Coca leaves are kept as a bolus weighing about 15 g in the mouth for about 2–3 hours and this is changed three to four times a day. This is mostly true in men of poor socio-economic status, and younger men leaving the altiplano for the city tend to forsake the habit. The coca leaves are mixed with wood-ash (lejia) or small amounts of calcium carbonate (Baker and Mazes 1963). One might wonder what influence this widespread habit might have on the incidence of cancer in the mouth and pharynx. The surprising answer is that cancer rates at these sites are lower in La Paz than in other countries with the anomalous finding that the incidence in females is some three times greater than in males. However, Rios-Dalenz *et al.* (1981) point out that the small numbers of cases involved in their study invite caution in the inter-

Table **34.1** Average annual truncated incidence rate for various tumours in La Paz Bolivia (1978–79) and selected registries throughout the world (data from Waterhouse et al. 1976; after Rios-Dalenz et al. 1981)

Centre	All tumours		Stomach		Lung		Breast	Cervix uteri	Penis	Thyroid	
	M	F	M	F	M	F	F	F	M	M	F
Connecticut, USA	387.4	439.9	17.3	7.0	85.9	25.5	157.5	20.7	0.5	2.4	5.7
Sao Paulo, Brazil	360.4	380.1	77.9	29.2	41.1	8.9	112.1	66.0	4.0	2.6	5.6
Birmingham, UK	341.7	341.7	32.1	11.9	128.2	23.0	120.2	31.6	1.5	1.1	2.2
Miyagi, Japan	260.3	219.9	133.1	65.8	23.7	10.9	33.5	32.9	0.6	0.9	3.5
Cali, Colombia	237.9	405.5	71.1	35.6	24.4	10.1	58.2	148.8	2.4	4.9	10.2
Ibadan, Nigeria	158.3	257.4	17.0	17.5	2.7	2.4	33.7	55.9	0.5	0.9	3.5
La Paz, Bolivia	158.2	365.4	25.9	18.1	13.7	3.2	47.7	151.4	1.2	1.6	8.0

Average annual truncated incidence rate per 100 000 patients * for tumours of

* Patients are between 35 and 64 years old.

pretation of their observations and that there is a need for further investigation of a larger number of cases. Far from predisposing to cancer of the oral cavity it would appear that Aymara communities have excellent dental and oral hygiene and show little in the way of dental disease (Palomino 1978).

THE ALIMENTARY TRACT

The rates of oesophageal, gastric, and colonic carcinoma in La Paz in the period studied were generally lower than those of other countries (Rios-Dalenz *et al.* 1981). In contrast to the situation in the oral cavity, oesophageal cancer rates in men in the Bolivian capital are much higher than in women. Gastric carcinoma has a low rate in La Paz which is in contradistinction to what occurs in the Indian populations in other areas of the Andes (Correa *et al.* 1976). The population of La Paz appears to be protected like the Mexicans. It has been speculated that the protecting factor is chilli peppers which are eaten by the citizens of La Paz with their meals and are known to have a high content of vitamins, particularly of ascorbic acid. The incidence of colonic and rectal carcinoma is low in La Paz as is that of predisposing conditions such as ulcerative colitis and adenomatous polyps.

GALL BLADDER AND EXTRAHEPATIC BILE DUCTS

In striking contrast the incidence of biliary tract cancer in the women of La Paz is the highest in the world (Table 34.2). Even in men, the rate is ex-

ceeded only by non-Jewish Israelis (Table 34.2). This finding is consistent with the reports of high mortality rates from cancer of the gall bladder and bile ducts in other predominantly Indian populations such as those of Mexico and Guatemala (Puffer and Griffith 1968). It is intriguing to speculate as to whether this incidence of gall bladder cancer is due to genetic or environmental, cultural influences.

The age- and population-standardized incidence rates for cancer of the gall bladder in Bolivia were 5.3/100 000 per year for males and 10.3/100 000 per year for females during the period 1978–80. Comparable rates (per 100 000 per year) in the United States were 1.0 for males and 2.1 for females. Corresponding figures for cancer of the extrahepatic bile ducts in Bolivia were 1.1 for males and 4.1 for females, and in the United States were 1.6 for males and 1.0 for females. In other words the overall incidence of cancer of the gall bladder in Bolivia is five times that of the United States. In contrast, cancer of the extrahepatic ducts has a female distribution in Bolivia but a male predisposition in the United States. The excess of cases in Bolivia cannot be explained solely by difference in the age and sex distribution of the populations. It can be only partially explained by differences in racial distribution. There may be other aetiological factors at high altitude such as differences in diet or other environmental features. The suggestion has been made that in Bolivia there is a high incidence of gall stones containing appreciable levels of the

Table 34.2 Selected truncated incidence rate per 100 000 of cancer of the gall bladder and bile ducts (after Rios-Dalenz *et al.* 1981)

	Incidence per 100 000	
	M	**F**
La Paz, Bolivia	13.7	28.5
New Mexico USA, Indians	4.6	21.1
Israel, non-Jews	14.5	18.7
Israel, all Jews	9.1	16.8
Warsaw, Poland	5.0	16.1
Cali, Colombia	5.2	9.3
Sao Paulo, Brazil	4.5	6.7
Miyagi, Japan	6.8	5.8
Connecticut, USA	2.4	2.9
Ibadan, Nigeria	0.6	2.6
Birmingham, UK	2.2	2.2

toxic glycolithocolic acid which remains because sulfation is deficient (Rios-Dalenz *et al.* 1983).

NASAL CAVITY AND PARANASAL SINUSES

Any visitor to La Paz will be impressed by the nasal congestion and irritation brought about by the combination of the extremely low humidity and the inhaled dust from the arid surroundings. The persistent irritation brings in its train an excess production of viscid mucus that hardens. Attempts to clear this readily induce haemorrhage, which leaves sharp-edged haematomas in the nasal cavity. Added to this chronic irritation is the possibility of substances of unknown carcinogenic potential in the ubiquitous dust. One recalls the zeolites in the dust of Capodocia in Turkey that lead to the appearance of pleural mesothelioma in the local residents. With this background it is not surprising that tumours of the nasal cavity and paranasal sinuses have an unexpectedly high frequency in La Paz (Table 34.3). The rate in females is the highest on record while that in males is also very high. Most of these tumours originated in the maxillary sinuses. The predominant histological type was the squamous cell carcinoma followed by undifferentiated carcinoma.

At the time of the study incidence rates for cancer of the lung and larynx were at the lower end of the scale, but in recent years the smoking of cigarettes has become increasingly common, especially in women. A vigorous anti-smoking campaign is now in progress in the city.

CANCER IN WOMEN

Female breast cancer rates in La Paz are low. Cancer of the body of the uterus and ovary, and pro-static cancer in males are also relatively low on the international scale but in a position occupied by other Latin American population such as that of Brazil. In contrast the incidence of cervical cancer in La Paz is very high. Little is known about aetiological factors associated with this tumour in the city. Its high incidence coincides with the well-known inverse relation with social class since most people in La Paz have limited economic resources. Other known risk factors, such as early starts of sexual activity and multiplicity of partners, have not been investigated in La Paz.

CANCER OF THE TESTIS

Cancer of the testis has an unexpectedly high frequency in La Paz as shown in Table 34.4 which includes the highest rates on record. The incidence rates in other Latin American countries are lower than the average throughout the world. This suggests that the high rate in Bolivia is due to some local environmental aetiology at high altitude. It has been suggested that testicular cancer may be associated with elevated temperature of the testicle brought about by heavy clothing used by the population as protection against cold weather (Lin and Kessler 1979). On the Bolivian altiplano the Indians use thick, long flannel underwear.

SKIN

Cancer of the skin is of low frequency in general at high altitude as we have pointed out in Chapter 25 and so it comes as no surprise to find that cutaneous cancer is of low frequency in La Paz. It seems likely that, as with the Quechua Indians of the Peruvian altiplano (Chapter 25), skin pigmentation and clothing may be protective factors for the Aymara in La

Table 34.3 Selected (highest) truncated incidence rates per 100 000 of cancer of the nasal cavity and paranasal sinuses (after Rios-Dalenz *et al.* 1981)

	Incidence per 100 000	
	M	F
La Paz, Bolivia	4.7	4.1
Osaka, Japan	5.2	2.5
Ibadan, Nigeria	5.1	3.4
Miyagi, Japan	4.2	2.6
Sao Paulo, Brazil	3.1	0.5
Newfoundland, Canada	2.9	0.6
Bombay, India	2.3	2.1

Table 34.4 Selected truncated incidence rates per 100 000 of testicular cancer (after Rios-Dalenz *et al.* 1981)

	Incidence per 100 000
Norway	6.5
La Paz, Bolivia	6.1
Alameda USA, White	6.1
Geneva, Switzerland	6.0
Saskatchewan, Canada	5.6
New Zealand, Maori	5.5
Connecticut, USA	3.4
Birmingham, UK	3.3
Alameda USA, Black	1.8
Sao Paulo, Brazil	1.6
Finland	1.5
Cali, Colombia	1.0
Miyagi, Japan	0.7
Ibadan, Nigeria	0.1

Paz against the excessive ultraviolet radiation found at high altitude.

CHEMODECTOMA

Chemodectomas occur more commonly in native highlanders than in sea-level subjects as we discuss at length in Chapter 7. This is almost certainly related to the progressive enlargement of the carotid bodies that occurs in response to the sustained stimulus of hypobaric hypoxia.

References

Baker, P. and Mazes, R.B. (1963). Calcium: unusual sources in the Highland Peruvian diet. *Science*, **142**, 1466

Correa, P., Cuello, C., Duque E., Burbario, L.C., Garcia, F.T., Bolano, E., Brown, C., and Haenszel W. (1976). Gastric cancer in Colombia. III Natural history of precursor lesions. *Journal of the National Cancer Institute*, **57**, 1027

Lin, R.S. and Kessler, L.J. (1979). Epidemiologic findings in testicular cancer. *American Journal of Epidemiology*, **110**, 357

Palomino, H. (1978). The Aymara of Western Bolivia. III Occlusion, pathology and characteristics of the dentition. *Journal of Dental Research*, **57**, 459

Puffer, R.R and Griffith, G.W. (1968). Características de la mortalidad urbana, *Pan American Health Organization Scientific Publication No. 151*. Washington, DC; Pan American Health Organization

Rios-Dalenz, J., Correa, P., and Haenszel, W. (1981). Morbidity from cancer in La Paz, Bolivia. *International Journal of Cancer*, **28**, 307

Rios-Dalenz, J., Takabayashi, A., Henson, D.E., Strom, B.L., and Soloway, R.D. (1983). The epidemiology of cancer of the extra-hepatic biliary tract in Bolivia. *International Journal of Epidemiology*, **12**, 156

Waterhouse, J., Muir, C., Correa, P., and Powell, J. (ed.) (1976). *Cancer Incidence in Five Continents*, Vol. III, IARC Scientific Publication No. 15. Lyon, France; IARC

35

Adaptation to hypobaric hypoxia

Throughout this book we have been concerned with the multiple and varied manifestations of the acclimatization of man to high altitude. Acclimatization is a reversible, non-inheritable change in the anatomy or physiology of an organism that enables it to survive in an alien environment. However, not all species of animal living at high altitude are of equal biological status and they adjust to the environmental stresses in different ways. Indigenous mountain species have developed different characteristics to enable them to survive and to thrive in the hypobaric hypoxia by the process of adaptation. Adaptation is the development of biochemical, physiological, and anatomical features that are heritable and of genetic basis, enabling the species to explore the environmental to its best advantage. This chapter considers the features of genetic adaptation to high altitude.

HYPOXIC PULMONARY VASOCONSTRICTOR RESPONSE

When life evolved from the sea to the land, the single cardiac ventricle that had sufficed for fish to propel blood through the gill-capillaries and then through the tissues of the body was no longer adequate. Birds and mammals evolved a vascular system with two ventricles. One was specifically devoted to the pulmonary circulation where the low ancestral arterial pressure was retained. The other supplied the tissues of the body at a pressure six or more times higher, a feature of all warm-blooded vertebrates (Harris 1986). The two redesigned systems of circulation and ventilation met in a new organ, the lung, which provided a massive increase in the transport of respiratory gases required for physical exercise.

A single in-pouching of the pharynx developed into a tree-like structure of branching airways that ended in an alveolar-capillary membrane less than 1 μm thick (see Chapter 4). The total area of the exchange membrane was equal to that of a squash court and unmodified it would have acted like an immense sail that would have prevented any rapid

and purposeful displacements of the body (Harris 1986). In the event the exchange membrane was contained within a small organ, the lung, but the price of the to-and-fro motion of the air in small blind-ended airways was its susceptibility to obstruction. At the same time, blood flow was continuous so that it would continue to supply unventilated portions of lung, thereby reducing the oxygen content of the systemic arterial blood. This evolutionary difficulty appears to have been overcome by the development of a system that controlled the local resistance to flow through the pulmonary circulation according to the partial pressure of oxygen in the alveoli. Obstruction to an airway caused a decrease in the partial pressure of oxygen in its alveolar spaces that automatically shut down the local flow of blood and maintained the systemic arterial oxygen tension. Harris (1986) points out the astonishing similarity between the oxygen – dissociation curve for haemoglobin (see Chapter 5) and the pulmonary vasoconstrictor response (Fig. 35.1) and notes that it can

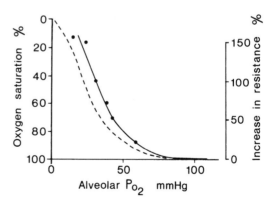

35.1 *The relation between the alveolar partial pressure of oxygen and the percentage increase in pulmonary vascular resistance is shown by a continuous line. (Data from Durand et al. (1970).) The oxygen dissociation curve for haemoglobin is superimposed as a discontinuous line. (After Harris (1986).)*

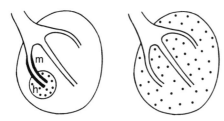

35.2 *Hypoxic pulmonary vasconstrictor response.*
(a) In mammals at low altitude an area of alveolar
hypoxia (h) in the lung brings about muscularization
(m) of pulmonary arterioles which constrict and shunt
blood away from the affected zone. (b) In contrast, at
high altitude the air in all the alveolar spaces is hypoxic
so that a vasoconstrictor response has no physiological
advantage. Indeed widespread muscularization of
arterioles throughout the lung would induce pulmonary
hypertension and carry with it the risk of producing lung
oedema.

hardly be by chance that the constrictor response co-incides so closely with the degree of unsaturation of the blood for a given partial pressure of oxygen.

This hypoxic pulmonary vasoconstriction evolved as a local homeostatic mechanism that proved advantageous to survival at sea level. However, at high altitude, where all the alveolar spaces contain hypoxic air, there is no advantage to be gained from shunting blood away from them (Fig. 35.2). Furthermore, the widespread pulmonary constriction induced by the hypoxia brings about pulmonary hypertension that may lead on to high-altitude pulmonary oedema (see Chapter 13). Hence the mechanism becomes disadvantageous at high altitude. This being so, one would expect the forces of natural selection to eliminate it in the mountain environment.

Man is thought to have lived in the Andes for about 35 000 years (see Chapter 3) and it would seem that this length of time is inadequate for the loss of the hypoxic pulmonary vasoconstrictor reflex, for we have already seen in Chapter 10 that the native Quechua highlander of the Andes develops mild pulmonary hypertension and muscularization of the terminal portion of the pulmonary arterial tree. In contrast to this, indigenous mountain species have been resident in the Andes and Himalaya for millennia and they appear to have lost the hypoxic pulmonary vasoconstrictor response through the forces of natural selection. Thus, one of the features of the animal adapted to high altitude is the thin-walled nature of the pulmonary arterial tree

and the absence of smooth muscle from the pulmonary arterioles.

PULMONARY VASCULATURE OF ADAPTED ANIMALS

In the llama (*Lama glama*) (Fig. 35.3) the media of the small pulmonary arteries is thin (Fig. 35.4) and there is no right ventricular hypertrophy, so that the left-to-right ventricular ratio is high (Heath *et al.* 1969, 1974; Harris *et al.* 1982; Table 35.1). The concept that the thin-walled pulmonary arterial tree of the llama is a manifestation of genetic adaptation to hypobaric hypoxia, representing a loss of the hypoxic pulmonary vasoconstrictor response, might be challenged by noting that this species is a high-altitude camelid and the camel family is characterized by a thin-walled pulmonary vasculature. This objection, however, is refuted by the finding of thin-walled pulmonary arteries in the yak (*Bos grunniens*; Fig. 35.5), which is a member of the cattle family living at high altitude. As already seen in Chapter 16, cattle (*B. taurus*) have a naturally muscular pulmonary vasculature that constricts vigorously in response to chronic alveolar hypoxia, leading to the development of brisket disease in calves in Utah. In contrast, we found the muscular pulmonary arteries of the yak to have a very thin media and its pul-

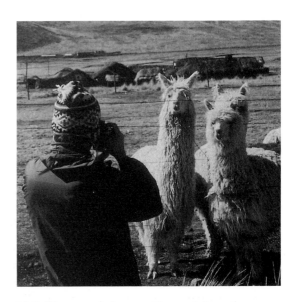

35.3 *Llamas and alpacas with one of the authors*
(D.R.W.) at La Raya (4200 m) in the Peruvian
Andes. In this indigenous mountain species the
pulmonary arteries are thin-walled and the pulmonary
arterioles are devoid of a muscular coat.

Table 35.1 Percentage medial thickness of pulmonary arteries and left-to-right ventricular ratios in indigenous mountain species

Species	Mean % medial thickness of pulmonary arteries	Left-to right ventricular ratios	Area	Altitude (m)	Reference
Llama	4.4	—	Cerro de Pasco, Peru	4330	Heath *et al.* (1969)
Llama	3.8	3.5	Rancas, Peru	4720	Heath *et al.* (1974)
Llama	4.9	3.0	Rancas, Peru	4720	Heath *et al.* (1974)
Llama	4.1	2.6	La Raya, Peru	4200	Harris *et al.* (1982)
Llama	5.8	3.0	La Raya, Peru	4200	Harris *et al.* (1982)
Alpaca	4.4	3.1	La Raya, Peru	4200	Harris *et al.* (1982)
Guanaco	6.0	3.1	London	0	Harris *et al.* (1982)
Guanaco	4.2	3.1	London	0	Harris *et al.* (1982)
Llama	4.6	3.7	London	0	Harris *et al.* (1982)
Yak	3.1	2.8	Nepal	4000	Heath *et al.* (1984)
Mountain-viscacha	5.0	3.1	La Raya, Peru	4200	Heath *et al.* (1981)
Mountain-viscacha	4.7	2.9	La Raya, Peru	4200	Heath *et al.* (1981)
Mountain-viscacha	5.1	3.6	La Raya, Peru	4200	Heath *et al.* (1981)
Mountain-viscacha	4.5	3.4	La Raya, Peru	4200	Heath *et al.* (1981)

monary arterioles to be devoid of muscle (Fig. 35.6; Heath *et al.* 1984; Table 35.1). This supports the concept of loss of hypoxic vasoconstrictor response as a feature of adaptation in high-altitude representatives of a zoological family. Another species that lives at altitudes exceeding 5000 m in the Andes is the mountain-viscacha (*Lagidium peruanum*; Fig. 35.7). It too has very thin-walled pulmonary arteries (Heath *et al.* 1981; Fig. 35.8; Table 35.1).

PULMONARY ARTERIAL PRESSURE OF ANIMALS ADAPTED TO HIGH ALTITUDE

The lack of medial hypertrophy in pulmonary arteries and of muscularization of pulmonary arterioles in indigenous mountain species, in contrast with man and cattle (see Chapter 10), is consistent with a low pulmonary arterial blood pressure and this is precisely what is found. Harris *et al.* (1982) carried out cardiac catheterizations on 12 llamas at La Raya (4200 m) in the Peruvian Andes and found the pulmonary arterial mean pressure to range from 8 to 18 mmHg (mean 14 mmHg; Fig. 35.9). Three

llamas from Regent's Park Zoo in London had pulmonary arterial mean pressures of 14, 9, and 3 mmHg respectively. In a single alpaca at 4200 m the pulmonary arterial mean pressure was 13 mmHg (Harris *et al.* 1982). In five yaks at Sakti (4500 m) in the Himalaya of Ladakh, Anand *et al.* (1986) found the pulmonary arterial mean blood pressure to be 20 mmHg. In contrast, the mean value in six yaks from Whipsnade Zoo at low altitude in England proved to be 19 mmHg. Clearly the hypoxic pulmonary vasoconstrictor response is greatly diminished.

DZOS AND STOLS

Although the pulmonary arterial pressure of yaks in Ladakh at an altitude of 4500 m does not differ from that found in yaks bred at low altitude, the pulmonary arterial resistance of highland cattle in the Himalaya is significantly higher (Table 35.2, p. 408). A matter of considerable biological interest is that the yak will breed easily with cattle. The cross between a cow and a yak produces an interbreed

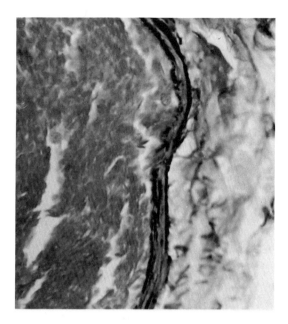

35.4 *Thin-walled pulmonary artery from a llama. The thin media is sandwiched between inner and outer elastic laminae. EVG, × 600.*

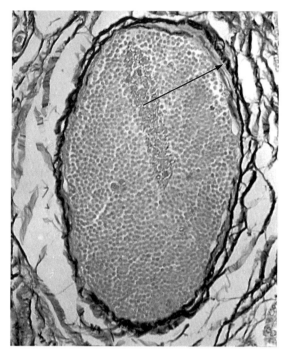

35.6 *Thin-walled pulmonary artery from a yak. The thin media (arrow) is sandwiched between inner and outer elastic laminae. EVG, × 315.*

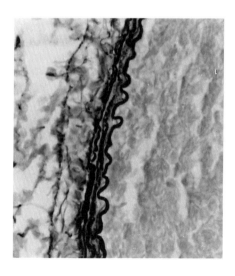

35.5 *Yak at Sakti (4500 m) in Ladakh, India. In this indigenous mountain species the pulmonary arteries are thin-walled and the pulmonary-arterioles are devoid of a muscular coat.*

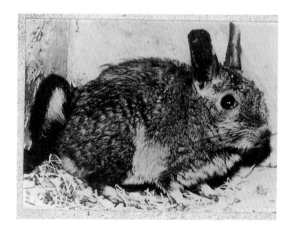

35.7 *Mountain-viscacha at La Raya, Peru (4200 m)*

called a dzo. Although the dzo is smaller than the yak, it preserves many of its body features. Thus its horns curve upwards (Fig. 35.10(a)), it has a short bushy tail (Fig. 35.10(b)), and shaggy hair hangs from its belly (Fig. 35.10(b)). It grunts like a yak. The male dzo (dzobi) is infertile and seldom survives

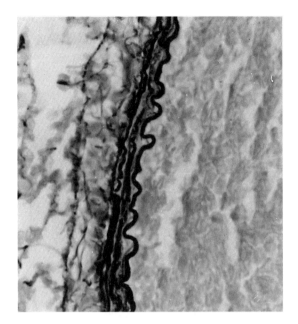

35.8 *Thin-walled elastic pulmonary artery from a mountain-viscacha. The thin media is sandwiched between inner and outer elastic laminae. EVG, × 600.*

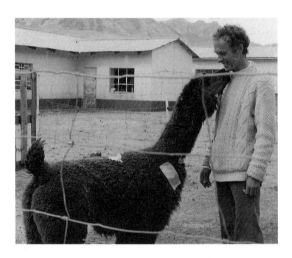

35.9 *Professor Peter Harris with an alpaca he had subjected to cardiac catheterization at La Raya (4200 m) in August 1979 during an expedition to the Peruvian Andes with the authors.*

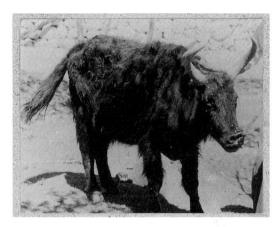

(a)

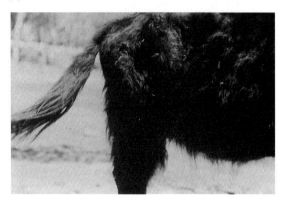

(b)

35.10 *Dzo at Sakti (4500 m). (a) General appearance with long upturned horns; (b) short bushy tail and shaggy body-hair and underbelly.*

more than a year. The female dzo (dzomo) is commonly mated with bulls to produce a further crossbreed, called a stol. The stol resembles a cow more closely. Its horns are shorter and tend to curve downwards (Fig. 35.11(a)), it has a long thin tail ex-

tending down to the hoof (Fig. 35.11(b)), and the belly is smooth (Fig. 35.11(b)). It moos like a cow.

It is clearly of interest to ascertain the pulmonary arterial pressure in these interbreeds. Anand *et al.* (1986) found that in dzos the pulmonary arterial resistance resembled that of the yaks and not that of cattle (Table 35.2). This suggests that the yak has adapted by attenuating the hypoxic vasoconstrictive response and that this trait is transmitted in a dominant fashion, as illustrated in Fig. 35.12(a). They found that for the stols the data separated in a fashion suggestive of a simple Mendelian inheritance. About half the stols resemble cattle, having presumably received the 'cattle' alleles in duplicate (Fig. 35.12(b)). The other half resembled yaks, having presumably received one 'cattle' and one (dominant) 'yak' allele (Fig. 35.12(b)). Their

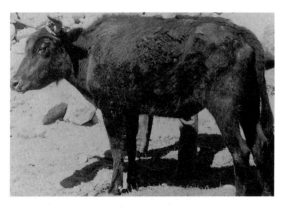

(a)

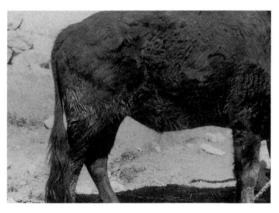

(b)

35.11 *Stol at Sakti (4500 m). (a) General appearance with short straight horns; (b) long thin tail and smooth underbelly.*

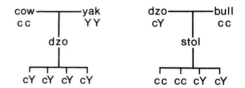

35.12 *(a) How the loss of hypoxic pulmonary vasoconstriction may be transmitted as an autosomal dominant. Cow × yak = dzo. (b) How the level of pulmonary arterial resistance in stols may be determined genetically on the basis of a simple Mendelian inheritance. Dzomo × bull = stol.*

level of pulmonary arterial pressure and resistance was more in keeping with cattle than yaks. However, the gar was only 1-year-old and it is conceivable that in this animal the effect of delayed involution of the pulmonary vasculature in early life was being manifested in maintaining a heightened pulmonary vascular resistance.

Anand *et al.* (1986) accept that their findings could be explained on a polygenic basis, but think it possible that the segregation of their data suggests the pattern of a single autosomal dominant. The number of animals involved in these experiments was small, and further breeding experiments would be needed to establish beyond doubt that the trait is under the control of a single locus.

PULMONARY CIRCULATION OF DOMESTIC ANIMALS AT HIGH ALTITUDE

We have made haemodynamic and histological measurements of the pulmonary circulation of breeds of goats and sheep at the relatively low altitude of Srinagar in Kashmir (1590 m) and the high altitude of Sakti in Ladakh (4500 m)(Anand *et al.* 1988). In Srinagar, '75% merino' sheep are bred for

findings in the single gar (a cross between a dzomo and a yak) they studied (Table 35.2) do not appear to fit in with their concept, in that in this animal the

Table 35.2 Pulmonary arterial pressure and resistance in indigenous Himalayan cattle, yaks, and their interbreeds at Sakti (4500 m) (after Anand *et al.* 1986)

Animal	Cross	Number studied	Pulmonary arterial mean pressure (mmHg)	Pulmonary arterial resistance (mmHg/l per min)
Highland cattle	—	6	27	1.92
Yak	—	5	20	0.58
Dzo	Cow × yak	5	21	0.79
Stol	Dzomo × bull	7	25	1.46
Gar	Dzomo × yak	1	25	2.53

wool and meat. In an attempt to improve the quality and quantity of wool of the indigenous Ladakhi sheep, while retaining their hardiness, the '75% merino' sheep from Srinagar have been transported to Ladakh and cross-bred with the indigenous Ladakhi sheep. Similar cross-breeding occurs between strains of low-altitude goats at Srinagar and indigenous high-altitude Ladakhi goats. These experiments in animal husbandry provided the opportunity to study how the pulmonary circulation of low-altitude sheep and goats responded to transportation to high altitude, the difference between indigenous high-altitude animals and their low-altitude counterparts moved to high altitude, and the effects of cross-breeding.

We found that the pulmonary arterial pressure was significantly higher in goats of low-altitude origin living at high altitude. The pulmonary arterial resistance was also increased in these animals, but did not reach a level of statistical significance. Although the pulmonary arterial pressure of the indigenous high-altitude goats was lower than that of the low-altitude goats living at high altitude, calculations of the pulmonary arterial resistance showed no important differences between the two groups or in their cross-breeds. The haemodynamic effects of high altitude on the sheep were more clear-cut. All breeds at high altitude had a significantly increased pulmonary arterial pressure and resistance irrespective of their origin. These results show that hypoxic pulmonary vasoconstriction affects sheep and probably goats at high altitude, although not nearly to the same extent as it affects cattle. At the same time, there is no evidence that the domestic breeds of sheep and goats at high altitude have selected out the capacity for hypoxic vasoconstriction in the way that seems to have occurred in the yak.

Morbid anatomical studies of the cardiac ventricles and histopathological investigations of the pulmonary vasculature in sheep and goats showed no effect of high altitude (Anand *et al.* 1988). The ratio of right-to-left ventricular weight was not increased and there was no measurable increase in the thickness of the walls of the muscular pulmonary arteries. It would seem likely that the minor degree of pulmonary hypertension was insufficient to give rise to any significant medial hypertrophy.

HAEMOGLOBIN LEVEL

An elevation of the haemoglobin level is a component of the process of acclimatization in man (see Chapter 5). This is not true of indigenous mountain species. In the Andes, alpacas, llamas, and vicuñas

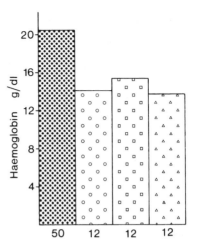

35.13 *Haemoglobin levels in the Quechua Indian and in three species of animals indigenous to the Andes: the alpaca; the llama; and the vicuña. The numbers of individuals studied are shown at the foot of each column. In this figure and in Figs 35.14–35.17 stippled columns represent values for highlanders, columns with open circles represent alpacas, columns with open squares llamas, and columns with open triangles vicuñas. (Figures 35.13–35.17 are based on data from Reynafarje (1966).)*

at altitudes between 4200 and 4300 m show striking differences in various haematological parameters, compared with Quechua Indians living at Morococha (4540 m) (Reynafarje 1966). Thus, haemoglobin levels and the haematocrit are significantly lower in these animals (Figs 35.13 and 35.14) suggesting that less is available for the transport of oxygen. Similarly, Sillau *et al.* (1976) found that in the alpaca the haemoglobin level was low at 11.8 g/dl, with a haematocrit of only 27%.

At the same time, these high-altitude camelids have a greater number of smaller red cells (Figs 35.15–35.17) which appears to increase the interface across which oxygen diffusion can take place. As with the case of the thin-walled pulmonary arteries of the llama, it has to be kept in mind that the smallness and the ellipsoidal shape of the erythrocytes may be a characteristic more of the camel family than of a high-altitude species (Bullard 1972). Nevertheless, the red cells of another indigenous mountains species, the yak, which is unrelated to camels, are also very small (Table 35.3). In contrast to man, but like other indigenous mountain species, the yak does not have a high level of haemoglobin (Table 35.3). Banchero *et al.* (1971) found that

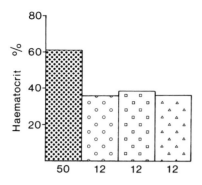

35.14 *Haematocrit percentages in the Quechua Indian and in the same three species of high-altitude animal.*

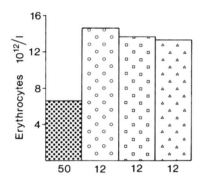

35.15 *Level of erythrocytes in the Quechua Indian and in the same three species of high-altitude animal.*

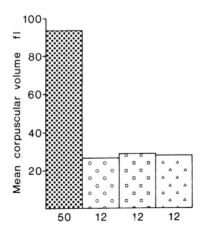

35.16 *Mean corpuscular volume in femtolitres (fl) in the Quechua Indian and in the same three species of high-altitude animal.*

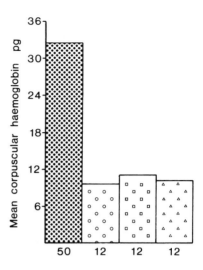

35.17 *Mean corpuscular haemoglobin concentration in picograms (pg) in the Quechua Indian and in the same three species of high-altitude animal.*

Table 35.3 Haematological observations on the yak (after Adams *et al.* 1975)

Subject	Value
White cell count (10^9 l^{-1})	8–10
Neutrophils (%)	35
Small lymphocytes (%)	55
Large lymphocytes (%)	6
Monocytes (%)	4
Eosinophils (%)	1 to 2
Basophils (%)	rare
Platelet count (10^9 l^{-1})	700
Hb level (at 4000 m) (g/dl)	13
Mean corpuscular volume (μm^3)	43
Mean corpuscular haemoglobin (pg)	16.2
Ratio of slow:fast Hb	38:62
2,3-DPG ($\mu mol/g$ Hb)	0.04
(Man: 2,3-DPG) ($\mu mol/g$ Hb)	(10.30)
P_{50} (mmHg)	26

llamas born at sea level show a very modest rise in haemoglobin level on residence at 3420 m for 10 weeks, and they presume that the mildness of the increase is due to the high systemic arterial saturation that this animal maintains in spite of a low arterial oxygen tension.

THE PIKA

The pikas (genus *Ochotona*) are widely distributed in the world, being found in such areas as Tibet, Nepal, Alaska, and the Colorado Rocky Mountains (Sakai *et al.* 1988). Fossils of *Ochotona* have been found on the northern edge of the Qinghai–Tibet plateau and dating suggests that this genus has been resident in the area for some 37 million years (Sakai *et al.* 1988). It would be anticipated that during this extraordinarily long period of time the pika would become genetically adapted to the hypobaric hypoxia of high altitude. Such is the case. Sakai *et al.* (1988) contrasted various physiological and haematological features of 52 adult pikas as contrasted with 28 adult Wistar albino rats at altitudes of 610, 2300, 3300 and 4460 m. Pulmonary arterial pressure in the pika increases with increasing altitude but this is less so than in rats and insignificant in extent. Pulmonary arterial pressure was 13.1 mmHg at 2300 m, 15.7 mmHg at 3300 m, and 17.2 mmHg at 4460 m. These figures were also reported by Tang *et al.* (1988). As a result there is much less increase in right-to-left ventricular weight compared to that which occurs in the rat (Sakai *et al.* 1988; Tang *et al.* 1988). Haematocrit in the pika increases from 37.45% at 2300 m to 44.6% at 3300 m but once again the rise is less than one finds in the rat. As a consequence blood viscosity is significantly lower in the pika than in the rat and shows no significant rise on ascent to higher altitude. Both the mean corpuscular volume and oxygen consumption are significantly lower in the pika compared to the rat. An expected association of these haemodynamic findings is that in *Ochotona curzoniae*, distributed on the Qinghai–Tibet plateau, the pulmonary arteries and veins are thin-walled and lack muscularity (Kou *et al.* 1988).

VENTILATION AND OXYGEN TRANSPORT

Banchero *et al.* (1971) studied the ventilatory response of three male llamas, 5–14 months old, who were born at sea level. The studies on the animals were made first at 260 m and then again after the llamas had been at 3420 m for 5 and 10 weeks. They found that, unlike man, the llama does not hyperventilate on exposure to the hypoxia of high altitude. In this respect it will be recalled (Chapter 7) that the carotid bodies of the alpaca, unlike those of man and cattle, do not enlarge at high altitude. Furthermore, they show a quiescent histological appearance with no suggestion of any form of hyperplasia. This observation on the ventilation of the llama in a hypoxic environment is in agreement with the data of Brooks and Tenney (1968), who found that llamas have a low hypoxic threshold so that the hypoxic ventilatory response occurs only when alveolar oxygen tension drops below 60 mmHg and arterial oxygen tension falls below 40 mmHg. When Sillau *et al.* (1976) studied oxygen transport in the alpaca at 3300 m and then after a sojourn of 3 months at sea level, they found a slight diminution of carbon dioxide tension at high altitude, indicating a slight degree of hyperventilation.

It would seem that, for any given altitude, and thus any given partial pressure of oxygen in inspired air, the llama operates at a lower arterial oxygen tension than man, but at levels of systemic arterial oxygen saturation that equal or exceed those found in man (Banchero *et al.* 1971). Hence with an arterial oxygen tension of 51 mmHg the llama does not show a sustained ventilatory response, maintaining a high systemic arterial oxygen saturation of 92%. Sillau *et al.* (1976) found virtually the same values for arterial oxygen tension and saturation in five alpacas at 3300 m. These features are explained by a higher affinity of llama and alpaca haemoglobin for oxygen and the shape of its oxygen–haemoglobin dissociation curve. When the llama ascends to altitude there is no decrease in the affinity of its haemoglobin for oxygen (P_{50} of 22.7 mmHg at sea level and P_{50} of 23.7 mmHg at 3420 m) (Banchero *et al.* 1971). There is no rightward shift in the oxygen–haemoglobin dissociation curve which remains to the left of that of man, with a P_{50} of 23.7 mmHg compared with 27.0 mmHg in man. In alpacas, P_{50} is 19.7 mmHg at sea level and 17.8 mmHg at 3300 m, figures even lower than those found in the llama (Reynafarje *et al.* 1975).

It was seen in Chapter 5 that, in the metabolism of glucose to pyruvate in the red blood cell, 2,3-DPG is formed and has a tendency to be bound by reduced haemoglobin, reducing its affinity for oxygen and producing a shift of the oxygen–haemoglobin dissociation curve to the right. However, in animals indigenous to high altitude such as the llama, vicuña, alpaca, and the yellow-bellied marmot, there is a shift of the oxygen–haemoglobin dissociation curve to the left. This suggests that successful genetic adaptation to high altitude in these animals does not involve an increase in concentration or action of this organic phosphate (Bullard 1972). These intraerythrocytic phosphates are present in normal amounts in the guanaco, but at extremely low levels in the yak (see Table 35.3). Considered below is their role in the affinity of haemoglobin for oxygen.

UNLOADING OF OXYGEN TO TISSUES

So far as the adaptation of the llama is concerned, the crux of the matter is that, although the haemoglobin concentration is lower, the oxygen extraction in resting conditions is, as in man, about 40–45 ml/l. (Banchero *et al.* 1971). Since the oxygen content of systemic arterial blood is lower because of the comparatively low haemoglobin concentration, the more efficient oxygen extraction implies diminished oxygen content and saturation of systemic venous blood. In the llama the enhanced affinity of the haemoglobin for oxygen does not diminish the unloading of oxygen to the tissues. There appears to be a very efficient utilization of oxygen by the tissues and the ability to operate at a mean venous oxygen tension lower than most other species, even at sea level (Banchero *et al.* 1971). In the alpaca mean venous oxygen tension is 26.2 mmHg and mean venous oxygen saturation is 62.8% (Sillau *et al.* 1976). Mechanisms for reducing the oxygen cascade such as hyperventilation (see Chapter 4) and increasing the haemoglobin concentration (see Chapter 5), which are so important in acclimatization in man, appear to play a very minor role in the adaptation of the llama to high altitude.

There are other aspects of the physiology of the alpaca that appear to aid diffusion of oxygen to the tissues. The muscle of the alpaca is said to have high concentrations of myoglobin, the significance of which has already been described in Chapter 6. The diameter of some of the muscle fibres of the alpaca is as low as 38 μm (Sillau *et al.* 1976) and we have already seen how this aids diffusion of oxygen to tissues when combined with increased capillary density (Chapter 6). Lactate dehydrogenase activity is said to be increased in alpaca tissue six times above that in man (Reynafarje *et al.* 1975).

CAUSE OF HIGH AFFINITY FOR OXYGEN OF HAEMOGLOBIN OF CAMELIDS AND GEESE ADAPTED TO HIGH ALTITUDE

The high oxygen affinity of haemoglobin and the resultant shift to the left of the oxygen–haemoglobin dissociation curve, which appear to be advantageous in adjusting to very high elevations and which are so characteristic of animals showing adaptation rather than acclimatization to this environment, could in theory arise in three distinct ways (Petschow *et al.* 1977; Fig. 35.18). First, the haemoglobin of the species concerned might have intrinsically a high affinity for oxygen. This appears to be the case in certain sheep (see Chapter 8). Secondly, the concentration of the intraerythrocytic organic phosphates

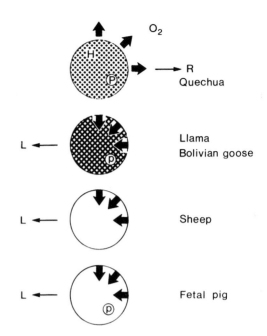

35.18 *How events in the red cell are thought to alter the affinity of haemoglobin for oxygen, thus determining the shift of the oxygen–haemoglobin dissociation curve and the impact of this on the processes of acclimatization and adaptation. (a) In the Quechua Indian, intraerythrocytic organic phosphates (P) such as 2,3-DPG maintain the haemoglobin (H) in its deoxy form, thus diminishing the affinity of haemoglobin for oxygen (represented by arrows), elevating the arterial oxygen tension, shifting the curve to the right (R), and aiding acclimatization. (b) Animals indigenous to high altitude such as the llama and Bolivian goose show a weak interaction between haemoglobin and intraerythrocytic phosphates (p), thus maintaining a high affinity of haemoglobin for oxygen which shifts the curve to the left (L) and aids adaptation (c). Some sheep possess a type of haemoglobin, HbA, which inherently has an increased affinity for oxygen, thus shifting the oxygen–haemoglobin dissociation curve to the left. (d) In the fetal pig there appear to be unusually low concentrations of intraerythrocytic organic phosphates that aid a high affinity of haemoglobin for oxygen and a leftward shift of the curve.*

such as 2,3-DPG, adenosine triphosphate, or inositol pentaphosphate that decrease the affinity of haemoglobin for oxygen might be low. This occurs in fetal as contrasted to adult pigs. Thirdly, the interaction of intraerythrocytic organic phosphates and haemoglobin might be reduced.

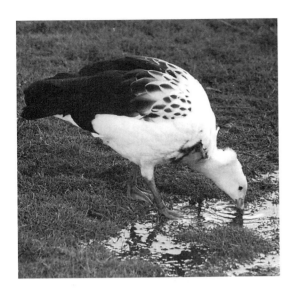

35.19 *The Bolivian goose (*Chloëphaga
melanoptera*).*

The third explanation appears to be the appropriate one for geese and camelids adapted to high altitude. The partial pressure of oxygen at 50% saturation of haemoglobin (P_{50}), and the concentration of various intraerythrocytic phosphate compounds, were measured by Petschow *et al.* (1977), in one species of goose from high altitude and two species from sea level. The high-altitude species chosen for study was the bar-headed goose (*Anser indicus*) which migrates across the Himalaya from India to Tibet at an altitude of 10 000 m where the ambient P_{O2} is some 50 mmHg (Swan 1970). A species from the Andes in which similar results might be anticipated is the Bolivian goose, *Chloëphaga melanoptera* (Fig. 35.19). The sea-level species studied were the Canada goose (*Branta canadensis canadensis*) and the greylag goose (*A. anser*). It was confirmed that there is a shift to the left of the oxygen–haemoglobin dissociation curve of the high-altitude species, the P_{50} for the bar-headed goose being 29.7 mmHg, whereas that for the Canada goose was 42.0 mmHg and that for the greylag goose was 39.5 mmHg. However, it also became apparent that this increased oxygen affinity of haemoglobin of the high-altitude bird was not due to its having a lower level within its erythrocytes of the organic phosphates listed above.

Indeed, while the concentration of such phosphates in the bar-headed goose was 7.2 μmol/ml RBC, that in the greylag goose was 7.9 μmol/ml

RBC and that in the Canada goose was 9.1 μmol/ml RBC. The levels of the individual organic phosphatess (IPP, ATP, ADP, and 2,3-DPG) were found to be very similar in high-altitude and sea-level species. Rather it became clear that the cause of the increased oxygen affinity of the haemoglobin of the Himalayan goose rested on the fact that it reacted more weakly with the organic phosphates than did the haemoglobin of the sea-level species.

The cause of the pronounced affinity of haemoglobin of camelids indigenous to high altitude was found to be of the same basis. Thus, Petschow *et al.* (1977) studied the haemoglobin of the guanaco (*Lama guanicoe*) and compared it with that of man. Once again the leftward shift of the dissociation curve was demonstrated, the P_{50} of the guanaco being 22.5 mmHg in contrast with the value of 26.8 mmHg found in man. In the guanaco, 2,3-DPG concentration is lowered by only some 20% compared with the levels of man. Once again the high affinity of guanaco blood for oxygen depends more on the weak interaction of the haemoglobin molecule and the organic phosphates.

MOLES AND HEDGEHOGS

Not all mammals perpetually subjected to hypoxia live at high altitude. The mole (*Talpa europaea*) is a sea-level mammal that spends more of its life underground in burrows, under conditions in which the tension of oxygen is reduced and that of carbon dioxide is increased. The haematological pattern of the mole shows several interesting divergences from that typical of most surface-dwelling mammals and particularly of that of the mole's closest British relative, the hedgehog (*Erinaceus europaeus*). In fact in many respects the blood of the mole resembles that of man fully acclimatized to high altitude.

The mole lives virtually its entire life underground and in its complex tunnel system it actively seeks food, eats, makes its nest, sleeps, breeds, and rears its young (Quilliam *et al.* 1971). It needs to emerge briefly only to drink or to collect nesting material. The metabolic requirements of this active animal are high and its respiratory rate is some 60 breaths per minute. Apart from the limited supply of fresh air through mole-holes in its deeper tunnels, especially during sleep it becomes directly dependent for its respiratory needs on soil air, that is, air trapped in the macropore spaces between soil crumbs and granules. These spaces occupy a tenth of total soil volume. Soil air is much richer in carbon dioxide and somewhat poorer in oxygen than is atmospheric air. Plant roots and soil organisms remove oxygen from, and respire carbon dioxide into, the macroscopic spaces of the soil. The normal atmospheric concentration of carbon dioxide is 0.03% (Chapter 2) and the average content of this gas in the soil exceeds this by a factor of some 50 times. The soil content of carbon dioxide of grassland was found to be 1.6% by Russell and Appleyard (1915). The oxygen content of the soil of grassland was reported by the same authors to be 18.4%; this contrasts with the figure of 20.93% for ambient air (Chapter 2). Such considerations do not take into account the role of soil water and water vapour which contains only dissolved carbon dioxide and nitrogen (Russell and Appleyard 1915) . The gaseous concentration of carbon dioxide locally could be less than theoretical calculations might suggest. Nevertheless, as Quilliam *et al.* (1971) point out, the mole may breathe in air whose composition approaches that of the expired air of man at sea level. These authors thought it probable that the mole has become adapted over the ages to its unique hypoxic environment. They studied various haematological features of the mole and contrasted them with findings in its free-living relative, the hedgehog, which breathes normal ambient air.

Quilliam *et al.* (1971) determined in the mole and hedgehog haemoglobin concentrations, packed cell volume, red cell counts, mean corpuscular volume and haemoglobin concentration, and reticulocyte counts. They also studied in both species the position of the oxygen dissociation curve. Some of their results are shown in Table 35.4. They show that, al-

though the total red cell counts are similar in both species, mole red cells are larger and carry a much greater weight of haemoglobin than do hedgehog red cells. Mole blood has a greater affinity than does normal human blood so that the oxygen dissociation curve is shifted to the left with a mean P_{50} of 16.0 mmHg compared to 26.6 mmHg in a normal lowlander.

It is clear that the mole has adapted to the chronic hypoxia of its underground life in much the same way as some species at high altitude. Thus as in the case of man at high altitude there is an elevated haemoglobin concentration, an increased packed cell volume, a rise in the red cell count, and a moderate reticulocytosis. However, the shift of its oxygen dissociation curve to the left is not typical of the rightward shift of the curve in acclimatized man (Chapter 5). It is more like the leftward shift of the species genetically adapted to hypobaric hypoxia such as we describe in this chapter. The haematological features of the mole are quite different from those of its free-living relative the hedgehog breathing in the ambient air of low altitude. In Chapter 5 we make the point that man does not include in his adaptation to hypobaric hypoxia the development of new haemoglobins. It is of interest that in the same way no difference between mole and hedgehog haemoglobins could be detected on electrophoresis.

References

Adams, W.H., Graves, I.L., and Pyakural, S. (1975). Hematologic observations on the yak.

Table 35.4 Haematological findings from three hedgehogs and three moles (mean values) compared with typical findings from human lowlanders and native highlanders (quoted by Wintrobe 1967); (after Quilliam *et al.* 1971)

Factor	Hedgehog	Mole	Lowlander	Highlander
Haemoglobin concentration (g/dl)	11.2	17.4	14.6	20.8
Packed cell volume (%)	34	49	46	60
Erythrocyte count ($\times 10^{12}$/l)	4.9	4.7	5.4	6.1
Mean corpuscular haemoglobin concentration ($\mu\mu$g)	23	36.5	29	34
Mean corpuscular volume (μ^3)	68	103	87	97.5
Reticulocyte count (%)	4.0	3.3	0.5	1.5
P_{50} at pH 7.4 and 37°C	...	16.0	26.6	31.2

Proceedings of the Society for Experimental Biology and Medicine, **148**, 701

Anand, I.S., Harris, E., Ferrari, R., Pearce, P., and Harris, P. (1986). Pulmonary haemodynamics of the yak, cattle and cross breeds are high altitude. *Thorax*, **41**, 696

Anand, I., Heath, D., Deen, M., Ferrari, R., Bergel, D., and Harris, P. (1988). The pulmonary circulation of some domestic animals at high altitude. *International Journal of Biometeorology*, **32**, 56

Banchero, N., Grover, R.F., and Will, J.A. (1971). Oxygen transport in the llama (*Lama glama*). *Respiration Physiology*, **13**, 102

Brooks, J.G. and Tenney, S.M. (1968). Ventilatory response of llama to hypoxia at sea level and high altitude. *Respiration Physiology*, **5**, 269

Bullard, R.W. (1972). Vertebrates at altitudes. In *Physiological Adaptations, Desert and Mountain* (M.K. Yousef, S.M. Horvath, and R.W. Bullard, Ed). New York; Academic Press, p. 209

Durand, J., Leroy Ladurie, M., and Ranson-Bitker, B. (1970). Effects of hypoxia and hypercapnia on the repartition of pulmonary blood flow in supine subjects. *Progress in Respiration Research*, **5**, 156

Harris, P. (1986). Evolution, hypoxia and high altitude. In *Aspects of Hypoxia* (D. Heath, ed.). Liverpool; Liverpool University Press, p. 209

Harris, P., Heath, D., Smith, P., Williams, D.R., Ramirez, A., Krüger, H., and Jones, D.M. (1982). Pulmonary circulation of the llama at high and low altitudes. *Thorax*, **37**, 38

Heath, D., Castillo, Y., Arias-Stella, J., and Harris, P. (1969). The small pulmonary arteries of the llama and other domestic animals native to high altitude. *Cardiovascular Research*, **3**, 75

Heath, D., Smith, P., Williams, D., Harris, P., Arias-Stella, J. and Krüger, H. (1974). The heart and pulmonary vasculature of the llama (*Lama glama*). *Thorax*, **29**, 463

Heath, D., Williams, D., Harris, P., Smith, P., Krüger, H., and Ramirez, A. (1981). The pulmonary vasculature of the mountain-viscacha (*Lagidium peruanum*). The concept of adapted and acclimatized vascular smooth muscle. *Journal of Comparative Pathology*, **91**, 293

Heath, D., Williams, D., and Dickinson, J. (1984). The pulmonary arteries of the yak. *Cardiovascular Research*, **18**, 133

Kou, X., Yang, Z., Zhan, X., Tang, G., Zhao, G., Li, Y., Su, M., Zhang, Y., and Sakai, A. (1988). The comparative study of the pulmonary blood vessel of Pika. In *High-Altitude Medical Science* (G. Ueda, S. Kusama, and N.F. Voelkel Ed.). Matsumoto, Japan; Shinshu University Press, p. 113

Petschow, D., Wurdinger, L., Baumann, R., Duhm, J., Braunitzer, G., and Bauer, C. (1977). Causes of high blood O_2 affinity of animals living at high altitude. *Journal of Applied Physiology*, **42**, 139

Quilliam, T.A., Clarke, J.A., and Salsbury, A.J. (1971). The ecological significance of certain new haematological findings in the mole and hedgehog. *Comparative Biochemistry and Physiology*, **40A**, 89

Reynafarje, C. (1966). Physiological patterns: hematological aspects. In *Life at High Altitudes*, Scientific Publication No. 140. Washington, DC; Pan American Health Organization, p. 32

Reynafarje, C., Faura, J., Villavicencio, D., Curaca, A., Reynafarje, B., Oyola, L., Contreras, L., Vallenas, E., and Faura, A. (1975). Oxygen transport of hemoglobin in high altitude animals (*Camelidae*). *Journal of Applied Physiology*, **38**, 806

Russell, E.J. and Appleyard, A. (1915). The atmosphere of the soil: its composition and the causes of variation. *Journal of Agricultural Science*, 7, 1

Sakai, A., Ueda, G., Yanagidaira, Y., Takeoka, M., Tang, G., and Zhang, Y. (1988). Physiological characteristics of Pika, Ochotona, as high-altitude adapted animals. In *High-Altitude Medical Science* (G. Ueda, S. Kusama, and N.F. Voelkel, Ed.). Matsumoto, Japan; Shinshu University Press, p. 99

Sillau, A.H., Cueva, S., Valenzuela, A., and Candela, E. (1976). O_2 transport in the Alpaca (*Lama pacos*) at sea level and at 3,300 m. *Respiration Physiology*, **27**, 147

Swan, L.W. (1970). Goose of the Himalayas. *Natural History*, **79**, 68

Tang, G., Yang, Z., Zhan, X., Kou, X.,. Long, W., Zhang, Y., and Sakai, A. (1988). Pulmonary circulation of the native species plateau pika at high altitude. In *High-Altitude Medical Science* (G. Ueda, S. Kusama, and N.F. Voelkel Ed.). Matsumoto, Japan; Shinshu, University Press, p. 108

Wintrobe, M.M. (1967). *Clinical Haematology*, 6th edn. London; Henry Kimpton

36

Life at high altitude

Most human beings and mammals on the planet live at sea level or at low altitude and their physiology is in harmony with the partial pressure of oxygen in the ambient air consequent upon the high barometric pressure. When they make temporary incursions into the high-altitude environment or seek to live there permanently, they have to adjust to the hypobaric hypoxia by various physiological mechanisms that often come to be associated with ultrastructural or histological changes. The rapid ascent of lowlanders or lowland animals to high altitude may induce diseases that may be incapacitating or even fatal. On the other hand, native highlanders born at high altitude come to terms from childhood with the environment, and genetic factors may be involved. In the case of indigenous mountain species, such genetic influences may be paramount. Clearly not all men and animals living at high altitude are of equal biological status and in this final chapter we shall review the various groups that have emerged throughout the book.

ACCLIMATIZATION

When man ascends to a higher altitude, many physiological adjustments take place very rapidly in response to the hypoxia. Examples are the increased secretion of erythropoietin and the formation of increased amounts of 2,3-DPG in the erythrocyte. At first the acclimatization is incomplete (lightly stippled subject in Fig. 36.1). However, the greater the elevation and the longer the exposure, the more complete does this *acquired acclimatization* become (fully stippled subject in Fig. 36.1).

Acclimatization is a reversible, non-inheritable change in the anatomy or physiology of an organism that enables it to survive in an alien environment. Acquired acclimatization in the lowlander is *qualitatively* identical with that which occurs in the highlander, but even after extended residence in the mountains it is *quantitatively* less complete than the *natural acclimatization* of the native highlander (Fig. 36.2). Thus, Hurtado (1966) (Fig. 36.3), at a meeting of the Pan American Health Organization

Advisory Committee on Medical Research stated: 'We observed that no matter how long a man from sea level stays at high altitude, his efficiency and his tolerance for maximal work were a great deal lower.' He found that the Quechua had a very high tolerance to maximal exercise on a treadmill at high altitude (Hurtado 1964). He thought a high work capacity is perhaps the best index of natural acclimatization. This view is supported by some Europeans like von Muralt (1966), who said at the same meeting: 'In the experience of every single European who has worked with Sherpas in the Himalayas, under any given conditions the Sherpa is superior to the European member of the party in physical performance except at the end.' In other words the acquired acclimatization of the lowlander is inferior to the natural acclimatization of the highlander, although its components are the same.

Apparently, however, von Muralt (1966) felt that the acquired acclimatization of the climber might also reach a high level. He said: 'In Switzerland too I think this fact can be corroborated. We have a group that we call Mountain Guides, the grandsons of the famous mountain guides who took Whymper and others up in the pioneer times of Alpine discovery. My personal experience with these men is that, under extreme conditions, their performance and resistance not only to hypoxia but also to cold and other difficulties are superior to what any sportsman can exhibit.'

THE FETUS AND ACCLIMATIZATION

At sea level the umbilical arterial oxygen tension is barely 20 mmHg, which corresponds to an atmospheric oxygen tension of about 60 mmHg which would be found at an elevation of 7500 m (see Chapter 23). Hence, even at sea level the fetus is hypoxaemic and lives under physiological conditions that in some ways resemble those experienced by the native highlander. However, the adjustment to the hypoxaemia of intrauterine life is not strictly comparable to that of acclimatization. One of the hallmarks of acclimatization is the production of increased red

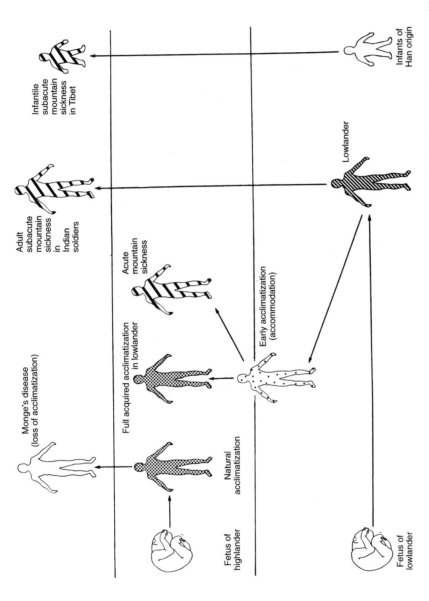

36.1 *Acclimatization, failure to achieve acclimatization, and loss of the condition in man. The upper and middle compartments represent life at high altitude, the lowest compartment life at sea level. The lowlander (hatched) ascending to high altitude passes through the various processes described in this book (lightly stippled) to reach the state of acquired acclimatization (stippled). This approaches but does not equal the level of natural acclimatization manifested by the Quechua Indian. Frequently the early stages of acclimatization do not proceed satisfactorily and the subject develops one of the various forms of acute mountain sickness (barred figure). The fetus is physiologically adjusted to the hypoxaemia of intrauterine life simulating high altitude, but this adjustment cannot be strictly compared to acclimatization (see text). On birth at high altitude the adjustment to hypoxia is usually maintained with a translation to the characteristic features of acclimatization. Some Chinese infants of Han origin in Tibet and young Indian soldiers stationed at very high altitudes in the Himalaya fail to achieve acclimatization (barred figures). On birth at sea level, adjustment to hypoxia is lost and the features of acclimatization do not develop. Quechuas ageing at high altitude may lose their natural acclimatization and develop chronic mountain sickness. (Monge's disease; open figure).*

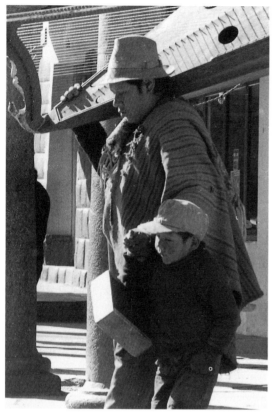

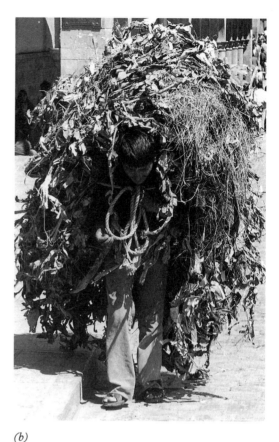

(a)   (b)

36.2 *Quechua Indians of Cuzco (3400 m) in the Andes. (a) Father (carrying Peruvian harp) and son exhibiting the features of* natural acclimatization *which enable them to lead an active life at high altitude. (b) Such acclimatization enables native highlanders to indulge in heavy work including carrying loads so large as almost to engulf them.*

cell mass, but the haemoglobin concerned is the adult form of HbA, which is retained in man for the transport and release of oxygen to the tissues (see Chapter 8). There is a shift of the oxygen–haemoglobin dissociation curve to the right, with increased levels of arterial oxygen tension being achieved at the expense of oxygen saturation of the haemoglobin.

In contrast to these features of acclimatization, the haemoglobin of the fetus is HbF which has a high affinity for oxygen, maintaining a high oxygen saturation of haemoglobin at the expense of arterial oxygen tension with a shift of the oxygen–haemoglobin dissociation curve to the left. Such features are more characteristic of the genetic adaptation of indigenous high-altitude species than of acclimatization. Hence

the position of the human fetus in relation to acclimatization is not straightforward (see Fig. 36.1).

On birth at high altitude the adjustment to hypoxia is usually maintained, with a translation to the recognizable features of acclimatization with increased levels of HbA and a loss of HbF. However, some Chinese infants of Han origin develop infantile subacute mountain sickness on ascent to live in Lhasa (3600 m) (see Fig. 36.1). On birth at sea level, adjustment to hypoxia is lost and the features of acclimatization do not develop.

ACUTE MOUNTAIN SICKNESS
In about half of all subjects ascending to high altitude the early stages of acclimatization are disturbed

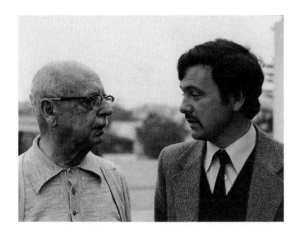

36.3 *Professor Alberto Hurtado (left), the 'father of high-altitude medicine', talking to one of the authors (D.R.W.) in Lima in August 1979.*

by the onset of acute mountain sickness (barred subject in Fig. 36.1). The symptoms of this illness do not appear to be due to hypoxia *per se*, but follow

several hours after exposure to significant high altitude. The hypobaric hypoxia appears to bring about maladjustments of physiological mechanisms, based on endocrinological disturbances, with the retention and redistribution of body water. Acute mountain sickness is not a phase of acclimatization but is an illness which may, moreover, progress into potentially fatal cerebral mountain sickness or high-altitude pulmonary oedema.

FAILURE TO ESTABLISH INITIAL ACCLIMATIZATION

Failure to acclimatize to the hypobaric hypoxia of high altitude occurs in both man (see Fig. 36.1) and cattle (Fig. 36.4). The bovine form, called 'brisket disease', is the better known and has been recognized as a distinct clinical entity for over 70 years (Chapter 16; see also Fig. 36.4). The human variety has been recognized in Chinese infants of Han origin in Tibet and designated 'subacute infantile mountain sickness' (Sui *et al.* 1988; see also Chapter 17 and Fig. 36.1). It has also been found as 'adult subacute mountain sickness' in young Indian soldiers in

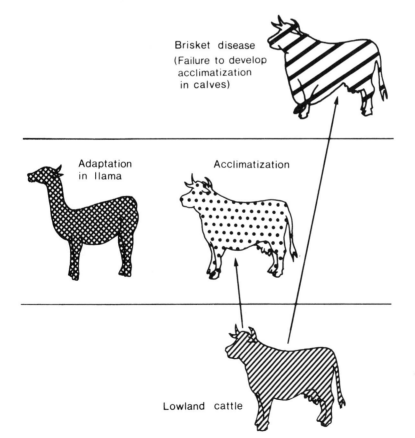

36.4 *Acclimatization and adaptation to high altitude in animals. Such species as cattle (hatched) have to undergo acclimatization (stippled) as in man. Susceptible calves in Utah may fail to gain acclimatization satisfactorily and develop brisket disease (barred figure). Indigenous mountain species such as the llama are genetically adapted to high altitude (cross-hatched).*

the Himalaya (Anand *et al.* 1990; Anand and Chandrashekhar 1992; see also Chapter 17 and Fig. 36.1). Both bovine and human forms of failure to achieve acclimatization occur in the young, being found in calves taken to graze in mountain ranges in Utah, in infants taken up to live in Lhasa (3600 m), and in young Indian soldiers stationed in the Himalaya. In the first two forms at least the target organ responsible for the failure to acclimatize is the pulmonary vasculature.

In cattle the pulmonary arterial tree is naturally highly muscular and susceptible to hypoxic constriction. In the infants affected by subacute mountain sickness both muscular pulmonary arteries and pulmonary arterioles appear to be very susceptile to hypoxic vasoconstriction and muscularization. In bovine and human varieties of failure to acclimatize to high altitude, genetic predisposition seems to be of importance. In those calves affected by brisket disease the pulmonary arterial tree appears to be genetically hypersensitive to hypoxia. Infants failing to acclimatize to hypobaric hypoxia in Lhasa are almost all of Han origin and the occurrence of the disease in Tibetan infants is exceptional. Brisket disease should not be misinterpretated as a bovine form of Monge's disease, for the condition in cattle represents a failure of the establishment of acclimatization (Fig. 36.4), whereas in man chronic mountain sickness is a breakdown in acclimatization already in existence for many years (see Fig. 36.1 and Chapter 15).

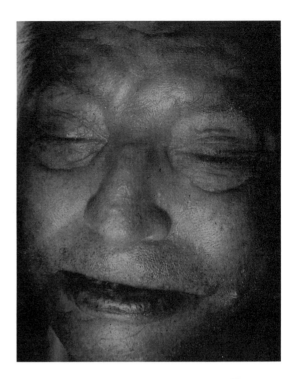

36.5 *A case of Monge's disease at necropsy. The characteristic swarthy, plethoric appearance is associated with very high levels of haemoglobin.*

from those of the acclimatized Quechua (Table 36.1). Hence successful adjustment to life at high

LOSS OF ACCLIMATIZATION

Some native highlanders, after having lived for many years above altitudes of about 4000 m, lose their acclimatization and develop chronic mountain sickness (Monge's disease). It is now considered that chronic mountain sickness may be an expression of ageing at high altitude (Fig. 36.5).

ADAPTATION

Some animal species such as the yak have lived for countless millennia at high altitude and have, through a process of natural selection, become fully adapted to the hypoxia of high altitude (Fig. 36.6). The process of *adaptation* (see Fig. 36.4) is the development of biochemical, physiological, and anatomical features that are heritable and of genetic basis, enabling the species to explore the environment of high altitude to its best advantage. Such indigenous mountain species as the llama, alpaca, vicuña, and guanaco exhibit features quite distinct

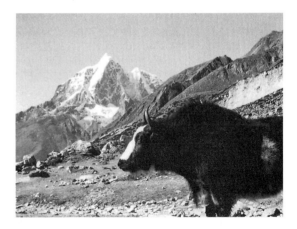

36.6 *Yak (*Bos grunniens*) in the Himalaya. In the background is Taweche (6710–7010 m). The yak is an indigenous mountain species and, unlike man and cattle, is adapted rather than acclimatized to high altitude.*

Table 36.1 Points of contrast between acclimatization in the Quechua Indian and adaptation in the llama at high altitude

Feature	Quechua	Llama
Major area where chronic oxygen deprivation is overcome	Diminution in magnitude of 'oxygen cascade' (see Chapter 4).	Increased extraction of oxygen from tissues (low P_{vo2}) (see Chapter 35)
Hyperventilation	Pronounced	Minimal or absent
Haematocrit	60%	30–40 %
2,3-DPG in red cell	Raised level	Weak reaction between haemoglobin molecule and intra erythrocytic phosphates
Shift of oxygen — haemoglobin dissociation curve	To right (P_{50} 26.8 mmHg)	To left (P_{50} 23.7 mmHg)
Carotid bodies	Enlarged	Not enlarged
Terminal portion of pulmonary arterial tree	Muscularized	Not muscularized
Right ventricle	Hypertrophied	Not hypertrophied

altitude can be made by the process of acclimatization or adaptation.

THE CONCEPT OF 'HIGH-ALTITUDE MAN'

So effectively does the native highlander cope with the chronic hypoxia of his mountain habitat that there has grown up the concept of a 'high altitude man' inherently more capable of surviving and living a normal active life at high altitude. The view of Monge (1948), based on his classic studies of the Quechua Indian, was that the indigenous races in mountainous areas became suited to high altitudes through an age-long process and that 'the Man of the Andes possesses biological characteristics distinct from those of sea-level man'. Such a viewpoint suggests that some features of native highlanders have a basis in heredity; this hypothesis conflicts with the definition of acclimatization. As noted above, von Muralt (1966) broadened this concept to include the Sherpa and hence the view grew up in one school of thought that there was an entity of a 'high-altitude man', the features of this native highlander being shared by the peoples of the Andes and of the Himalaya.

Chiodi (1966) doubted the traditional concept of Monge and concluded that 'there are few data on permanent biological features that would differenti-

ate an Andean man from his sea level peer'. He believed that many of the biological characteristics of 'the Man of the Andes' are features acquired through a given subject's long residence at high altitudes. It is instructive to examine this concept of 'high-altitude man' by comparing the characteristics of the Quechuas and Aymaras of the Andes with those of the Sherpas of the Nepal Himalaya.

Quechua and Sherpa

There are in fact many points of contrast between the highlanders of the Andes and of the Himalaya and some of these are given in Table 36.2. They are the result of several predisposing factors. The highlanders of the Himalaya are of a different ethnic background from those of South America and they appear to have been domiciled in their mountain home for very much longer. The Sherpas and Tibetans live at considerably lower altitudes than do the Quechuas and Aymaras in the Andes and this may account for the lower haemoglobin levels generally found in the Sherpa.

Studies of haematological parameters in Quechuas and Sherpas by Morpurgo *et al.* (1972, 1976) led them to the conclusion that differences between the two groups had a further significance, suggesting that, whereas the Andean Indians were acclimatized,

Table 36.2 Points of contrast between the Quechua and the Sherpa

Feature	Quechua	Sherpa	Relevant chapter for references
Chest	Prominent and barrel-shaped	Lack of classical prominent chest	3
Haemoglobin level	Very high levels especially above 4000 m	Normal to moderately elevated	5
Carotid body	Enlarged with prominent clusters of light chief cells	Enlarged with prominent dark cells	7
Position Hb/O$_2$ dissociation curve	Shift to right	Shift to left	5
Blood group	O	A, B	3
Length of domicile at high altitude	14 000 years	Many thousands of years	

the native highlanders of the Himalaya were in part adapted. In 1970 and 1972 Morpurgo and co-workers carried out work that appeared to demonstrate an increased Bohr effect in Quechua Indians, which they regarded as a feature of acclimatization. Subsequently, however, Winslow *et al.* (1985) were unable to substantiate these findings, as pointed out in Chapter 5. Further work by Morpurgo *et al.* (1976) was carried out in the small Nepalese villages in the Solu-Khumbu region (Kunde at 3800 m and Kumjung at 3900 m). They also studied Sherpas living permanently at 1200 m. They found that the Sherpas at high altitude had normal haematocrits, most values falling in the range of 41–50%, with haemoglobin levels in the range of 14.5–17.5 g/dl and a red cell count of 4.0–5.0 × 10^{12}/l. These results may be contrasted with those which we have quoted for the acclimatized Quechua (see Chapter 5). They found that the levels of 2,3-DPG were not raised in highland Sherpas compared with sea-level subjects. There was a pronounced shift of the oxygen–haemoglobin dissociation curve to the left, indicating an increased affinity of haemoglobin for oxygen. The mean P_{50} value in Sherpas living permanently at high altitudes was 22.6 mmHg, contrasted to 27.0 mmHg in sea-level Caucasians, and 36.7 mmHg in Sherpas living permanently at low altitudes. The mechanism of the shift to the left in the highland Sherpas was not clear. The presence of abnormal haemoglobins was excluded, since the electrophoretic patterns of European and Sherpa haemoglobins were indistinguishable.

Hence the investigations of Morpurgo *et al.* (1976) raised interesting questions. Not only did they reveal an absence of increased Bohr effect in Sherpas compared with Quechuas, but also showed a leftward shift of the oxygen–haemoglobin dissociation curve reminiscent of adaptation in indigenous high-altitude animals. Such findings are consistent with the view that the Quechuas are acclimatized, whereas the Sherpas are to some extent adapted to the hypobaric hypoxia of high altitude. Morpurgo and co-workers related this to the length of time the two peoples have been domiciled in the mountains. According to them, man migrated to America through the Bering Strait probably only 35 000 years ago, the colonization of the Peruvian Andes having taken place only over the past 14 000 years. In contrast, it seems likely that man has inhabited Central Asia including Tibet for close on half a million years. This is an interesting concept, but it is weakened by the failure of Winslow *et al.* (1985) to substantiate the increased Bohr effect in the Quechua. It seems to us that there are different types of native highlander whose characteristics are the result of the complex interaction between the genetic and environmental influences outlined in Chapter 3.

In progressing through the chapters of this book it will have become clear that adjustment to life at high altitude is complex, involving most sytems of the body. However, man and mammals ascending to, or living permanently at, high altitude are not of equal biological status.

References

Anand, I.S. and Chandrashekhar, Y. (1992). Subacute mountain sickness syndromes: role of pulmonary hypertension. In *Hypoxia and Mountain Medicine* (J.R. Sutton, G. Coates, and C.S. Houston, Ed.). Oxford; Pergamon Press, p. 241

Anand, I.S., Malhotra, R.M., Chandrashekhar, Y., Bali, H.K., Chauhan, S.S., Bhandari, R.K., and Wahi, P.I. (1990). Adult subacute mountain sickness — a syndrome of congestive heart failure in man at very high altitude. *Lancet*, **335**, 561

Chiodi, H. (1966). Acquired acclimatization to high altitude. In *Life at High Altitudes*, Scientific Publication No. 140. Washington, DC; Pan American Health Organization, p. 67

Hurtado, A. (1964). Acclimatization to high altitudes. In *The Physiological Effects of High Altitude* (W.H. Weihe, Ed.). Oxford; Pergamon Press, pp. 2, 344

Hurtado, A. (1966). In *Life at High Altitudes*, Scientific Publication No. 140. Washington; Pan American Health Organization, p. 68

Monge-M, C. (1948). *Acclimatization in the Andes*. Baltimore; Johns Hopkins Press

Morpurgo, G., Battaglia, P., Bernini, L., Paolucci, A.M., and Modiano, G. (1970). Higher Bohr effect in Indian natives of Peruvian Highlands as compared with Europeans. *Nature (London)*, **227**, 387

Morpurgo, G., Battaglia, P., Carter, N.D., Modiano, G., and Passi, G. (1972). The Bohr effect and the red cell 2,3-DPG and Hb content in Sherpas and Europeans at low and at high altitude. *Experientia*, **28**, 1280

Morpurgo, G., Arese, P., Bosia, A., Pescarmona, G.P., Luzana, M., Modiano, G., and Krishna Ranjit, S. (1976). Sherpas living permanently at high altitude: a new pattern of adaptation. *Proceedings of the National Academy of Sciences of the United States of America*, **73**, 747

Sui, G.J., Liu, Y.H. Cheng, X.S., Anand, I.S., Harris, E., Harris, P., and Heath, D. (1988). Subacute infantile mountain sickness. *Journal of Pathology*, **155**, 161

von Muralt, A. (1966). Acquired acclimatization to high altitudes. In *Life at High Altitudes*, Scientific Publication No. 140. Washington, DC; Pan American Health Organization, pp. 53, 69

Winslow, R.M., Monge, -C, C., Winslow, N.J., Gibson, C.G., and Whittembury, J. (1985). Normal white blood Bohr effect in Peruvian natives at high altitude. *Respiration Physiology*, **61**, 197

Index

(Note: Page numbers in bold type indicate illustrations. HAPO = high-altitude pulmonary oedema. HA = high altitude)